# The Clinician's Handbook of Natural Medicine

SECOND EDITION

# The Clinician's Handbook of Natural Medicine

SECOND EDITION

Joseph E. Pizzorno Jr, ND

Michael T. Murray, ND

Herb Joiner-Bey, ND

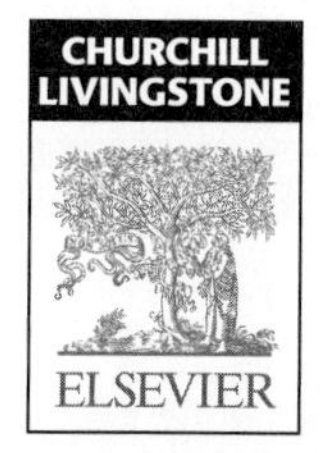

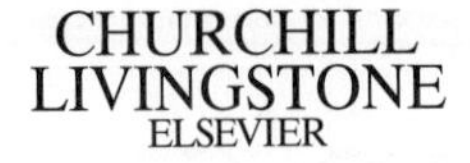


11830 Westline Industrial Drive
St. Louis, Missouri 63146

THE CLINICIAN'S HANDBOOK OF NATURAL MEDICINE, SECOND EDITION
ISBN: 978-0-443-06723-5



**Library of Congress Control Number: 2007933363**

*Vice President and Publisher:* Linda Duncan
*Acquisitions Editor:* Kellie White
*Developmental Editor:* Kelly Milford
*Publishing Services Manager:* Patricia Tannian
*Project Manager:* Claire Kramer
*Designer:* Gene Harris



Printed in the United States of America

Last digit is the print number: 9 8 7 6 5 4 3 2 1

*In loving memory of the late*

Dr. Bill Mitchell,

*whose faith, passion, dedication, vision, and compassion*
*made him the living embodiment*
*of the spirit and essence of naturopathic holistic healing*

# Preface

We are excited to see the continuing blossoming of natural medicine by many names. No matter the term used (e.g., *integrative, holistic,* or *functional*), the philosophical precepts kept alive in the culture by natural medicine physicians are informing and transforming medicine. Treating the person, rather than the disease, seems an obvious concept, yet it has struggled to be heard. As Dr. Bastyr taught us as students, "Despite the obstacles, the truth of our medicine will win out."

*The Clinician's Handbook of Natural Medicine,* second edition, was created as a companion to the *Textbook of Natural Medicine,* third edition. It was written for several audiences: students, clinicians, and researchers. For the busy clinician it provides concise guidance for the care of patients who may have one or more of over 80 of the most common diseases effectively treated with natural medicine. Although Sections 4 and 6 of the *Textbook* provide an in-depth discussion of the pathophysiology, causes, documented natural medicine interventions, and full references for these diseases, the *Handbook* provides only the most pertinent information needed for intervention for the typical patient. Together, these books provide the clinician with the best of both worlds: easily accessible advice for quick guidance, for the less complicated patient, and in-depth understanding when needed. (Of course, the *Textbook* also contains considerable additional information in its other four sections.)

For students, this resource helps them understand more deeply the patient who has the disease. One of the challenges for those learning natural medicine is the pitfall of "green drug" medicine; that is, simply substituting an herb or a natural therapy for the synthetic drug to treat the symptoms. Our best practice of medicine is to understand the true causes of disease and then to help the patient restore normal function. By carefully studying the unique flowcharts offered by the *Handbook,* the student can more profoundly understand the uniqueness of each patient. The guidance on when to refer to (or use, depending on the student's training and licensure) more conventional approaches will also help the students recognize the limitations of natural therapies.

For the researcher wanting to truly evaluate the efficacy of natural medicine, we hope the flowcharts in the *Handbook* will help him or her progress beyond the false homogeneity of disease. Although the standardization of disease works for symptom relief–oriented health care, it is an oversimplification and is inconsistent with the curative medicine we believe is possible. With recognition that multiple interventions are needed for each disease, depending on the patient, algorithms can be developed that lead to more accurate research on how we actually care for patients.

Each chapter of the *Handbook* is composed of several parts: Diagnostic Summary, General Considerations, Flowchart, Therapeutic Considerations, and Therapeutic Approach. We believe that this format is unique, and we are unaware of any other textbook in which the flowchart approach is used to provide guidance for integrative and natural medicine care.

The Flowchart separates the diagnostic and therapeutic deliberation into three phases: (1) determine the need for conventional intervention, (2) minimize obstacles to healing, and (3) tailor natural interventions to patient needs. The first phase is provided to assist the clinician in understanding which patients may immediately require a more conventional intervention or whose condition has progressed beyond the capabilities of natural therapies. The other phases present the most relevant diagnostic and therapeutic differentiations needed to determine which cause(s) must be controlled and which interventions are needed to provide each patient highly personalized natural medicine care. Carefully following this thoughtfully constructed logic chain will efficiently provide key therapeutic insights.

The astute reader may notice a few inconsistencies between the recommendations found in the *Handbook* and the *Textbook*. Because the *Handbook* was written approximately 3 years after the *Textbook*, we have worked to ensure that the latest research has been incorporated.

This second edition closely follows the format of the first edition. The main differences are the inclusion of several additional diseases and a conceptual flowchart showing the philosophical precepts of the "therapeutic order" to further assist the clinician's understanding of where the patient is in the disease and healing process.

We are excited to provide clinicians with this special resource, which we believe will substantially aid their efforts to provide their patients with the best care possible.

*Joseph E. Pizzorno Jr, ND*
*Michael T. Murray, ND*
*Herb Joiner-Bey, ND*

## ACKNOWLEDGMENTS

Most of all I would like to acknowledge that inner voice that has guided me in my life, providing me with inspiration, strength, and humility at the most appropriate times. My motivation has been largely the good that I know can come from using natural medicine appropriately. It can literally change people's lives. I know it changed mine.

There are many things that I am thankful for. I am especially thankful for my wife and best friend, Gina. I have also been blessed by having wonderful parents whose support and faith have never waned. I now have the opportunity to carry on their legacy of love with my own children, Alexa, Zachary, and Addison.

In addition to my family, those people who have truly inspired me include Dr. Ralph Weiss, Dr. Ed Madison, Dr. Bill Mitchell, Dr. Gaetano Morello, my classmates and the entire Bastyr University community, and all the special people I am lucky enough to call friends who have helped me on my life's journey.

And finally, I am deeply honored to have Dr. Joe Pizzorno and Dr. Herb Joiner-Bey, not only as my coauthors, but also as truly valued friends.

*Michael T. Murray, ND*

I would like to acknowledge all my students over the years for the health and healing they have brought to millions of people. You made the hard work of creating Bastyr University worth every sacrifice.

Dr. Michael Murray, with your many books and tireless teaching to the public, you have played a major role in transforming medicine. I am speechless with your accomplishments.

I would like to again acknowledge our new coauthor, Dr. Herb Joiner-Bey. His conversion of the much more complex *Textbook of Natural Medicine* into this concise, insightful, and extremely accessible resource is very impressive, and his expansion of this work to the second edition a true gift to all.

As ever, this work would not have been possible without the love and care of my family: Lara, my dear wife, and Galen and Raven, my beloved children. Thank you for bringing such joy and fullness to my life.

*Joseph E. Pizzorno Jr, ND*

I wish to extend to Dr. Joseph Pizzorno and Dr. Michael Murray my deep appreciation for the high honor and privilege of preparing the second edition of this handbook, based on the third edition of their *Textbook of Natural Medicine*. Because of my declining visual acuity, the challenges of preparing this new edition have been far greater than encountered for the first. It is with deep gratitude that I wish to thank Ms. Kim Fons, developmental editor, and Elsevier for their patience, understanding, and generosity in providing whatever support they could to make my task easier. It is also with great appreciation that I wish to thank Dr. Pizzorno for his gracious willingness to lighten my load by preparing a number of the chapters himself. Thank you so very much, Kim and Joe. Without your help, this project could not have been finished in a timely fashion.

*Herb Joiner-Bey, ND*

Finally, we would like to acknowledge the outstanding professional staff at Elsevier, whose creative talents and expertise have been indispensable to the publishing of this book. Thank you to Kellie White and Claire Kramer. We especially appreciate you, Kim Fons—though you've moved on to other endeavors, your help and encouragement for Herb were far beyond the call of duty. (We still miss you too, Inta Ozols.)

# Contents

The Therapeutic Order in Naturopathic Medicine — 1
Acne Vulgaris and Acne Conglobata — 3
Affective Disorders — 8
Alcoholism — 26
Alzheimer's Disease — 36
Angina Pectoris — 48
Aphthous Stomatitis (Aphthous Ulcer/Canker Sore/Ulcerative Stomatitis) — 56
Asthma — 60
Atherosclerosis — 73
Atopic Dermatitis (Eczema) — 90
Attention Deficit Hyperactivity Disorder in Children — 97
Bacterial Sinusitis — 107
Benign Prostatic Hyperplasia — 112
Cancer: Integrated Naturopathic Support — 119
Carpal Tunnel Syndrome — 136
Celiac Disease — 142
Cellulite — 147
Cervical Dysplasia — 152
Chronic Candidiasis — 161
Chronic Fatigue Syndrome — 167
Congestive Heart Failure — 177
Cystitis — 183
Dermatitis Herpetiformis — 191
Diabetes Mellitus — 194

Endometriosis 226
Epilepsy 233
Erythema Multiforme 246
Fibrocystic Breast Disease 249
Fibromyalgia Syndrome 255
Gallstones 267
Glaucoma: Acute (Angle Closure) and Chronic (Open-Angle) 275
Gout 281
Hair Loss in Women 289
Hepatitis 294
Herpes Simplex 303
HIV/AIDS 308
Hypertension 337
Hyperthyroidism 351
Hyperventilation Syndrome/Breathing Pattern Disorders 361
Hypoglycemia 367
Hypothyroidism 377
Immune Support 387
Infectious Diarrhea 394
Inflammatory Bowel Disease 406
Insomnia 424
Intestinal Protozoan Infestation 433
Irritable Bowel Syndrome 436
Kidney Stones 442
Leukoplakia 451
Lichen Planus 454
Macular Degeneration 459
Male Infertility 465
Menopause 476
Menorrhagia 492

Migraine Headache 502
Multiple Sclerosis 521
Nausea and Vomiting of Pregnancy 533
Obesity 538
Osteoarthritis 552
Osteoporosis 565
Otitis Media 581
Parkinson's Disease 588
Pelvic Inflammatory Disease 605
Peptic Ulcers 618
Periodontal Disease 625
Pneumonia: Bacterial, Mycoplasmal, and Viral 633
Porphyrias 640
Premenstrual Syndrome 650
Proctologic Conditions 664
Psoriasis 684
Rheumatoid Arthritis 693
Rosacea 708
Seborrheic Dermatitis 713
Senile (Aging-Related) Cataracts 717
Streptococcal Pharyngitis 725
Trichomoniasis 729
Urticaria 736
Uterine Fibroids 748
Vaginitis and Vulvovaginitis 756
Varicose Veins 772
Index 779

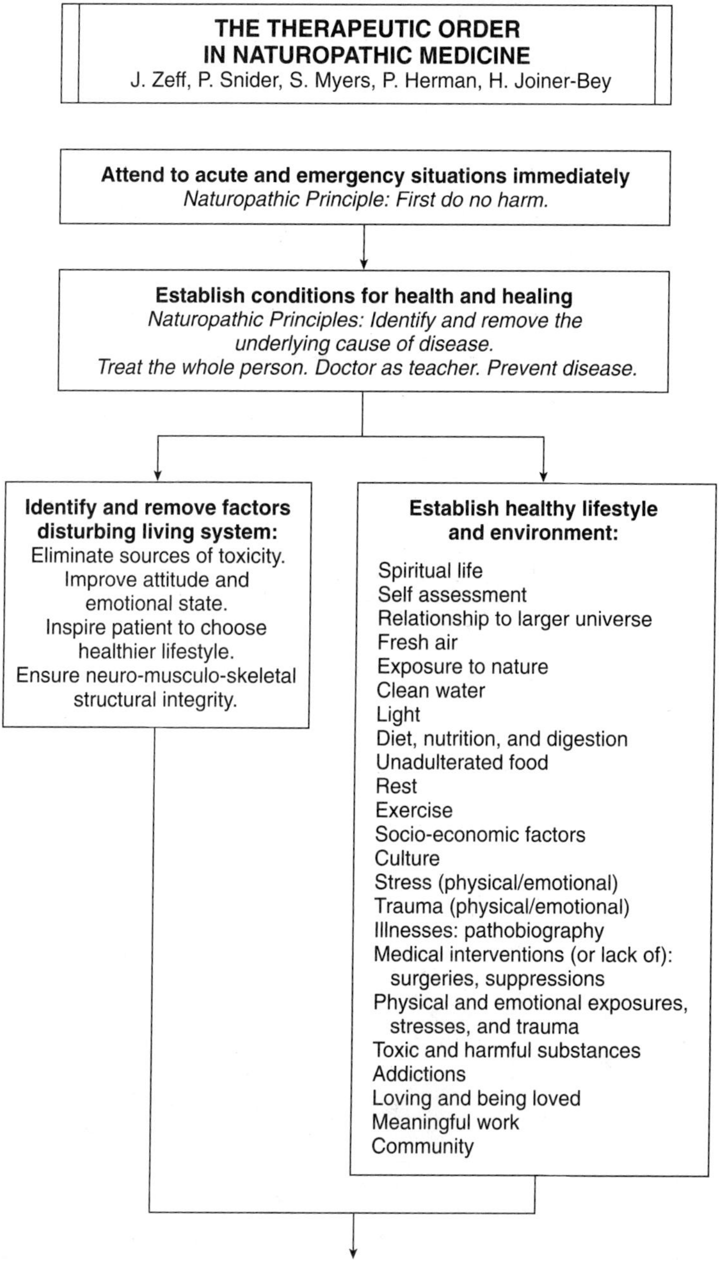

# THE THERAPEUTIC ORDER IN NATUROPATHIC MEDICINE

J. Zeff, P. Snider, S. Myers, P. Herman, H. Joiner-Bey

**Attend to acute and emergency situations immediately**
*Naturopathic Principle: First do no harm.*

↓

**Establish conditions for health and healing**
*Naturopathic Principles: Identify and remove the underlying cause of disease.*
*Treat the whole person. Doctor as teacher. Prevent disease.*

↓

**Identify and remove factors disturbing living system:**
Eliminate sources of toxicity.
Improve attitude and emotional state.
Inspire patient to choose healthier lifestyle.
Ensure neuro-musculo-skeletal structural integrity.

**Establish healthy lifestyle and environment:**

Spiritual life
Self assessment
Relationship to larger universe
Fresh air
Exposure to nature
Clean water
Light
Diet, nutrition, and digestion
Unadulterated food
Rest
Exercise
Socio-economic factors
Culture
Stress (physical/emotional)
Trauma (physical/emotional)
Illnesses: pathobiography
Medical interventions (or lack of):
surgeries, suppressions
Physical and emotional exposures,
stresses, and trauma
Toxic and harmful substances
Addictions
Loving and being loved
Meaningful work
Community

↓

## THE THERAPEUTIC ORDER IN NATUROPATHIC MEDICINE

J. Zeff, P. Snider, S. Myers, P. Herman, H. Joiner-Bey

**Mobilize self-healing processes:**
*Naturopathic Principles: The healing power of nature.*
*Treat the whole person. Identify and treat the cause of disease.*
Constitutional hydrotherapy
Classical homeopathy
Traditional Chinese medicine
Spiritual healing

↓

**Repair weakened tissues:**
*Naturopathic Principles: The healing power of nature.*
*Treat the whole person. Identify and treat the cause of disease.*
Improve digestion
Optimize elimination
Optimize metabolism
Modulate immune function as indicated
Normalize inflammatory responses
Correct endocrine imbalances
Support natural regeneration function
Guide patient in harmonizing with life-force

↓

**Treat specific tissue pathological states:**
*Naturopathic Principles: First, do no harm.*
*Treat the whole person. Prevent future disease.*
Preferred order of interventions:
Natural modalities
Pharmaceuticals
Surgery, chemotherapy, radiotherapy

# Acne Vulgaris and Acne Conglobata

## DIAGNOSTIC SUMMARY

- Open comedones: dilated follicles with central dark, horny plugs (blackheads)
- Closed comedones: small follicular papules with (red papules) or without (whiteheads) inflammatory changes
- Superficial pustules: collections of pus at follicular opening
- Nodules: tender collections of pus deep in dermis
- Cysts: nodules that fail to discharge contents to the surface
- Large, deep pustules: nodules that break down adjacent tissue, leading to scars

## GENERAL CONSIDERATIONS

Most common skin problem. Lesions are mainly on the face, but also back, chest, and shoulders. More common in males; onset during puberty but later for conglobata. Acne vulgaris onset from increased size of pilosebaceous glands and sebum secretion by androgenic stimulation. Severity and progression arise from interactions of hormones, keratinization, sebum, and bacteria.

- **Progression**: hyperkeratinization of upper portion of follicle, blockage of canal, dilation and thinning, formation of comedones (open or closed based on degree of keratinization and blockage of duct), purulent exudate in pustules and cysts.
- **Bacteria**: normal skin species (*Propionibacterium acnes* [*Corynebacterium acnes*] and *Staphylococcus albus*). *P. acnes* releases lipases, hydrolyzing sebum triglycerides into free fatty acid lipoperoxides, promoting inflammation.
- **Inducing compounds and habits**: corticosteroids, halogens, isonicotinic acid, diphenylhydantoin, lithium carbonate, machine oils, coal tar derivatives, chlorinated hydrocarbons, cosmetics, pomades, overwashing, and repetitive rubbing.
- **Endocrinologic aspects**: androgen-dependent condition. Androgens control sebaceous secretion and exacerbate follicular

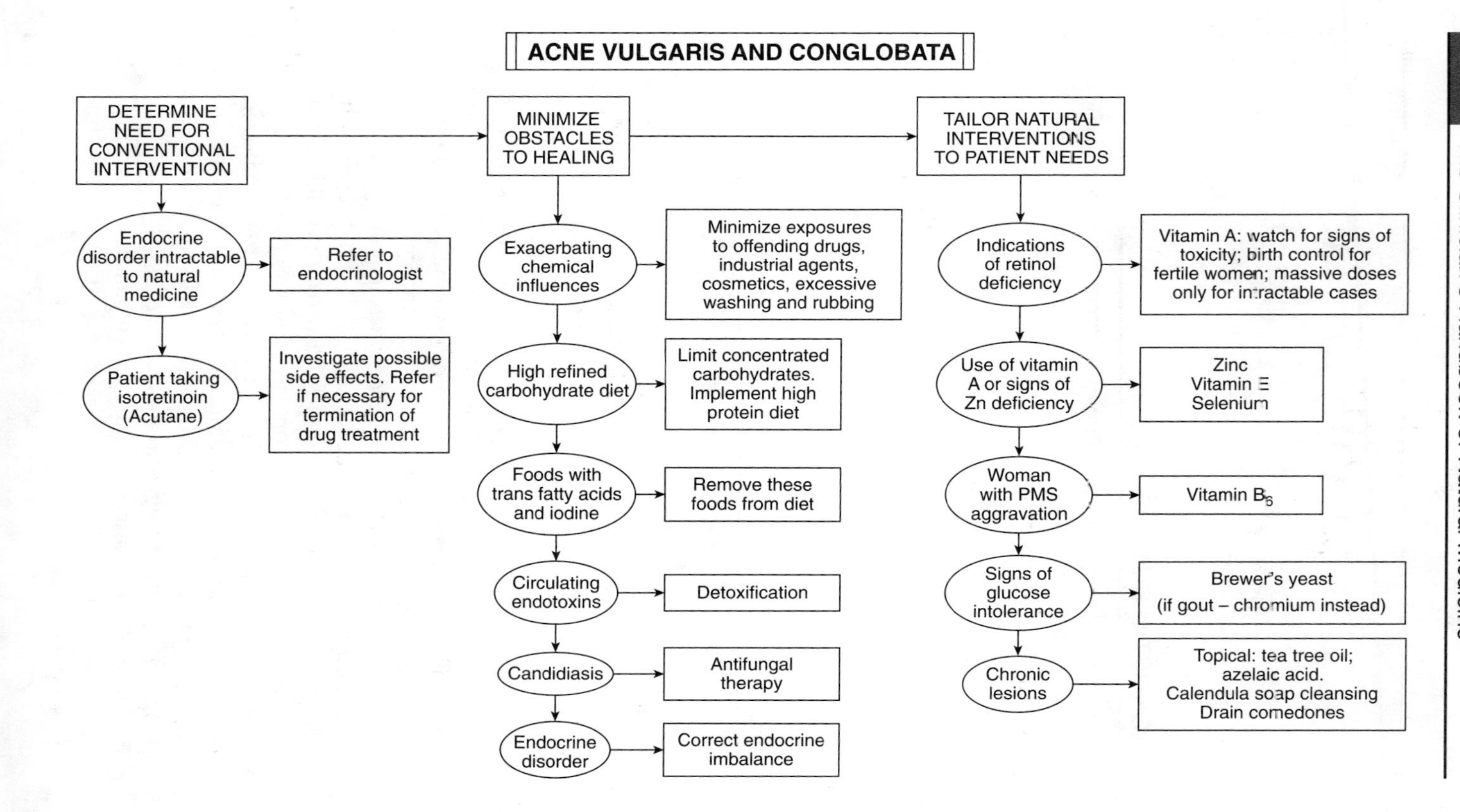
ACNE VULGARIS AND CONGLOBATA
DETERMINE NEED FOR CONVENTIONAL INTERVENTION
Endocrine disorder intractable to natural medicine
Refer to endocrinologist
Patient taking isotretinoin (Acutane)
Investigate possible side effects. Refer if necessary for termination of drug treatment
MINIMIZE OBSTACLES TO HEALING
Exacerbating chemical influences
Minimize exposures to offending drugs, industrial agents, cosmetics, excessive washing and rubbing
High refined carbohydrate diet
Limit concentrated carbohydrates. Implement high protein diet
Foods with trans fatty acids and iodine
Remove these foods from diet
Circulating endotoxins
Detoxification
Candidiasis
Antifungal therapy
Endocrine disorder
Correct endocrine imbalance
TAILOR NATURAL INTERVENTIONS TO PATIENT NEEDS
Indications of retinol deficiency
Vitamin A: watch for signs of toxicity; birth control for fertile women; massive doses only for intractable cases
Use of vitamin A or signs of Zn deficiency
Zinc
Vitamin E
Selenium
Woman with PMS aggravation
Vitamin B6
Signs of glucose intolerance
Brewer's yeast
(if gout – chromium instead)
Chronic lesions
Topical: tea tree oil; azelaic acid.
Calendula soap cleansing
Drain comedones

hyperkeratinization. Endocrine disorders producing excess androgens induce acne development: idiopathic adrenal androgen excess, 21-hydroxylase, polycystic ovaries, free testosterone (T), DHEA, DHEA sulfate, deficient sex-hormone binding globulin. Skin of patient with acne has greater activity of 5-alpha-reductase, elevating more active male hormone DHT locally in skin tissue.

## THERAPEUTIC CONSIDERATIONS

### Nutrition

- **Diet/incidence ratio**: linked to Western diet. Recommend high-protein diet (45% protein, 35% carbohydrate [CHO], 20% fat) to decrease 5-alpha-reductase activity and increase cytochrome P-450 degradation of estradiol. High CHO diet (10% protein, 70% CHO, 20% fat) has opposite effect. Limit foods high in iodine and milk (high hormone content); eliminate trans fats and high-fat foods.
- **Sugar, insulin, and chromium**: insulin efficacy in treating acne suggests cutaneous glucose intolerance and/or insulin insensitivity. Impaired skin glucose tolerance suggests that acne may be called "skin diabetes." Eliminate concentrated CHOs to minimize immunosuppression. High-chromium yeast improves glucose tolerance and may help acne.
- **Vitamin A**: retinol reduces sebum production and hyperkeratinization of sebaceous follicles. Effective at toxic dosage of 300,000-400,000 IU q.d. × 5-6 months. Toxicity: cheilitis (chapped lips) and xerosis (dry skin), especially in dry weather; headache then fatigue, emotional lability, and muscle and joint pain. Lab tests are unreliable to monitor toxicity—serum vitamin A correlates poorly with toxicity, whereas SGOT and SGPT are elevated only in symptomatic patients. Massive doses are teratogenic—women of child-bearing age must use birth control during and for at least 1 month after treatment. Reserve massive doses for intractable cases, in which it should not be used alone.
- **Zinc**: vital to acne treatment. Involved in production of local hormones and retinol-binding protein, wound healing, tissue regeneration, and immune function. Absorption characteristics of Zn salts used may affect results; requires 12 weeks to show good results. Prefer Zn picolinate, acetate, or monomethionine. Zn is essential to normal skin function (e.g., Zn-deficient syn-

drome acrodermatitis enteropathica). Zn is essential for retinol-binding protein and serum retinol levels. Low Zn levels increase 5-alpha reduction of T, and high Zn inhibits this reaction. Serum Zn is lower in 13- and 14-year-old males than in any other age group.

- **Vitamin E and selenium**: vitamin E regulates retinol levels. Male patients with acne have decreased RBC glutathione peroxidase, which normalizes with vitamin E and selenium. Acne of men and women improves with this treatment—inhibiting lipid peroxide formation—suggesting use of other free-radical quenchers.
- **Pyridoxine**: helpful for women with premenstrual acne because of effect on steroid hormone metabolism. $B_6$ deficiency causes increased uptake and sensitivity to T. In some patients thyroid therapy markedly improves acne.
- **Pantothenic acid**: Active in synthesis of cholesterol and steroids. High dosages (10 g q.d. in four divided doses combined with cream consisting of 20% by weight pantothenic acid applied four to six times a day for 1-2 weeks) induce regression of lesions without side effects.

Miscellaneous factors: patients with acne have elevated circulating endotoxins, which can elevate copper/zinc ratio and enhance tissue destruction by alternate complement pathway and fibrin formation.

### Topical Treatments

Goal is to reduce bacteria and inflammation.

- **Tea tree oil (*Melaleuca alternifolia*)**: from leaves of small trees in New South Wales, Australia; antiseptic properties; ideal skin disinfectant. Effective against wide range of organisms (including 27 of 32 strains of *P. acnes*); good penetration without skin irritation. Therapeutic uses are based on antiseptic and antifungal properties; prefer strong solutions (up to 15% tea tree oil) for best results; occasionally produces contact dermatitis.
- **Azelaic acid**: natural 9-carbon dicarboxylic antibiotic against *P. acnes*. Twenty percent azelaic acid cream has an effect in all forms of acne. Must be applied b.i.d. to affected areas for 4 weeks and must be continued for 6 months. Twenty percent azelaic acid cream is as effective as 5% benzoyl peroxide, 4% hydroquinone cream, 0.05% tretinoin, 2% erythromycin, and 0.5-1 g/day oral tetracycline at ameliorating comedonal, papulopustular, and nodulocystic acne but less effective than oral isotretinoin 0.5-1

mg/kg q.d. at reducing conglobate acne; few side effects; no overt systemic toxicity; plus lower incidence of allergic sensitization, exogenous ochronosis, and residual hypopigmentation—better clinical choice.

## THERAPEUTIC APPROACH

Beware of side effects seen in patients using pharmaceutical Accutane (isotretinoin, a derivative of vitamin A): intracranial hypertension, depression, and suicidal ideation.

Rule out treatable underlying causes and hormonal abnormalities; consider consequences of long-term antibiotics—candidiasis (*Textbook,* "Chronic Candidiasis").

- **Diet**: eliminate refined and/or concentrated CHOs and foods containing trans fats and iodine.
- **Supplements**:
  —Vitamin A: 100,000 IU q.d. for 3 months (monitor closely for side effects)
  —Vitamin E: 400 IU q.d.
  —Vitamin C: 1000 mg q.d.
  —Zinc: 50 mg q.d. (picolinate, acetate, or monomethionine)
  —Selenium: 200 μg q.d.
  —Brewer's yeast: 1 tbsp b.i.d. (patients with gout—use chromium instead)
- **Physical medicine**: sun or UV lamp
- **Topical medicine:**
  —Tea tree oil (5%-15%) preparations
  —Azelaic acid (20%) preparations
  —Daily cleansing with calendula soap
  —Drainage of comedones with comedo extractor

# Affective Disorders

## DIAGNOSTIC SUMMARY

**Depression** (major or unipolar depression)—DSM-IV criteria:

- Poor appetite with weight loss or increased appetite with weight gain
- Insomnia or hypersomnia
- Physical hyperactivity or inactivity
- Loss of interest or pleasure in usual activities, decrease in sexual drive
- Loss of energy and feelings of fatigue
- Feelings of worthlessness, self-reproach, or inappropriate guilt
- Diminished ability to think or concentrate
- Recurrent thoughts of death or suicide

Presence of five of these for at least 1 month indicates clinical depression; presence of four means depression probable.

**Dysthymia**: patient depressed most of the time at least 2 years (1 year for children or adolescents) plus at least three of following:

- Low self-esteem, lack of self-confidence
- Pessimism, hopelessness, despair
- Lack of interest in ordinary pleasures and activities
- Withdrawal from social activities
- Fatigue, lethargy
- Guilt, ruminating about past
- Irritability, excessive anger
- Lessened productivity
- Difficulty in concentrating or making decisions

**Manic phase**: mood typically elation but irritability and hostility not uncommon; inflated self-esteem, grandiose delusions, boasting, racing thoughts, decreased need for sleep, psychomotor acceleration, weight loss from increased activity and lack of attention to dietary habits.

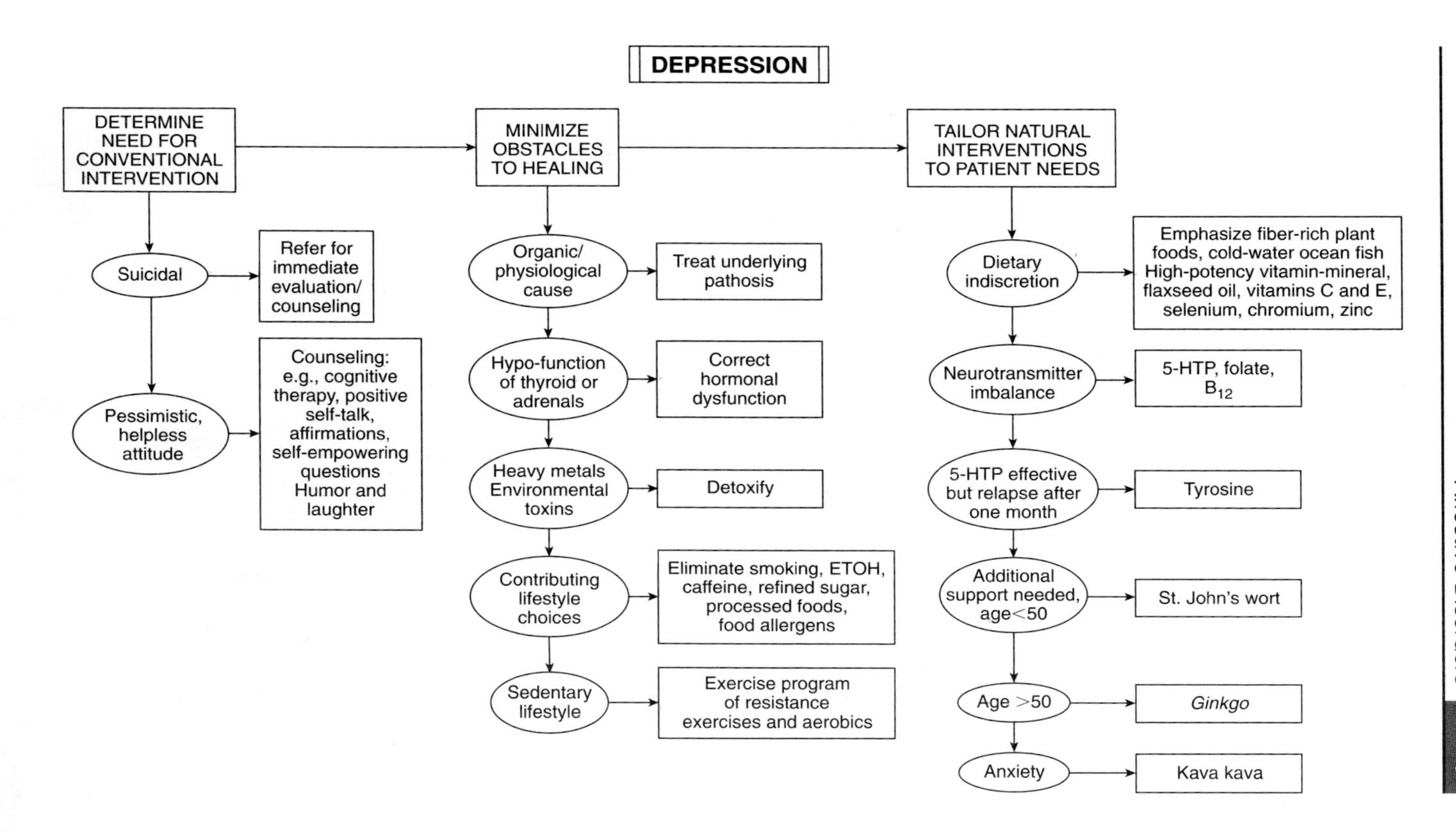
DEPRESSION
DETERMINE NEED FOR CONVENTIONAL INTERVENTION
Suicidal
Refer for immediate evaluation/ counseling
Pessimistic, helpless attitude
Counseling: e.g., cognitive therapy, positive self-talk, affirmations, self-empowering questions Humor and laughter
MINIMIZE OBSTACLES TO HEALING
Organic/ physiological cause
Treat underlying pathosis
Hypo-function of thyroid or adrenals
Correct hormonal dysfunction
Heavy metals Environmental toxins
Detoxify
Contributing lifestyle choices
Eliminate smoking, ETOH, caffeine, refined sugar, processed foods, food allergens
Sedentary lifestyle
Exercise program of resistance exercises and aerobics
TAILOR NATURAL INTERVENTIONS TO PATIENT NEEDS
Dietary indiscretion
Emphasize fiber-rich plant foods, cold-water ocean fish High-potency vitamin-mineral, flaxseed oil, vitamins C and E, selenium, chromium, zinc
Neurotransmitter imbalance
5-HTP, folate, $B_{12}$
5-HTP effective but relapse after one month
Tyrosine
Additional support needed, age<50
St. John's wort
Age >50
*Ginkgo*
Anxiety
Kava kava

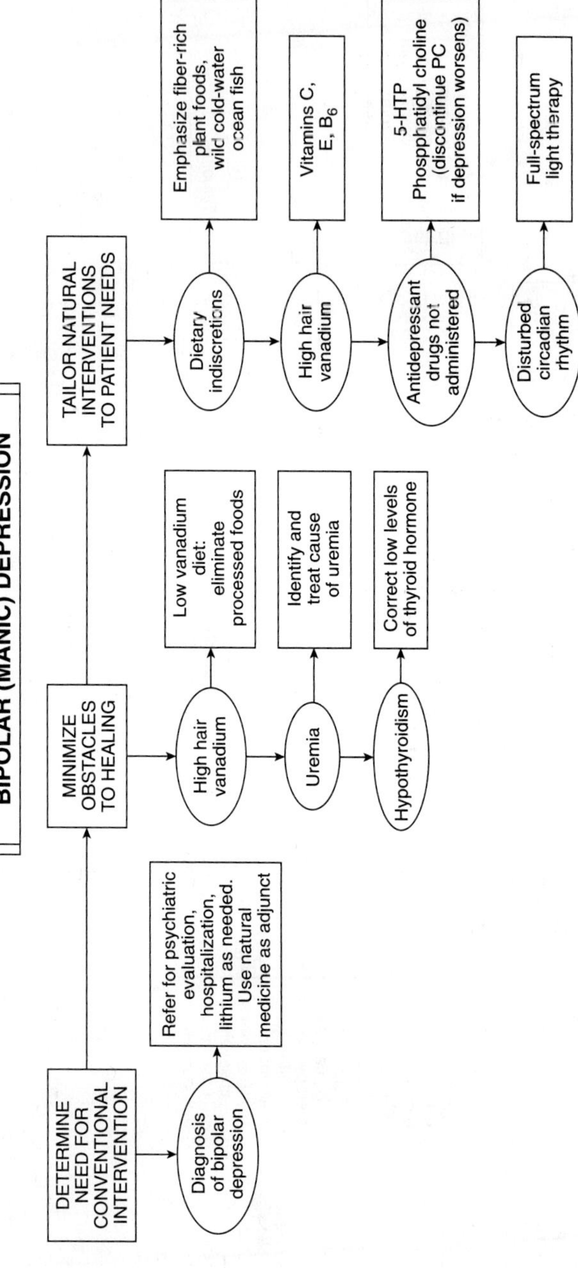
BIPOLAR (MANIC) DEPRESSION
DETERMINE NEED FOR CONVENTIONAL INTERVENTION
Diagnosis of bipolar depression
Refer for psychiatric evaluation, hospitalization, lithium as needed. Use natural medicine as adjunct
MINIMIZE OBSTACLES TO HEALING
High hair vanadium
Low vanadium diet: eliminate processed foods
Uremia
Identify and treat cause of uremia
Hypothyroidism
Correct low levels of thyroid hormone
TAILOR NATURAL INTERVENTIONS TO PATIENT NEEDS
Dietary indiscretions
Emphasize fiber-rich plant foods, wild cold-water ocean fish
High hair vanadium
Vitamins C, E, $B_6$
Antidepressant drugs not administered
5-HTP Phospphatidyl choline (discontinue PC if depression worsens)
Disturbed circadian rhythm
Full-spectrum light therapy

**Seasonal affective disorder**: regularly occurring winter depression frequently associated with summer hypomania.

**Introduction:** affective disorders = mood disturbances; mood = prolonged emotional tone dominating outlook; transient moods (sadness, grief, elation, etc.) part of daily life—demarcation of "pathologic" difficult to determine; depression and mania, alone or in alternation, are the most common disorders and depression alone is much more common; unipolar = depression alone; bipolar = either mania alone or mania alternating with depression.

- **Eight factors modify functional state of brain and affect mood and behavior**: genetic inheritance; age of neuronal development (age-specific variability); functional plasticity of brain during development; motivational state affected by biologic drives, channeling behavior toward goals by priorities or prejudicing context of incoming information; memory-stored information and processing strategies; environment that adjusts incoming input according to momentary significance; brain disease or lesion causing aberrant function; metabolic or hormonal system or biochemical environment of central nervous system (CNS).

**Chapter focus:** nutritional, environmental, and lifestyle factors affecting mood and therapies to alter brain neurotransmitter levels.

## DEPRESSION

### General Considerations

- **Five theoretical models**: "aggression turned inward" (apparent in many cases but no substantial proof); "loss model" (depression = reaction to loss of person, thing, status, self-esteem, or habit pattern); "interpersonal relationship" (depressed person uses depression to control other people, including doctors, by pouting, silence, or ignoring something or someone); "learned helplessness" (habitual feelings of pessimism and hopelessness); "biogenic amine" hypothesis (biochemical derangement of biogenic amines). Learned helplessness model (Martin Seligman, PhD) is most useful.
- **Biogenic amine model**: dominant medical conception of depression. Counseling is valuable, especially with clear psychological etiology.

- **Learned helplessness (Seligman)**: Animals and human beings can be experimentally conditioned to feel and act helpless. Animals conditioned to be helpless have alteration of brain monoamine content; teaching them how to gain environmental control normalizes brain chemistry. Altered brain monoamines in animals with learned helplessness mirror altered brain monoamine biochemistry in human beings during depression. This model revolutionized psychopharmacology; animals conditioned to be helpless and then given antidepressant drugs unlearn helplessness and exercise control over environment. Antidepressants restore monoamine balance and, thereby, alter behavior. Helping patients gain control over their lives produces greater brain biochemical changes than drugs. Powerful technique—teach optimism. Determining factor for person's reaction to uncontrollable events = "explanatory style" (how patient explains events to self). Optimistic people are immune to helplessness and depression; they have positive, optimistic explanatory style. Pessimists are susceptible to depression when "bad" things happen; they have negative, fatalistic explanatory style. Direct correlation between level of optimism and risk for depression and other illnesses.

## Therapeutic Considerations

Ascertain what nutritional, environmental, social, and psychological factors are involved. Rule out simple organic factors known to contribute to depression: nutrient deficiency or excess, drugs (prescription, illicit, alcohol, caffeine, nicotine, etc.), hypoglycemia, consumption, hormonal derangement, allergy, environmental factors, microbial factors.

Psychiatry focuses on manipulating neurotransmitters rather than identifying and eliminating psychological factors. Regardless of whether there is underlying organic cause, always recommend counseling for patients with depression.

- **Counseling**: most merit and support in medical literature—cognitive therapy—as effective as antidepressants for moderate depression with lower rate of relapse. Patient is taught new skills to change the way he or she consciously thinks about failure, defeat, loss, and helplessness. Five basic tactics: (1) recognize negative automatic thoughts when patient feels worst, (2) dispute negative thoughts by focusing on contrary evidence, (3) generate different explanation to dispute negative thoughts, (4) avoid rumination (constant churning of negative thoughts in mind) by consciously controlling thoughts, (5) question negative thoughts and beliefs and replace with empowering positive thoughts and beliefs. Does not involve long psychoanalysis—solution oriented.

- **Organic/physiological causes**: preexisting physical condition, diabetes, heart disease, lung disease, rheumatoid arthritis, chronic inflammation, chronic pain, cancer, liver disease, multiple sclerosis, prescription drugs, antihypertensives, antiinflammatories, birth control pills, antihistamines, corticosteroids, tranquilizers and sedatives, premenstrual syndrome, stress or low adrenal function, heavy metals, food allergies, hypothyroidism, hypoglycemia, nutritional deficiencies, sleep disturbances.
- **Conduct comprehensive clinical evaluation**: ascertain nutritional, environmental, social, and psychological factors; rule out organic factors: nutrient deficiency or excess, drugs (prescription, illicit, alcohol, caffeine, nicotine), hypoglycemia, hormonal derangement, allergy, environmental factors, microbes; counseling recommended regardless of underlying organic cause.

### Hormonal Factors

The focus of this text is on thyroid and adrenal hormones.

- **Thyroid**: depression = early manifestation of thyroid disease: subtle decreases in thyroid hormone can be symptomatic. Whether hypothyroidism results from depression-induced hypothalamic-pituitary-thyroid dysfunction or from thyroid hypofunction is uncertain, but it may be a combination. Screen for hypothyroidism, particularly with suggestive symptoms (e.g., fatigue).
- **Stress and adrenal function**: adrenal dysfunction associated with depression can result from stress. Adrenal stress index measures cortisol and DHEA in saliva. Depression signs: elevated morning cortisol and decreased DHEA. Cortisol elevation reflects disturbed hypothalamic-pituitary-adrenal (HPA) axis and is the basis of the dexamethasone suppression test (DST). HPA dysregulation affecting mood = excessive cortisol independent of stress responses, abnormal nocturnal cortisol release, and inadequate suppression by dexamethasone. CNS effects of increased endogenous cortisol = depression, mania, nervousness, insomnia, and schizophrenia (high levels). Glucocorticoid effects on mood are related to induction of tryptophan oxygenase, shunting

tryptophan to kynurenine pathway at the expense of serotonin and melatonin synthesis.

- **Tests of hypothalamic-pituitary function**: DST and thyroid stimulation test—determine if mood is caused by hypothalamic dysfunction and categorize psychiatric illness (e.g., severe major affective disorders vs. severe psychotic disorders). DST—little clinical value for screening and no better than urinary free cortisol. Thyroid hormone assays do not detect all cases of hypothyroidism—not an effective screening procedure. Thyroid stimulation test (TRH) is more sensitive, diagnosing subclinical hypothyroidism. TRH test has wide clinical utility because thyroid dysfunction is implicated in many disorders.
  TRH grading system for hypothyroidism is as follows:
  —Grade 3 (subclinical hypothyroidism, 4%): patients without classic hypothyroid signs; normal T3RU, T4, and TSH; abnormal TSH response to TRH test
  —Grade 2 (mild hypothyroidism, 3.6%): mild isolated clinical signs or symptoms; normal T3RU and T4; baseline TSH elevated; abnormal TRH test
  —Grade 1 (overt hypothyroidism, 1%): classic hypothyroid signs and symptoms; abnormal lab values (reduced T3RU and T4, increased TSH, abnormal TRH response)

### Environmental Toxins

- **Heavy metals** (Pb, Hg, Cd, As, Ni, Al), solvents (cleaning materials, formaldehyde, toluene, benzene, etc.), pesticides, herbicides—affinity for nervous tissue; associated symptoms = depression, headache, mental confusion, mental illness, tingling in extremities, abnormal nerve reflexes, other signs of impaired nervous function (*Textbook,* "Environmental Medicine" and "Metal Toxicity: Assessment of Exposure and Retention").
- **Detailed medical history and hair mineral analysis** screen for environmental toxins. If hair mineral analysis is inconclusive, a more sensitive test is the 8-hour lead mobilization test—chelating agent EDTA (edetate calcium disodium)—measure lead excreted in urine for 8 hours after injection of EDTA.

### Lifestyle Factors

Eliminate smoking, excess alcohol consumption, sugar abuse, caffeine. Add regular exercise and healthful diet—better clinical results than antidepressants with no side effects or monetary cost.

- **Smoking:** major factor contributing to premature death. Nicotine stimulates adrenal secretion (cortisol) = feature of depression. Cortisol and stress activate tryptophan oxygenase, reducing tryptophan delivery to the brain. Brain serotonin depends on amount of tryptophan delivered—cortisol reduces levels of serotonin and melatonin. Cortisol downregulates brain serotonin receptors, reducing sensitivity to available serotonin. Smoking induces relative vitamin C deficiency; vitamin C helps detoxify smoke. Low levels of brain vitamin C can cause depression and hysteria.
- **Alcohol**: brain depressant; increases adrenal hormone output; interferes with brain cell processes; disrupts sleep cycles; leads to hypoglycemia and craving for sugar, which aggravates hypoglycemia and mental and emotional problems.
- **Caffeine**: stimulant. Intensity of response varies greatly—people prone to depression or anxiety are sensitive to caffeine. "Caffeinism" = clinical syndrome of nervousness, palpitations, irritability, and recurrent headache. Students with moderate to high coffee intake score higher on depression scale and have lower academic performance than low users. Patients with depression have high caffeine intake (more than 700 mg/day). Caffeine intake is positively correlated with degree of mental illness in patients with psychiatric disorders. Caffeine plus refined sugar is worse than either alone—combination has clinical link to depression. Average American intake: 150-225 mg caffeine q.d. = 1-2 cups coffee. Some people are more sensitive to effects than others, even small amount in decaf. Patients with psychological disorders should avoid caffeine completely.
- **Exercise**: most powerful natural antidepressant. Benefit in heart health may be related as much to improved mood as to cardiovascular fitness. Profound antidepressive effects—decreased anxiety, depression, and malaise plus higher self-esteem and more happiness; increases endorphins, which are directly correlated with mood. Sedentary men are more depressed, perceive greater life stress, have higher cortisol and lower beta-endorphins than joggers. Depression is responsive to exercise, firming up biochemical link between physical activity and depression; improves self-esteem and work behavior; can be as effective as antidepressant drugs and psychotherapy. Best exercises = strength training (weight lifting) or aerobics (walking briskly, jogging, bicycling, basketball, cross-country skiing, swimming, aerobic dance, and racquet sports).

## Nutrition

Any single nutrient deficiency can alter brain function, inducing depression or anxiety. Nutrition powerfully influences cognition, emotion, and behavior. Even in the absence of lab validation of deficiency, nutritional supplementation can be of benefit. Full-range high-potency multiple vitamin = foundation. Nutrient deficiencies are common in depressed individuals; most common = folate, $B_{12}$, and $B_6$.

**Behavioral Effects of Some Vitamin Deficiencies**

| Deficient Vitamin | Behavioral Effects |
|---|---|
| Thiamin | Korsakoff's psychosis, mental depression, apathy, anxiety, irritability |
| Riboflavin | Depression, irritability |
| Niacin | Apathy, anxiety, depression, hyperirritability, mania, memory deficits, delirium, organic dementia, emotional lability |
| Biotin | Depression, extreme lassitude, somnolence |
| Pantothenic acid | Restlessness, irritability, depression, fatigue |
| Vitamin $B_6$ | Depression, irritability, sensitivity to sound |
| Folic acid | Forgetfulness, insomnia, apathy, irritability, depression, psychosis, delirium, dementia |
| Vitamin $B_{12}$ | Psychotic states, depression, irritability, confusion, memory loss, hallucinations, delusions, paranoia |
| Vitamin C | Lassitude, hypochondriasis, depression, hysteria |

- **Diet**: brain requires constant sugar supply; hypoglycemia must be avoided. Hypoglycemia symptoms: psychological disturbances (e.g., depression, anxiety, irritability), fatigue, headache, blurred vision, excessive sweating, mental confusion, incoherent speech, bizarre behavior, convulsions. Hypoglycemia is common in depressed individuals; eliminate refined carbohydrates; health promotion diet rich in whole, natural, unprocessed foods, especially high in plant foods (fruits, vegetables, whole grains, beans, seeds, nuts).
- **Folate and $B_{12}$**: function together in many pathways. Folate deficiency is the most common nutrient deficiency worldwide;

31%-35% of patients with depression are folate deficient, 35%-92.6% among the elderly. Depression is the most common symptom of folate deficiency. $B_{12}$ deficiency is less common but can also cause depression, especially in the elderly. Folate, $B_{12}$, and SAM (S-adenosyl-methionine) are "methyl donors"; SAM is the major methyl donor in the body. Antidepressant effects of folate = increasing brain SAM. The key brain compound dependent on methylation is tetrahydrobiopterin (BH4), a coenzyme in the manufacture of monoamine neurotransmitters (e.g., serotonin and dopamine) from respective amino acids. Patients with recurrent depression have reduced BH4 synthesis, probably from low SAM levels. BH4 synthesis is stimulated by folate, $B_{12}$, and C; supplementation can increase BH4 and serotonin content. Folate dosages as antidepressant are very high: 15-50 mg is safe (except in epilepsy) and is as effective as antidepressant drugs. Dosages of 800 μg folate and 800 μg $B_{12}$ are sufficient to prevent deficiencies. Folate supplements should always be accompanied by $B_{12}$ to prevent masking $B_{12}$ deficiency.

- **Vitamin $B_6$**: low in patients with depression, especially women on birth control pills or Premarin; essential to manufacture of all monoamines; dosage = 50-100 mg q.d.
- **Zinc**: cofactor in 70 metalloenzymes. Severe deficiency symptoms: bullous-pustular dermatitis, diarrhea, alopecia, recurrent infections. Derangement of Zn homeostasis is linked to mood disorders. Antidepressant drugs increase Zn in hippocampus of patients with depression with low baseline Zn. Zn may act as antagonist of NMDA glutamate receptor. Small study: Zn reduces scores on Hamilton and Beck depression scales in patients taking antidepressant drugs. Balance with copper during long-term use.
- **Selenium**: Se levels are low in alcoholics. Low Se status encourages depressed mood; high dietary Se or supplementation improves mood. Low Se is linked to depression, anxiety, confusion, hostility. Alcoholism combined with depression in the same person increases risk for suicide.
- **Chromium**: increased sugar intake is correlated with depression. Cr may balance insulin levels. Atypical depression (one fifth of all depressive illness) is characterized by mood reactivity, increased appetite and weight gain, hypersomnia, leaden paralysis, interpersonal rejection sensitivity, earlier onset, greater chronicity, disability, and suicidality than other forms of depression. Cr picolinate may help some atypical patients with depression

at 400 to 600 μg daily. Mechanism of action: alteration of brain serotonin levels and increasing insulin insensitivity.

- **Omega-3 fatty acids:** insufficiency linked to depression; affect phospholipid composition of neuronal cell membranes. The brain is the richest source of phospholipids in the body; lack of essential fatty acids (EFAs) (omega-3 oils) and excess saturated fats induce formation of cell membranes less fluid than optimal and impair membrane regulation of passage of molecules into and out of cell, disrupting homeostasis and proper nerve cell function, impacting behavior, mood, and mental function. Biophysical properties, including fluidity of brain cell membranes, influence neurotransmitter synthesis, signal transmission, neurotransmitter binding and uptake, and activity of monoamine oxidase—factors implicated in depression. Omega-3 EFAs may inhibit development of depression as they do cardiovascular disease. Lowering plasma cholesterol by diet and medications increases suicide, homicide, and depression. The quantity and type of dietary fats consumed alter biophysical and biochemical properties of cell membranes. Dietary efforts to lower cholesterol tend to increase the n-6/n-3 ratio and decrease eicosapentaenoic acid and docosahexanoic acid. Decreased consumption of omega-3 EFAs correlates with increasing rates of depression. Consistent association between depression and coronary artery disease, also linked to omega-3 deficits.
- **Food allergies**: depression and fatigue are linked to food allergies; "Allergic toxemia" is a syndrome with symptoms of depression, fatigue, muscle and joint aches, drowsiness, difficulty concentrating, and nervousness.

## Monoamine Metabolism and Precursor Therapy

Monoamine precursors (tryptophan, 5-hydroxytryptophan [5-HTP], and tyrosine) offer natural alternative to monoamine oxidase (MAO) inhibitors and tricyclics for influencing monoamine metabolism.

- **Tryptophan catastrophe**: for more than 30 years, L-tryptophan has been used by millions in the United States and around the world safely and effectively for insomnia and depression. In October 1989, one Japanese manufacturer, Showa Denko, the largest supplier to the United States (50%-60%), produced batches contaminated with substances now linked to eosinophiliamyalgia syndrome (EMS) caused by changes in the bacteria used to produce L-tryptophan and the filtration process. Patients with EMS have the following signs and symptoms: eosinophils >1000/ $mm^3$ (twice normal); allergic and inflammatory symptoms from release of histamine by eosinophils: severe muscle and joint pain, high fever, weakness, swelling of arms and legs, skin rashes, and shortness of breath. EMS affected 144 of every 50,000 men and 268 of every 50,000 women, or 1 in 250 people taking contaminated L-tryptophan. Only those with an abnormal activation of kynurenine pathway reacted to the contaminant; kynurenine and its metabolites (quinolic acid) are linked to other EMS-related illnesses (e.g., Spain's 1991 toxic oil syndrome, one of the largest food-related epidemics ever); people who took multiple vitamin preparation were somewhat protected against EMS; vitamins ($B_6$ and niacin) shunted tryptophan away from the kynurenine pathway or contaminants were somehow metabolized by vitamin-dependent enzymes.

- **L-Tryptophan**: increases brain serotonin and melatonin. Many depressed individuals have low tryptophan and serotonin. Supplementation provides mixed clinical results; only two of eight studies indicated superiority compared with placebo, but nine of 11 studies indicated equivalence to antidepressant drugs. Factors to consider: study size, severity of depression, duration, and dosage. Hormones (estrogen and cortisol) and tryptophan itself stimulate tryptophan oxygenase, which converts tryptophan to kynurenine with less tryptophan delivered to brain. Summary: L-tryptophan only modestly effective when used alone; must be used with $B_6$ and niacinamide to block kynurenine pathway; better results with 5-HTP.
- **5-HTP**: cannot be converted to kynurenine and easily crosses the blood-brain barrier. Only 3% of oral L-tryptophan is converted to serotonin, whereas more than 70% of oral 5-HTP is converted. 5-HTP causes increased endorphins and catecholamine; equipotency with serotonin reuptake inhibitors and tricyclics; advantages: less expensive, better tolerated, fewer and milder side effects.
- **Phenylalanine and tyrosine**: phenylalanine is hydroxylated to tyrosine and degraded to phenylketonic acids, but also decarboxylated to phenylethylamine (PEA). PEA is an amphetamine-like endogenous stimulatory/antidepressive substance in human beings. (PEA = biogenic amine in high concentrations in chocolate.) Low urinary PEA is found in patients with depression, high

levels in schizophrenics. D-Phenylalanine and L-phenylalanine increase urinary and CNS PEA. Phenylalanine is a tyrosine hydroxylase inhibitor; shunting phenylalanine to PEA synthesis occurs with supplementation. Tyrosine increases trace amines (octopamine, tyramine, and PEA), enhances catecholamine synthesis, stimulates thyroid hormone synthesis. L-Dopa alone is ineffectual in affective disorders. Central norepinephrine turnover is decreased in patients with depression—may result from low serum tyrosine seen in some depressed individuals. Brain tyrosine is best determined by ratio of serum tyrosine to sum of its brain-uptake competitors (leucine, isoleucine, valine, tryptophan, and phenylalanine). Tyrosine ratios increase with high-protein meals. Tyrosine supplements increase urine 3-methoxy-4-hydroxyphenethylene glycol (MHPG), the principal breakdown product of norepinephrine in CNS and a biochemical marker for determining which amino acid to supplement. Phenylalanine and tyrosine are encouraging alternatives to tricyclics and MAO inhibitors. Van Praag study: 20% of patients who responded well to 5-HTP relapsed after 1 month despite the fact that blood 5-HTP and presumably brain serotonin remained the same as when experiencing benefit; other monoamine neurotransmitters (dopamine and norepinephrine) declined; patients responded to supplemental tyrosine.

- **SAM**: involved in methylation of monoamines, neurotransmitters, and phospholipids. The brain manufactures SAM from methionine; SAM synthesis is impaired in patients with depression. SAM supplementation in patients with depression increases serotonin, dopamine, and phosphatides and improves binding of neurotransmitters to receptors, increasing serotonin and dopamine activity and improving neuron membrane fluidity and clinical symptoms. SAM is an effective natural antidepressant but expensive; oral dosage 400 mg q.i.d. (1600 mg total). Better tolerated with quicker action than tricyclics; study comparing SAM to tricyclic desipramine: 62% of SAM patients and 50% of desipramine patients significantly improved. Regardless of type of treatment, patients with 50% decrease in Hamilton Depression scale had significant increase in plasma SAM. No significant side effects with oral SAM; nausea and vomiting in some people. Start dosage at 200 mg b.i.d. first day, 400 mg b.i.d. day 3, 400 mg t.i.d. day 10, and 400 mg q.i.d. after 20 days. Bipolar (manic) patients should not take SAM—susceptible to hypomania or mania.

- Botanical medicines
  - ***Hypericum perforatum*** (St. John's wort): extracts standardized for hypericin and hyperforin = most thoroughly researched natural antidepressants. Mechanisms of action may include serotonin reuptake modulation, increases in interleukin-6 activity, and agonist action of sigma receptors. Improves many symptoms: depression, anxiety, apathy, sleep disturbances, insomnia, anorexia, feelings of worthlessness. Advantages over antidepressant drugs are fewer side effects, lower cost, and greater patient tolerance. Beware of hyperforin's enhancement of drug degradation, including contraceptives, by liver cytochrome p450 enzymes (*Textbook, "Hypericum perfatum* [St. John's Wort]").
  - ***Piper methysticum* (Kava kava)**: approved in Germany, United Kingdom, Switzerland, and Austria for treatment of nervous anxiety, insomnia, depression, and restlessness based on detailed pharmacologic data and favorable clinical studies; efficacy compares favorably with benzodiazepines without drug side effects (impaired mental acuity, addictiveness). Prefer extracts standardized for kavalactones (30%-70%). High incidence of improper dosing of kava extract; know how to use this botanical properly for best efficacy; most useful for depression with severe anxiety (*Textbook, "Piper methysticum* [Kava]").
  - ***Ginkgo biloba***: leaf extract standardized to 24% ginkgo flavonglycosides and 6% terpenoids; exerts good antidepressant effects, especially for those older than 50; improves mood in patients with cerebrovascular insufficiency; can be used with antidepressant drugs and may enhance their efficacy in patients older than 50. Counteracts one of the major brain chemistry changes associated with aging—reduction in number of serotonin receptors. Mechanism of effect: correcting or preventing impaired receptor synthesis or changes in cerebral neuronal membranes or receptors as a result of free radical damage; increases protein synthesis and acts as a potent antioxidant (*Textbook, "Ginkgo biloba* [Ginkgo Tree]").

## Therapeutic Approach

Accurately determine which factors contribute to patient's depression; balance errant neurotransmitter levels and optimize patient's nutrition, lifestyle, and psychological health.

- **Diet**: increase fiber-rich plant foods (fruits, vegetables, grains, legumes, raw nuts and seeds); avoid caffeine, nicotine, other stimulants, sugar, and alcohol; identify and control food allergies; increase consumption of small wild cold-water fish to at least twice per week.

- **Lifestyle**: refer to counselor or counsel patient to develop positive, optimistic mental attitude—help patient set goals, use positive self-talk and affirmations, identify self-empowering questions, and find ways to inject humor and laughter into life. Exercise at least 30 minutes at least three times a week; apply relaxation/stress reduction techniques 10 to 15 minutes daily.
- **Supplements**:
  - High-potency multiple vitamins and minerals
  - Vitamin C: 500-1000 mg t.i.d.
  - Vitamin E: 200-400 IU q.d.
  - Selenium: 200 μg q.d.
  - Chromium: 400-600 μg q.d.
  - Zinc: 25 mg q.d.
  - Flaxseed oil: 1 tbsp q.d.
  - 5-HTP: 100-200 mg t.i.d.
  - Folic acid and vitamin $B_{12}$: 800 μg of each q.d.
- **Botanical medicines:**
  —Younger than 50: St. John's wort extract (0.3% hypericin, 4% hyperforin): 300 mg t.i.d.; severe cases, St. John's wort in combination with 5-HTP
  —Older than 50: *Ginkgo biloba* extract (24% ginkgo flavonglycosides, 6% terpenoids), 80 mg t.i.d.; severe cases, use in combination with St. John's wort and/or 5-HTP
  —Significant anxiety: kava extract (standardized to kavalactones): 45-70 mg kava lactones t.i.d.

## BIPOLAR (MANIC) DEPRESSION AND HYPOMANIA

### Diagnostic Summary

Diagnostic criteria for bipolar depression—at least three of following symptoms:

- Excessive self-esteem or grandiosity
- Reduced need for sleep
- Extreme talkativeness, excessive telephoning
- Extremely rapid flight of thoughts along with the feeling that the mind is racing
- Inability to concentrate, easily distracted

- Increase in social or work-oriented activities, often with a 60-80 hour work week
- Poor judgment, as indicated by sprees of uncontrolled spending, increased sexual indiscretions, and misguided financial decisions

## General Considerations

Bipolar depression is characterized by periods of major depression alternating with periods of elevated mood. If elevated mood is relatively mild and lasts 4 days or less, it is called hypomania. Mania is longer and more intense. Full-blown manic attack requires hospitalization: loss of self-control, may hurt themselves or others. Standard treatment is lithium—stabilizes mood, prevents manic phase—used either alone or with antidepressant. Antidepressant drugs can occasionally induce mania and hypomania; difficult to control lows in bipolar depressives with drugs.

## Therapeutic Considerations

Initially hospitalize 2 weeks under sedation with antipsychotic drugs until blood lithium levels are acceptable. Refer for conventional therapy until mood stabilizes. Principles outlined for depression also apply to mania; seriousness of condition—use nutritional therapy as adjunct rather than primary therapy. Selective serotonin reuptake inhibitors are helpful in combination with lithium; 5-HTP and St. John's wort may be useful as adjuncts to lithium but without side effects.

- **Tryptophan**: effective doses are generally quite large: 12 g q.d. L-tryptophan. Better choice is 5-HTP, in combination with lithium, at 100 mg t.i.d.
- **Phosphatidylcholine (PC)**: large amounts of PC (15-30 g q.d. in both pure form and lecithin)—better results for mania than monoamine precursors. Lithium promotes increased CNS cholinergic activity by inhibition of choline flux across the blood-brain barrier; mania is associated with reduced CNS cholinergic activity. Using PC to increase CNS choline may improve symptoms in some patients.
- **Omega-3 fatty acids**: One 4-month, double-blind, placebo-controlled study found marked therapeutic efficacy and no side effects. Dosage: 9.6 g/day of omega-3 fatty acids. Benefits: longer period of remission and may inhibit neuronal signal transduction pathways in a manner similar to that of lithium carbonate and valproate.

- **Vanadium**: increased Va found in hair of manic patients; levels normalize with recovery. Patients with depression have normal hair Va, with whole blood and serum Va elevated and returning to normal on recovery. Vanadate ion is a strong inhibitor of Na+K+-ATPase; lithium reduces this inhibition. Therapies to reduce vanadate to less-inhibitory vanadyl form include ascorbic acid, methylene blue, and EDTA separately and in combination. Ascorbic acid (3 g q.d.) provides significant clinical improvement. Low-vanadium diet—low-Va foods (1-5 ng/g) include fats, oils, fresh fruits, vegetables; range of 5-30 ng/g includes whole grains, seafood, meat, dairy; range of 11 to 93 ng/g includes prepared foods (peanut butter, white bread, breakfast cereals). Other correctable factors known to inhibit Na+K+-ATPase are uremia, hypothyroidism, and catecholamine insensitivity. Vitamins E and $B_6$ increase Na+K+-ATPase activity in vitro; vitamin E also stabilizes membranes.
- **Circadian rhythms**: patients with manic depression have disturbed circadian rhythms, seasonal patterns of exacerbations, and supersensitivity to light. Alteration of circadian light-dark cycles with light therapy may help (see the section on seasonal affective disorder below).

### Therapeutic Approach

Same dietary and lifestyle guidelines as for depression.

- **Diet**: low-vanadium diet—eliminate all refined and processed foods; promote fresh fruits and vegetables.
- **Supplements**:
  —Phosphatidylcholine: 10-25 g q.d. (PC may induce depression in some patients; if this occurs, discontinue immediately)
  —Vitamin C: 3-5 g q.d. in divided doses
  —Vitamin E: 400-800 IU q.d.
  —Pyridoxine: 100 mg q.d.

## SEASONAL AFFECTIVE DISORDER (SAD)

### General Considerations

Associated with winter depression and summer hypomania. Typically patients feel depressed, slow down, oversleep, overeat, and crave carbohydrates in winter. In summer, they feel elated, active, energetic.

## Therapeutic Considerations

- **Melatonin**: light exposure is the main contributing factor. Key hormonal changes are reduced melatonin from pineal and increased cortisol from adrenals. Melatonin supplementation may improve SAD; it increases brain melatonin and suppresses cortisol secretion.
- **Light therapy**: full-spectrum light therapy has antidepressive effects in SAD and clinical depression by restoring pineal melatonin synthesis and secretion and reestablishing circadian rhythm. Place full-spectrum fluorescent tubes in regular fluorescent fixtures (eight tubes total). Patients sit 3 feet away from light from 05.00-08.00 hours (5-8 AM) and 17.30-20.30 hours (5:30-8:30 PM). Patients are free to engage in activities as long as they glance at the light at least once per minute. Protocol restricts social life; replacing standard bulbs with full-spectrum light may help.
- ***Hypericum perforatum***: St. John's wort extract (standardized to 0.3% hypericin, 4% hyperforin) (*Textbook, "Hypericum perforatum* [St. John's Wort]") at dosage of 300 mg t.i.d. improves SAD but is more effective in combination with light therapy. Beware of enhanced drug degradation by liver cytochrome p450 enzymes.

## Therapeutic Approach

Extend light exposure on winter days; use full-spectrum lighting throughout indoor environment; nighttime melatonin (3 mg 45 min before retiring); daytime St. John's wort or 5-HTP.

# Alcoholism

## DIAGNOSTIC SUMMARY

- Alcohol dependence manifested when alcohol is withdrawn: tremulousness, convulsions, hallucinations, delirium
- Alcoholic binges, benders (48 hours or more of drinking associated with failure to meet usual obligations), or blackouts
- Evidence of alcohol-induced illnesses: cirrhosis, gastritis, pancreatitis, myopathy, polyneuropathy, cerebellar degeneration
- Physical signs of excess alcohol consumption: alcohol odor on breath, flushed face, tremor, ecchymoses
- Psychological/social signs of excess alcohol consumption: depression, loss of friends, arrest for driving while intoxicated, surreptitious drinking, drinking before breakfast, frequent accidents, unexplained work absences.

## GENERAL CONSIDERATIONS

World Health Organization definition: consumption exceeding limits accepted by culture or that injures health or social relationships

- **Consequences**: increased mortality: 10-12 years lower life expectancy; twice death rate in men, three times in women; six times the suicide rate; major factor in four leading causes of death in men aged 25-44 (accidents, homicides, suicides, cirrhosis); economic toll; health effects: metabolic damage to every cell; intoxication; abstinence and withdrawal syndromes; nutritional deficiency diseases; cerebellar degeneration; cerebral atrophy; psychiatric disorders; esophagitis, gastritis, ulcer; increased risk of cancer of mouth, pharynx, larynx, esophagus; pancreatitis; liver fatty degeneration and cirrhosis; arrhythmias; myocardial degeneration; hypertension; angina; hypoglycemia; decreased protein synthesis; increased serum and liver triglycerides; decreased serum testosterone; myopathy; osteoporosis; rosacea, spider veins; coagulation disorders.

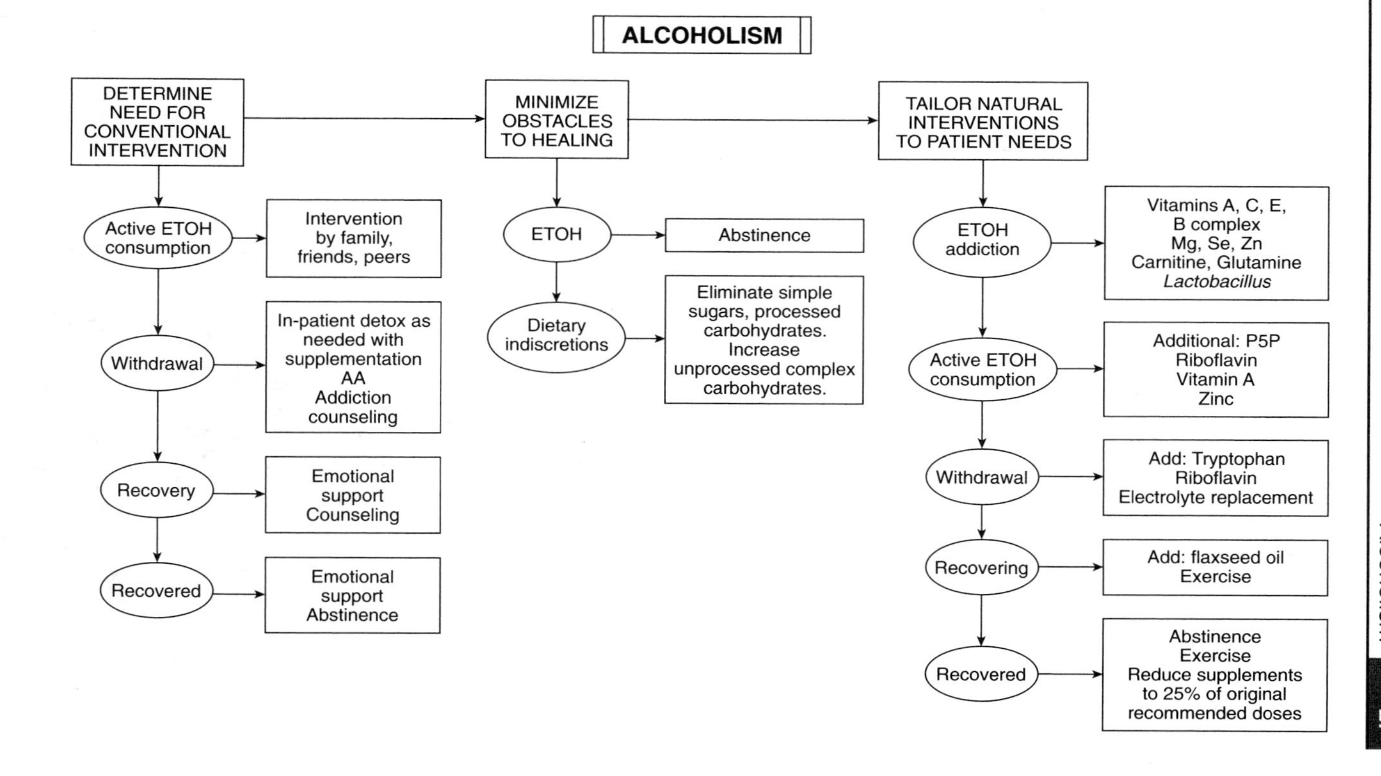
ALCOHOLISM
DETERMINE NEED FOR CONVENTIONAL INTERVENTION
MINIMIZE OBSTACLES TO HEALING
TAILOR NATURAL INTERVENTIONS TO PATIENT NEEDS
Active ETOH consumption
Intervention by family, friends, peers
Withdrawal
In-patient detox as needed with supplementation AA Addiction counseling
Recovery
Emotional support Counseling
Recovered
Emotional support Abstinence
ETOH
Abstinence
Dietary indiscretions
Eliminate simple sugars, processed carbohydrates. Increase unprocessed complex carbohydrates.
ETOH addiction
Vitamins A, C, E, B complex Mg, Se, Zn Carnitine, Glutamine Lactobacillus
Active ETOH consumption
Additional: P5P Riboflavin Vitamin A Zinc
Withdrawal
Add: Tryptophan Riboflavin Electrolyte replacement
Recovering
Add: flaxseed oil Exercise
Recovered
Abstinence Exercise Reduce supplements to 25% of original recommended doses

- **Effects on fetus**: growth retardation; mental retardation; fetal alcohol syndrome; teratogenicity.
- 18 million alcoholics in United States; often a "hidden" disease disguised by sympathetic family and friends.

The brief Michigan alcoholism screening test (MAST) indicates alcoholism by a score of greater than 5:

| | | |
|---|---|---|
| 1. Do you feel you are a normal drinker? | Yes (0) | No (2) |
| 2. Do friends or relatives think you are a normal drinker? | Yes (0) | No (2) |
| 3. Have you ever attended a meeting of Alcoholics Anonymous (AA)? | Yes (5) | No (0) |
| 4. Have you ever lost friends, girlfriends, or boyfriends because of drinking? | Yes (2) | No (0) |
| 5. Have you ever gotten into trouble at work because of drinking? | Yes (2) | No (0) |
| 6. Have you ever neglected your obligations, your family, or your work for 2 or more days in a row because you were drinking? | Yes (2) | No (0) |
| 7. Have you ever had delirium tremens (DTs), severe shaking, heard voices, or seen things that were not there after heavy drinking? | Yes (2) | No (0) |
| 8. Have you ever gone to anyone for help about your drinking? | Yes (5) | No (0) |
| 9. Have you ever been in a hospital because of drinking? | Yes (5) | No (0) |
| 10. Have you ever been arrested for drunk driving or driving after drinking? | Yes (2) | No (0) |

- **Etiology**: obscure; multifactorial: genetic, physiologic, psychological, and social factors equally important; 35% of alcoholics start between ages 15 and 19 years, 80% before age 30; most common in men; female/male ratio is rising to 1:2. Women become addicted at lower intake than men.

Antibody-mediated mechanisms may play a role in pathogenesis. Incidence of alcoholism is four to five times more common in biologic children of alcoholics than of nonalcoholic parents. Association with genetic markers: color vision, nonsecretor ABH, HLA-$B_{13}$, and low platelet monoamine oxidase. Biochemical studies show importance of alcohol dehydrogenase polymorphism in racial susceptibility to alcoholism.

## Intoxication and Withdrawal

- **Intoxication signs**: central nervous system depression: drowsiness, errors of commission, disinhibition, dysarthria, ataxia, and nystagmus; 15 mL pure ETOH (1 oz whiskey, 4 oz wine, or 10 oz beer) raises blood ETOH level by 25 mg/dL in 70-kg person; effects of varying levels of blood ETOH are as follows:

| Blood Level (mg/dl) | Effect |
|---|---|
| <50 | No significant motor dysfunction |
| 100 | Mild intoxication: decreased inhibitions, slight visual impairment, slight muscular incoordination, slowing of reaction time; legally intoxicated in most jurisdictions |
| 150 | Ataxia, dysarthria, slurring of speech, nausea and vomiting |
| 350 | Marked muscular incoordination, blurred vision, approaching stupor |
| 500 | Coma and death |

- **Withdrawal symptoms**: 1-3 days after last drink; anxiety, tremulousness, mental confusion, tremor, sensory hyperactivity, visual hallucinations, autonomic hyperactivity, diaphoresis, dehydration, electrolyte disturbances, seizures, and cardiovascular abnormalities.

## Metabolic Effects of Alcohol and Alcoholism

- **Ethanol metabolism**: factors influencing ETOH catabolism are rate of ETOH absorption, concentration and activity of liver alcohol dehydrogenase (ADH) and aldehyde dehydrogenase (ALDH), and NADH/NAD+ ratio in liver mitochondria. Availability and regeneration of NAD+ are rate-limiting factors for ETOH oxidation. ETOH is converted to acetaldehyde by ADH, with cofactor NAD+. Aldehyde is responsible for harmful effects and addictive process; high blood aldehyde found in alcoholics and relatives after ETOH consumption—either increased ADH activity or depressed ALDH activity in people susceptible to alcoholism. Acetaldehyde is converted by ALDH to acetate, with little entering Krebs cycle; most is converted to long-chain fatty acids, leading to fatty liver.

- **Fatty liver**: in all alcoholics, even with minimal consumption; severity proportional to duration and degree of ETOH excess. Pathogenesis arises from increased endogenous fatty acid synthesis, diminished triglyceride utilization, impaired lipoprotein excretion, direct damage to endoplasmic reticula by free radicals produced by ethanol metabolism, and high-fat diet typical of alcoholics. Leptin is peptide hormone helping regulate appetite and energy metabolism. Circulating leptin levels are increased in a dose-dependent manner in chronic alcoholism regardless of nutritional status. Elevated leptin contributes to liver pathology: increased fibrosis, a known factor in liver steatosis.
- **Hypoglycemia**: ETOH induces reactive hypoglycemia and produces craving for foods that quickly elevate blood sugar (sugar and ETOH). Sugar aggravates reactive hypoglycemia, particularly with ETOH-induced impairment of gluconeogenesis. Hypoglycemia aggravates mental and emotional problems of alcoholics and withdrawal with sweating, tremor, tachycardia, anxiety, hunger, dizziness, headache, visual disturbance, decreased mental acuity, confusion, depression.

## THERAPEUTIC CONSIDERATIONS

### Nutrition

Nutritional problems are related to ETOH and fact that alcoholics tend not to eat. ETOH is substitute for food.

- **Zinc**: ADH and ALDH are Zn-dependent enzymes, with ALDH more sensitive to deficiency. Short- and long-term ETOH abuse induces Zn deficiency from decreased dietary intake, decreased ileal absorption (interference with Zn-binding ligand, picolinic acid, and nonspecific mucosal damage), hyperzincuria. Higher hair Zn and Cu are found in male alcoholics. Hair Cu is related to amount of ETOH consumed; hair Zn is higher with distilled beverages; observations may indicate abnormal metabolism and loss of these minerals. Low serum Zn is associated with impaired ETOH metabolism, risk of cirrhosis, and impaired testicular function. Zn supplementation, particularly with ascorbate, greatly increases ETOH detox and survival in rats.

- **Vitamin A**: deficiency is common in alcoholics and works with zinc deficiency to produce major complications of alcoholism. Mechanism is reduced intestinal absorption of A and Zn, with impaired liver function (reduced extraction of Zn, mobilization of retinol-binding protein [RBP], and storage of vitamin A), results in reduced blood Zn, vitamin A, RBP, and transport proteins and a shift to nonprotein ligands. Effects: reduced tissue A and Zn, abnormal enzyme activities and glycoprotein synthesis, and impaired DNA/RNA metabolism with increased kidney Zn loss. Results: symptoms of alcoholism—night blindness, skin disorders, liver cirrhosis, reduced skin healing, decreased testicular function, impaired immunity. Endocrine influences: supplementation with A inhibits ETOH consumption in female, but not male, rats, and the effect is inhibited by exogenous testosterone; ovariectomized and adrenalectomized rats show decreased preference for ETOH; corticosterone injections increase preference. Supplementation in alcoholic corrects A deficiency: improved night blindness and sexual function. *Caution*: excessive amounts of A are contraindicated because ETOH-damaged liver loses ability to store A; risk of vitamin A toxicity at dosage greater than dietary allowance of 5000 IU daily.
- **Antioxidants**: ETOH increases lipid peroxidation, causing increased lipoperoxide in liver and serum. Alcoholics are deficient in antioxidants and nutrients: E, Se, and C. Significant correlation between serum lipid peroxide, SGOT activity, and liver cell necrosis. Antioxidants, before or simultaneous with ETOH intake, inhibit lipoperoxide formation and prevent fatty liver infiltration. Effective antioxidants: C, E, Zn, Se, and cysteine.
- **Carnitine (Crn)**: common lipotropic agents (choline, niacin, cysteine) are indicated but of little value. Crn significantly inhibits ETOH-induced fatty liver disease. Long-term ETOH abuse causes functional Crn deficiency. Crn facilitates fatty acid transport and oxidation in mitochondria; high liver Crn is needed for increased fatty acid produced from ETOH. Crn supplements reduce serum triglycerides and SGOT levels while elevating HDL.
- **Amino acids (AAs)**: chromatography patterns are aberrant in alcoholics; normalization greatly assists alcoholics (liver is the primary site for AA metabolism). AAs are particularly indicated in hepatic cirrhosis and depression. Branched-chain amino acids (BCAAs) (valine, isoleucine, leucine) inhibit hepatic encephalopathy and protein catabolism (sequelae of cirrhosis). Deranged neurotransmitter profiles (from very low plasma tryptophan)

cause depression, encephalopathy, and coma—aggravated by low-protein diet in standard therapy for cirrhosis and avoided by free-form AAs without risk of hepatic encephalopathy (see chapter on affective disorders—depression). Individualized approach indicated because of differences in nutritional status, biochemistry, and amount of liver damage. AA chromatography is helpful for best results.

- **Vitamin C**: deficiency of ascorbate found in 91% of patients with alcohol-related diseases. C helps ameliorate effects of ETOH toxicity in human beings and guinea pigs (species unable to synthesize own ascorbate). Direct correlation between WBC ascorbate (good index of body ascorbate status), rate of ETOH blood clearance, and activity of hepatic ADH. C is strong reducing agent: acts as electron donor similar to NAD in ETOH metabolism, increasing ETOH conversion to acetaldehyde and catabolism of acetaldehyde.
- **Selenium**: plasma, serum, WBC, and RBC Se is lower in alcoholics. Low Se encourages depression, anxiety, confusion, and hostility; supplementation improves mood. Alcoholism and depression in same patient increase risk for suicide. Se supplementation is warranted to ameliorate untoward comorbid psychological and physical profiles.
- **B vitamins**: alcoholics are deficient in most B vitamins. Mechanisms: low dietary intake, deactivation of active form, impaired conversion to active form by ETOH or acetaldehyde, impaired absorption, decreased storage capacity. ETOH decreases absorption and utilization of B vitamins by liver and/or increases urinary excretion of B vitamins (especially folate). $B_1$ deficiency is the most common (55%) and most serious, leading to beriberi and Wernicke-Korsakoff syndrome and greater intake of ETOH. ($B_1$ deficiency may predispose for alcoholism.) Functional $B_6$ deficiency is also common, leading to impaired conversion to active form, pyridoxal-5-phosphate, and enhanced degradation.
- **Magnesium**: deficiency common in alcoholics (60%), strongly linked to delirium tremens, and major reason for increased cardiovascular disease in alcoholics. Deficiency is caused by reduced intake plus ETOH-induced renal hyperexcretion, which continues during withdrawal despite hypomagnesiemia. Alcoholic cardiomyopathy has been linked to $B_1$ deficiency but may instead be from Mg deficiency.
- **Essential fatty acids (EFAs)**: ETOH interferes with EFA metabolism; ETOH abuse may produce symptoms of EFA deficiency.

ETOH abuse in rhesus monkeys leads to alcoholic amblyopia, a rare neuropathy characterized by blurred vision, diminished retinal function, and reduced visual acuity. DHA deficits found in brain and retinal tissues.

- **Glutamine**: supplementation (1 g q.d.) reduces voluntary ETOH consumption in uncontrolled human studies and experimental animal studies. This preliminary research is 40+ years old, but there has been no follow-up despite efficacy, safety, and low cost.

## Psychosocial Aspects

Physicians must be nonjudgmental, but not passive, in their attitude toward their patients. Alcoholism is a chronic, progressive, addictive, and potentially fatal disease. Social support for patient and family is essential. Success is often proportional to involvement of Alcoholics Anonymous (AA), counselors, and social agencies. Maintain close working relationships with experienced counselors, AA, Al-Anon, and Ala-Teen. *Requirements for successful initiation of treatment*: patient realization that he or she has ETOH problem; education of patient and/or family about physical and psychosocial aspects of alcoholism; and immediate patient involvement in treatment program. *Elements of successful programs*: strict control of ETOH plus replacement with another addiction that is nonchemical; time consuming; and heavily supported by family, friends, and peers; strict abstinence safest and most effective choice.

**Depression**: common in alcoholics; leads to high suicide rate. Many are depressed first then become alcoholic (primary depressives); others are alcoholic first then develop depression in context of alcoholism (secondary depressives). Alterations in serotonin metabolism and availability of precursor (tryptophan) are implicated in some forms of depression; other forms are linked to catecholamine metabolism and tyrosine availability. Alcoholics have severely depleted tryptophan, leading to depression and sleep disturbances. ETOH impairs tryptophan transport into brain. Enzyme tryptophan pyrolase is rate limiting in tryptophan catabolism and more active in rats during ETOH withdrawal. Plasma tryptophan is depleted in withdrawing alcoholics but normalizes after 6 days of treatment and abstinence. Brain tryptophan uptake is also influenced by competition from AAs sharing the same transport (tyrosine, phenylalanine, valine, leucine, isoleucine, methionine), which are elevated in malnourished alcoholics. Depressed alcoholics have lowest ratios of tryptophan to these AAs; AAs that lower ratio are catecholamine precursors (tyrosine and phenylalanine). Elevated plasma catecholamines are common in alcoholics and may contribute to depression. Taurine is also low in depressed alcoholics, with lowest levels in psychotic alcoholics.

### Miscellaneous Factors

- **Intestinal flora**: severely deranged in alcoholics. Endotoxin-producing bacteria may colonize small intestine, inducing malabsorption of fats, carbohydrates, protein, folate, and $B_{12}$. ETOH increases intestinal permeability to endotoxins and macromolecules, increasing toxic and antigenic effects, contributing to complications of alcoholism. Addictive tendency of food allergies may contribute to ETOH cravings.
- **Exercise**: graded, individualized fitness program improves likelihood of maintaining abstinence. Regular exercise alleviates anxiety and depression and enables better response to stress and emotional upset.
- ***Silybum marianum* (milk thistle)**: flavonoid complex (silymarin) effective in treatment of full spectrum of ETOH-related liver disease; extends life span of alcoholics. Silymarin can improve immune function in patients with cirrhosis.

## THERAPEUTIC APPROACH

Alcoholism is difficult to treat; little documented long-term success, except for AA (overall success of AA is highly controversial); requires integrated, whole-person, stage-oriented program designed for four stages of alcoholism: (1) active consumption, (2) withdrawal, (3) recovery, (4) recovered. Recovery stage = period between withdrawal and full reestablishment of normal metabolism. Complete diagnostic workup required because of high risk for wide variety of clinical and subclinical diseases. Therapeutic support is needed in all stages.

- **Diet**: stabilize blood sugar; eliminate simple sugars (sucrose, fructose, glucose; fruit juice; dried fruit; low-fiber fruits: grapes and citrus); limit processed carbohydrates (white flour, instant potatoes, white rice, etc.); increase unprocessed complex carbohydrates (whole grains, vegetables, beans, etc.).

- **Supplements**:
  —Vitamin A: 5000 IU q.d.
  —B complex: 20 times the RDA
  —Vitamin C: 1 g b.i.d.
  —Vitamin E: 400 IU q.d. D-alpha-tocopherol
  —Magnesium: 250 mg b.i.d.
  —Selenium: 200 μg q.d.
  —Zinc: 30 mg q.d. picolenate
  —Carnitine: 500 mg b.i.d. L-carnitine
  —Glutamine: 1 g q.d.
  —*Lactobacillus acidophilus*: 1 tsp q.d.
- **Exercise**: graded program using heart rate response to determine intensity; five to seven times weekly for 20-30 minutes at intensity raising heart rate to 60%-80% of age group maximum.
- **Counseling**: AA and experienced counselor with alcohol addiction expertise.
- **Additional recommendations for four stages**:
  1. *Active ETOH consumption*: family, peers, social group support to elicit patient's recognition of ETOH problem and willingness to enter treatment program; additional supplements: pyridoxal-5-phosphate (20 mg q.d.), riboflavin (100 mg q.d.), vitamin A (50,000 IU q.d.), zinc (30 mg q.d.).
  2. *Withdrawal*: symptom severity variable, proportional to degree of dependence and duration of disease. Milder cases—within a few hours after cessation of drinking and resolves within 48 hours; more severe cases—in patients older than 30 and develop after 48 hours of abstinence—need in-patient facility, additional supplements (obtain institutional permission before admission): tryptophan (3 g q.d.); riboflavin (100 mg q.d.); electrolyte replacement as needed.
  3. *Recovering*: strong emotional support network; involve patient in intense, people-oriented activities; help patient reject ETOH as destructive response to stress and develop more effective ways of handling adversity; additional supplement: flaxseed oil (1 tbsp t.i.d.).
  4. *Recovered*: maintain emotional support network; continue total abstinence; slowly reduce supplement doses, after 6 months of abstinence, to 25% of above recommendations.

# Alzheimer's Disease

## DIAGNOSTIC SUMMARY

- Progressive mental deterioration, loss of memory and cognitive functions, inability to carry out activities of daily life
- Characteristic symmetrical, usually diffuse, EEG pattern
- Diagnosis usually made by exclusion
- Definitive diagnosis can be made only by postmortem biopsy of brain, demonstrating atrophy, senile plaques, and neurofibrillary tangles

## GENERAL CONSIDERATIONS

Alzheimer's disease (AD) is a neurodegenerative disorder of progressive deterioration of memory and cognition or dementia. Five percent of U.S. population older than 65 have severe dementia; another 10% have mild to moderate dementia. Frequency rises with increasing age: 50%-60% of all cases of dementia (senile and presenile) are caused by AD. "The disease of the twentieth century": tenfold increase in AD in U.S. population older than age 65.

### Neuropathology

Distinctive neuropathologic features: plaque formation, amyloid deposition, neurofibrillary tangles, granulovascular degeneration, massive loss of telencephalic neurons; particularly evident in cerebral cortex and hippocampal formation. Clinical features are believed to arise from cholinergic dysfunction by reduced activity of enzyme choline acetyltransferase (which synthesizes acetylcholine) and neuronal transfer of choline.

### Etiology

Genetic factors play a major role: amyloid precursor gene on chromosome 21 (close association between Down's syndrome and AD); presenilin genes on 14 and 1; apolipoprotein E (*ApoE*) gene on 19;

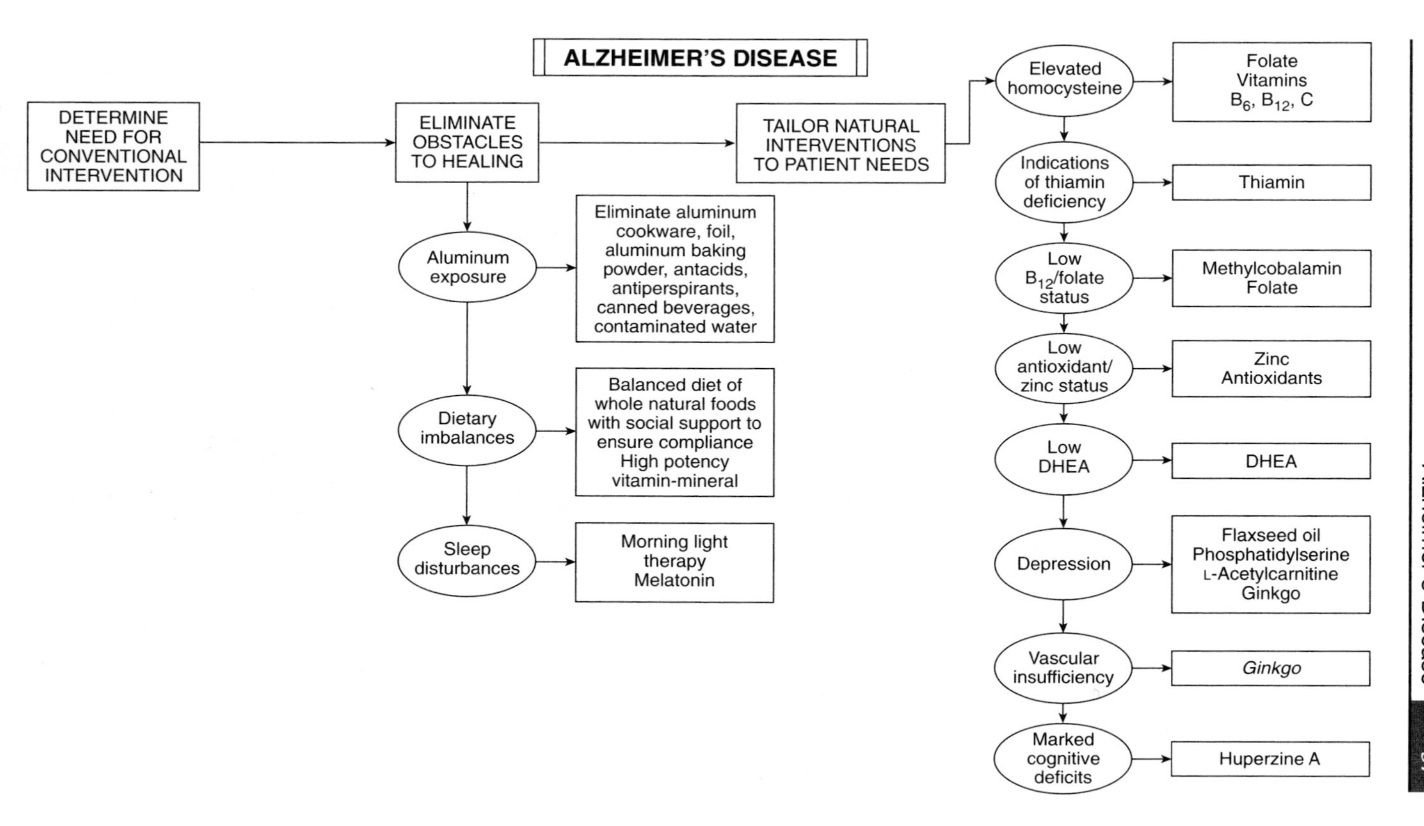
ALZHEIMER'S DISEASE
DETERMINE NEED FOR CONVENTIONAL INTERVENTION
ELIMINATE OBSTACLES TO HEALING
TAILOR NATURAL INTERVENTIONS TO PATIENT NEEDS
Aluminum exposure
Eliminate aluminum cookware, foil, aluminum baking powder, antacids, antiperspirants, canned beverages, contaminated water
Dietary imbalances
Balanced diet of whole natural foods with social support to ensure compliance
High potency vitamin-mineral
Sleep disturbances
Morning light therapy
Melatonin
Elevated homocysteine
Folate
Vitamins $B_6$, $B_{12}$, C
Indications of thiamin deficiency
Thiamin
Low $B_{12}$/folate status
Methylcobalamin
Folate
Low antioxidant/zinc status
Zinc
Antioxidants
Low DHEA
DHEA
Depression
Flaxseed oil
Phosphatidylserine
L-Acetylcarnitine
Ginkgo
Vascular insufficiency
*Ginkgo*
Marked cognitive deficits
Huperzine A

mutations on 21, 14, and 1;—rare and associated with symptoms before age 50. The most significant genetic finding is the link with *ApoE*; *ApoE* of e4-type is linked to much greater risk; e2-type is linked to greater protection.

Genetically linked aberrant immune system regulation of inflammation may contribute. Innate immune function in brain normally removes plaque. Long-term excessive reaction to immune protofibrils of amyloid proteins can promote AD. Immunotherapeutic trials resulted in both beneficial and adverse effects. Antioxidants protect against untoward immune processes; consider natural anti-inflammatories used for cardiovascular disease.

- **Lifestyle factors**: diet—excess saturated or trans fatty acids may predispose neurons to aluminum-induced toxicity. Sleep—abnormal sleep-wake cycles and decreased morning light exposure (see melatonin, later).
- **Other factors**: traumatic head injury; long-term exposure to aluminum, silicon, environmental neurotoxins, and free radicals; increased oxidative damage.
- **Homocysteine**: increased plasma (and perhaps urine) homocysteine is a strong, independent risk factor for dementia and AD, just as it is for atherosclerosis. Plasma level greater than 14 μmol/L nearly doubles risk of AD. Control homocysteine with folate and vitamins $B_{12}$, $B_6$, and C.
- **Aluminum** (AL): concentrated in neurofibrillary tangles and significantly contributes to AD; strong affinity for and cofactor with paired helical filament tau (PHFt) involved in forming neurofibrillary tangles. AL selectively binds to PHFt, induces PHFt aggregation, and retards brain's ability to break down PHFt. Long-term exposure of animals to ecologic doses of AL induces ghostlike neurons with cytoplasmic and nuclear vacuolations, with AL deposits; neuritic plaques in hippocampus; amyloid deposits in cerebrovasculature; behavorial changes reminiscent of AD. Brain and serum AL levels increase with age as AD incidence increases with age. Patients with AD have much higher AL than normal people and patients with other dementias (ETOH, atherosclerosis, stroke). Efforts to remove AL help but probably are too late, after disease is well established. Even in those without mental disease, elevated AL is linked with poorer mental function. Sources of AL are water supply (immediately enters brain tissue), food, antacids, antiperspirants.

## DIAGNOSTIC CONSIDERATIONS

Only 50% of patients with dementia have AD; comprehensive diagnostic workup paramount. Diagnosis depends on clinical judgment. *Workup:* detailed history; neurologic and physical exam; psychological evaluation with particular attention to depression; general medical evaluation revealing subtle metabolic, toxic, or cardiopulmonary disorders inducing confusion in elderly; neurophysiology tests to document the type and severity of cognitive impairment; social worker mobilization of community resources; lab tests (ECG, EEG, CT scan, MRI).

- **Diagnostic process**: exclude other possible diagnoses.
  —*Step 1*: diagnose dementia accurately. (10%-50% error rate when diagnosis is based only on first evaluation. Avoid

**Causes and Mechanisms of Development of Senile Dementia**

| Etiology | Pathogenesis |
|---|---|
| **Degenerative Etiology** | Disturbances of gene expression and thus of protein metabolism |
| Altered genetic code | Disturbance of the synthesis of specific proteins |
| Alzheimer's disease | Reduction in acetylcholine synthesis resulting from decreased ChAc activity |
| Huntington's chorea | Disturbance of the GABAergic system |
| Idiopathic dementia, localized form | Decline in cognitive function |
| Parkinson's disease | Reduction in dopamine turnover |
| Pick's disease | Reduction in cholinergic activity |
| Loss of neuronal redundancy | Disturbance of cerebral metabolism after infection or trauma; reduction in cholinergic activity caused by loss of neurons and synapses |
| Cerebrovascular disease | |
| Chronic meningitis | |
| Tuberculosis, mycotic | |
| Encephalopathy after head injury (boxers) | |
| Viral encephalopathy | |
| Encephalomyelitis | |
| Epileptic dementia | |

*Continued*

### Causes and Mechanisms of Development of Senile Dementia—cont'd

| Etiology | Pathogenesis |
|---|---|
| **Nutritive Etiology** | |
| Chronic alcoholism | |
| Diabetes mellitus | |
| Disturbances of electrolyte metabolism | |
| Hypoglycemia | Insulin, starvation |
| Hyponatremia | Diuretics |
| Hypothyroidism | |
| Korsakoff syndrome | Thiamine transketolase deficiency |
| Nicotinamide deficiency | |
| Vitamin B deficiency | Disturbances of energy formation |
| **Toxic Etiology** | |
| Addiction to barbituates, psychotropic drugs, etc. | |
| Chronic CO intoxication | |
| Chronic $CO_2$ intoxication | |
| Mycotoxins | |
| Renal/hepatic encephalopathy | |
| Vincristine intoxication | |

misdiagnosing pseudodementing functional illness. Depression mimics dementia in the elderly.
—*Step 2*: do careful neurologic exam to reveal (a) focal, circumscribed brain disease; (b) diffuse, bilateral brain dysfunction; or (c) no evidence of neurologic dysfunction. Routine neurologic exam recognizes (a) and (c) but not diffuse brain dysfunction displaying subtle indications: patient's level of consciousness, attentiveness to examiner, comprehension, performance of tasks, facial expressions, quality of speech, posture, respiratory rhythm, and gait.

- **Signs of diffuse brain dysfunction**: persistent glabella-tap response (light tapping above bridge of nose produces blink that normally fatigues rapidly); corneomandibular reflex (ipsilateral strong blink and contralateral movement of chin from firm stimulus applied quickly to cornea); sucking reflex; snout reflex; palmomental reflex (ipsilateral contraction of mentalis muscle in response to stimulating thenar eminence); grasp reflex.

- **Recognizing reversible causes for diagnosed dementia**: drug toxicity, metabolic and nutritional disorders (hypoglycemia; thyroid disturbances; deficiencies of vitamin $B_{12}$, folate, or thiamine), hyperhomocysteinemia, neurosyphilis, disorders causing dementia (Huntington's chorea, cerebral vascular disease, normal pressure hydrocephalus, intracranial masses).
- **Recommended lab tests in dementia**: CBC (anemia, infection); RPR (syphilis); electrolyte (metabolic dysfunction); liver function tests (hepatic dysfunction); BUN (renal dysfunction); TSH, $T_4$, $T_3$, $T_3U$ (thyroid dysfunction); serum $B_{12}$ and RBC folate (deficiency); plasma and urine homocysteine, urinalysis (renal/hepatic dysfunction); hair mineral analysis (heavy metal intoxication); ECG (heart function); EEG (focal vs. diffuse pathosis); CT scan (atrophy, intracranial mass).

**Recommended Laboratory Tests in Dementia**

| Test | Rationale |
|---|---|
| CBC | Anemia, infection |
| VDRL or RPR | Syphilis |
| Electrolytes | Metabolic dysfunction |
| Liver function tests | Hepatic dysfunction |
| BUN | Renal dysfunction |
| TSH, $T_4$, $T_3$, $T_3U$ | Thyroid dysfunction |
| Serum $B_{12}$ and RBC folate | Deficiency |
| Urinalysis | Renal/hepatic dysfunction |
| Hair mineral analysis | Heavy metal intoxication |
| ECG | Heart function |
| EEG | Focal vs. diffuse |
| CT scan | Atrophy, intracranial mass |

- **EEG**: an important tool in differentiating dementias. Normal EEG does not rule out dementia, particularly in early stages, but provides valuable information. AD has characteristic sym-

metrical diffuse slowing of EEG. EEG differentiates focal (e.g., intracranial mass or vascular disease) and diffuse (e.g., metabolic disorders or normal pressure hydrocephalus) dysfunction.
- **CT scan**: rules out high incidence (4%-5%) of silent brain tumors or other lesions (e.g., subdural hematoma); limited use in AD. Brain atrophy is normal part of aging.
- **MRI**: useful diagnostic information in minutes; noninvasive; characterizes neuronal markers and neurotransmitters (glutamate, GABA).
- **Fingerprint patterns**: abnormal in Alzheimer's and Down's; increased number of ulnar loops on fingertips, with concomitant decrease in whorls, radial loops, and arches. Ulnar loops (pointing toward ulnar bone, away from thumb) frequently are found on all 10 fingertips. Radial loops (pointing toward thumb), when they occur, are shifted away from index and middle fingers—where they most commonly occur—to ring and little fingers. Appearance of Alzheimer fingerprint pattern warrants immediate aggressive preventive approach.

## THERAPEUTIC CONSIDERATIONS

Prevention by (1) addressing suspected pathophysiology and (2) using natural measures to improve mental function in early stages; in advanced stages natural measures are of only limited benefit.

- **Diet**: recommend small, wild, ocean fish and high monounsaturated fatty acids of Mediterranean diet. Emphasize whole foods high in synergistic proportions of antioxidants. Minimize saturated fat, trans fatty acids. Antioxidant deficits may lead to increased serum and brain AL and transition metal ions, increasing oxidative stress and inflammation. Apply cardioprotective risk reduction factors—whole grains and vegetables.
- **Estrogen**: promoted to offer protection and therapeutic benefits, but epidemiologic and clinical evidence is weak—no major gender differences in rate or severity of AD; particularly problematic because of long-term adverse effects that outweigh benefits.
- **Aluminum**: avoid all known sources of AL—antacids, antiperspirants, AL-containing baking powder, cookware, foil food wrap, canned beverages, nondairy creamers, table salt additives. Citric acid and calcium citrate supplements increase AL absorption (but not Pb) from water and food. AL absorption is decreased by Mg (competes for absorption at intestinal mucosa and blood-

brain barrier). Recommend Mg-rich diet: unprocessed whole foods (avoid milk and dairy), vegetables, whole grains, nuts, and seeds.

## Nutrition

Directly related to cognition in the elderly; nutrient deficiency common.

- **Antioxidants**: oxidative damage plays a major role in AD. Antioxidant nutrients offer significant protection. Antioxidants (e.g., vitamins C and E) protect against inflammation and oxidative stress and slow progression of Parkinson's in patients not yet on medications. Digestive dysfunction is common among elderly; fat malabsorption, including vitamin E, leads to neuronal symptoms of vitamin E deficiency: ataxia, proprioceptive and vibratory sense impairment, and gait disturbance. Vitamin E RDA is 15 mg (22 IU). Vitamin E (2000 IU/day) slows progression of moderately severe AD dementia; better results when vitamin C used concurrently with antioxidants started earlier in disease process. These antioxidants improve cognition even if no dementia or cognitive impairment is apparent. Vitamin E improves response of patients taking pharmaceutical drug donepezil for AD. Antioxidants support mitochondrial function and presenilin despite genetic predisposition to decline.
- **Thiamin (vitamin $B_1$)**: deficiency rather uncommon (except alcoholics), but many elderly do not get even RDA (1.5 mg). $B_1$ potentiates and mimics brain neurotransmitter of memory, acetylcholine. $B_1$ (3-8 g/day) improves mental function in AD and age-related impaired mental function (senility) without side effects.
- **Vitamin $B_{12}$**: deficiency induces impaired nerve function, causing numbness, paresthesiae, or burning feeling in feet, impaired mental function that mimics AD in the elderly. $B_{12}$ deficiency is common in the elderly and a major cause of depression in this age group. Best test is serum cobalamin or urine methylmalonic acid; plasma homocysteine indicates $B_{12}$ and folate status. $B_{12}$ declines with age and deficiency is found in 3%-42% of persons aged 65 and over. Untreated deficiency affects neurologic and cognitive function. $B_{12}$ screening tests are indicated in elderly given positive cost-benefit ratio. Urinary methylmalonic acid assay is the best: sensitive, noninvasive, and relatively convenient for patient. Correcting $B_{12}$ deficiency improves mental

function and quality of life. Low $B_{12}$ levels are common in patients with AD. High homocysteine levels increase AD risk. $B_{12}$ and/or folate supplements may completely reverse some patients, but generally there is little improvement in patients with AD symptoms longer than 6 months because of irreversible changes. Active forms in body: methylcobalamin and adenosylcobalamin.

- **Zinc**: common nutrient deficiency in the elderly and possible major factor in AD development. Enzymes involved in DNA replication, repair, and transcription are Zn dependent. Long-term Zn deficiency may cause cascading effects of error-prone/ineffective DNA-handling enzymes in nerve cells. Zn is required by antioxidant enzymes (superoxide dismutase). Levels of Zn in brain and cerebrospinal fluid in patients with AD are markedly decreased. There is a strong inverse correlation between serum Zn and senile plaque count. Supplementation is beneficial in AD. "The zinc paradox": Zn is neurotoxic at high concentrations and accumulates at sites of degeneration. Total tissue Zn is markedly reduced in brains of patients with AD. Much higher concentration of copper-zinc superoxide dismutase in and around damaged brain tissue of patients with AD suggests increased Zn in damaged areas from body's efforts to neutralize free radicals by increasing local production of dismutases. Possible corollary: higher focal Zn results in increased amyloid formation when free radical scavenging is inadequate.
- **Phosphatidylcholine (PC)**: dietary PC can increase brain acetylcholine (Ach) in normal patients. AD is characterized by decreased cholinergic transmission. PC supplementation would seem beneficial in AD but basic defect in cholinergic transmission in AD = impaired enzyme acetylcholine transferase, which combines choline (provided by PC) with acetyl moiety to form neurotransmitter Ach. Providing more choline (by PC) will not increase enzyme activity. Mild to moderate dementia may be helped by high-quality PC (15-25 g q.d.); discontinue if no noticeable improvement within 2 weeks.
- **Phosphatidylserine (PS)**: the major phospholipid in the brain; helps determine integrity and fluidity of cell membranes. Deficiency of methyl donors (*S*-adenosyl-methionine [SAM], folate, $B_{12}$) or essential fatty acids may inhibit production of PS. Low brain PS is linked to impaired mental function and depression in the elderly. PS is useful in treating depression and/or impaired mental function in the elderly, including AD (100 mg t.i.d.).

- L-**Acetylcarnitine (LAC)**: thought to be much more active than other forms of carnitine in brain disorders; close structural similarity to Ach; mimics Ach and benefits patients with early-stage AD and elderly with depression or impaired memory; powerful antioxidant within neurons; stabilizes cell membranes; improves energy production within neurons; delays progression of AD (2 g b.i.d.); also beneficial for non-AD mild mental deterioration in the elderly (1500 mg q.d.); enhances effect of acetylcholinesterase inhibitors in patients with AD unresponsive to drugs alone (2 g q.d.).

## Other Therapies

- **DHEA (dehydroepiandrosterone)**: the most abundant steroid hormone in the bloodstream, with extremely high brain levels. Levels decline dramatically with aging—symptomatic, including impaired mentality. DHEA itself has no known function but is a source for all endogenous steroids (e.g., sex hormones and corticosteroids). Declining DHEA is linked to diabetes, obesity, hypercholesterolemia, heart disease, and arthritis. DHEA may enhance memory and cognition. Dosages: men over 50 years, 25-50 mg q.d.; women, 15-25 mg; men and women aged 70+ years: 50-100 mg q.d. Excessive dosing causes acne and, in women, menstrual irregularities. Use lab assessment before prescribing and as tool to monitor and modulate therapy.
- **Melatonin**: synthesized from serotonin, released by pineal gland. Master hormone normalizes circadian rhythms and sleep cycles; powerful antioxidant for cancer therapies; protects neurons from heavy metal cobalt damage (Co found in high levels in patients with AD). Melatonin inhibits induction of oxidative damage and beta-amyloid release; may be preventive treatment because Co is essential nutrient, as in $B_{12}$. Dose of 3 mg at 8 PM increased sleeping time, decreased nightime activity, improved congnitive and noncognitive functions. Morning light therapy induces greater improvement.

## Botanical Medicines

- ***Ginkgo biloba* extract (GBE)**: standardized to 24% ginkgo flavonglycosides/6% terpenoids; great benefit in senility and AD; increases brain functional capacity; normalizes Ach receptors in hippocampus of aged animals, increasing cholinergic transmission (*Textbook, "Ginkgo biloba* [Ginkgo Tree]"). GBE (240 mg q.d.) only helps reverse or delay mental deterioration in early stages of AD; may help patient maintain normal life, avoid nursing home; improves Clinical Global Impressions scale (120 mg q.d.), stabilizes AD, and significantly improves mental function without side effects; equally as effective as second-generation cholinesterase inhibitors (tacrine, donepezil, rivastigmine, metrifonate) in treating mild to moderate AD and with lower dropout rate among patients; reverses mental deficits caused by vascular insufficiency or depression; must be taken consistently for at least 12 weeks to determine efficacy.

- **Huperzine A (HupA)**: alkaloid isolated from moss *Huperzia serrata*, long used in China for fever and inflammation, but no antipyretic or antiinflammatory properties in experimental models; potent inhibitor of acetylcholinesterase; more selective and much less toxic than conventional drugs (physostigmine, tacrine, donepezil); used by more than 100,000 people since early 1990s with no serious adverse effects; considerable benefit for dementia; 200 μg b.i.d. improves memory, cognition, and behavior in AD.
- ***Bacopa monniera* (BM)**: Ayurvedic botanical used for memory enhancement, epilepsy, insomnia; mild sedative; reduces memory dysfunction in rat models of AD; inhibits in vitro formation of reactive species and DNA damage from toxins, mimicking effect of excess nitric oxide exposure on neurons.
- **Kempo**: ancient Japanese botanical medicine; normalizes neurons subjected to stress-induced damage of brains with genetically induced propensity for seizures; suppresses effects on amyloid beta protein–induced neuron death.
- ***Galanthus nivalis*** (snowdrop): contains alkaloid galanthamine; inhibits cholinesterases. Huperazine A (see above) shares common binding sites with galanthamine.

## THERAPEUTIC APPROACH

Goal is prevention or starting therapy as soon as dementia is noted.

- Dietary and lifestyle recommendations:
  —Avoid aluminum (antiperspirants, antacids, beverage cans, cookware)
  —Follow general healthful dietary and lifestyle plan
  —Increase whole foods: wild small ocean fish, cereals, vegetables, and monounsaturated fats

—Decrease total calories and unhealthy fats
—Morning light therapy

- Supplements:
  —High-potency multiple vitamin/mineral supplement
  —Vitamin C: 500-1000 mg t.i.d.
  —Vitamin E: 400-800 IU q.d.
  —Flaxseed oil: 1 tbsp q.d.
  —Thiamin: 3-8 g q.d.
  —Phosphatidylserine: 100 mg t.i.d.
  —L-Acetylcarnitine: 500 mg t.i.d.
  —Methylcobalamin: 1000 μg b.i.d.
- Botanical medicine:
  —*Ginkgo biloba* extract (24% ginkgo flavonglycosides/6% terpenoids): 80 mg t.i.d.
  —Hup A: 200 μg b.i.d.

# Angina Pectoris

## DIAGNOSTIC SUMMARY

- Squeezing pain or pressure in the chest appearing immediately after exertion. Other precipitating factors include emotional tension, cold weather, or a large meal. Pain may radiate to the left shoulder blade, left arm, or jaw. The pain typically lasts for only 1-20 minutes.
- Stress, anxiety, and high blood pressure typically are present.
- The majority demonstrate an abnormal electrocardiographic reading (transient ST-segment depression) in response to light exercise (stress test).

## GENERAL CONSIDERATIONS

Angina pectoris results when oxygen supply and, occasionally, other nutrients, are inadequate for metabolic needs of heart muscle. Primary cause is atherosclerosis; also platelet aggregation, coronary artery spasm, nonvascular mechanisms (e.g., hypoglycemia), and increased metabolic need (e.g., hyperthyroidism). Primary lesion of atherosclerosis is atheromatous plaque blocking coronary arteries; symptomatic after major coronary artery is more than 50% blocked, transient platelet aggregation (*Textbook,* "Atherosclerosis"), and coronary artery spasm.

- **Prinzmetal's variant angina**: most common form of coronary artery spasm, not caused by plaque, occurs at rest or at odd times during day or night; more common in women younger than 50.
- **Magnesium insufficiency–induced coronary artery spasm**: more common in men than in women; important cause of MI and significant in angina pectoris.

## DIAGNOSTIC CONSIDERATIONS

Diagnosis frequently made by history alone. Workup: 12-lead ECG at rest, chest radiograph, ECG stress test or 24-hour Holter monitor

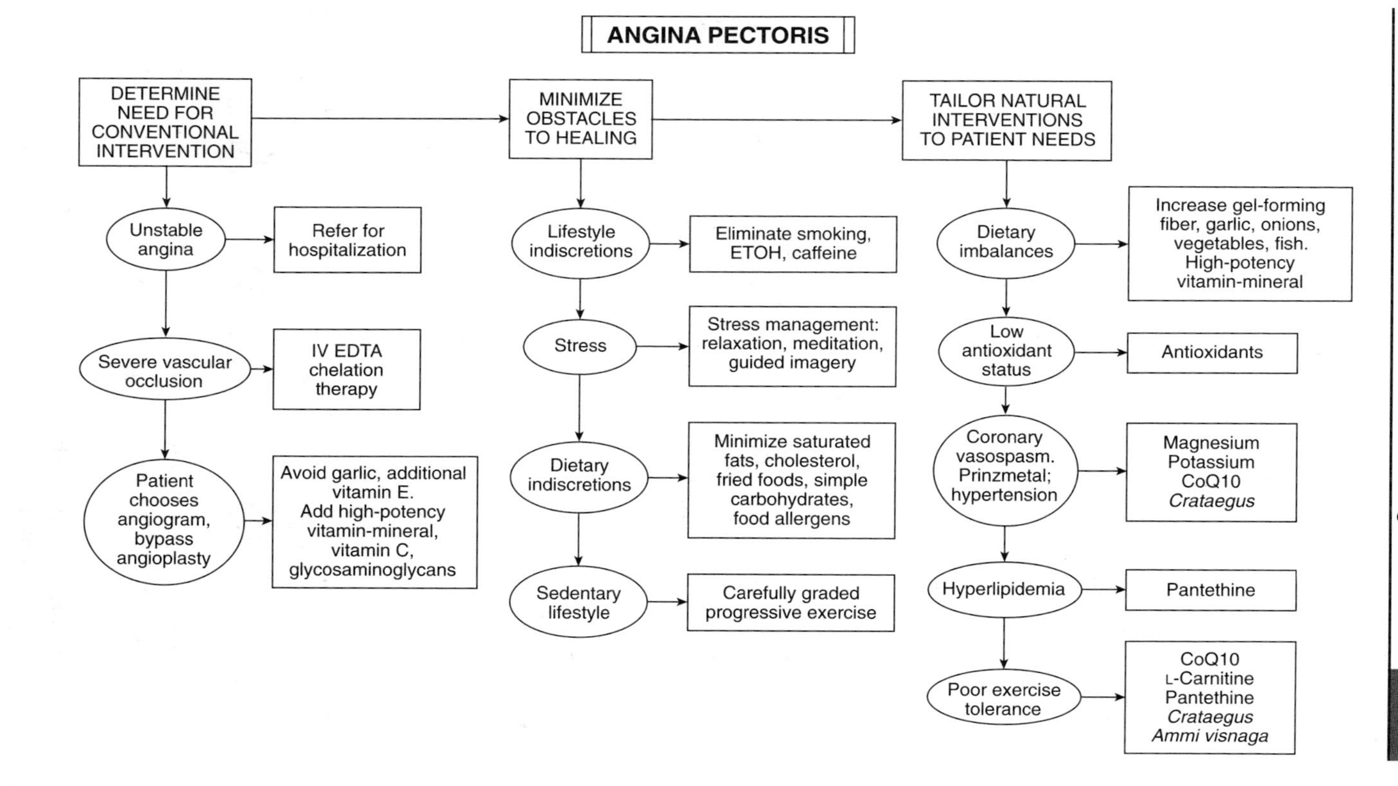
ANGINA PECTORIS
DETERMINE NEED FOR CONVENTIONAL INTERVENTION
Unstable angina
Refer for hospitalization
Severe vascular occlusion
IV EDTA chelation therapy
Patient chooses angiogram, bypass angioplasty
Avoid garlic, additional vitamin E. Add high-potency vitamin-mineral, vitamin C, glycosaminoglycans
MINIMIZE OBSTACLES TO HEALING
Lifestyle indiscretions
Eliminate smoking, ETOH, caffeine
Stress
Stress management: relaxation, meditation, guided imagery
Dietary indiscretions
Minimize saturated fats, cholesterol, fried foods, simple carbohydrates, food allergens
Sedentary lifestyle
Carefully graded progressive exercise
TAILOR NATURAL INTERVENTIONS TO PATIENT NEEDS
Dietary imbalances
Increase gel-forming fiber, garlic, onions, vegetables, fish. High-potency vitamin-mineral
Low antioxidant status
Antioxidants
Coronary vasospasm. Prinzmetal; hypertension
Magnesium Potassium CoQ10 *Crataegus*
Hyperlipidemia
Pantethine
Poor exercise tolerance
CoQ10 L-Carnitine Pantethine *Crataegus* *Ammi visnaga*

(ambulatory ECG). ECG changes seen with angina provide evidence of previous MI, and ST-segment and T-wave changes occurring during attacks of pain—displacement of ST segment with or without T-wave inversion. Hypoglycemia-induced angina does not manifest with rate or ST-segment abnormalities.

## THERAPEUTIC CONSIDERATIONS

Angina pectoris is a serious condition requiring careful treatment and monitoring. Prescription medications may be necessary; condition controllable with help of natural measures. Significant blockage of coronary artery: IV EDTA chelation, angioplasty, or coronary artery bypass may be appropriate. Two primary therapeutic goals: improve energy metabolism within heart and improve blood supply to heart. Heart uses fats as major metabolic fuel; defects in fat metabolism in heart greatly increase risk of atherosclerosis, MI, and angina attacks. Impaired use of fatty acids by heart results in accumulation of fatty acids within heart muscle, causing extreme susceptibility to cellular damage and MI. Carnitine, pantetheine, and coenzyme Q10 (CoQ10) are essential to fat metabolism and extremely beneficial in angina; prevent accumulation of fatty acids within heart muscle by improving conversion of fatty acids into energy.

### Coronary Angiogram, Artery Bypass Surgery, and Angioplasty

Angiogram (cardiac catheterization) is a radiographic procedure; dye is injected into coronary arteries to highlight blockages, subsequently treated by surgery. To date, no study has demonstrated a mortality benefit of percutaneous transluminal coronary angioplasty (PTCA) or cardiac revascularizations (also known as coronary artery bypass graft [CABG] operations) over nonsurgical interventions in patients with stable coronary artery disease.

Medicine, Angioplasty, or Surgery Study (MASS-II) showed no difference in cardiac death or acute MI among patients in CABG, PCTA, or medical treatment groups. But there was greater need for additional revascularization in patients who underwent PCTA. Medical treatment is a reasonable alternative for patients with multivessel CAD.

- **Angiograms**: landmark study of patients told they needed angiograms to determine degree of blockage and need for bypass surgery or angioplasty. Noninvasive tests (exercise stress test, echocardiogram, 24-hour Holter monitor) revealed that 80% did not need catheterization. These patients had an annual fatal MI rate over a 5-year period much lower than mortality rates for surgical procedures. Noninvasive testing to determine the functional state of the heart is far more important in determining indicated therapy than is dangerous search for blocked arteries. If heart is dysfunctional, *then* angiogram is indicated to ascertain need for surgery. Blockages found by angiogram are usually not relevant to risk of MI.

- **Coronary Artery Surgery Study (CASS)**: patients with heart disease who had healthy hearts, but one, two, or all three major heart vessels blocked, did surprisingly well without surgery. Regardless of number or severity of blockages, each group had the same low annual death rate of 1%. Severity of blockage does not estimate reduction in blood flow; no correlation between blood flow and severity of blockage; angiogram did not provide clinically relevant information. Critical factor: how well left ventricle is working, not degree of blockage or number of arteries affected. Bypass only helpful when ejection fraction is <40%. (Greater than 50% is adequate for circulatory needs.) Studies: 61% of patients who underwent bypass surgery had nervous system disorders as a result; 2%-5% die during or soon after operation; 10% have MIs.
- **Dietary and lifestyle changes**: significantly reduce risk of MI and other causes of death from atherosclerosis (*Textbook,* "Atherosclerosis"). Nutritional supplements and botanical medicines improve heart function in even the most severe angina cases. IV EDTA chelation: controversial, but clinical research has proven its efficacy.
- **When cardiac procedure is unavoidable, goal is to prevent damaging effects and restenosis**: high-potency multiple vitamin-mineral, additional vitamin C (500 mg t.i.d.+) and CoQ10 (100 mg q.d. 2 weeks before surgery and for 3 months after); garlic and high dosages vitamin E (>200 IU) to be avoided before surgery because of inhibition of platelet aggregation. Vitamin C plummets by 70% 24 hours after bypass surgery and persists for 2 weeks. After surgery, vitamin E and carotene levels do not change significantly—fat-soluble and retained longer; vitamin C depletion may deteriorate wound repair and defenses against free radicals and infection; CoQ10 can prevent oxidative damage during reperfusion. (Return of blood after bypass surgery induces

oxidative damage to vascular endothelium and myocardium, increasing risk for subsequent coronary artery disease.) CoQ10 (150 mg q.d. for 7 days before surgery) prevents reperfusion injury and lowers incidence of ventricular arrhythmias during recovery period. Mixture of purified *bovine aortic glycosaminoglycans* (dermatan sulfate, heparin sulfate, hyaluronic acid, chondroitin sulfate) (100 mg q.d.) helps prevent reperfusion injury and restore structural integrity of endothelium.

## Nutritional Supplements

**Antioxidant supplements**: plasma level of antioxidants is more predictive of unstable angina than is severity of atherosclerosis. They prevent tolerance to oral nitrate treatment for angina. Nitrate tolerance is linked to increased vascular superoxide that degrades nitric oxide formed from nitroglycerine, lowering cGMP (intracellular regulator and vasorelaxant). Vitamin C is main aqueous antioxidant and scavenger of superoxide; vitamin E is main lipid-phase antioxidant. High-dose vitamins C and E can prevent nitrate tolerance.

- **Carnitine (Crn)**: vitamin-like compound that transports fatty acids across mitochondrial membrane and stimulates metabolism of long-chain fatty acids by mitochondria. Crn deficiency decreases mitochondrial fatty acid levels and energy production. Normal heart function depends on adequate Crn. The normal heart stores more Crn than it needs; heart ischemia induces decreased Crn and energy production in heart and increased risk for angina and heart disease. Crn (900 mg q.d.) improves angina and heart disease, allows heart muscle to use limited oxygen more efficiently, improves exercise tolerance and heart function. Crn is an effective alternative to drugs (beta-blockers, calcium-channel antagonists, and nitrates), especially in patients with chronic stable angina pectoris. Crn (40 mg/kg per day) may prevent production of toxic fatty acid metabolites that activate phospholipases, disrupt cell membranes, impair heart contractility and compliance, and increase susceptibility to irregular beats and eventual death of heart tissue.
- **Pantethine**: stable form of pantethine is active form of pantothenic acid, a fundamental component of coenzyme A (CoA). CoA transports fatty acids within cell cytoplasm and mitochondria. Pantethine reduces hyperlipidemia (pantothenic acid does not); 900 mg pantetheine q.d. reduces serum triglyceride and cholesterol while increasing HDL with no toxicity; inhibits cho-

lesterol synthesis and accelerates fatty acid breakdown in mitochondria. Heart pantethine decreases during ischemia.

- **CoQ10 (ubiquinone)**: essential component of mitochondrial energy production; synthesized within body; synthesis impaired by nutritional deficiencies, genetic or acquired defect, or increased tissue need. Angina, hypertension, mitral valve prolapse, and congestive heart failure require increased tissue levels of CoQ10; elderly have increased CoQ10 needs. CoQ10 decline with age contributes to age-related decline in immunity. CoQ10 deficiency is common in patients with heart disease. High metabolic activity of heart tissue causes unusual susceptibility to CoQ10 deficiency. CoQ10 reduces frequency of anginal attacks by 53% in stable patients and increases treadmill exercise tolerance.
- **Magnesium**: deficiency may play a major role in angina, including Prinzmetal's. Deficiency produces coronary vasospasms; may be cause of nonocclusive MI. Sudden MI in death of men is linked to much lower heart $Mg^{2+}$ and $K^{+}$ than that of matched controls. Researchers recommend Mg as treatment of choice for angina because of coronary vasospasm; helps manage arrhythmias and angina from atherosclerosis. IV Mg during first hour after acute MI reduces immediate and long-term complications and death rates; beneficial effects of Mg in acute MI: improves energy production within the heart; dilates coronary arteries, improves heart oxygenation; reduces peripheral vascular resistance (decreasing demand on heart); inhibits platelet aggregation; reduces size of infarct; and improves heart rate and arrhythmias.

## Botanical Medicines

- ***Crataegus* spp. (hawthorn)**: Berry and flowering tops extracts reduce angina attacks, lower blood pressure and serum cholesterol levels; improve blood and oxygen supply of heart by dilation of coronary vessels; improve metabolic processes in heart; improve cardiac energy metabolism, enhancing myocardial function with more efficient use of oxygen; interact with key enzymes to enhance myocardial contractility (*Textbook, "Cratageus oxyacantha* [Hawthorn]").
- ***Ammi visnaga* (khella)**: ancient Mediterranean medicinal plant used historically to treat angina and other heart ailments. Constituents dilate coronary arteries; mechanism of action similar to calcium-channel blocking drugs. Constituent *khellin* is extremely effective in relieving angina symptoms, improving exercise tolerance, and normalizing ECGs. Higher doses (120-150 mg q.d.) of

pure khellin are linked to mild side effects (anorexia, nausea, dizziness). Most clinical studies used high doses; several studies used only 30 mg khellin q.d., which offered good results with fewer side effects. Khella extracts standardized for khellin content (12%) are preferred at dose of 250-300 mg q.d. Khella works synergistically with hawthorn.

## Other Therapies

- **Acupuncture**: improves angina, reducing nitroglycerin use, decreasing number of angina attacks, and improving exercise tolerance and ECG readings.
- **Relaxation and breathing exercises**: improve angina symptoms when anxiety is significant contributor. In cardiac syndrome X, a form of angina in human beings with otherwise normal coronary arteries, transcendental meditation (20 minutes b.i.d. silently chanting mantra with eyes closed) reduces anginalike chest pain and normalizes ECGs.
- **IV EDTA chelation therapy**: alternative to bypass surgery or angioplasty; may be more effective and is definitely safer and less expensive. EDTA is amino acid–like molecule that binds with minerals (e.g. Ca, Fe, Cu, and Pb) and carries them to kidneys for excretion; commonly used for Pb poisoning but found to help atherosclerosis in late 1950s; Dr Norman Clarke treated patients with angina, cerebral vascular insufficiency, and occlusive peripheral vascular disease; 87% showed symptomatic improvement. Patients with blocked leg arteries, particularly diabetics, avoided amputation. EDTA chelates out excess Fe and Cu that stimulate free radicals in presence of oxygen. Free radicals damage endothelium, causing atherosclerosis. Giving too much EDTA or giving it too fast is dangerous, possibly resulting in kidney failure; but no deaths or significant adverse reactions in more than 500,000 patients treated under controlled protocols; improves blood flow throughout body: recommended for angina, peripheral vascular disease, and cerebral vascular disease; substantiated by numerous FDA-approved studies. Insufficient evidence to ascertain efficacy or lack thereof for improving clinical outcomes of patients with atherosclerotic cardiovascular disease. (Contact American College of Advancement in Medicine [ACAM], 23121 Verdugo Drive, Suite 204, Laguna Hills, CA 92653; 1-800-532-3688 [outside California] or 1-800-435-6199 [inside California].)

## THERAPEUTIC APPROACH

Primary therapy is prevention because angina usually is secondary to atherosclerosis. Once developed, restore proper blood supply to heart and enhance energy production within heart. Unstable angina (progressive increase in frequency and severity of pain over several days, increased sensitivity to precipitating factors, and prolonged coronary pain) mandates hospitalization.

- **Diet**: increase fiber, especially gel-forming and mucilaginous fibers (ground flaxseed, oat bran, pectin). Increase onions, garlic, vegetables, small wild ocean fish. Decrease saturated and trans fats, cholesterol, sugar, animal proteins. Avoid fried foods and food allergens. Patients with reactive hypoglycemia: eat small, frequent regular meals and avoid simple carbohydrates (sugar, honey, dried fruit, fruit juice, etc.).
- **Lifestyle**: stop smoking, ETOH use, coffee intake. Decrease stress by progressive relaxation, meditation, or guided imagery. Carefully follow graded, progressive, aerobic exercise (30 min three times weekly); start with walking.
- **Nutritional supplements**:
  —Vitamin C: 500-1500 mg q.d.
  —Vitamin E: 400-800 IU q.d. (prefer mixed tocopherols emphasizing gamma-tocopherol)
  —Coenzyme Q10: 150-300 mg q.d. (Note: CoQ10 blood levels must reach greater than 2.5 μg\mL for efficacy)
  —L-Carnitine: 500 mg t.i.d.
  —Pantetheine: 300 mg t.i.d.
  —Magnesium (aspartate, citrate, or other Krebs cycle intermediates): 200-400 mg t.i.d.

### Botanical Medicines

- *Crataegus oxyacantha* (t.i.d.):
  —Berries or flowers (dried): 3-5 g or as a tea
  —Tincture (1:5): 4-6 ml (1-1.5 tsp)
  —Fluid extract (1:1): 1-2 ml (0.25-0.5 tsp)
  —Solid extract (10% procyanidins or 1.8% vitexin-4′-rhamnoside): 100-250 mg
- *Ammi visnaga* (t.i.d.):
  —Dried powdered extract (12% khellin content): 100 mg.

# Aphthous Stomatitis (Aphthous Ulcer/Canker Sore/Ulcerative Stomatitis)

## DIAGNOSTIC SUMMARY

- Single or clustered, shallow, painful ulcers found anywhere in the oral cavity.
- Lesions are from 1-15 mm in diameter, have fairly even borders, are surrounded by an erythematous border, and are often covered by a pseudomembrane.
- Lesions usually resolve in 7-21 days but are often recurrent.

## GENERAL CONSIDERATIONS

Recurrent aphthous stomatitis (RAS) (also called canker sores or ulcertive stomatitis) is a common condition (20% of population). Etiology: food sensitivities (e.g., gluten), stress, and/or nutrient deficiency. Lesions are mucosal ulcerations with mixed inflammatory cell infiltrates; T-helper cells predominate in preulcerative and healing phases; T-suppressor cells predominate in ulcerative phase. Lesions = mucosal ulcerations with mixed inflammatory cell infiltrates; T-helper cells predominate in preulcerative and healing phases; T-suppressor cells predominate in ulcerative phase. Cause: dysregulation of immune system in the oral mucosa. Key features of immune dysfunction: lymphomononuclear infiltrate and hemagglutination antibodies against oral mucosa; reduced response of lymphocytes to mitogens; increased circulating immune complexes; alterations in natural killer cell activity; increased adherence of neutrophils; release of tumor necrosis factor-alpha; mast cell involvement.

## THERAPEUTIC CONSIDERATIONS

- **Food and environmental allergens**: association of RAS with increased serum antibodies to food antigens and atopy strongly

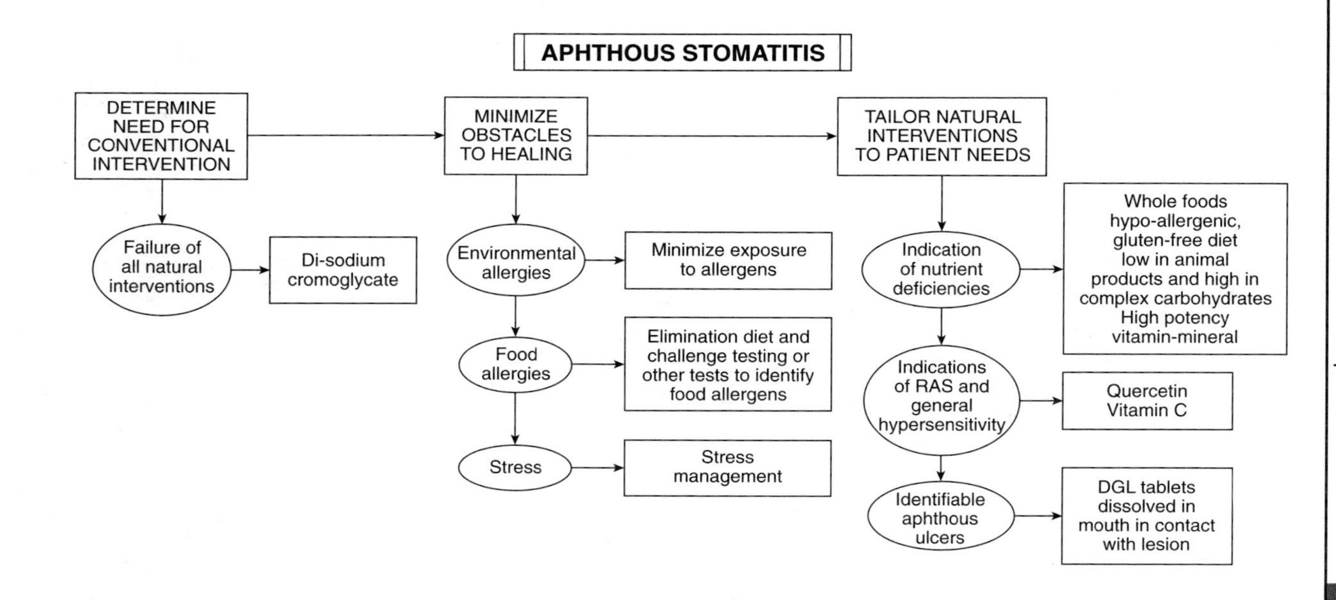
APHTHOUS STOMATITIS
DETERMINE NEED FOR CONVENTIONAL INTERVENTION
Failure of all natural interventions
Di-sodium cromoglycate
MINIMIZE OBSTACLES TO HEALING
Environmental allergies
Minimize exposure to allergens
Food allergies
Elimination diet and challenge testing or other tests to identify food allergens
Stress
Stress management
TAILOR NATURAL INTERVENTIONS TO PATIENT NEEDS
Indication of nutrient deficiencies
Whole foods hypo-allergenic, gluten-free diet low in animal products and high in complex carbohydrates High potency vitamin-mineral
Indications of RAS and general hypersensitivity
Quercetin Vitamin C
Identifiable aphthous ulcers
DGL tablets dissolved in mouth in contact with lesion

suggests that allergic reaction is involved. IgE-bearing lymphocytes are increased in aphthous lesions; mast cells are increased in tissue from prodromal stages of recurrent ulcers. Mast cell degranulation is important in producing lesion. Elimination diet gives good results. Allergen does not have to be food; frequent allergens inducing RAS are benzoic acid, cinnamaldehyde, nickel, parabens, dichromate, sorbic acid; allergen elimination usually brings complete resolution or significant improvement.

- **Gluten sensitivity**: gluten sensitivity is the primary cause of RAS in many cases. Incidence of RAS is increased in patients with celiac disease. Jejunal biopsy of patients with RAS reveals villous atrophy typical of celiac disease plus signs of immunologic reactions to food antigens. Gluten may act directly on oral mucosa or produce functional changes in small intestine distinct from those of celiac disease. Gluten-sensitive enteropathy induces nutritional deficiencies. Withdrawing gluten causes complete remission of RAS in patients with celiac disease and some improvement in other patients. Even without villous atrophy, gluten sensitivity can produce RAS. Measure alpha-gliadin antibodies in any patient presenting with RAS.
- **Stress**: precipitating factor in RAS, suggesting breakdown in host protective factors.
- **Nutrient deficiency**: oral cavity often is the first place where nutritional deficiency is visible—high turnover of mucosal epithelium. Thiamin ($B_1$) deficiency is the most significant. Low levels of transketolase ($B_1$-dependent enzyme) found in RAS compared with controls. Nutrient deficiencies are much more common in those with RAS: 14.2% deficient in Fe, folate, $B_{12}$, or combination of these nutrients; 28.2% deficient in $B_1$, $B_2$, or $B_6$; when deficiencies are corrected, majority are completely remitted. Zinc (50 mg elemental) daily for 1 month has reduced aphthae and prevented reappearance for 3 months. Low nutrient status may explain why patients with RAS have increased oxidant/antioxidant status: decreased catalase and glutathione peroxidase activities and antioxidant potential levels in the erythrocytes and decreased antioxidant potential and increased malondialdehyde in plasma. Enzymatic and nonenzymatic antioxidant defense systems are impaired in patients with RAS.
- **Quercetin**: inhibits mast cell degranulation, basophil histamine release, and formation of other mediators of inflammation. Antiallergy drug disodium cromoglycate has similar structure and function and is effective in treating RAS. Quercetin increased

number of ulcer-free days with mild symptomatic relief. Other flavonoids (acacetin, apigenin, chrysin, and phloretin, but not catechin, flavone, morin, rutin, or taxifolin) have antiallergy effects similar to the drug.

- **Deglycyrrhizinated licorice (DGL)**: may be effective in promoting healing of RAS lesions. Solution of DGL used as mouthwash (200 mg powdered DGL dissolved in 200 mL warm water q.i.d.)—75% of patients had 50%-75% improvement within 1 day, followed by complete healing of ulcers by third day; DGL tablets may be more convenient and effective. Let them melt in the mouth directly adjacent to the lesions.

## THERAPEUTIC APPROACH

No single factor is solely responsible for initiating aphthous lesions, but underlying tendency to ulceration may be facilitated in expression by these factors. The underlying problem may be gluten sensitivity plus nutrient deficiencies. Use antiinflammatory nutrients.

- **Diet**: low in animal products, high in complex carbohydrates, free of known allergens and all gluten sources (i.e., grains).
- **Supplements**:
  —Vitamin C 1000 mg q.d.
  —High-potency multiple vitamin/mineral.
  —DGL: one to two 380-mg chewable tablets held in direct contact with the lesion.

# Asthma

## DIAGNOSTIC SUMMARY

- Recurrent attacks of dyspnea, cough, and expectoration of tenacious mucoid sputum
- Prolonged expiration phase with generalized wheezing and musical rales
- Eosinophilia, increased serum IgE, positive food and/or inhalant allergy tests

## GENERAL CONSIDERATIONS

Bronchial asthma is a hypersensitivity disorder characterized by bronchospasm, mucosal edema, and excessive excretion of a viscous mucus that can lead to ventilatory insufficiency. Its prevalence is approximately 3% of the U.S. population, and although it occurs at all ages, it is most common in children younger than 10. There is a 2:1 male/female ratio in children that equalizes by the age of 30.

- **Major factors**: hypersensitivity of airways; beta-adrenergic blockade; cyclic nucleotide imbalance in airway smooth muscle; release of inflammatory mediators from mast cells. Rate in United States is rising rapidly, especially in children; reasons for this are increased stress on immune system (greater chemical pollution in air, water, and food; insect allergens from mites and cockroaches; earlier weaning of and introduction of solid foods to infants; food additives; higher incidence of obesity; genetic manipulation of plants—food components with greater allergenic tendencies).
- **Multiple genetic variables increasing susceptibility**: deficiency in glutathione S-transferase M1 (gene responding to oxidative stress) increases susceptibility; this suggests need for antioxidants. ADAM33 gene on chromosome 20p13 is linked to airway remodeling (see mediators later) and corticosteroid resistance. Genes on chromosomes 7 and 12 are also implicated.

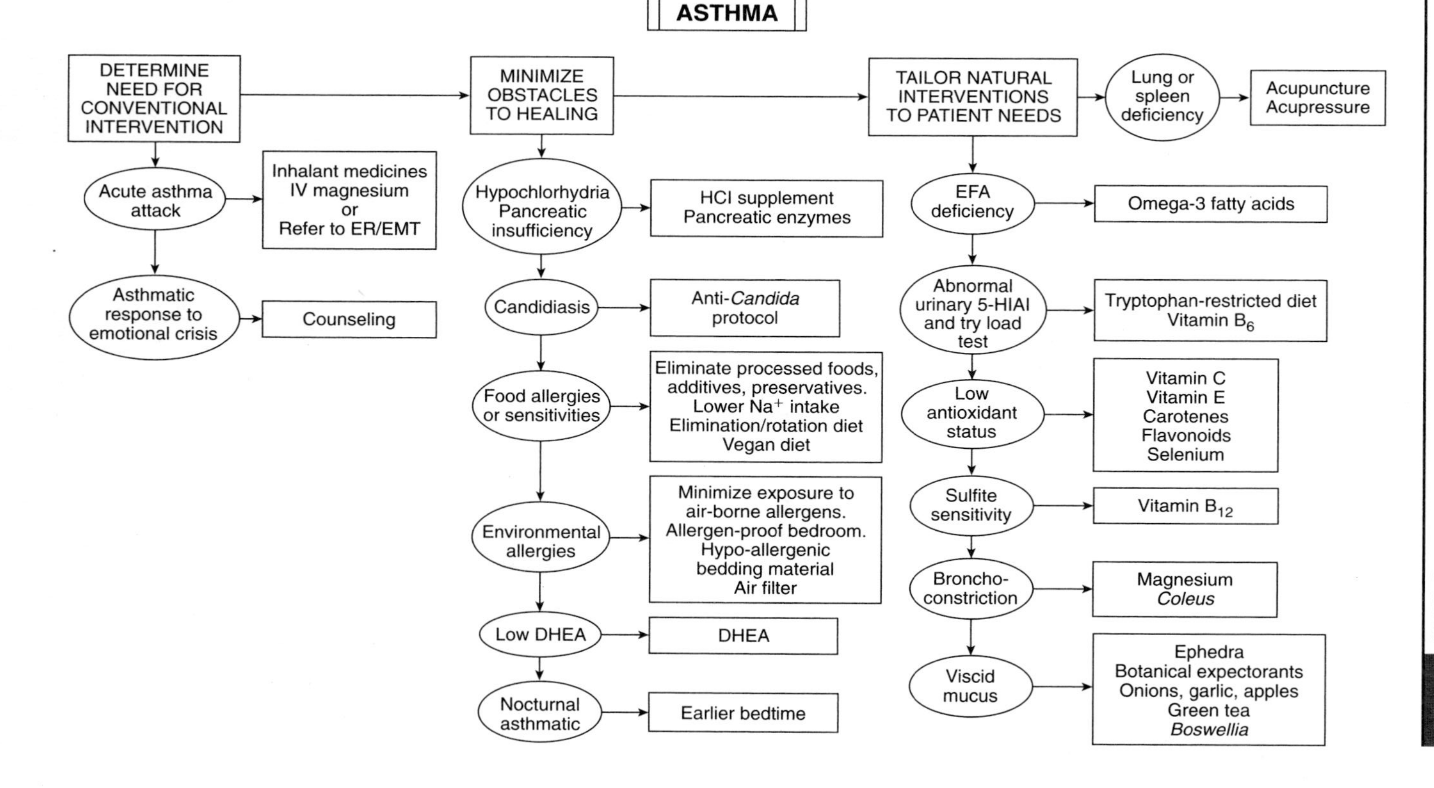
ASTHMA
DETERMINE NEED FOR CONVENTIONAL INTERVENTION
Acute asthma attack
Inhalant medicines
IV magnesium
or
Refer to ER/EMT
Asthmatic response to emotional crisis
Counseling
MINIMIZE OBSTACLES TO HEALING
Hypochlorhydria
Pancreatic insufficiency
HCl supplement
Pancreatic enzymes
Candidiasis
Anti-*Candida* protocol
Food allergies or sensitivities
Eliminate processed foods, additives, preservatives.
Lower $Na^+$ intake
Elimination/rotation diet
Vegan diet
Environmental allergies
Minimize exposure to air-borne allergens.
Allergen-proof bedroom.
Hypo-allergenic bedding material
Air filter
Low DHEA
DHEA
Nocturnal asthmatic
Earlier bedtime
TAILOR NATURAL INTERVENTIONS TO PATIENT NEEDS
Lung or spleen deficiency
Acupuncture
Acupressure
EFA deficiency
Omega-3 fatty acids
Abnormal urinary 5-HIAI and try load test
Tryptophan-restricted diet
Vitamin $B_6$
Low antioxidant status
Vitamin C
Vitamin E
Carotenes
Flavonoids
Selenium
Sulfite sensitivity
Vitamin $B_{12}$
Broncho-constriction
Magnesium
*Coleus*
Viscid mucus
Ephedra
Botanical expectorants
Onions, garlic, apples
Green tea
*Boswellia*

- Major categories:
  —extrinsic or atopic: immunologically mediated with increased serum IgE
  —intrinsic: bronchial reaction due, not to antigen-antibody stimulation, but factors such as chemicals, cold air, exercise, infection, agents that activate alternative complement pathway, and emotional upset.

## Causes

**Inflammation and Th1/Th2 balances**: imbalances in T-helper cell immune responses comprise mechanism of immune system–mediated airway inflammation. $CD4^+$ T-helper cell categories: Th1 and Th2. Th1 cells release interferons and IL2, increasing immune response of cancer, MS, viruses, and type IV hypersensitivity. Th2 cells facilitate release of IL4, IL6, IL9, IL13, and IgE; eosinophilia; and activated B-cell humoral immunity. Related disorders: asthma, atopic syndromes, and allergies. Asthmatics have normal Th1 gene expression, but upregulated Th2 genes, causing Th2 dominance. Genetics, fungi, heavy metals, nutrition, viruses, and pollution are factors in this upregulation. "Hygiene hypothesis"—minimizing exposure to infectious agents by hygienic lifestyle choices favors Th2 dominance of immune responses to allergens, encouraging asthma and atopic diseases.

- **Mediators**: extrinsic and intrinsic factors involving Th2 imbalances trigger cytokine-activated release of mast cell mediators of bronchoconstriction and mucus secretion. Preformed mediators are histamine, chemotactic peptides (eosinophilotactic factor [ECF] and high-molecular weight neutrophil chemotactic factor [NCF]), proteases, glycosidases, and heparin proteoglycan. Membrane-derived agents are lipoxygenase products (leukotrienes [LT] and slow-reacting substance of anaphylaxis [SRS-A]), prostaglandins (PG), thromboxanes (TX), and platelet-activating factor (PAF). Effects of mediators are bronchoconstriction (histamine, $LTC_4$, $LTD_4$, $LTE_4$, $PGF_{2alpha}$, $PGD_2$, PAF), mucosal edema (histamine, $LTC_4$, $LTD_4$, PAF), vasodilation ($PGD_2$, $PGE_2$), mucous plugging (histamine, hydroxy-eicosatetraenoic acid [HETE], $LTC_4$), inflammatory cell infiltrate (NCF, ECF-A, HETE, $LTB_4$, PAF), and epithelial desquamation (proteases, glycosidases, lysosomal enzymes, and basic proteins from neutrophils and eosinophils). Mediators cause airway remodeling in chronic asthma, affecting epithelium and mesenchymal tissues. Induced growth factors encourage fibroblasts, smooth muscle proliferation, and matrix protein deposits, thickening the wall.

- **Mild episodic asthma versus moderate to severe sustained asthma**: latter has subacute and chronic bronchial inflammation with infiltration of eosinophils, neutrophils, and mononuclear cells. Episodic is caused by bronchial smooth muscle contraction.
- **Lipoxygenase products**: leukotrienes are most potent chemical mediators in asthma. SRS-A ($LTC_4$, $LTD_4$, $LTE_4$) is 1000 times more potent a bronchoconstrictor than histamine. Asthmatics have imbalance in arachidonic acid metabolism, causing relative increase in lipoxygenase products; platelets from asthmatics show 40% decrease in cyclooxygenase metabolites and 70% increase in lipoxygenase products. Imbalance is aggravated in "aspirin-induced asthma"—aspirin and NSAIDs inhibit cyclooxygenase while promoting lipoxygenase, shunting arachidonic acid to lipoxygenase pathway and excessive leukotrienes. Tartrazine (yellow dye #5) is cyclooxygenase inhibitor and induces asthma, especially in children. Tartrazine is antimetabolite of vitamin $B_6$.
- **Autonomic nervous system** (parasympathetic vs. sympathetic innervation): $beta_2$-adrenergic receptors are localized in lung tissue and react to catecholamines. Parasympathetic vagus nerve stimulation releases acetylcholine (Ach), which binds to receptors on smooth muscle, forming cGMP. Increased cGMP and/or relative deficiency in cAMP causes bronchoconstriction and degranulation of mast cells and basophils. Decreased sympathetic activity or diminished $beta_2$-receptor numbers or sensitivity also promotes the cyclic nucleotide imbalance. Some mediators block $beta_2$ receptors and elevate cGMP.
- **Adrenal gland**: cortisol activates beta receptors. Epinephrine (Epi) is the prime stimulator of beta receptors. Asthmatic attacks may be induced by relative deficiency of cortisol and Epi (which stimulate $beta_2$ receptors to catalyze formation of cAMP from AMP), leading to decreased cAMP/cGMP ratio and bronchial constriction.
- **Pertussis vaccine**: among children breastfed from first day of life, fed exclusively breast milk for first 6 months and weaned after 1 year, the relative risk of developing asthma is 1% in children receiving no immunizations, 3% in those receiving vaccinations other than pertussis, and 11% for those receiving pertussis. In a group of 203 not immunized to pertussis, 16 developed

whooping cough compared with only 1 of 243 in the immunized group.

- **Influenza vaccine**: although the relatively new cold-adapted trivalent intranasal influenza virus vaccine was deemed safe for children and adolescents, increased relative risk of 4.06 for asthma and reactive airway disease arose in children age 18 to 35 months.

## THERAPEUTIC CONSIDERATIONS

### General

- **Hypochlorhydria**: 80% of tested asthmatic children had inadequate gastric acid secretion; hypochlorhydria and food allergies are predisposing factors for asthma.
- **Increased intestinal permeability**: "leaky gut" permits increased food antigen load, overwhelming immune system, increasing risk of additional allergies and exposure to bronchoconstrictive compounds.
- Identify offending foods:
  —***Candida albicans***: GI overgrowth implicated as causative factor in allergic conditions, including asthma. Acid protease produced by *C. albicans* is the responsible allergen.
  —**Food additives**: must be eliminated: coloring agents, azo dyes (tartrazine [orange], sunset yellow, amaranth and new coccine [both red]) and non–azo dye pate blue. Most common preservatives are sodium benzoate, 4-hydroxybenzoate esters, and sulfur dioxide. Sulfite sources are salads, vegetables (particularly potatoes), avocado dip served in restaurants, wine, and beer. Molybdenum deficiency may cause sulfite sensitivity; sulfite oxidase is the enzyme that neutralizes sulfites and is molybdenum dependent.
  —**Salt**: Increased intake worsens bronchial reactivity and mortality from asthma. Bronchial reactivity to histamine is positively correlated with 24-hour urinary Na and rises with increased dietary Na.
- **Estrogen and progesterone**: For women with severe asthma, consider decreasing hormonal fluctuations. Estrogen and progesterone are smooth muscle relaxants. Airways of premenopausal and postmenopausal women may respond differently to exogenous HRT and need assessment independent of this intervention. During premenstrual and menstrual phases, when hormones are

low, asthmatic women have episodes and are hospitalized with decreased pulmonary function. Stabilizing hormone fluctuations (by pregnancy or oral contraceptives) improves pulmonary function and reduces need for medication. Liver detox and botanicals are safer methods to balance hormones. If these fail, natural HRT may be less risky (*Textbook,* "Asthma" and "Menopause").

- **DHEA**: decreased levels are common in postmenopausal women with asthma compared with matched controls. Transdermal 17b-estradiol (E2) and medroxyprogesterone acetate increase serum DHEAs in asthmatics, with no change in controls. Therapeutic benefit of DHEA in asthma is undemonstrated, but its importance to immune function suggests possible positive effects.
- **Melatonin**: concern exists that elevated melatonin may contribute to airway inflammation in nocturnal asthmatics and inflammation in RA. In nocturnal asthmatics, peak serum melatonin is inversely correlated with overnight change in forced expiratory volume but not in nonnocturnal asthmatics or healthy controls. Release of melatonin is delayed in nocturnal asthmatics. Supplementation plus earlier bedtime may regulate late melatonin peaking and mitigate symptoms. Avoid giving melatonin to asthmatics, especially nocturnal type, until further study is completed.

## Diet

- **Beneficial foods**: antioxidants in fruit and vegetables lower risk of poor respiratory health. Fruit high in vitamin C lowers prevalence of asthma symptoms and improves lung function in children. Even small increases in fruit intake are beneficial. Fish lowers airway hyperreactivity in children and increases lung function in adults. Fruit decreases phlegm. Fruit (>180 g/day), whole grains (>45 g/day), and moderate ETOH (1-3 glasses/day) have increased forced expiratory volume by 139 mL and lowered by 50% the prevalence of COPD symptoms. Apples and red wine (moderate) antioxidants decrease asthma severity.
- **Food allergy** (*Textbook,* "Food Allergy Testing"): immediate onset sensitivities can be caused by (decreasing order of frequency) egg, fish, shellfish, nuts, peanuts. Delayed onset can arise from (decreasing order of frequency) milk, chocolate, wheat, citrus, food colorings. Elimination diets identify allergens and treat asthma, especially in infants. Avoiding common allergens during infancy (first 2 years) reduces allergic tendencies in high-risk children (strong familial history).

- **Breastfeeding**: can prevent asthma. Children not breastfed are more likely to become asthmatic. Vitamin C in breast milk correlates with maternal intake; low maternal intake results in low infant intake, increasing susceptibility to oxidative stress. Applying preventive interventions (house dust control; avoidance of pets, tobacco smoke, day care during first year; breastfeeding exclusively or partially hydrolyzed whey formula until age 4 months) for infants with atopic family history lowers risk for asthma at ages 1 and 2 years. A 90% reduction in recurrent wheezing has also been noted.
- **Vegan diet**: long-term trial (eliminating all animal products) significantly improved 92% of 25 patients who completed the study (nine dropped out) based on vital capacity, forced expiratory volume at 1 second ($FEV_1$), physical working capacity, haptoglobin, IgM, IgE, cholesterol, and triglycerides. Vegan diet also reduces tendency for infectious disease. Seventy-one percent of patients responded in 4 months; 1 year was required for 92%. Diet excludes all meat, fish, eggs, dairy products, chlorinated tap water (drink spring water only), coffee, ordinary tea, chocolate, sugar, and salt. Herbal spices are allowed; water and herbal teas allowed up to 1.5 L q.d. Vegetables used freely are lettuce, carrots, beets, onions, celery, cabbage, cauliflower, broccoli, nettles, cucumber, radishes, Jerusalem artichokes, all beans except soya and green peas. Potatoes are allowed in restricted amounts. Fruits used freely: blueberries, cloudberries, raspberries, strawberries, black currants, gooseberries, plums, pears. Apples and citrus fruits are not allowed. Grains are restricted or eliminated. Beneficial effects of vegan diet are elimination of food allergens, altered prostaglandin metabolism, increased intake of antioxidants and Mg. Avoid dietary sources of arachidonic acid (animal products). Inflammatory PGs and LTs made from arachidonic acid intensify asthmatic reactions. Vegan diet reduces health care costs (corticosteroids, other drugs, therapies) and increases patients' sense of responsibility for their own health.

## Nutrition

- **Omega-3 essential fatty acids (n-3 EFAs)**: children who eat fish more than once a week have one third the asthma risk of those who do not. Fish oil supplements with EPA and DHA improve airway hyperresponsiveness to allergens and respiratory function. Benefits are from increasing ratio of n-3 to n-6 EFAs in cell membranes, reducing arachidonic acid. n-3 EFAs shift LT synthesis from inflammatory 4-series to less inflammatory 5-series, improving asthma symptoms. Benefits may take as long as 1 year before apparent from turnover of cellular membranes toward n-3s.

- **Tryptophan metabolism and pyridoxine (vitamin $B_6$) supplementation**: asthmatic children have metabolic defect in tryptophan metabolism and reduced platelet transport for serotonin. Tryptophan is converted to serotonin (bronchoconstrictor in asthmatics). Serotonin is high in blood and sputum of asthmatics, causing elevated urinary 5-hydroxyindole acetic acid (5-HIAI), the breakdown product of serotonin. Urinary 5-HIAI correlates well with symptom severity. Patients benefit from tryptophan-restricted diet or $B_6$ supplements. Plasma and RBC pyridoxal phosphate in asthmatics is much lower than in controls. Fifty to 100 mg oral $B_6$ b.i.d. greatly decreases frequency and severity of wheezing and attacks and dosages of bronchodilators and corticosteroids. $B_6$ fails to improve well patients dependent on steroids, but $B_6$ is indicated in patients on theophylline. Theophylline depresses P5P; $B_6$ supplements reduce side effects of theophylline (headache, nausea, irritability, sleep disorders). Tryptophan load test (*Textbook,* "5-Hydroxytryptophan") may determine appropriateness and level of $B_6$ supplementation needed. Urinary excretion of kynurenic and xanthurenic acids increases in patients responding to $B_6$.
- **Antioxidants**: increased prevalence of asthma is explained by reduced intake of antioxidants. Patients in acute asthmatic distress have lowered serum total antioxidants. Genetics may influence antioxidant need. Fifty mg/day vitamin E and 250 mg/day vitamin C can protect children against ozone diminishing of pulmonary function. Antioxidants help maintain lung redox state that prevents oxidants from stimulating bronchoconstriction and increasing hyperreactivity to other agents. Analgesics (e.g., acetaminophen, which depletes antioxidant glutathione) must be used cautiously in asthmatics.
- **Vitamin C**: the major antioxidant in extracellular fluid lining airway surfaces. Children of smokers have a higher rate of asthma (smoke depletes respiratory vitamins C and E), and symptoms in adults appear increased by exposure to environmental pro-oxidants and decreased by C supplements. Nitrogen oxides are oxidants from endogenous and exogenous sources. Vitamin C protects against nitrogen oxide lung damage in lab animals. Asthmatics have much lower serum and WBC ascorbate.

Clinically asthmatics have higher need for C. Seven of 11 studies showed significant improvements in respiratory measures and symptoms using 1-2 g vitamin C q.d. High-dose C therapy may lower histamine; histamine initially amplifies immune response by increasing capillary permeability and smooth muscle contraction, then suppresses accumulated WBCs to contain inflammation. Vitamin C prevents histamine secretion by WBCs and increases histamine detox. Vitamin C will only lower blood histamine if taken over time.

- **Flavonoids**: key antioxidants that inhibit histamine release from mast cells and basophils stimulated by antigens, phospholipase $A_2$ in neutrophils, lipoxygenase, anaphylactic contraction of smooth muscle, phosphodiesterase in lung (increasing cAMP), biosynthesis of SRS-A, and Ca influx. Quercetin spares vitamin C and stabilizes mast cell membranes. Sources are quercetin supplements, grape seed, pine bark, green tea, or *Ginkgo biloba*. Proanthocyanidins from grape seed or pine bark have affinity for lungs (*Textbook*, "Flavonoids—Quercetin, Citrus Flavonoids, and Hydroxyethylrutosides").
- **Carotenes**: powerful antioxidants that increase integrity of respiratory epithelium; act as substrates for lipoxygenase, possibly competing with arachidonic acid, decreasing inflammatory leukotriene formation.
- **Vitamin E**: antioxidant inhibitor of lipoxygenase and phospholipase.
- **Selenium**: Reduced Se levels are found in asthmatics. Glutathione peroxidase (Se-dependent metalloenzyme) reduces hydroperoxy-eicosatetraenoic acid (HPETE) to HETE, thereby reducing leukotriene formation. Decreased glutathione peroxidase is common in asthmatics.
- **Vitamin $B_{12}$**: mainstay in childhood asthma for Jonathan Wright, MD. Weekly 1000 μg IM injections improve symptoms—less shortness of breath on exertion and improved appetite, sleep, and general condition. $B_{12}$ is especially effective in sulfite-sensitive patients; offers best protection when given orally (1-4 mg) before challenge; forms sulfite-cobalamin complex, blocking sulfite effect.
- **Magnesium**: IV Mg (2 g of Mg sulfate infused every hour up to total of 24.6 g) well proven and clinically accepted to halt acute asthma attack as well as acute exacerbations of COPD. IV Mg is only necessary in emergency: acute MI or asthma. Oral Mg is effective to optimize body Mg stores—6 weeks needed to elevate tissue Mg. Supplementation is warranted because dietary Mg

intake is independently related to lung function and asthma severity.

## Botanical Medicines

Misuse of botanicals in asthma can exacerbate symptoms, leading to hospitalization. Historical herbals for asthma are *Ephedra sinica* (*Ma huang*) in combination with herbal expectorants, such as *Glycyrrhiza glabra* (licorice), *Grindelia camporum* (grindelia), *Euphorbia hirta* (euphorbia), *Drosera rotundifolia* (sundew), and *Polygala senega* (senega). Ephedra alkaloids are effective bronchodilators for mild to moderate asthma and hay fever. Peak bronchodilation occurs in 1 hour and lasts 5 hours after administration.

- ***Glycyrrhiza glabra*** **(licorice root)**: documented antiinflammatory and antiallergic (*Textbook,* "*Glycyrrhiza glabra* [Licorice]"). Primary active constituent is glycyrrhetinic acid; inhibits phospholipase $A_2$, which cleaves arachidonic acid from membrane phospholipid, initiating eicosanoid synthesis. Licorice is also an expectorant.
- ***Lobelia inflata*** **(Indian tobacco)**: alkaloid lobeline is an efficient expectorant. Lobelia has a long history of use in asthma but promotes bronchoconstriction and is respiratory stimulant in vitro. It binds to nicotine Ach receptors in ganglions, promoting release of Epi and NE that provide therapeutic effects. It is effective alone but traditionally is used in combination with other botanical agents (*Capsicum frutescens* and *Symphlocarpus factida*).
- ***Capsicum frutescens*** **(cayenne)**: capsaicin induces long-lasting desensitization of airway mucosa to mechanical and chemical irritants. Capsaicin depletes substance P (which increases vascular permeability and flow) in respiratory nerves. Substance P is an undecapeptide linked to neurogenic inflammation by direct effect and synergy with histamine on peripheral nervous system. Respiratory and GI tracts have many substance P–containing neurons, believed to contribute to atopy (asthma and atopic dermatitis).
- ***Zizyphi fructus*** **(jujube plum)**: traditional Chinese herb for treatment of asthma and allergic rhinitis that contains 100-500 nmol cAMP/g of dry weight, a concentration 10 times more than that of any other plant or animal tissue reported. It contains beta-adrenergic receptor stimulator that also raises cAMP.
- ***Thea sinensis*** **(green tea)**: adjunctive in asthma containing methylxanthine and antioxidant constituents (*Textbook,* "Asthma").
- **Allium family**: onions and garlic may block biosynthesis of arachidonic acid metabolites by inhibiting cyclooxygenase

pathways, which generate $TxA_2$, $PGD_2$ and $PGE_2$. Onion contains quercetin plus benzyl and other isothiocyanates (mustard oils).

- ***Tylophora asthmatica***: Ayurvedic medicine for asthma and other respiratory disorders whose mode of action is unknown but thought to be attributable to alkaloids (e.g., tylophorine), which have antihistamine, antispasmodic activity and inhibit mast cell degranulation. Good results—a dose of 200 mg tylophora leaves b.i.d. for 6 days improves symptoms and respiratory function during treatment and for 2 weeks thereafter. Incidence of side effects (nausea, partial diminution of taste for salt, slight mouth soreness) 16.3% in tylophora group and 6.6% in placebo group. Benefits of tylophora are short lived.
- ***Ginkgo biloba***: unique terpenes (ginkgolides) antagonize PAF; key mediator in asthma, inflammation, and allergies. Ginkgolides compete with PAF for binding sites and inhibit events induced by PAF. Ginkgo improves respiratory function and reduces bronchial reactivity. Dosage = 120 mg pure ginkgolides q.d.; dosage very expensive using 24% ginkgo flavonglycoside and 6% terpenoid ginkgo biloba extract.
- ***Aloe vera***: may be effective for patients not dependent on corticosteroids. The extract is produced from supernatant of fresh leaves stored in dark at 4° C for 7 days to increase polysaccharide fraction. One gram of this extract produces 400 mg neutral polysaccharides versus 30 mg produced from leaves not subjected to cold or dark. At 5 mL of 20% solution of aloe vera extract in saline b.i.d. for 24 weeks: 40% of patients without steroid dependence felt much better. Mechanism of action may be restoring protective mechanisms, with augmentation of immune system.
- ***Coleus forskohlii***: forskolin increases intracellular cAMP, relaxing bronchial muscles and relieving respiratory symptoms (*Textbook, "Coleus forskohlii"*). Studies used inhaled doses of pure *forskolin*; efficacy of oral *C. forskohlii* extract has yet to be determined. Historical use and additional mechanisms of action recommend its use.
- ***Boswellia***: Ayurvedic botanical that inhibits leukotriene biosynthesis. It has reduced bronchial asthma 70% in 40 patients treated with gum resin at 300 mg t.i.d. for 6 weeks compared with improvement in 27% of controls. Effects—disappearance of dyspnea and rhonchi; reduced number of attacks; increased forced expiratory volume, vital capacity and peak expiratory flow rates; and decreased eosinophilia and sedimentation rates.

**Acupuncture and acupressure**: chronic asthma is linked to lung or spleen deficiency. Acute symptoms arise from environmental invasion by cold wind or internal condition of lung heat (inflammation and eosinophilia). Chronic asthma indicates lung weakness, or weakness of spleen, which nourishes lung qi. Grief weakens lung qi. As adjuncts to standard care for chronic asthma, acupuncture (20 treatments) induces 18.5-fold improvement (St. George's Respiratory Questionnaire); daily self-administered acupressure for 8 weeks induces 6.57-fold improvement with 11.8-fold improvement in irritability domain score.

## THERAPEUTIC APPROACH

Underlying defects and initiating factors must be determined and resolved: (1) defect allowing sensitization; (2) metabolic defect causing excessive inflammatory response; (3) triggering allergens with lifestyle, diet, and environment changes to avoid them; (4) modulating inflammatory process to limit severity; (5) effective treatment for bronchoconstriction of acute attack.

- **Environment**: minimize exposure to airborne allergens (pollen, dander, dust mites). Avoid dogs, cats, carpets, rugs, upholstered furniture, surfaces where allergens can collect. Ensure bedroom is allergen proof; encase mattress in allergen-proof plastic; wash sheets, blankets, pillow cases, and mattress pads weekly. Consider Ventflex (hypoallergenic synthetic) bedding material. Install air purifier, such as HEPA (high-efficiency particulate arresting) attachable to central heating and air-conditioning system.
- **Diet**: eliminate all food allergens, additives, and bananas if they aggravate condition. Patient with many food allergies may need 4-day rotation diet (*Textbook,* "Rotation Diet Master Chart, Plans I and II"). Mild tryptophan reduction is helpful—essential if there is a metabolic defect in the tryptophan metabolism. Use garlic and onions liberally unless patient reacts to them. If patient willing, or asthma unresponsive, try vegan diet (for 4+ months), with possible exception of small wild cold-water ocean fish. Encourage moderate fruit consumption, especially apples.
- **Supplements** (adult doses; rule out potential allergens in supplements):
  —Vitamin $B_6$: 25-50 mg b.i.d.
  —Vitamin $B_{12}$: 1000 μg q.d. (oral) or weekly IM; evaluate for efficacy after 6 weeks

—Vitamin C: 10-30 mg/kg body weight in divided doses
—Vitamin E: 200-400 IU q.d.
—Magnesium: 200-400mg t.i.d.
—Quercetin: 400 mg 20 minutes before meals
—Grape seed extract (95% PCO content): 50-100 mg t.i.d.
—Carotenes: 25,000-50,000 IU q.d.
—Selenium: 200 μg q.d.

- Botanical medicines:
  —*Ephedra sinica*: extract providing 12.5-25.0 mg ephedrine b.i.d./t.i.d.; crude herb: 500-1000 mg t.i.d.; can be combined with herbal expectorants indicated above.
  —*Glycyrrhiza glabra*: powdered root (1-2 g); fluid extract (1:1): 2-4 mL; solid (dry powdered) extract (4:1): 250-500 mg
  —*Camellia sinensis*: liberal use (green tea only)
  —*Tylophora asthmatica*: 200 mg leaves or 40 mg dry ETOH extract b.i.d.
  —*Coleus forskohlii* (standardized to 18% forskolin): 50 mg (9 mg forskolin) b.i.d. or t.i.d.
- **Counseling**: important for patients who respond to emotional crisis with asthmatic attacks and children with moderate to severe asthma, who may develop behavioral problems.
- **Acupuncture/acupressure**: regular acupuncture and home acupressure treatments.
- **Acute attack**: medical emergency; IV Mg or refer patient to ER/EMT immediately.

# Atherosclerosis

## DIAGNOSTIC SUMMARY

- High blood pressure, weak pulse, and wide pulse pressure
- Symptoms and signs depend on arteries involved and degree of obstruction: angina, leg cramps (intermittent claudication), gradual mental deterioration, weakness or dizziness; may be asymptomatic
- Diagonal earlobe crease

## GENERAL CONSIDERATIONS

Largely a disease of diet and lifestyle. Underlying pathosis in cardiovascular disease (CVD), heart disease, or coronary artery disease (CAD); myocardial, pulmonary, and cerebral infarction. CAD is the leading and stroke the third leading cause of death in the United States.

- An artery has three major layers:
  - —Intima (internal lining) = layer of endothelial cells; glycosaminoglycans (GAGs) line exposed endothelial cells to protect them from damage and promote repair; beneath surface cells, internal elastic membrane: layer of GAGs and ground substance compounds.
  - —Media = smooth muscle cells, interposed GAGs and other ground substance.
  - —Adventitia = external elastic membrane of connective tissue, including GAGs.
- **Process of atherosclerosis**: lesions initiated in response to injury to intima: weakening of GAG layer, leaving endothelial cells exposed to damage (free radicals, immune complexes, inflammation mediators). Sites of injury are more permeable to plasma constituents (lipoproteins). Binding lipoproteins to GAGs disintegrates ground substance matrix, increasing affinity for cholesterol; monocytes, T-lymphocytes, and platelets adhere to lesion, releasing growth factors stimulating smooth muscle cell

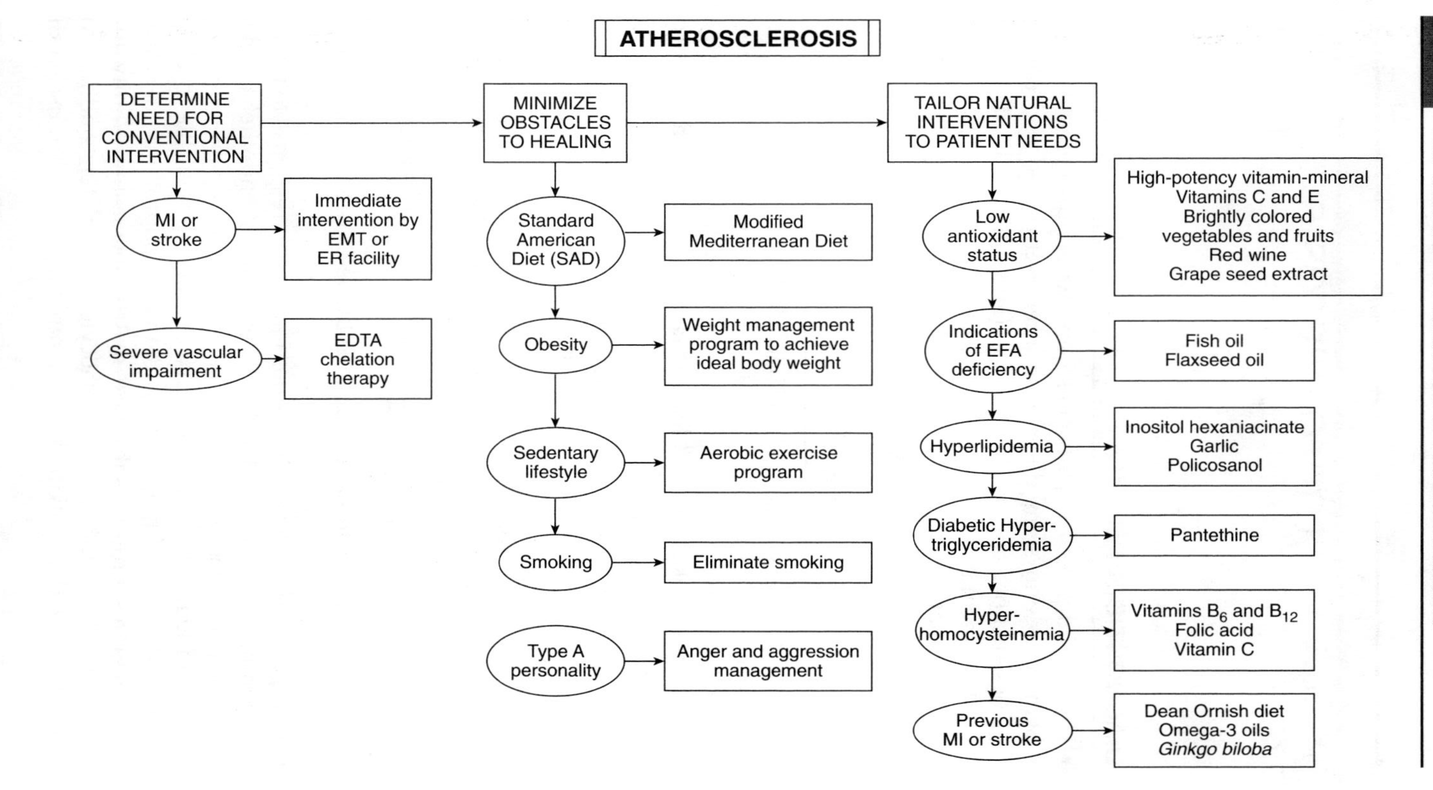
ATHEROSCLEROSIS
DETERMINE NEED FOR CONVENTIONAL INTERVENTION
MI or stroke
Immediate intervention by EMT or ER facility
Severe vascular impairment
EDTA chelation therapy
MINIMIZE OBSTACLES TO HEALING
Standard American Diet (SAD)
Modified Mediterranean Diet
Obesity
Weight management program to achieve ideal body weight
Sedentary lifestyle
Aerobic exercise program
Smoking
Eliminate smoking
Type A personality
Anger and aggression management
TAILOR NATURAL INTERVENTIONS TO PATIENT NEEDS
Low antioxidant status
High-potency vitamin-mineral
Vitamins C and E
Brightly colored vegetables and fruits
Red wine
Grape seed extract
Indications of EFA deficiency
Fish oil
Flaxseed oil
Hyperlipidemia
Inositol hexaniacinate
Garlic
Policosanol
Diabetic Hyper-triglyceridemia
Pantethine
Hyper-homocysteinemia
Vitamins $B_6$ and $B_{12}$
Folic acid
Vitamin C
Previous MI or stroke
Dean Ornish diet
Omega-3 oils
*Ginkgo biloba*

migration from media into intima and replication. Smooth muscle cells dump debris into intima, developing plaque. Fibrous cap (collagen, elastin, GAGs) forms over intimal surface. Fat and cholesterol deposits accumulate. Plaque grows until artery is blocked. Blockage can be 90% before symptomatic.

- **Causative risk factors**:
  - —Major factors: hypercholesterolemia, hypertension, smoking, diabetes, physical inactivity
  - —Other risk factors: low antioxidant status, low essential fatty acids (EFAs), elevated C-reactive protein (CRP), low magnesium and potassium, increased platelet aggregation, insulin resistance, increased fibrinogen formation, elevated homocysteine, hypothyroidism, "type A" personality.
- **Clinical evaluation**: lab tests (total cholesterol, LDL, HDL, lipoprotein(a) [Lp(a)], fibrinogen, homocysteine, ferritin [iron-binding protein], lipid peroxides); exercise stress test, electrocardiogram (ECG), echocardiogram.

### Risk Factors

- **Smoking**: most important risk factor for coronary heart disease (70% greater risk than nonsmokers). Smokers die 7 to 8 years sooner than nonsmokers. Smoking is the single major cause of cancer death in the United States (twice the risk). Tobacco smoke contains more than 4000 chemicals, with more than 50 carcinogens that damage intima directly or damage LDL, which damages arteries. Toxins travel on plasma cholesterol; elevated LDL worsens damaging effects. Damaged LDL impairs feedback mechanisms in liver that control how much cholesterol is manufactured. Smoking promotes platelet aggregation, elevated fibrinogen, and hypertension. Environmental (secondary/passive) smoke increases heart disease mortality and morbidity rates. Best results occur when people quit "cold turkey."
- **Hypercholesterolemia**: Recommended levels—total cholesterol <200 mg/dL; LDL <130 mg/dL; HDL >35 mg/dL; triglycerides <150 mg/dL. VLDL and LDL transport triglycerides and cholesterol from liver to body cells; HDL returns fats to liver. Ratio of total cholesterol to HDL and ratio of LDL to HDL = cardiac risk factor ratios: reflect whether cholesterol is being deposited into tissues or broken down and excreted. Total cholesterol: HDL ratio should be <4.2 and LDL/HDL ratio should be <2.5. For every 1% drop in LDL, myocardial infarction (MI)

### Tips to Help Patients Stop Smoking

- List reasons why you want to quit smoking; review them daily.
- Set specific day to quit; tell 10 friends; then **do it**.
- Discard all cigarettes, butts, matches, and ashtrays.
- Use substitutes: raw vegetables, fruits, gum. Play with pencil to occupy fingers.
- Take one day at a time.
- 40 million Americans have quit; so can you!
- Visualize yourself as a nonsmoker with more money, pleasant breath, unstained teeth, and sense of self-control.
- Join a support group; contact local American Cancer Society chapter.
- Relax: use deep breathing exercises.
- Avoid situations you associate with smoking.
- Reward yourself daily in a positive way with money saved.

risk drops 2%; for every 1% increase in HDL, MI risk drops 3%-4%. Lp(a) is a plasma lipoprotein similar to LDL but with adhesive protein called apolipoprotein(a) [Apo(a)]. Elevated plasma Lp(a) is an independent risk factor for CHD, especially with elevated LDL. High Lp(a) has 10 times the risk of elevated LDL [LDL lacks adhesive Apo(a)]. Lp(a) <20 mg/dL is linked with low risk, 20-40 mg/dL moderate risk, and >40 mg/dL extremely high risk.

- **Genetic inherited diseases**: Familial hypercholesterolemia (FH), familial combined hyperlipidemia (FCH), and familial hypertriglyceridemia (FT) are common (1 in every 500 people). FH involves defect in liver receptor protein that removes LDL from blood and helps decrease cholesterol synthesis. LDL receptors are damaged by aging and diseases (diabetes). Diet high in saturated fat and cholesterol decreases number of LDL receptors, reducing feedback telling liver cells no more cholesterol is needed. Lifestyle and dietary changes increase function and/or number of LDL receptors. FCH defect is accelerated production of VLDL in liver. Patients may have only hypertriglyceridemia, or only hypercholesterolemia, or both. FT has only hypertriglyceridemia with low HDL. FT defect involves VLDL particles, made by liver, larger than normal and carrying more triglycerides. FT is worse in diabetes, gout, and obesity.
- **Hypertension**: Sign of considerable atherosclerosis and most significant risk factor for stroke.

- **Diabetes**: Atherosclerosis causes many chronic complications of diabetes, including twofold to threefold higher risk of premature death from heart disease or stroke. CVD causes 55% of deaths in diabetics (see Handbook chapter on diabetes; *Textbook,* "Diabetes Mellitus").
- **Physical inactivity**: Physical activity protects against CVD and improves CVD risk factors: blood pressure, blood lipids, insulin resistance, and obesity; therapeutic for stable angina, prior MI, peripheral vascular disease, heart failure, or recovery from cardiovascular event.
- **Chronic inflammation**: Inflammatory mediators influence atheroma development. CRP is an acute-phase reactant reflecting degrees of inflammation and an independent risk factor for CAD; it is a stronger predictor of CVD than is LDL. Screening for both is more prognostic than either alone. Elevated CRP is linked to insulin resistance and metabolic syndrome (syndrome X), found in 60 million U.S. adults. Diagnostic criteria for metabolic syndrome include at least three of following risk factors in one person:
  —Central obesity (waist/hip ratio >1.0 for men; >0.8 for women)
  —Dyslipidemia (high triglycerides >150 mg/dL; low HDL [male <40 mg/dL, female <50 mg/dL])
  —Hypertension (130/85 mm Hg or higher)
  —Insulin resistance or glucose intolerance (fasting blood sugar >101 mg/dL)
  —Prothrombotic state (e.g., high blood fibrinogen or plasminogen activator inhibitor)
  —Proinflammatory state (e.g., elevated high-sensitivity CRP)

## THERAPEUTIC CONSIDERATIONS

- **Diet**: Reduce saturated and trans fats. Increase vegetables, fruit, and fiber. Support cell membranes with monounsaturated and omega-3 fats. Prevent oxidative and free radical damage with antioxidants and phytochemicals.
- **"Mediterranean diet"**: eat minimally processed foods, use olive oil as fat source, and eat seasonally fresh and locally grown plant food (fruit, vegetables, breads, pasta [prefer whole grain], potatoes, beans, nuts, and seeds), fresh fruit as dessert (concentrated sugars or honey only a few times per week), low to moderate amounts dairy (cheese, yogurt), fish, poultry and eggs (1-4 times weekly),

low amounts of red meat, low to moderate wine (prefer red) at meals. Benefits include reduced CRP and inflammatory mediators, improved endothelial function, and weight management.

- **Olive oil and omega-3s**: Olive oil (monounsaturated fats and antioxidants) lowers LDL and triglycerides, increases HDL, prevents free radical damage to LDL. Omega-3 eicosapentaenoic acid (EPA) and docosahexaenoic acid (DHA) reduce cardiovascular risk. EPA/DHA have little effect on cholesterol but they lower triglycerides, reduce platelet aggregation, improve endothelial function and arterial flexibility, improve blood and oxygen supply to the heart, and lower blood pressure. Level of EPA and DHA within red blood cells is more predictive of heart disease than CRP; total, LDL, or HDL cholesterol; or homocysteine. Lab parameter: **Omega-3 index** ≥8% indicates greatest protection; index ≤4% indicates least. Total of combined 1000 mg of EPA and DHA daily achieves target omega-3 index ≥8%. Raising long-chain omega-3 fatty acids reduces overall cardiovascular mortality rate by 45%. Cretans and Japanese who inhabit Kohama have lowest rate of MIs from a high intake of alpha-linolenic acid.
- **Nuts and seeds**: reduce CVD risk. Substituting nuts for equivalent amount of carbohydrate reduces risk by 30%. Substituting fat from nuts for saturated fats (meat, dairy) reduces risk by 45%. Nuts lower cholesterol and provide L-arginine, precursor of nitric oxide (endothelium-derived relaxing factor), which improves blood flow, normalizes blood clotting, and reduces blood viscosity. Walnuts contain antioxidants and alpha-linolenic acid (LNA); they improve endothelial cell function (vasodilation and reduced vascular cell adhesion molecule-1) and reduce total cholesterol (TC) (–4.4%) and LDL (–6.4%).
- **Vegetables, fruits, red wine**: Antioxidants in carotene- or flavonoid-rich foods reduce risk. High blood antioxidants are linked with lower CRP. Tomato products supply carotene lycopene, which protects against LDL-oxidation and MI better than beta-carotene. Red wine ("French paradox") contains antioxidant flavonoids and polyphenols, which protect LDL and reduce inflammatory mediators. Moderate alcohol intake positively affects HDL/LDL ratio, CRP, and fibrinogen. Benefit of alcohol on CVD must be counterbalanced by its addictive and psychologic effects.
- **Lower TC and LDL**: reduces CVD risk. Statin drugs arose from traditional Chinese medicine, red yeast (*Monascus purpureus*) fermented on rice, producing monacolins (e.g., lovastatin or monacolin K). FDA has ruled that red yeast rice products can only be

sold if they are free of monacolins. Diversifying cholesterol-lowering components in same dietary protocol increases efficacy and offers results comparable to statin drugs. Natural agents that potentiate statin therapy are niacin, phytosterols, phytostanols, and policosanol. Patients taking statins need coenzyme Q10 (CoQ10) because 3-hydroxy-3methylglutaryl coenzyme A reductase is required for synthesis of CoQ10. Statins lower CoQ10, causing fatigue, muscle pain, and rhabdomyolysis. CoQ10, in subjects on statins, reduces markers of oxidative damage. Statins lower CRP by 13% to 47%, but vitamin E (800 IU q.d.) lowers CRP by 49% and niacin (1500 mg at night) lowers it by 20%.

- **Soluble fiber**: Legume, fruit, and vegetable fibers lower cholesterol, especially viscous/gel-forming soluble fiber, in a dose-dependent way. Normal or low cholesterol levels show little change. For high cholesterol (>200 mg/dL), 3 g soluble oat fiber lowers TC by 8%-23%. For each 1% drop in cholesterol, heart risk decreases 2%. Three grams of fiber are in one bowl of oat bran cereal or oatmeal. Oatmeal fiber content (7%) is less than that of oat bran (15%-26%), but polyunsaturated fatty acids, higher in oats, also help reduce cholesterol. Recommend daily intake of 35 g of fiber from the fiber-rich foods.
- **Lifestyle**: get regular aerobic exercise, avoid smoking, reduce or eliminate coffee (caffeinated and decaf).
- **Margarine, trans fatty acids, and partially hydrogenated oils**: raise LDL, lower HDL, interfere with EFA metabolism, and are suspected of carcinogenicity; restrict both butter and margarine; use natural polyunsaturated oils to meet EFA requirements: 1 tbsp high-quality flaxseed oil.
- **Cold-water fish and flaxseed oil**: cold-water ocean fish are sources of longer-chain omega-3 EFAs (EPA and DHA); lower cholesterol and triglycerides; preferably fish oils lab certified against lipid peroxides, small wild cold-water fish, and flaxseed oil.
- **Dietary animal protein**: the body handles animal proteins differently from plant proteins; high intake of animal protein is linked to heart disease, cancer, hypertension, kidney disease, osteoporosis, and kidney stones; vegetarian diet linked to reduced risk. Limit animal protein to <4-6 oz/day, preferably fish, skinless poultry, and lean cuts.
- **Olive and canola oil**: best oils for cooking; composed of oleic acid and monounsaturated oil; resistant to heat and light damage; LDL largely composed of oleic acid is less susceptible to peroxidation.

- **Refined carbohydrates**: significant factor in atherosclerosis; high sugar intake elevates triglyceride, cholesterol, and insulin; elevated insulin is linked to elevated cholesterol, triglycerides, blood pressure, and CVD; limit sources of refined sugar; serum cholesterol is lowest among adults eating whole grain cereal for breakfast.

## Nutritional Supplements

- **Niacin**: lowers LDL by 16% to 23%; raises HDL by 20% to 33%; lowers Lp(a) by 35%, and lowers triglyceride, CRP and fibrinogen; the only lipid-lowering agent proven to reduce overall mortality rate. Effects are long lasting, with better overall results despite the fact that some patients are unable to tolerate full dosage because of skin flushing. Benefits: 33% increase in HDL, 35% reduction in Lp(a). Side-effects of high doses are skin flushing 20-30 minutes after ingestion, gastric irritation, nausea, and liver damage. Older sustained-release, timed-release, or slow-release forms were more toxic to the liver; newer forms are well tolerated, even when used with statins. Inositol hexaniacinate lowers cholesterol, improves blood flow in intermittent claudication, is better tolerated, and induces less flushing. Niacin can impair glucose tolerance—use with caution in diabetics. Avoid with liver disease or elevated liver enzymes—use policosanol, gugulipid, garlic, or pantethine. Check cholesterol and liver function every 3 months. Dose at night because most cholesterol synthesis occurs while sleeping. Begin niacin dosing at 100 mg t.i.d. and carefully increase dosage over 4-6 weeks to full therapeutic dose of 1.5-3 g q.d. in divided doses. Sustained-release or inositol hexaniacinate dosing: begin with 500 mg at night for 2 weeks, then increase to 1500 mg q.d. If LDL is not lowered wihtin 1 month, increase dose to 3000 mg q.d.
- **Phytosterols and phytostanols**: Structural similarity to cholesterol allows them to displace cholesterol from intestinal micelles. These compounds are added to functional foods (margarine, orange juice, etc.) and supplements. Daily intake of 2 g of stanols or sterols reduces LDL by 10%. Higher intake adds little additional benefit. Effects of sterols and stanols are additive with diet or drug interventions; adding sterols or stanols to statins is more effective than doubling statin dosing alone. Best responders have high cholesterol absorption and low cholesterol biosynthesis. Phytosterols and phytostanols also have antiplatelet and antioxidant effects. At higher doses, they may reduce carotenoid absorp-

tion, which can be partially reversed by increased intake of vegetables and fruits.

- **Pantethine:** stable form of pantetheine, the active form of vitamin $B_5$ (pantothenic acid), the most important component of coenzyme A, involved in transport of fatty acids within cell cytoplasm and mitochondria. Pantethine has significant lipid-lowering activity, whereas pantothenic acid has very little. Dose = 900 mg q.d. Effects: reduces triglycerides by 32%, TC by 19%, LDL by 21%; increases HDL by 23%; especially useful for hyperlipidemia in diabetics; virtually no toxicity. The mechanism of action inhibits cholesterol synthesis and accelerates use of fat as energy source.
- **Vitamin C**: levels correspond to TC and HDL; the higher the ascorbate content of blood, the lower the TC and triglycerides and the higher the HDL. For each 0.5 mg/dL increase in blood ascorbate, HDL is increased 14.9 mg/dL in women and 2.1 mg/dL in men; most significant effects of high-dosage vitamin C may be reducing Lp(a) and antioxidant activity; reduces Lp(a) by 27%.

## Botanical Medicines

- ***Allium sativum* (garlic) and *Allium cepa* (onion)**: Increase onion consumption. Garlic at daily dose of 10 mg allicin or total allicin potential of 4000 μg lowers TC by 10%-12%, LDL and triglycerides by 15% each, and increases HDL by 10%. Garlic greatly improves LDL/HDL ratio. Garlic dosage = 10 mg alliin or total allicin potential of 4000 μg q.d. (German Commission E says 4000 mg fresh garlic q.d. = 1-4 cloves (*Textbook, "Allium cepa* [Onions]" and "*Allium sativum* [Garlic]").
- **Policosanol**: Mixture of fatty substances from wax of sugar cane (*Saccharum officinarum*) that lowers cholesterol and triglycerides and improves LDL/HDL ratio within first 6-8 weeks at dosage of 5-20 mg/day. Dosing 10 mg at night drops LDL by 20%-25% within 6 months. At 20 mg, LDL drops by 25%-30%. HDL increases by 15%-25% after 2 months. Reduces platelet aggregation without affecting coagulation, prevents smooth muscle cell proliferation into arterial intima, and acts as antioxidant preventing LDL oxidation (*Textbook,* "Policosanol"). Dosage: 5-20 mg at evening meal; adjust dosing based on cholesterol checks every 8 weeks.
- **Gugulipid**: standardized extract of mukul myrrh tree (*Commiphora mukul*) of India; active components = Z-guggulsterone and E-guggulsterone; lowers TC by 14%-27% in 4-12 weeks, LDL by 25%-35%, and triglyceride by 22%-30%; raises HDL by 16%-20%;

lipid reductions comparable to lipid-lowering drugs but without side effects. Mechanism of action: increases liver metabolism of LDL; guggulsterone increases liver uptake of LDL from blood; prevents formation of atherosclerosis and helps regress preexisting plaques in animals; mildly inhibits platelet aggregation and promotes fibrinolysis; may prevent stroke or embolism. Dosage based on guggulsterone content—gugulipid standardized to 25 mg guggulsterone per 500 mg tablet t.i.d.; no significant side-effects with purified gugulipid; crude guggul (e.g., gum guggul) is associated with side-effects (skin rashes, diarrhea, etc.) (*Textbook*, "*Commiphora mukul* [Mukul Myrrh Tree]").

## Comparing Natural Cholesterol-Lowering Agents

**Comparative Effects on Blood Lipids of Several Natural Compounds**

| | Niacin | Garlic | Policosanol | Pantethine |
|---|---|---|---|---|
| Total cholesterol (% decrease) | 18 | 10 | 24 | 19 |
| LDL cholesterol (% decrease) | 23 | 15 | 25 | 21 |
| HDL cholesterol (% increase) | 32 | 31 | 15 | 23 |
| Triglycerides (% decrease) | 26 | 13 | 5 | 32 |

- **Niacin**: plus dietary and lifestyle improvements produce best overall effect; dosing at 1500 mg to 3000 mg at night reduces TC by 50%-75 mg/dL in patients above 250 mg/dL within 2 months. If above 300 mg/dL, it may take 4-6 months. After TC is below 200 mg/dL, reduce niacin to 500 mg t.i.d. for 2 months. If TC rises above 200 mg/dL, increase niacin to 1000 mg t.i.d. If TC remains below 200 mg/dL, withdraw niacin completely; recheck TC in 2 months; restore niacin if above 200 mg/dL.
- **Policosanol**: Add policosanol if after 4 months TC remains above 250 mg/dL; use policosanol for patients who cannot tolerate niacin.
- **Gugulipid**: added to above protocol if after 4 months TC remains >250 mg/dL; gugulipid also used for rare patient who cannot tolerate inositol hexaniacinate.

- **Pantethine**: for hypertriglyceridemia and cases of hyperlipidemia in diabetics (high-dose niacin adversely affects blood sugar control in some diabetics); normalizes platelet lipid composition and function and blood viscosity.
- **Elevated Lp(a)**: Both niacin and vitamin C reduce Lp(a) by 35% and 27%, respectively.
- **Rule out hypothyroidism** in all cases of hyperlipidemia, especially Lp(a). Overt hypothyroidism predisposes to CVD because of increased LDL and decreased HDL. Subclinical hypothyroidism (normal triiodothyronine and FTI with raised thyroid-stimulating hormone) is linked to significantly elevated LDL and Lp(a) (*Textbook,* "Hypothyroidism").

## GENERAL THERAPEUTIC CONSIDERATIONS

**Antioxidant status**: Antioxidant nutrients (lycopene, lutein, Se, vitamins E and C) protect against heart disease and slow the aging process. Lipids are particularly susceptible to free radical damage, forming lipid peroxides and oxidized cholesterol, which damage artery walls and accelerate atherosclerosis. Antioxidants block formation of damaging compounds. Combination antioxidants provide greater protection than any single nutritional antioxidant. Most antioxidants require "partner" antioxidants for optimal efficient effect. The two primary antioxidants are vitamins C ("aqueous phase") and E ("lipid phase") (*Textbook,* "Atherosclerosis").

**Phytochemicals** (carotenes [lycopene and lutein] and flavonoids) and plant antioxidants potentiate vitamin/mineral antioxidants. Beta-carotene may protect endothelium, but lycopene and lutein are protectively incorporated into LDL. Lutein may be the best carotene against atherosclerosis. Lycopene, beta-carotene, and cryptoxanthin infuse larger, less-dense LDL particles; lutein and zeaxanthin prefer smaller, more dense LDL particles that are more easily oxidized.

**Multiple vitamin/mineral supplement**: lowers CRP. Serum vitamins $B_6$ and C levels are inversely associated with CRP level.

- **Vitamin E:** easily incorporated into LDL molecule. The higher the dosage of vitamin E, the greater the degree of protection against LDL oxidative damage. Doses of 400-800 IU (prefer mixed tocopherols emphasizing gamma fraction) are required for significant effects; reduces LDL peroxidation and increases plasma

LDL breakdown; inhibits excessive platelet aggregation; increases HDL; increases fibrinolytic activity; reduces CRP; improves endothelial cell function; improves insulin sensitivity and plasma lipids in non–insulin dependent diabetes mellitus. Vitamin E levels may be part of the "French paradox" and be more predictive of MI or stroke than TC; plays major role in treating heart disease, recovery from stroke, and peripheral vascular diseases (e.g., intermittent claudication). Vitamin E and CoQ10 work synergistically and regenerate each other; work better together than alone for CRP, LDL oxidation, and aorta lipid peroxidation.

- **Selenium**: Se is also needed for optimal antioxidant effects as a component of antioxidant enzyme glutathione peroxidase. Low Se status is linked to CAD.
- **Vitamin C**: first line of water-soluble antioxidants; partners are fat-soluble vitamin E and carotenes; works with antioxidant enzymes (glutathione peroxidase, catalase, and superoxide dismutase). Regenerates (with CoQ10) oxidized vitamin E, thus potentiating antioxidant benefits of vitamin E; prevents LDL oxidation, even in smokers; significantly reduces risk of death from MI and stroke; lowers standardized mortality ratio up to 48%, equivalent to increased longevity of 5-7 years for men and 1-3 years for women. The higher the blood level of vitamin C, the lower are levels of TC and triglycerides and the higher is HDL. Vitamin C lowers risk for CVD by acting as an antioxidant, strengthening arterial collagen, lowering TC and Lp(a), lowering blood pressure, raising HDL, promoting fibrinolysis, reducing markers of inflammation, and inhibiting platelet aggregation.
- **Red wine**: flavonoids in red wine protect against LDL oxidation; serum antioxidant capacity effects; there is significantly better protection from consuming 1000 mg vitamin C than one glass of either red or white wine.
- **Grape seed and pine bark extracts**: plant flavonoids called proanthocyanidins (or procyanidins); most potent proanthocyanidins are mixtures of proanthocyanidin dimers, trimers, tetramers, etc., called procyanidolic oligomers (PCOs). Commercial PCO sources are extracts from grape seeds and bark of maritime (Landes) pine. Uses of PCO extracts: vascular disorders (venous insufficiency, varicose veins, capillary fragility, diabetic retinopathy, macular degeneration). PCOs have greater antioxidant effect than vitamins C and E. They prevent damage to cholesterol and arterial lining, lower blood choles-

terol in animals, and shrink size of arterial cholesterol deposits. PCOs inhibit platelet aggregation and vasoconstriction in animals.

## Miscellaneous Risk Factors

**Excessive platelet aggregation**: independent risk factor for MI and stroke. Aggregated platelets release compounds that promote atherosclerotic plaque or they can form obstructing clot. Adhesiveness of platelets is determined by type of fats in diet and level of antioxidants. Saturated fats and cholesterol increase platelet aggregation, whereas omega-3 (medium- and long-chain) and monounsaturated fats have the opposite effect.

- **Essential fatty acids**: people who consume diets rich in omega-3 oils from fish or vegetable sources have reduced risk of heart disease; highest degree of coronary artery disease found in individuals with lowest concentration of omega-3 oils in their fat tissues; individuals with lowest degree of coronary artery disease have highest concentration of omega-3 oils; omega-3 fatty acids lower LDL and triglycerides, inhibit excessive platelet aggregation, lower fibrinogen levels, and lower systolic and diastolic blood pressure in hypertensives; lowest rate of MI among people with high intake of alpha-linolenic acid (omega-3); oleic acid–containing oils (canola and olive oil) generate LDL that is less susceptible to peroxidation.
- **Vitamin $B_6$**: Antioxidant nutrients, flavonoids, and $B_6$ inhibit platelet aggregation, lower blood pressure and homocysteine. Pyridoxine inhibits platelet aggregation by 41%-48%, prolongs bleeding and coagulation time, but not over physiologic limits, and has no effect on platelet count. Pyridoxine lowers total plasma lipids and cholesterol with inverse, graded relation between serum pyridoxal-5-phosphate (P5P) and both CRP and fibrinogen. Low P5P increases CAD risk that adds to risk from elevated CRP or increased LDL/HDL ratio.
- **Garlic**: inhibits platelet aggregation, increases microcirculation of the skin, and decreases plasma viscosity.

**Fibrinogen**: Elevated fibrinogen is a major primary risk factor for CVD with stronger link to CVD deaths than cholesterol. Natural therapies (e.g. exercise, omega-3 oils, niacin, and garlic) promoting fibrinolysis can prevent MI and stroke. Mediterranean diet alone reduces fibrinogen and is linked to 20% lower CRP, 17% lower interleukin-6, 15% lower homocysteine, and 6% lower fibrinogen.

**Hyperhomocysteinemia**: Homocysteine is an intermediate in conversion of methionine to cysteine. Functional deficiency in folate, $B_6$, or $B_{12}$ induces increase in homocysteine, promoting atherosclerosis by directly damaging artery, reducing vessel integrity, and interfering with formation of proper collagen. Homocysteine is an independent risk factor for MI, stroke, and peripheral vascular disease. Elevation is found in 20%-40% of patients with heart disease. Folic acid (400 μg q.d.) alone could reduce number of MIs by 10%. Folate, $B_{12}$, and $B_6$ work synergistically for proper homocysteine metabolism.

**"Type A" personality**: extreme sense of time urgency, competitiveness, impatience, and aggressiveness is linked to a twofold increase in CAD. Regular expression of anger is damaging to cardiovascular system. Positive correlation between serum cholesterol and aggression: the higher the aggression, the higher the cholesterol; negative correlation between LDL/HDL ratio and controlled affect: the greater the ability to control anger, the lower the LDL/HDL ratio. Those who learn to control anger reduce risk for heart disease. Unfavorable lipid profile is linked to aggressive (hostile) anger coping style.

## Other Nutritional Factors

- **Magnesium (Mg) and potassium (K)**: absolutely essential to cardiovascular functioning; prevent heart disease and stroke. Mg and/or K supplementation is effective for angina, arrhythmias, CHF, and hypertension (K, *Textbook*, "Atherosclerosis"). Average U.S. Mg intake = 143-266 mg q.d., but Mg RDA = 350 mg for men and 300 mg for women. Mg sources are whole foods: tofu, legumes, seeds, nuts, whole grains, and green leafy vegetables. Mg deficiency contributes to atherosclerosis and CVD by generating a proinflammatory, prothrombotic, and proatherogenic environment that leads to endothelial dysfunction. People dying of MI have low heart Mg. IV Mg is a treatment measure in acute MI; during first hour after hospital admission it reduces immediate and long-term complications and death rates. Benefits of Mg for MI: improves heart energy production, dilates coronary arteries, reduces peripheral vascular resistance, inhibits platelet aggregation and blood clotting, reduces size of infarct, and improves heart rate and arrhythmias.

### Preventing Recurrent Heart Attack

Primary prevention of subsequent cardiovascular events is by controlling major risk factors: hyperlipidemia, hypertension, smoking, diabetes, and physical inactivity.

- **Aspirin (ASA)**: statistically significant reduction in mortality rate; reduces mortality rate from all causes and cardiovascular deaths. Mortality rate for all causes is reduced by 30% with ASA at doses of 326-1500 mg q.d. ASA is linked with risk of gastrointestinal bleeding from peptic ulcer at all dosage levels. Dosage necessary for prevention of stroke = 900 mg.
- **Natural alternatives to aspirin**: Dietary modifications are more effective in preventing MI recurrence than ASA and can reverse blockage of clogged arteries. Dean Ornish diet: low-fat vegetarian for 1 year (fruits, vegetables, grains, legumes, and soybean products with no animal products except egg white and 1 cup nonfat milk or yogurt daily) provides 10% fat, 15%-20% protein, and 70%-75% complex carbohydrate. Stress reduction techniques include breathing exercises, stretching, meditation, imagery for 1 h daily plus exercise at least 3 hours per week. Ornish regimen induces regression in atherosclerosis of coronary vessels. American Heart Association's dietary recommendations are ineffective. People consuming a diet rich in omega-3 oils have significantly reduced risk of heart disease. The highest degree of CAD is in individuals with the lowest omega-3 levels in fat tissues; individuals with lowest degree of CAD have highest omega-3 levels. Omega-3 fatty acids from plant sources (alpha-linolenic acid) offer the same protection as increased fish intake. Lyon Heart Study (Mediterranean/Cretan diet): whole-grain bread, root vegetables, green vegetables, fish, less meat (beef, lamb, pork replaced with poultry), fruit, and butter and cream replaced with canola and olive oil.
- **GAGs**: mixture of purified bovine GAGs native to aorta tissue (dermatan sulfate, heparin sulfate, hyaluronic acid, chondroitin sulfate, and related hexosaminoglycans) inhibit platelet aggregation; protect and promote normal artery and vein function; effective in treating cerebral and peripheral arterial insufficiency, venous insufficiency and varicose veins, hemorrhoids, vascular retinopathies including macular degeneration, and postsurgical edema; value primarily for patients recovering from MI or stroke, angiograms, coronary artery bypass surgery, or

angioplasty; dosage = 100 mg q.d.; less-impressive results in treating atherosclerosis with chondroitin sulfate at 3 g q.d. (1 g with meals t.i.d.).

- **Preventing a subsequent stroke**: *Ginkgo biloba* extract, standardized to 24% *Ginkgo* flavonglycosides and 6% terpenoids, improves cerebral vascular insufficiency, short-term memory loss, depression, dizziness, ringing in ears, and headache. *Ginkgo* enhances stroke recovery.

### Other Considerations

- **Angiography, coronary artery bypass surgery, or angioplasty**: procedures used far more frequently than justified by appropriateness and efficacy (*Textbook,* "Atherosclerosis").
- **Intravenous ethylenediamine tetraacetic acid chelation therapy**: *Textbook,* "Atherosclerosis."
- **Earlobe crease**: presence of diagonal earlobe crease has been considered a sign of cardiovascular disease since 1973. The earlobe is richly vascularized, and decreased blood flow over extended period collapses vascular bed, causing diagonal crease. This sign has 82% accuracy in predicting heart disease, with false-positive rate of 12% and false-negative rate of 18%; it is highly correlated with demonstrable heart disease and, less strongly, with previous MI. It is seen more commonly with advancing age, until age 80 years, when incidence drops dramatically. The link to heart disease is age independent. Its presence does not prove heart disease but strongly suggests it. Correlation does not hold true with Asians, Native Americans, and children with Beckwith's syndrome.

## THERAPEUTIC APPROACH

Tailor interventions to individual patient needs.

- **Modified Mediterranean diet**: reduce saturated fat and cholesterol by reducing or eliminating animal products. Increase fiber-rich plant foods (fruits, vegetables, grains, legumes, raw nuts, and seeds). Increase omega-3 and monounsaturated fats. Maintain low glycemic load.
- **Lifestyle recommendations**: Achieve ideal body weight. Engage in regular aerobic exercise. Avoid smoking. Eliminate coffee (caffeine and decaf). Drink 1.4+ L water daily.

- **Supplements**:
  —High-potency multiple vitamin/mineral
  —Vitamin C: 500-1000 mg t.i.d.
  —Vitamin E: 400-800 IU q.d. (mixed tocopherols emphasizing gamma fraction)
  —Fish oil: providing 1000 mg combined EPA/DHA q.d.
  —Inositol hexaniacinate: 500 mg t.i.d. with meals for 2 weeks, then increase to 1000 mg t.i.d. with meals.
  —Garlic: providing 4000 μg allicin q.d. (or equal to 4000 mg of fresh raw garlic)
  —Diabetics: pantethine 300 mg t.i.d.

# Atopic Dermatitis (Eczema)

## DIAGNOSTIC SUMMARY

- Chronic, pruritic, inflammatory skin condition
- Skin is dry and hyperkeratotic
- Lesions include excoriations, papules, eczema (patches of erythema, exudation, and scaling with small vesicles formed within the epidermis), and lichenification (hyperpigmented plaques of thickened skin with accentuated furrows)
- Scratching and rubbing lead to lichenification, most commonly in the antecubital and popliteal flexures
- Personal or family history of atopy

## GENERAL CONSIDERATIONS

Common condition (2.4%-7% of population).

- **Immediate hypersensitivity disease**: serum immunoglobulin E is elevated in 80% of patients. All patients have positive skin, radioallergosorbent test, and other allergy tests. Positive family history in two thirds of patients. Many develop allergic rhinitis and/or asthma. Most improve with elimination diet.
- **Physiologic and anatomic abnormalities of skin**: type of abnormality determines manner in which atopic dermatitis (AD) is manifested in each patient: lowered threshold to itch stimuli (substance P excess?); hypersensitivity to alpha-adrenergic agonists and cholinergic agents by partial beta-adrenergic blockade (receptor site insensitivity); dry, hyperkeratotic skin with decreased water-holding capacity (dry: zinc or thyroid deficiency; hyperkeratotic: vitamin A deficiency?); tendency to lichenify in response to rubbing and scratching (membrane fragility?); skin heavily colonized by bacteria (coagulase-positive *Staphylococcus aureus*) (immune dysfunction).
- **Dennie's sign**: accentuated double pleat below margin of lower eyelid and tendency toward vasoconstriction provoked by physical pressure ("white dermatographism").

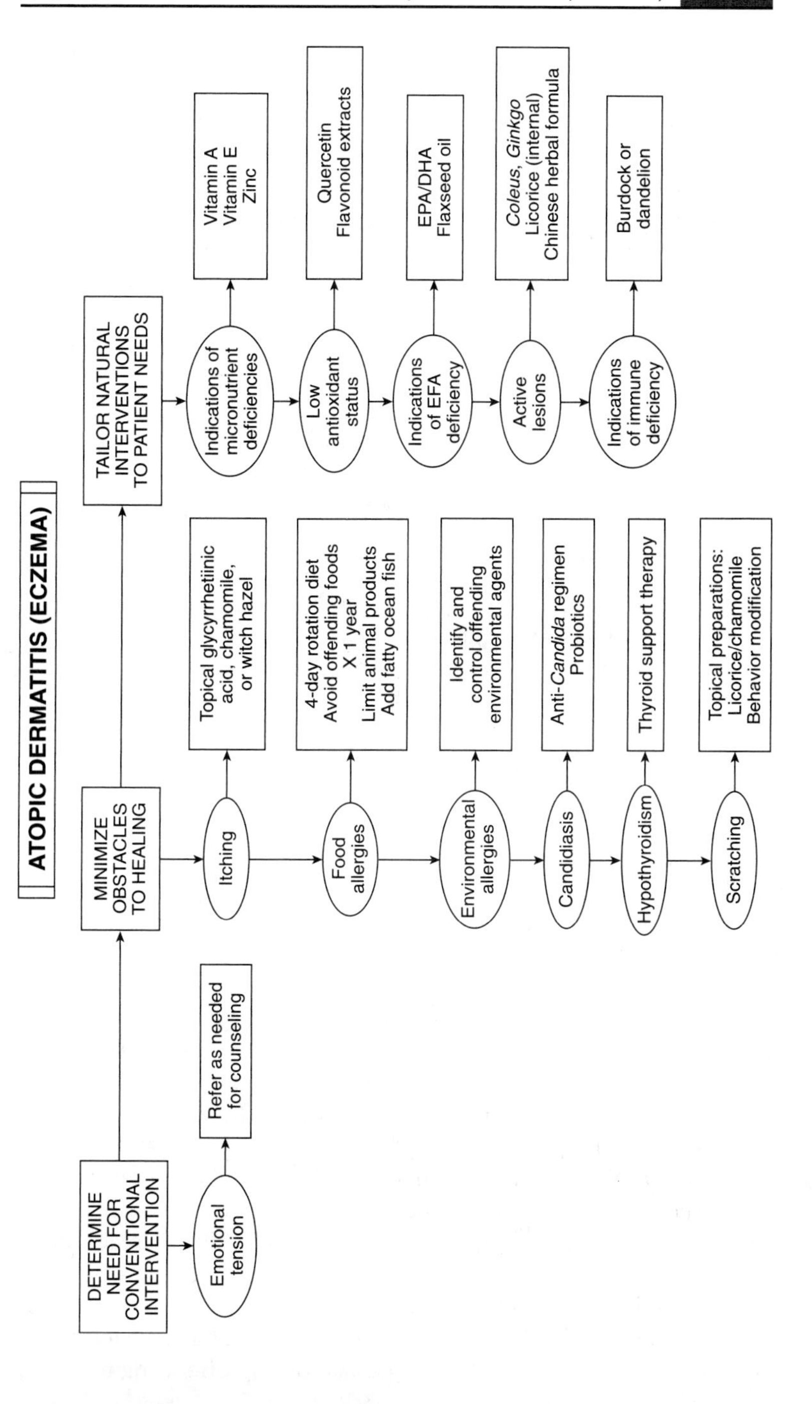
ATOPIC DERMATITIS (ECZEMA)
DETERMINE NEED FOR CONVENTIONAL INTERVENTION
Emotional tension
Refer as needed for counseling
MINIMIZE OBSTACLES TO HEALING
Itching
Topical glycyrrhetiinic acid, chamomile, or witch hazel
Food allergies
4-day rotation diet
Avoid offending foods X 1 year
Limit animal products
Add fatty ocean fish
Environmental allergies
Identify and control offending environmental agents
Candidiasis
Anti-*Candida* regimen
Probiotics
Hypothyroidism
Thyroid support therapy
Scratching
Topical preparations: Licorice/chamomile
Behavior modification
TAILOR NATURAL INTERVENTIONS TO PATIENT NEEDS
Indications of micronutrient deficiencies
Vitamin A
Vitamin E
Zinc
Low antioxidant status
Quercetin
Flavonoid extracts
Indications of EFA deficiency
EPA/DHA
Flaxseed oil
Active lesions
*Coleus*, *Ginkgo*
Licorice (internal)
Chinese herbal formula
Indications of immune deficiency
Burdock or dandelion

- **Predictors of severity in children**: eczema starting during the first year of life, a history of atopy (asthma, hay fever, or both), and urban living (independent of ethnicity) increase risk of severe disease.
- **Immunologic abnormalities**: leukocytes have decreased cyclic adenosine monophosphate (cAMP) from increased cAMP-phosphodiesterase activity and decreased prostaglandin precursors. Decreased intracellular cAMP increases histamine release and decreases bactericidal activity.
- **Defect in serum bactericidal activity** (alternate complement pathway [ACP]): inulin-containing herbs (burdock root [*Arctium lappa*] and dandelion root [*Taraxacum officinale*]) may restore bactericidal activity and increase cAMP. Inulin activates ACP.
- **Predominance of pathogenic *Staphylococcus aureus*** in skin flora in 90% of patients, increasing susceptibility to *Staphylococcus* infections.
- **Cell-mediated immunity defects**: increase susceptibility to cutaneous herpes simplex, vaccinia, molluscum contagiosum, and verruca vulgaris infections. Others include reduced delayed-type hypersensitivity, cutaneous anergy, and decreased in vitro lymphocyte reactivity to mitogens and antigens. Cell-mediated defects normalize during remission and become abnormal again during recurrences.

## THERAPEUTIC CONSIDERATIONS

- **Food allergy**: plays a major role in AD (*Textbook*, "Atopic Dermatitis [Eczema]"). Breastfeeding acts as prophylaxis against AD (and allergies in general). Breastfed infants develop AD as a result of transfer of antigens in breast milk. Mothers should avoid common food allergens (milk, eggs, peanuts, fish, soy, wheat, citrus, and chocolate). In older or formula-fed infants, milk, eggs, and peanuts are the most common foods inducing AD. Virtually any food can be offending agent. Food allergy is best diagnosed by elimination diet and challenge. Lab methods to identify food allergens in eczema: enzyme-linked immunosorbent assay for immunoglobulin (Ig) E and IgG4 (*Textbook*, "Food Reactions"). Food allergies are linked to "leaky gut," that is, increased gut permeability with increased antigen load on immune system and developing additional allergies. Eliminating allergenic foods can stop development of new allergies. Avoiding offending foods for

1 year may eradicate allergy; loss rate after 1 year is 26% for five major allergens (egg, milk, wheat, soy, peanut) and 66% for other foods.

- ***Candida albicans***: gastrointestinal overgrowth is a causative factor in allergies, including AD. Elevated anti-*Candida* antibodies are common in atopy. Severity of lesions correlates with level of IgE antibodies to *Candida*; anti-*Candida* therapy (*Textbook*, "Atopic Dermatitis [Eczema]") may significantly improve AD. Intestinal flora play major role in AD; probiotics are especially indicated. *Lactobacillus rhamnosus* GG, alone or with *Lactobacillus reuteri*, reduces severity in infants with AD and cow's milk allergy. Positive effect of probiotics is more pronounced in patients with allergic constitution (positive skin prick test).
- **Essential fatty acids and prostaglandin metabolism**: AD patients have altered essential fatty acid (EFA) and prostaglandin metabolism: increased linoleic acid levels with decreased longer-chain polyunsaturated fatty acids (gamma-linolenic acid and arachidonic acid) and omega-3s (eicosapentaenoic acid [EPA] and docosahexaenoic acid [DHA]). Proportions of linoleic acid in total plasma lipids and phospholipids are greater, and those of oleic acid lower, than normal in AD patients. Ratio of omega-3 to omega-6 fatty acids is lower in AD patients. Lack of significant decreases in proportions of dihomo-gamma-linolenic acid and arachidonic acid observed in plasma lipids of AD patients suggests that delta-6-desaturase is not impaired. Fish oil, providing EPA and DHA, or simply eating more wild fatty fish (mackerel, herring, salmon) increases omega-3 fatty acids in membrane phospholipids. Degree of clinical improvement correlates with increased DHA in serum phospholipids; fish oils are more effective in raising DHA than is flaxseed oil; EPA/DHA supplements or increasing consumption of wild cold-water fish may produce better results than flaxseed oil.
- **Inhibiting excess histamine release**: agents that stimulate cAMP production and/or inhibit cAMP phosphodiesterase reduce inflammatory process in AD by reducing shunting to histamine. *Coleus forskohlii* strongly enhances cAMP. Many botanicals inhibit diesterase; licorice (*Glycyrrhiza glabra*) shows marked activity. Flavonoids also inhibit cAMP phosphodiesterase: quercetin and hyperoside, the flavones orientin and vitexin, and the flavanone naringen. The common flavanol, rutin, has <1/10 activity of quercetin. Flavonoid extracts from *Vaccinium myrtillus*, *Rosa damascena*, *Ruta graveolens*, *Prunus spinosa*, and *Crataegus pentagyna* are

the most potent inhibitors of cAMP phosphodiesterase and also inhibit mast cell degranulation. Flavonoid-rich extracts (grape seed, pine bark, green tea, *Ginkgo biloba*) may prove helpful. *Ginkgo* terpenes (ginkgolides) antagonize platelet-activating factor (PAF), a key mediator in AD. PAF plays central role in neutrophil activation, increasing vascular permeability and smooth muscle contraction (bronchoconstriction), and reducing coronary blood flow. Ginkgolides compete with PAF for binding sites. Mixtures of ginkgolides and *Ginkgo biloba* extract (standardized to 24% *Ginkgo* flavonglycosides and 6% terpenoids) demonstrate significant antiallergy effects.
- **Zinc**: low Zn is common in AD. EFA metabolism is essential in AD (Zn required for delta-6-desaturase).
- **Vitamin E**: 400 IU q.d. for 8 months significantly improved 60% of patients, with significant reductions in serum IgE.

### Botanical Medicines

Two categories: internal and external.

- **Licorice (*Glycyrrhiza glabra*)**: useful in either application. Internally, licorice has antiinflammatory and antiallergic effects (*Textbook*, "*Glycyrrhiza glabra* [Licorice]").
- **Chinese herbal formula**: used in double-blind crossover trials. It contains licorice, plus *Ledebouriealla seseloides, Potentilla chinensis, Clematis chenisis, Clematis armandi, Rehmania glutinosa, Paeonia lactiflora, Lophatherum gracile, Dictamnus dasycarpus, Tribulus terrestris,* and *Schizonepeta tenuiflora*. The formula induces significant objective and subjective improvement in adults and children but many patients reported unpalatability of decoction. Pill or capsule forms many be available in the future. Base dosage on level of delivered licorice. Topical licorice commercial preparations featuring pure glycyrrhetinic acid have effects similar to topical hydrocortisone for eczema, contact and allergic dermatitis, and psoriasis.

### Miscellaneous Factors

- **Hypothyroid** patients with eczema respond well to thyroid.
- **Scratching**: is extremely detrimental in AD; breaks skin, aiding bacterial ingress, and promotes lichenification. Factors that limit itching promote healing and prevent recurrence. Some behavior modification techniques help reduce exacerbation of symptoms caused by scratching.

- **Emotional tension**: aggravates itching in AD. AD patients show higher anxiety, hostility, and neurosis than matched controls. Psychotherapy has reduced use of corticosteroids in some patients for up to 2 years.

### Environmental Considerations

Environmental sensitivities (e.g., dust mite [*Dermatophagoides pteronyssinus*] and detergents) may play a role in AD.

- **Dust mites**: concurrent asthma and/or rhinoconjunctivitis may benefit from dust mite reduction the most—changing mattress covers and bedding and using air filters. Skin sensitivity: replace clothing and personal soaps with hypoallergenic brands.
- **Microwave**: continuous mobile phone use for 1 hour increases allergic response to dust and pollen in adults with eczema. Microwaves also increase plasma substance P and vasoactive intestinal peptide in patients with AD.
- **Essential oils**: Repeated airborne exposure (by aroma lamp) to lavender, jasmine, and rosewood essential oils was factor in one case. Natural substances may also encourage allergic reactions. Choose all-natural therapies carefully and monitor closely.

## THERAPEUTIC APPROACH

Relieve and prevent itching while treating underlying metabolic abnormalities. Detect and control food and environmental allergens. Normalize prostaglandin metabolism; balance immune system.

- **Diet**: 4-day rotation diet, eliminating all major allergens (milk, eggs, peanuts in 81% of cases). As patient improves, slowly reintroduce allergens and reduce stringency of rotation diet. Limit animal products; add wild fatty fish (salmon, mackerel, herring, halibut).
- **Supplements**:
  —Vitamin A: 50,000 IU q.d.
  —Vitamin E: 400 IU q.d. mixed tocopherols
  —Zinc: 50 mg q.d., decrease as condition clears
  —Quercetin: 200-400 mg t.i.d. 5-10 min before meals
  —EPA and DHA: 540 and 360 mg q.d., respectively (or flaxseed oil 10 g q.d.)
  —Evening primrose oil: 3000 mg q.d.
  —Probiotics: 1-10 billion viable *Lactus acidophilus* and *Bifidobacterium bifidum* cells daily

- **Botanicals** (t.i.d.):
  —*Arctium lappa* or *Taraxacum officinale*: dried root, 2-8 g by infusion or decoction; fluid extract (1:1), 4-8 mL (1-2 tsp); tincture (alcohol-based tinctures of dandelion are not recommended because of the extremely high dosage required); juice of fresh root, 4-8mL (1-2 tsp); powdered solid extract (4:1), 250-500 mg.
  —*Coleus forskohlii* extract standardized to 18% forskolin: 50 mg (providing 9 mg of forskolin).
  —Glycyrrhiza glabra: powdered root, 1–2 g; fluid extract (1:1), 2-4 mL; solid (dry powdered) extract (4:1), 250-500 mg.
- **Topical treatment**: glycyrrhetinic acid-containing commercial preparations; chamomile preparations (*Textbook*, "Psoriasis"); witch hazel preparations.
- **Helpful tips**: avoid sweating and rough-textured clothing. Wash clothing with mild soaps only and rinse thoroughly. Avoid exposure to chemical irritants. Local application of soothing lotions ameliorates itching (zinc oxide), but minimize greasy preparations that block the sweat ducts.
- **Psychologic**: Determine if patient has significant anxiety, hostility, or neurosis. Refer to counselor for therapy as needed.

# Attention Deficit Hyperactivity Disorder in Children

## DIAGNOSTIC SUMMARY

A neurobehavioral disorder that begins in early childhood with persistence into adolescence and adulthood, characterized by the following:

- One or more symptoms of disabling inattentiveness, hyperactivity, and/or impulsivity
- Commonly accompanied by comorbid conditions such as mood disorders or learning disabilities

## GENERAL CONSIDERATIONS

DSM-IV defines attention deficit–hyperactivity disorder (ADHD) by developmentally inappropriate inattention and impulsivity with or without hyperactivity. Incidence is 5%-15% of school-age children, causing 50% of referrals to childhood diagnostic clinics. All forms of the disorder are properly referred to as ADHD, with three main subtypes: inattention, hyperactivity, and combined. Challenges include academic impairment, risk of injuries, and self-esteem and socialization issues. Problems in adolescence and adulthood: psychologic disorders, substance abuse, traffic accidents, financial problems, vocational underachievement, social dysfunction, and difficulties with the law. Yet personal success is possible.

### Executive Control

ADHD is linked to diminished function of polysynaptic dopaminergic circuits of executive centers in the brain's prefrontal cortex. Executive centers inhibit impulses and maintain sustained attention. Brains of those with ADHD are morphologically and metabolically abnormal in the prefrontal executive centers. Disturbances in dopaminergic and norepinephrine activity are implicated. Decreased sensitivity of dopaminergic (D4) receptor and

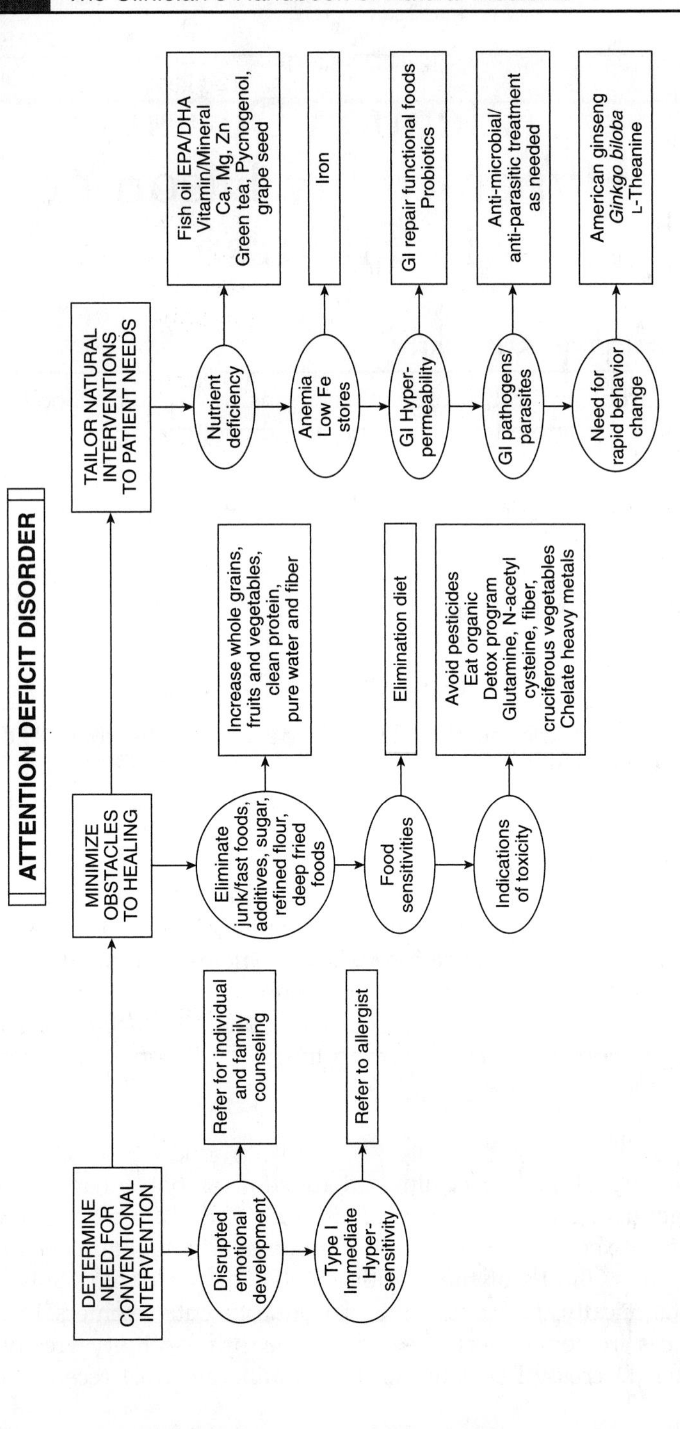
ATTENTION DEFICIT DISORDER
DETERMINE NEED FOR CONVENTIONAL INTERVENTION
Disrupted emotional development
Refer for individual and family counseling
Type I Immediate Hyper-sensitivity
Refer to allergist
MINIMIZE OBSTACLES TO HEALING
Eliminate junk/fast foods, additives, sugar, refined flour, deep fried foods
Increase whole grains, fruits and vegetables, clean protein, pure water and fiber
Food sensitivities
Elimination diet
Indications of toxicity
Avoid pesticides
Eat organic
Detox program
Glutamine, N-acetyl cysteine, fiber, cruciferous vegetables
Chelate heavy metals
TAILOR NATURAL INTERVENTIONS TO PATIENT NEEDS
Nutrient deficiency
Fish oil EPA/DHA
Vitamin/Mineral
Ca, Mg, Zn
Green tea, Pycnogenol, grape seed
Anemia Low Fe stores
Iron
GI Hyper-permeability
GI repair functional foods
Probiotics
GI pathogens/ parasites
Anti-microbial/ anti-parasitic treatment as needed
Need for rapid behavior change
American ginseng
Ginkgo biloba
L-Theanine

heightened dopamine reuptake by presynaptic dopamine transporter result in diminished dopaminergic activity within executive centers.

### Reward Deficiency Syndrome

Decreased dopamine activity may be a primary factor in addiction. ADHD is closely associated with addiction. Dopamine D2 receptor is central to brain reward mechanisms, which convey a sense of reward or satisfaction. D2 dysfunction leads to substance seeking (alcohol, drug, tobacco, food) and other behaviors (sexual addiction, pathologic gambling). Need for "neurologic satisfaction" may explain euphoria seeking—high-risk sports, criminal activities—and low tolerance to boredom.

### Minimal Brain Dysfunction

ADHD is associated with other cognitive deficits. Approximately 50% of ADHD patients have definable learning disabilities and measurable cognitive disturbances. Diminished nonverbal working memory impairs sense of time and decreases ability to hold events or tasks in the mind. The results are tardiness, missed appointments, procrastination, poor task planning, and failure to meet deadlines. Reduced serotonergic neuronal activity leads to depression or aggressive behavior. Antidepressants improve behavior in many cases.

### Genetics

Inherited predisposition to ADHD is polygenetic. Defects in genes encoding for both D2 and D4 dopamine receptors in ADHD create a state of dopamine insensitivity in affected brain regions. ADHD also is linked to genetic polymorphisms with increased activity of presynaptic dopamine transporter (increasing dopamine uptake). Other genetic factors: inherited allergic states, decreased immune competence, and genetic polymorphisms impairing capacity to detoxify drugs, heavy metals, and xenobiotics.

## THERAPEUTIC CONSIDERATIONS

### Environmental Neurotoxins

Effects may begin at or even before conception. Maternal-fetal transport of neurotoxicants (metals, solvents, pesticides, polychlorinated biphenyls, alcohol, drugs of abuse) occurs during pregnancy. Exposed mother with body burden of neurotoxic substances may exhibit ADHD symptoms. ADHD in her is acquired, not inherited. Children are susceptible to neurotoxicants after delivery.

### Maternal Tobacco and Drug Use

These are linked to higher risk of ADHD; 25% of all behavioral disorders in children are linked to smoking in pregnancy.

### Lead and Other Heavy Metals

Roughly 2% of American children younger than 6 years have lead (Pb) toxicity at a level that impairs cognition and disturbs behavior (>10 μg/dL whole blood lead). Low-level Pb intoxication is linked to addiction and impulsivity, suggesting neurologic changes of reward deficiency syndrome. Calcium (Ca) edetate chelation may be helpful. Mercury, cadmium, aluminum, pesticides, and polychlorinated biphenyls (PCBs) in dental amalgams, food, air, and drinking water may synergistically impair neurologic function and development. Autistic children have elevated body burdens of heavy metals.

### Neurotoxins

Autistic children also have organic xenobiotics. Functional liver detoxification testing (caffeine, acetaminophen, aspirin clearance) is also abnormal. Autism may primarily be a neurotoxicologic disorder from fetal and infant exposure to xenobiotics, while the blood-brain barrier is poorly developed, combined with inherited insufficiency of liver detoxification mechanisms. ADHD and autism may be part of the same spectrum of disorders and may share many etiologic features.

### Nutrient Deficiencies

- **Essential fatty acids**: ADHD children have reduced tissue docosahexaenoic acid (DHA). Brain essential fatty acids (EFAs) are critical in neuronal structure and function. Eicosapentaenoic acid (EPA), DHA, and arachidonic acid (AA) are components of brain and peripheral neuron structure, help normalize immune response, and regulate allergy and inflammation. DHA is crucial to fetal and childhood brain and retinal development. DHA levels are high at neuronal synapses, facilitating impulse transmission and neurotransmitter concentrations. Dopamine-producing nerve endings are 80% DHA. DHA is high in retina, supporting normal vision. DHA deficiency increases permeability of blood-brain barrier, critical to brain defense against neurotoxic xenobiotics. Primary effect of xenobiotics may be oxidative destruction and depletion of membrane EFAs. Bottle-fed children have twice the risk of developing ADHD as breastfed infants. Infant formulas do not provide DHA; breast milk contains DHA. Western diets are low in EFAs. ADHD children have impaired ability to synthesize DHA, AA, and gamma-linolenic acid (GLA) from vegetable oil precursors and increased oxidative destruction of omega-3 fatty acids. EFA deficiency is linked to diuresis and renal Ca loss. Increased thirst and enuresis associated with ADHD may be correctable by reducing food allergens. EFA deficiency in ADHD may be connected to food hypersensitivity. Atopy and food allergy require increased EFAs. Trans fatty acids arise from hydrogenation of vegetable oils, impair fetal/childhood brain development, and block enzymatic conversion of vegetable EFAs into GLA, AA, EPA, and DHA.

- **Magnesium**: low in serum, red blood cells, and hair of ADHD children. Behavior improves when supplemented.
- **Zinc**: children with low serum zinc (Zn) have lower free fatty acid levels, suggesting abnormalities in fatty acid metabolism may be liked to Zn deficiency. Low hair Zn correlates with poorer response to amphetamine treatment. Zn can reduce hyperactivity.
- **Iron**: helps regulate dopaminergic activity. Supplementating nonanemic ADHD children can diminish ADHD symptoms within 30 days.
- **B vitamins**: low vitamin $B_1$ levels have been observed in ADHD children.
- **Diet**: improved behavior and school performance have been noted in children with a junk food diet—sucrose, artificial flavors, artificial colors, and preservatives—replaced by nutrient-dense foods. High glycemic diets correlate with high tissue cadmium and poor cognition in children. ADHD children have impaired catecholamine control of blood sugar with worsened behavior after sucrose challenge.

## Food Allergy and Gastrointestinal Function

### Food Allergy

ADHD may be connected to atopy and food allergy and intolerance. Electroencephalographic changes occur immediately after ingesting sensitizing food. Allergies are associated with higher incidence of recurrent otitis media, which is associated with increased risk of ADHD. Both food allergy and ADHD patients have sleep disturbances. Heavy snoring and sleep apnea occur in atopic and food-allergic children, which may worsen ADHD. Low allergy potential (oligoantigenic) diet improves sleep in ADHD children. Enzyme-potentiated desensitization (EPD) to a broad range of food antigens improves behavior in ADHD children. EPD and methylphenidate (Ritalin) are equally effective in reducing ADHD symptoms.

Mediators of inflammation (histamine, bradykinins, interleukins, tumor necrosis factor-alpha, prostaglandin $E_2$, neuropeptides) appear in blood immediately after exposure to sensitizing food, affecting cerebral vasculature to produce migraine headaches and seizures. Oligoantigenic diet reduces these symptoms. Neuroactive peptides from food and endogenous opioids are implicated in etiology of autism. Neuroactive opioid peptides (exorphins) are in cow's milk and wheat gluten and are released from immune cells by sensitizing food. Allergy or EFA deficiency may allow neuroactive peptides increased access to brain. Gut-derived inflammatory mediators disrupt blood-brain barrier. ADHD may arise from barrier breakdown combined with increased toxic neuroactive substances (*Textbook,* "Attention Deficit Hyperactivity Disorder in Children").

## Intestinal Hyperpermeability

Sensitizing foods may induce gut mucosal inflammation and edema, maldigestion and malabsorption, causing nutritional insufficiencies and hyperpermeability, allowing macromolecular transport through mesenteric lymphatics and portal vein. Gut lymphatics and liver Kupffer cells engage antigenic debris. Released cellular messengers and inflammatory mediators (histamine, bradykinins, tumor necrosis factor) increase permeability of blood-brain barrier. Macromolecules escaping liver first pass may directly affect the brain. Intestinal permeability testing is a marker for food allergies and helps monitor progress. Intestinal hyperpermeability is associated with autism, eczema, arthritis, and gastrointestinal (GI) diseases. Decreased gut permeability may accompany disease improvement. The hormone secretin improves behavior and cognition in autistic children. The mechanism is unknown. Intravenous secretin in autistic children improves GI function and decreases urinary microbial organic acid derivatives.

## Gastrointestinal Dysbiosis

Intestinal hyperpermeability is linked to antibiotics. Antimicrobials are used for recurrent otitis in ADHD, disrupting gut flora. Normal flora help maintain mucosal barrier, act as first line of defense, and develop immune tolerance to dietary components. Bifidobacteria and lactobacilli may normalize altered permeability (*Textbook*, "Probiotics"). Adherence of beneficial bacteria to mucosa triggers generation of secretory immunoglobulin A (IgA), preventing ingress of antigens. Inadequate secretory IgA may be a factor in ADHD. Probiotics also may generate signaling molecules to gut-associated lymphoid tissue to establish tolerance to food antigens. Probiotics can ameliorate food allergy, desensitizing patients to offending foods. Some flora may modify immunomodulatory properties of food proteins by enzymatic hydrolysis. Symbiotic microbes neutralize microbial toxins and carcinogens and inhibit pathogenic bacteria (e.g., *Helicobacter pylori*). Neurotoxic endotoxins in urine and breath of neuropsychologic patients include d-lactic acid, tartaric acid, ethanol, arabinose, dihydroxyphenyl-propionic acid, ammonia, benzodiazepine receptor ligands, and methane. Bacterial beta-glucuronidase deconjugates steroids intended for fecal excretion, increasing aggressive behavior in ADHD children. Microbial endotoxins and enzymes degrade mucosa, causing microbial translocation, mucosal inflammation, and hyperpermeability. Stool pathogens in ADHD patients (protozoa, *Candida albicans*) are associated with allergic response, atopy, reactive arthritis, synovitis, and autoimmune colitis. Certain bacterial pathogens increase the pathogenicity of protozoa. *Klebsiella pneumoniae*, *Citrobacter freundii*, and *Pseudomonas*, also found in stools of ADHD patients, are linked to tropical malabsorption syndrome or tropical sprue, causing nutrient malabsorption (*Textbook*, "Bacterial Overgrowth of the Small Intestine Breath Test"). *Klebsiella* is linked to autoimmunity, and ADHD is associated with antineural antibodies. Autoimmune cross-reactivity between bacterial and neuronal antigens may contribute to ADHD.

## Immune System Impairment

Immune dysfunction may be a problem in ADHD. Cellular and humoral immunity are abnormal in ADHD children. Plasma complement is low. Immune dysfunction in ADHD may be inherited or acquired from malnutrition, toxins, or atopy. Autoimmunity also may be involved. Antineural antibodies occur in blood and cerebrospinal fluid. Gut mucosal immunity may be impaired; stool secretory IgA tends to be low, increasing susceptibility to gut pathogens and food allergens.

### Drug Therapy

**Conventional approach**: monotherapy with stimulant drugs. Stimulants work by blocking dopamine reuptake in nerve endings by way of dopamine transporter. Other treatments: antidepressants, antihypertensives, and the norepinephrine reuptake inhibitor atomoxetine. Drugs improve behavior and cognition in 75% of children during trials; success is less common in clinical practice and prognosis does not improve. Adverse effects and long-term impact on brain and cardiovascular health are unknown. Cerebral atrophy occurs in young adults treated with stimulants as children. Nonstimulant atomoxetine (Strattera) may be hepatotoxic. Selective serotonin reuptake inhibitors are problematic in children and adolescents.

### Cognitive Behavior Therapies

Conduct thorough neurobehavioral and cognitive assessment. Gifted children can be mistaken for ADHD. Mood disorders, learning disabilities, and abuse or trauma need specific psychotherapeutic interventions. Cognitive behavioral therapies at school and home can be effective.

### Neurofeedback

Electroencephalographic biofeedback provides real-time feedback about brainwave activity from electronic instruments, allowing self-regulation of brainwave intensity and frequency. ADHD patients have cortical slowing and diminished brainwave intensity in the prefrontal region and frontal lobes. Neurofeedback trains patients to increase brainwave patterns that reduce cortical slowing. Neurofeedback can be as effective as methylphenidate and permits cessation of drug in children without loss of treatment effect. Many expensive treatments are required. Home equipment is available and affordable.

## THERAPEUTIC APPROACH

**Reasonable approach**: multimodal, addressing as many factors as practical. Basic workup: rule out common disorders that present as ADHD. Differential diagnosis: celiac disease, depression, Pb poisoning, sleep apnea, visual or auditory impairment. Contributing factors (intestinal hyperpermeability; food sensitivities; iron, magnesium [Mg], Zn, and omega-3 deficiency) can be lab tested or treated empirically if finances are constrained.

- **Step 1**: Help parents eliminate junk and fast foods, food additives, sugar, refined flour, and fried foods while increasing whole grains, fruits and vegetables, clean protein, pure water, and fiber.
- **Step 2**: Nutritional supplements—pharmaceutical-grade fish oil or DHA/EPA concentrate; high-potency multivitamin/trace mineral supplement; Ca, Mg, Zn (additional iron is beneficial in anemic children and adolescents or for low iron stores); antioxidants (e.g., green tea extract, Pycnogenol, or grape seed extract).
- **Step 3**: GI rehabilitation to reduce hyperpermeability, improve nutrient absorption, increase immune response to gut pathogens, and diminish hypersensitivities. Mnemonic ANT PIE (*a*bstain, *n*ourish, *t*oxins/detoxification, *p*robiotics, *i*dentify, *e*liminate).
  —*A*bstain from junk foods, fried foods, sugar, foods that harm or irritate the gut, unnecessary drugs, excess alcohol.
  —*N*ourish GI tract with nutrients that support gut healing. Use functional foods combining hypoallergenic protein and nutrients helpful for GI healing.
  —*T*oxins/detoxification: avoid pesticides by eating organic. Consume nutrients that improve detoxification efficiency (L-glutamine, *N*-acetyl cysteine, fiber, cruciferous vegetables). Exercise regularly and reduce stress.
  —*P*robiotics improve GI microecology and immune response to gut pathogens, reduce immune hypersensitivity, and stimulate gut repair.
  —*I*dentify allergenic and intolerable foods and gut pathogens. Identify food allergies (type I/immediate hypersensitivity) by using skin prick testing, radioallergosorbent test, or enzyme-linked immunosorbent assay testing for IgE anti-food antibodies. Refer to allergists for definitive testing, patients with type I hypersensitivity, indicated by postprandial lip swelling, urticaria, wheezing, and so forth to prevent anaphylaxis. Identify delayed hypersensitivity (type III mediated) with elimination test diet followed by reintroductions of individual foods eliminated. Test for IgG anti-food antibodies before any dietary manipulation. Identify intestinal parasites, yeast, and pathogenic bacteria by stool testing, *Candida* and *Helicobacter pylori* serology, breath testing, and urinary organic acids.
  —*E*liminate allergenic and intolerable foods by using elimination diet or lab testing. Treat gut pathogens, parasites, and *Candida* overgrowth.

- **Step 4**: Nutraceuticals can improve behavior and cognition, especially if parents are pressured to medicate a child. A combination of standardized extracts of American ginseng and *Ginkgo biloba* improves behavior and school performance in ADHD children. L-theanine, an amino acid found in green tea, reduces anxiety, increases concentration, improves sleep quality, stabilizes mood without sedation, and improves cerebral dopaminergic activity. It is patented for treating ADHD in Japan and the European Union, and it is an approved food additive and nutritional supplement in the United States and Canada.

# Bacterial Sinusitis

## DIAGNOSTIC SUMMARY

- History of acute viral respiratory infection, dental infection, or nasal allergy
- Nasal congestion and purulent discharge
- Fever, chills, and frontal headache
- Pain, tenderness, redness, and swelling over the involved sinus
- Transillumination shows opaque sinus
- Chronic infection may produce no symptoms other than mild postnasal discharge, a musty odor, or a nonproductive cough.

## GENERAL CONSIDERATIONS

Predisposing factor is viral upper respiratory infection (common cold). Allergic rhinitis and other factors interfering with normal protective mechanisms may precede viral infection and are predisposing factors. Any factor inducing mucous membrane edema may obstruct meatal drainage. Transudate serves as medium for bacteria. Streptococci, pneumococci, staphylococci, and *Haemophilus influenzae* are the most common. Allergy is common in chronic sinusitis; 25% of chronic maxillary sinusitis involves underlying dental infection. Vasoconstrictors and antihistamines give transient relief but prolonged use is contraindicated—reflex reaction after long-term administration.

## THERAPEUTIC CONSIDERATIONS

- **Antibiotics**: their value is limited and efficacy is controversial. Analysis of clinical trials: Antibiotic treatment in acute maxillary sinusitis in general practice population is not sufficiently based on evidence. They are warranted in severe or unresponsive cases. Newer, more potent antibiotics (lactam antibiotics) are more effective than penicillin, amoxicillin, and other less-potent antibiotics. Even less evidence exists of significant benefit in

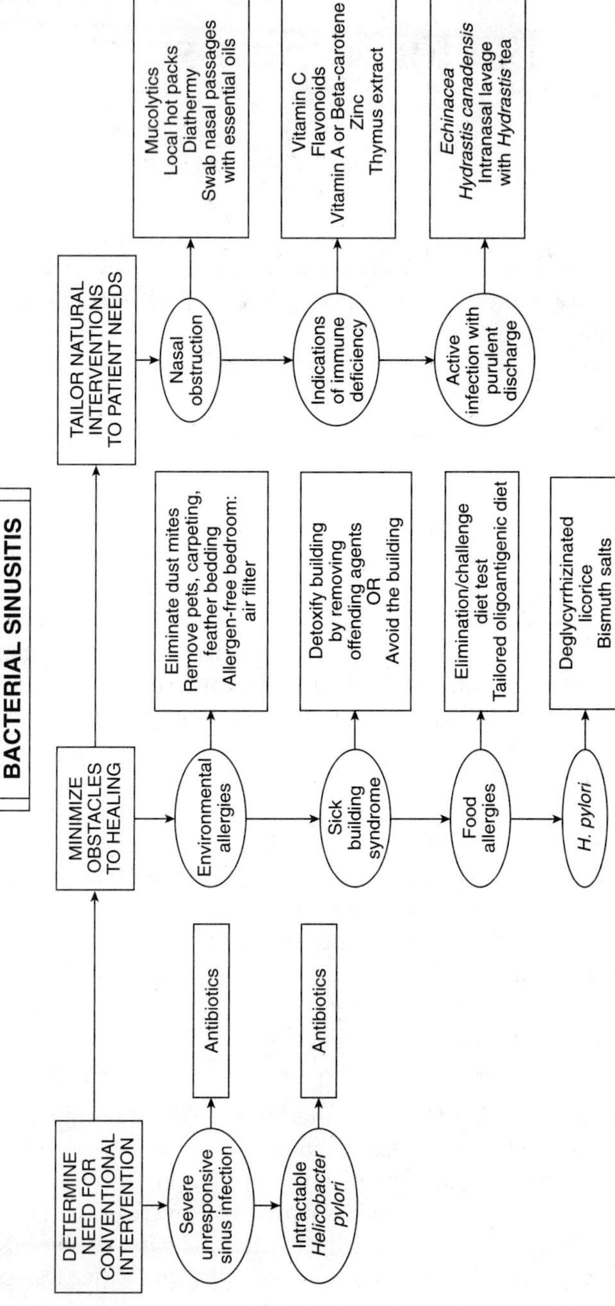
BACTERIAL SINUSITIS
DETERMINE NEED FOR CONVENTIONAL INTERVENTION
Severe unresponsive sinus infection
Antibiotics
Intractable *Helicobacter pylori*
Antibiotics
MINIMIZE OBSTACLES TO HEALING
Environmental allergies
Eliminate dust mites
Remove pets, carpeting, feather bedding
Allergen-free bedroom: air filter
Sick building syndrome
Detoxify building by removing offending agents
OR
Avoid the building
Food allergies
Elimination/challenge diet test
Tailored oligoantigenic diet
*H. pylori*
Deglycyrrhizinated licorice
Bismuth salts
TAILOR NATURAL INTERVENTIONS TO PATIENT NEEDS
Nasal obstruction
Mucolytics
Local hot packs
Diathermy
Swab nasal passages with essential oils
Indications of immune deficiency
Vitamin C
Flavonoids
Vitamin A or Beta-carotene
Zinc
Thymus extract
Active infection with purulent discharge
*Echinacea*
*Hydrastis canadensis*
Intranasal lavage with *Hydrastis* tea

children. Overuse of antibiotics in children with sinusitis or otitis media can generate antibiotic-resistant bacterial pathogens. In chronic sinusitis, antibiotics are of little or no benefit. Addressing underlying cause (respiratory or food allergens) and providing supportive therapy (saline nasal sprays, immune-enhancing herbs, and natural decongestants) is the most rational approach.

- **Allergy**: approximately 84% of those with chronic sinusitis have allergies.
- **Screen chronic sinusitis patients** aggressively for environmental and food allergies. Control the patient's environment. Eliminate dust mites by washing at temperature of at least 58° C, using air-filtering vacuum cleaner and air cleaner with high-efficiency particulate air filter, and keeping humidity <50%. Remove all pets, carpeting, and feather bedding, if necessary.

**Mucolytics**: mucociliary clearance depends on mucus properties and volume, ciliary function, and mucociliary interactions. In chronic sinusitis, mucus viscoelasticity is higher than optimal for mucociliary clearance. Mucolytics (*N*-acetylcysteine [NAC], proteolytic enzymes) can reduce viscoelasticity. NAC is a commonly used agent. Free NAC sulphydryl group interacts with disulphide bonds of mucus glycoproteins, breaking protein network into less-viscous strands. Use nasal NAC 10% solution diluted with saline, sodium bicarbonate, and sterile water or use oral supplement. Enzymes (trypsin, chymotrypsin, serratia peptidase, bromelain, streptokinase) may break down proteins at inflammation site, exert antimicrobial effects, or act on peptide region of mucus glycoproteins when administered topically. The ratio of viscosity to elasticity influences mucociliary transport. *Serratia* peptidase is rapidly effective for a variety of acute or chronic ear, nose, and throat disorders, including sinusitis. Oral bromelain also is beneficial for chronic sinusitis.

- **Sick building syndrome**: environmental chemicals within buildings can induce lethargy, headache, and blocked or runny nose—symptoms of chronic sinusitis.
- ***Helicobacter pylori***: in atopic patients with symptoms of peptic ulcer, urticaria, sinusitis, and exercise-induced anaphylaxis increased when patients were positive for *H. pylori*. *H. pylori*–specific immunoglobulin (Ig) E and IgG reactivity was identified, with endoscopy confirming *H. pylori* in stomachs or sinuses of those with *H. pylori* antibodies. Antibiotic therapy for *H. pylori*–

induced ulcers resolves allergy symptoms in a significant number of such patients.

## THERAPEUTIC APPROACH

- **Therapeutic goals**: in acute sinusitis, reestablish drainage and clear acute infection.
- **Methods**: local heat application, local use of volatile oils, antibacterial botanicals, and immune system support (*Textbook*, "Bacterial Sinusitis"):
  —Isolate and eliminate food or air-borne allergens and correct underlying problem allowing allergy to develop (*Textbook*, "Food Reactions").
  —Acute phase: eliminate common food allergens (milk, wheat, eggs, citrus, corn, and peanut butter) pending definitive diagnosis.
  —Local applications of heat may alleviate short- and long-term symptoms of allergic rhinitis.
- Supplements:
  —Vitamin C: 500 mg t.i.d.
  —Bioflavonoids: 1000 mg q.d.
  —Vitamin A: 5000 IU q.d. (or beta-carotene 25,000 IU q.d.)
  —Zinc: 30 mg q.d.
  —Thymus extract: 120 mg pure polypeptides with molecular weights <10,000 or 500 mg crude polypeptide fraction q.d.
  —*N*-acetyl-cysteine: 200 mg t.i.d.
  —*Serratia* peptidase or bromelain:
    - Bromelain (1200-1800 milk clotting unit [MCU]): 250 mg t.i.d.
    - *Serratia* peptidase (enteric coated): 50 mg t.i.d. between meals
- Botanicals
  —*Echinacea* species (t.i.d.): dried root (or as tea), 0.5–1 g; freeze-dried plant, 325-650 mg; juice of aerial portion of *E. purpurea* stabilized in 22% ethanol, 2-3 mL; tincture (1:5), 2-4 mL; fluid extract (1:1), 2-4 mL; solid (dry powdered) extract (6.5:1 or 3.5% echinacoside), 150-300 mg
  —*Hydrastis canadensis*: dosage based on berberine content, preferably standardized extracts: dried root or as infusion (tea), 2-4 g; tincture (1:5): 6-12 mL (1.5-3 tsp); fluid extract (1:1), 2-4 mL (0.5-1 tsp); solid (powdered dry) extract (4:1 or 8%-12% alkaloid content), 250-500 mg

- Local treatment:
  - —Intranasal douche with *Hydrastis* tea
  - —Swab passages with oil of bitter orange, menthol, or eucalyptus packs over sinuses (care should be taken to avoid irritation)
  - —Hot packs
  - —Diathermy: 30 minutes (discontinue if pain increases without drainage)

# Benign Prostatic Hyperplasia

## DIAGNOSTIC SUMMARY

- Symptoms of bladder outlet obstruction: progressive urinary frequency, urgency and nocturia, hesitancy, and intermittency with reduced force and caliber of urine
- Enlarged, nontender prostate
- Uremia if prolonged obstruction

## GENERAL CONSIDERATIONS

- **Affects more than 50% of men in their lifetime**: incidence increases with advancing age: 5%-10% at age 30 years, more than 90% among those older than 85 years.
- **Genetic predisposition**: hereditary benign prostatic hyperplasia (BPH; early-onset enlarged prostate) is autosomal dominant or codominant. More common late-onset BPH has weaker genetic aspect. Alleles of genes coding for cytochrome P450c17alpha enzyme, which mediates sex steroid synthesis, are implicated in BPH and prostate cancer. Hereditary BPH may be recalcitrant to natural means alone; late-onset type may be more responsive. Treatments described below modify sex steroid metabolism and decrease symptoms; they are recommended for both types of BPH.
- **Androgen-dependent disorder of metabolism**: free testosterone decreases with age; prolactin, estradiol, sex hormone–binding ligand, luteinizing hormone, and follicle-stimulating hormone increase. Synthesis of potent androgen dihydrotestosterone (DHT) from testosterone by 5-alpha-reductase increases and hydroxylation metabolism of testosterone and DHT decreases from inhibition by elevated estrogens.
- **Ultimate effect**: increased intraprostatic DHT. Prostatic androgen receptors have a fivefold greater affinity for DHT than testosterone. BPH tissue has three- to fourfold greater net ability to increase tissue levels of DHT.

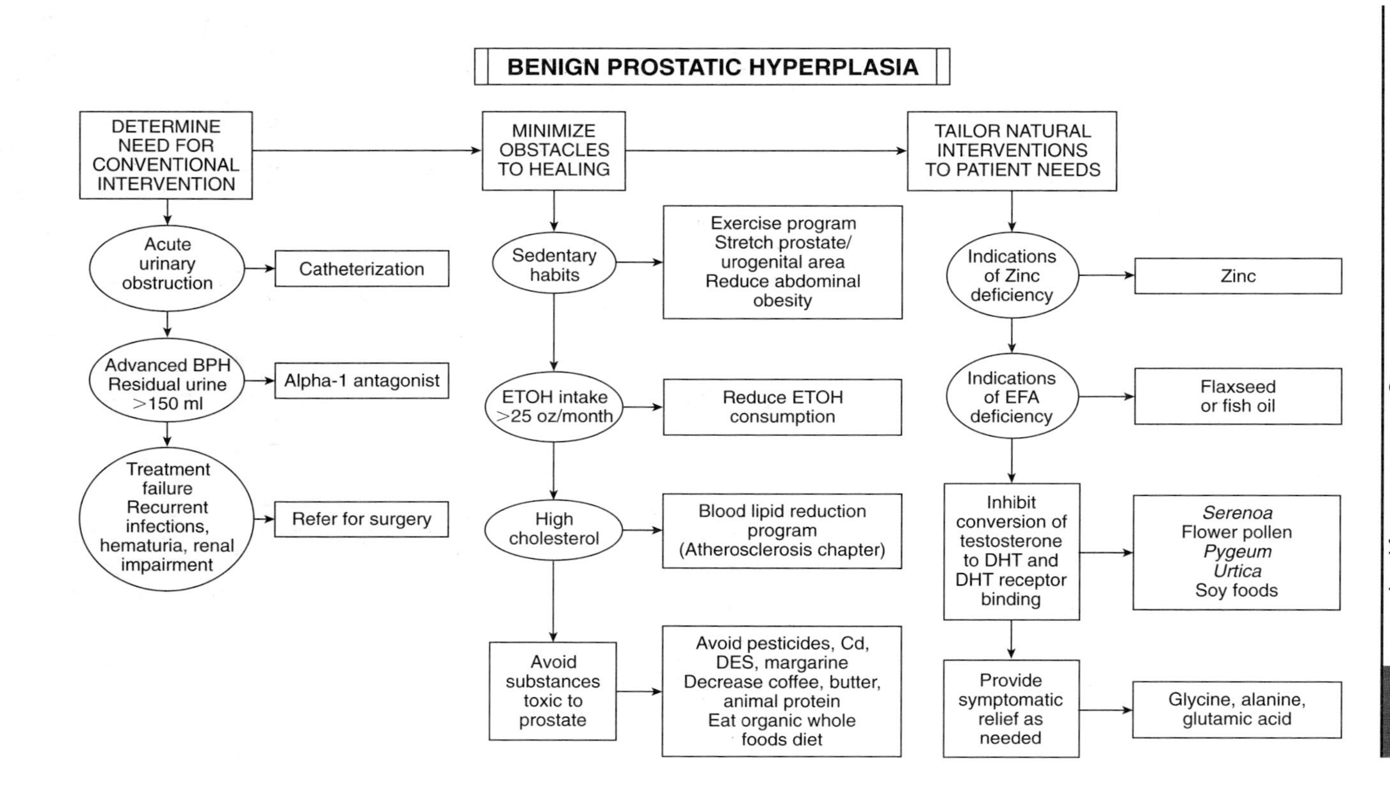
BENIGN PROSTATIC HYPERPLASIA
DETERMINE NEED FOR CONVENTIONAL INTERVENTION
Acute urinary obstruction
Catheterization
Advanced BPH Residual urine >150 ml
Alpha-1 antagonist
Treatment failure Recurrent infections, hematuria, renal impairment
Refer for surgery
MINIMIZE OBSTACLES TO HEALING
Sedentary habits
Exercise program Stretch prostate/urogenital area Reduce abdominal obesity
ETOH intake >25 oz/month
Reduce ETOH consumption
High cholesterol
Blood lipid reduction program (Atherosclerosis chapter)
Avoid substances toxic to prostate
Avoid pesticides, Cd, DES, margarine Decrease coffee, butter, animal protein Eat organic whole foods diet
TAILOR NATURAL INTERVENTIONS TO PATIENT NEEDS
Indications of Zinc deficiency
Zinc
Indications of EFA deficiency
Flaxseed or fish oil
Inhibit conversion of testosterone to DHT and DHT receptor binding
Serenoa Flower pollen Pygeum Urtica Soy foods
Provide symptomatic relief as needed
Glycine, alanine, glutamic acid

## DIAGNOSTIC CONSIDERATIONS

- BPH originates in periurethral and transition zones of prostate as early as the third decade of life.
- Develops from microscopic to palpable enlargement with age and androgen influence.
- Symptomatic in only 50% to 60% of men with macroscopic enlargement. Many men symptomatic without macroscopic enlargement; hyperplasia constricts urethral lumen.
- Digital palpation for diagnosis is unreliable; half of men with palpable enlargement are symptomatic, and half without palpable enlargement are symptomatic.

### Urine and Blood Tests

- Dipstick or microscopic urinalysis to screen for infection or hematuria.
- Serum creatinine to check kidney function.
- Prostate-specific antigen (PSA) and rectal exam for men age 50 years and older. Black men and men with a first-degree relative with prostate cancer are at higher risk; screen them at age 45 years.
- PSA: Normal is <4 ng/mL. PSA greater than 4.0 should be referred to a urologist. Elevation >10 is highly indicative of prostate cancer (90% of cases). Cancer may be present without PSA elevation. Mid-range elevations can occur with BPH, prostatitis, urinary retention, ejaculation, and exercise.

## THERAPEUTIC CONSIDERATIONS

- **Natural course of untreated disease process**: bladder outlet obstruction, urinary retention, kidney damage. Effective treatment, including surgery if needed, is critical.
- **Surgery**: may be indicated in patients who have failed medical therapy or have recurrent infection, hematuria, or renal insufficiency. Transurethral resection of the prostate (TURP) has high rate of morbidity (sexual dysfunction, incontinence, and bleeding). Thermal microwave and laser, to reduce hyperplastic tissue, are also available. These newer procedures are less expensive than TURP with fewer complications, but subsequent therapies are often required.
- **Lifestyle and exercise**: BPH is inversely association with physical activity and is linked to abdominal obesity. Increasing caloric

intake increases BPH risk. Higher caloric intake does not increase BPH risk when accompanied by increased physical activity. Benefits of physical activity: increases blood flow to tissues, facilitating waste removal; decreases sympathetic stress responses, relaxing prostatic tissue; reduces abdominal obesity; decreases lower torso pressure; relaxes prostate and rectal region; and improves blood flow through tissues.

## Dietary and Nutritional Factors

- **Nutrition**: avoid pesticides; decrease coffee and butter; avoid margarine and trans fat; increase fruit, zinc, and essential fatty acids; keep cholesterol levels <200 mg/dL.
- **Diet**: higher intake of animal protein is associated with higher risk of BPH. Eat high-quality, organic, plant-derived and wild cold water fish–based protein sources in moderate amounts.
- **Zinc**: reduces size of prostate and symptoms in most patients. Intestinal uptake is impaired by estrogens (increased in men with BPH) and enhanced by androgens. Zinc (Zn) inhibits 5-alpha-reductase and inhibits specific binding of androgens to the cytosol and nuclear receptors. Zn also inhibits prolactin secretion, reducing prostatic androgen uptake. Zn is concentrated in prostate glands of BPH patients, perhaps as a protective mechanism to modulate 5-alpha-reductase.
- **Alcohol**: beer raises prolactin levels. Higher alcohol intake—especially beer, wine, and sake—may be associated with BPH. Other studies indicate an inverse association between alcohol intake and BPH surgery, and higher BPH rates correlate with coronary disease. In men at higher risk for coronary artery disease from high LDL, alcohol may be protective overall by reducing LDL.
- **Essential fatty acids**: can improve symptoms in many patients; may correct underlying essential fatty acid deficiency because prostatic and seminal lipid levels and ratios are often abnormal. Use antioxidants to protect against peroxidation.
- **Amino acids**: combination of glycine, alanine, and glutamic acid (two 6-grain capsules t.i.d. for 2 weeks, one capsule t.i.d. thereafter) relieves many symptoms. The mechanism of action is unknown; amino acids may act as inhibitory neurotransmitters, reducing feelings of full bladder.
- **Cholesterol**: metabolites are cytotoxic and carcinogenic and accumulate in hyperplastic or cancerous prostate tissue. Epoxy-

cholesterols degenerate epithelial cells, triggering increased hyperplastic regeneration.

- **Soy**: rich in phytosterols (e.g., beta-sitosterol) that decrease cholesterol and improve BPH (20 mg beta-sitosterol t.i.d.). A 3.5-oz serving of soybeans, tofu, or other soy food provides 90 mg beta-sitosterol. Soy is associated with decreased risk of prostate cancer because of the isoflavonoids genistein and daidzein (phytoestrogens) acting on estrogen receptors and inhibiting 5-alpha-reductase. Recommend food sources of phytotherapeutic isoflavones (e.g., soy and *Trifolium praetense* [red clover]) for BPH, especially during watchful waiting stage.
- **Pesticides and other contaminants**: increase 5-alpha reduction of steroids.
- **Diethylstilbestrol**: produces changes in rat prostates histologically similar to BPH.
- **Cadmium**: antagonist of zinc that increases activity of 5-alpha-reductase, but effects on BPH are unclear.

## Botanical Medicines

- **Order of relative efficacy**: *Serenoa* > cernilton > *Pygeum* > *Urtica*. Each plant has a slightly different mechanism of action.
- **Therapy must be tailored** to individual patient needs.
- **Chance of clinical success** determined by the degree of obstruction indicated by residual urine volume: levels <50 mL, excellent; 50-100 mL, quite good; 100-150 mL, tougher to improve within 4-6 weeks; >150 mL, botanicals not likely to improve symptoms significantly.
- ***Serenoa repens* (saw palmetto)**: Liposterolic extract of fruit of palm significantly improves signs and symptoms. It inhibits DHT binding to receptors, inhibits 5-alpha-reductase, and interferes with intraprostatic estrogen receptors. *Serenoa* decreases urinary tract symptom scores and nocturia and improves urinary tract symptoms self-rating scores and peak urine flow. Matched with men taking DHT inhibitor finasteride (Proscar), men taking *Serenoa* experienced similar improvements in urinary symptom scores and peak urine. Adverse effects are mild and infrequent; erectile dysfunction appears more frequently with finasteride (4.9%) than with *Serenoa* (1.1%). Mild gastrointestinal upset can be overcome by taking *Serenoa* with food. *Serenoa* is better tolerated and less expensive and has no known drug interactions and nominal side effects. Approximately 90% of mild to moderate cases improve in all symptoms (especially nocturia) within 4-6 weeks.

- **Cernilton flower pollen extract**: approximately 70% overall success rate in 35 years of European experience; 70% reduction in nocturia and diurnal frequency; significant reductions in residual urine volume; some antiinflammatory action; contractile effect on bladder while relaxing urethra; inhibits growth of prostate cells. However, more recent research suggests cernilton may not improve urine flow rates, residual volume, or prostate size, but it does improve self-rated urinary symptom scores and nocturia compared with placebo and an amino acid mixture.
- ***Pygeum africanum***: African evergreen tree whose bark was used historically for urinary tract disorders. Bark components are fat-soluble sterols and fatty acids. All research is based on extract standardized to 14% triterpenes, including beta-sitosterol and 0.5% *N*-docosanol. It is effective in reducing symptoms and signs, especially in early cases. *Serenoa* gives greater relief, is better tolerated, and induces higher urine flow rate with less residual urine. But serenoa does not produce effects that *Pygeum* has on prostate secretion. *Pygeum* may inhibit endothelin growth factor, basic fibroblast growth factor, and insulinlike growth factor-I, linked to prostatic overgrowth.
- ***Urtica dioica* (stinging nettles)**: fewer studies; more effective than placebo; interacts with binding of DHT to cytosolic and nuclear receptors. Both *Serenoa* and *Urtica* offer clinical benefit equal to that of finasteride. *Urtica* lignans may modulate hormonal effects because of affinity for sex hormone–binding globulin.

## THERAPEUTIC APPROACH

- **Therapeutic goals**: normalize prostate nutrient levels; restore steroid hormones to normal levels; inhibit excessive conversion of testosterone to DHT; inhibit DHT receptor binding; and limit promoters of the hyperplastic process (e.g., prolactin).
- **Severe BPH**: acute urinary retention may require catheterization; for relief, advanced case may not quickly respond to natural therapy and may require short-term $alpha_1$ antagonist or surgery.
- **Lifestyle**: increase exercise. Ensure proper stretching of prostate and urogenital area to increase blood flow.
- **Diet**: initially higher in vegetable protein, lower in carbohydrates and animal fats, higher in unsaturated oils. After patient responds, adopt a less-strict, balanced, organic, whole foods diet. Limit alcohol

and coffee. Avoid drug-, pesticide-, and hormone-contaminated foods. Limit cholesterol-rich foods. Eat soy foods regularly.

- **Supplements:**
  —Zinc: 50 mg/day (picolinate preferred, maximum of 6 months; monitor copper status)
  —Flaxseed oil: 1 tbsp twice daily (with antioxidants)
  —Glycine: 200 mg/day
  —Glutamic acid: 200 mg/day
  —Alanine: 200 mg/day
- **Botanicals:**
  —*Serenoa* extract (standardized at 85%-95% liposterols): 160 mg b.i.d.
  —Flower pollen extract (e.g., Cernilton): 63 mg b.i.d. to t.i.d.
  —*Pygeum* extract (standardized at 14% triterpenes): 100-200 mg q.d.
  —*Urtica* extract: 120 mg b.i.d.

# Cancer: Integrated Naturopathic Support

## DIAGNOSTIC SUMMARY

Cancer is a group of more than 200 individual diseases characterized by uncontrolled growth, proliferation, and spread of abnormal cells. Diagnosis and treatment vary depending on type of cancer cells and location, extent of total tumor burden, health and performance status of the patient, prior treatments administered, and which conventional treatment regimens are currently considered standard of care.

## GENERAL CONSIDERATIONS

Prevention should take precedence over treatment. Occurrence involves two compounding factors: genetic susceptibility and environmental exposure to carcinogens. Environmental factors contribute more than half of risk for the 11 most common cancers. Naturopathy reduces lifestyle-based risk factors and counteracts some genetic factors.

Sensitive screening and diagnostic testing are needed to diagnose in early, more curable stages. Roles of naturopathy include the following:

- Preventing disease and screening for pathology
- Testing and evaluating suspicious lesions
- Reducing side effects of conventional therapies
- Improving tumor kill from conventional therapies
- Improving environment that allowed malignancy
- Supporting patient metabolically while starving tumor
- Slowing or stopping abnormal cell division
- Promoting normal cell differentiation and apoptosis
- Reducing metastasis and angiogenesis
- Enhancing cell-to-cell communication
- Using natural antitumor agents
- Blocking hormonal stimulation of tumors by normalizing hepatic clearance

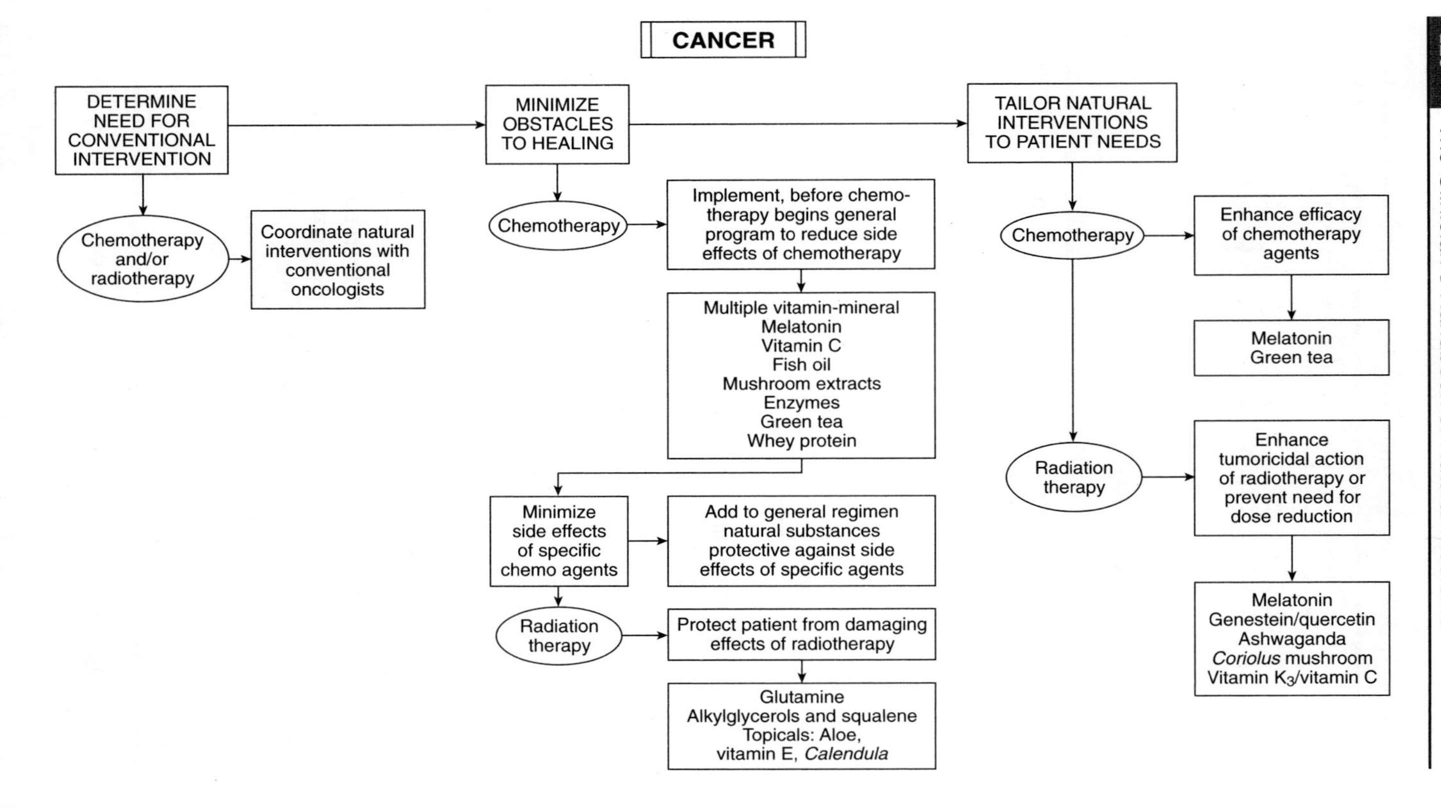

CANCER
DETERMINE NEED FOR CONVENTIONAL INTERVENTION
Chemotherapy and/or radiotherapy
Coordinate natural interventions with conventional oncologists
MINIMIZE OBSTACLES TO HEALING
Chemotherapy
Implement, before chemotherapy begins general program to reduce side effects of chemotherapy
Multiple vitamin-mineral
Melatonin
Vitamin C
Fish oil
Mushroom extracts
Enzymes
Green tea
Whey protein
Minimize side effects of specific chemo agents
Add to general regimen natural substances protective against side effects of specific agents
Radiation therapy
Protect patient from damaging effects of radiotherapy
Glutamine
Alkylglycerols and squalene
Topicals: Aloe, vitamin E, *Calendula*
TAILOR NATURAL INTERVENTIONS TO PATIENT NEEDS
Chemotherapy
Enhance efficacy of chemotherapy agents
Melatonin
Green tea
Radiation therapy
Enhance tumoricidal action of radiotherapy or prevent need for dose reduction
Melatonin
Genestein/quercetin
Ashwaganda
*Coriolus* mushroom
Vitamin $K_3$/vitamin C

- Supporting healthy immune response
- Supporting secondary prevention for patient after treatment
- Dealing with death and dying for those who succumb
- Encouraging prevention and screening for family members of patient

### Stages of Cancer Development

- **Initiation**: damage to cellular DNA leading to mutations and resulting in development of cancerous cell.
- **Promotion**: factors in cellular environment (free radicals, xenobiotic chemicals, hormones) "feed" cancerous cell growth into a tumor.
- **Progression**: tumor metastasizes to other parts of body.

### Cell Cycle

The cell cycle is usually divided into the following four or five phases:

- **G0 phase**: resting state, or gap phase. Many cells spend most of their time in this phase either at rest or performing assigned duties. Generally resistant to chemotherapy.
- **G1 phase**: gap 1 phase, or interphase. Cells synthesize RNA and prepare for cell division.
- **S phase**: synthesis phase. Cells duplicate DNA to create daughter cells.
- **G2 phase**: gap 2 phase. DNA synthesis completed. Microtubules of mitotic spindles produced.
- **M phase**: mitosis. Division of DNA and cellular proteins into two daughter cells. Return to G0 or resting phase.

### Chemotherapy Agent Efficacy According to Cell Cycle Phase

Certain chemotherapeutic agents work best in particular phases of cell cycle:

- **G1**: asparaginase
- **S phase**: antimetabolites, procarbazine, topotecan, topoisomerase I inhibitors
- **G2 phase**: etoposide, bleomycin, paclitaxel, and topoisomerase II inhibitors
- **M phase**: vinca alkaloids

### Types of Cancer

- **Sarcomas**: cells of mesenchymal origin (e.g., bone, muscle, fibrous tissue)
  —**Bone**: e.g., osteosarcoma
  —**Soft tissues**: e.g., leiomyosarcoma.
- **Leukemia**: white blood cell–producing tissues (bone marrow)
  —Chronic lymphocytic leukemia
  —Chronic myelogenous leukemia
  —Acute lymphocytic leukemia
  —Acute myelogenous leukemia
- **Lymphoma**: lymphatic system, especially lymph nodes
  —Hodgkin's disease
  —Non-Hodgkin's lymphoma
- **Cell type**: T cell or B cell
  —Physical form: follicular, diffuse
  —Degree of indolence or aggressiveness

### Staging

Staging expresses extent of spread to make treatment decisions, evaluate responses, and make survival prognoses. Usually based on anatomic spread, but certain cancers have other pertinent characteristics (e.g., any breast cancer of inflammatory subtype is stage IV regardless of spread; in colon cancer depth of penetration through colon wall is critical).

### Complete Staging Description

- Origin of tumor
- Histologic type and grade
- Extent of spread of tumor and locations of metastatic lesions
- Functional status of patient
- TNM score includes size of tumor (T), number of involved lymph nodes (N), and presence or absence of distant metastasis (M). For example, breast cancer with primary tumor 2.5 cm, positive lymph nodes in ipsilateral axilla, and no metastasis would be T2, N1, M0.
- Staging designation
  —**Stage 0**: in situ or noninvasive
  —**Stage I**: small localized disease
  —**Stage II**: larger disease but localized; may involve small number of local lymph nodes

—**Stage III**: regionally advanced
—**Stage IV**: advanced metastasis

## Tumor Markers

Tumor markers are tissue proteins in blood whose elevation indirectly reveals cancer progression. Caveats include the following:

- Most are not useful as screening tests. Noncancerous tissue can also secrete higher amounts of these markers in conditions such as inflammation and infection.
- Tumor may express different marker than typical for that tumor type.
- Most useful: monitoring response to treatment or disease progression.
- Raw number is less important than direction of change.

**Common Tumor Markers**

| Tumor Marker | Typical Tumor Types |
|---|---|
| CEA | Colorectal, breast, small cell lung |
| PSA | Prostate (some breast) |
| CA-15-3 | Breast |
| CA 19-9 | Pancreas, hepatic, biliary, gastric, colon |
| CA27-29 | Breast |
| CA-125 | Ovarian |
| Beta-HCG | Testis, trophoblastic neoplasia |
| $Beta_2$ microglobulin | Multiple myeloma, lymphoma |
| Thyroglobulin | Thyroid |

## Performance Indexes

Indicate level of health of patient. Most commonly used are Karnofsky score and Eastern Cooperative Oncology Group (ECOG) score. Based on patient's ability to perform daily activities, need for assistance, and need for medical treatment. Reflect patient vitality and ability to withstand and respond to further treatment. Patients with similar stages of disease but radically different performance indexes may have quite different outcomes.

**Comparison of Karnofsky and ECOG scoring**

| Karnofsky Score | Description | ECOG Score |
|---|---|---|
| 100 | Asymptomatic | 0 |
| 90 | Normal activity, minor disease signs | 1 |
| 80 | Some disease signs with exertion | 1 |
| 70 | Cares for self; unable to do active work | 2 |
| 60 | Requires occasional assistance; in bed less than 50% of day | 2 |
| 50 | Requires considerable assistance and medical care | 3 |
| 40 | Disabled; requires special assistance; in bed more than 50% of day | 3 |
| 30 | Severely disabled; hospital indicated | 4 |
| 20 | Quite ill; requires active supportive treatment; bedridden | 4 |
| 10 | Moribund | 4 |
| 0 | Deceased | 5 |

## Tumor Response Criteria and Terminology

Tumor response does not always mean cure or even an improvement in survivability. Cytotoxic therapy selects for resistant clones of tumor cells, which will over time no longer respond to treatment.

- **Cure**: treatment that allows patient to live as long as an age-matched cohort or die of other causes, even if some disease remains.
- **Remission**: complete disappearance of all detectable tumors. Millions of tumor cells may remain. Remission is a better term than "cure."
- **Complete response**: complete disappearance of all evidence of disease for at least 2 measurement periods at least 4 weeks apart.
- **Partial response**: decrease of at least 50% in diameter of all measurable lesions with no new lesions for at least 4 weeks.
- **Stable disease**: less than 50% up to an increase of 25% in measurable lesions.

- **Progression**: increase of more than 25% or appearance of new lesions.
- **Palliation**: treatment not aimed at cure, simply reduction of symptoms or transient extension of life for brief period.

## THERAPEUTIC CONSIDERATIONS

When making therapeutic decisions, results must be at least as good as those of conventional therapies to justify declining those therapies. This advice may determine whether a patient lives or dies. Make recommendations based on hard data, not on theory, anecdote, or opinion.

### Goals of Naturopathic Oncology Support

- Improve nutrition
- Selectively starve tumor
- Inhibit metastasis
- Reduce side effects of treatment
- Maximize tumor kill from conventional therapies
- Support normal cell division
- Remove tumor promoters
- Use antitumor herbs and nutrients (avoid waste of money on worthless products)
- Support immune function
- Support positive attitude and healthy lifestyle
- Regular secondary cancer screening after completion of treatment

### Stages of Clinical Care

Typical clinical pattern in most cancer cases includes the following:

1. Detection of abnormality suggestive of cancer.
2. Evaluation of suspicious finding with imaging studies; biopsy of questionable lesion; diagnosis of malignancy; staging.
3. Surgery to remove or debulk tumor. If inoperable, neoadjuvant chemotherapy before surgery to shrink tumor and make surgery less invasive.
4. Chemotherapy, radiation, hormones, or biologic response modifiers.
5. Monitor for recurrence. Biologic response modifiers based on type of cancer.

## Goals of Natural Therapies

- Reduce surgical complications
- Improve healing and recovery
- Support formation of healthy scar and connective tissue

Patients may be debilitated by disease or previous treatments; may need more aggressive support. Surgery may allow spread of tumor cells during perioperative period.

## Natural Medicine Support for Surgery

General preoperative guidelines (begin 2 weeks before surgery):

- **Avoid**: alcohol, recreational drugs, tobacco, sugar, fried foods, anything capable of causing increased bleeding (e.g., aspirin, ginkgo biloba, garlic, fish oil). Any drugs or herbs that may react with anesthesia (e.g., kava, *Hypericum*, valerian). Discontinue at least 5 days before surgery. Taper off caffeine slowly to avoid withdrawal headaches.
- **Increase**: fiber, protein (1-2 g/kg body weight), vegetables, fresh fruit, fluids, essential fatty acids, probiotics, vitamin C with bioflavonoids.

## Preoperative Nutritional Support

- Fractionated citrus pectin (6 g b.i.d.) to inhibit micrometastases.
- Gotu kola to reduce adhesions; three cups tea daily.
- High-potency multiple vitamin.
- Vitamin A (25,000-50,000 IU/day, 5000 IU in pregnancy) to support healing.
- Vitamin C (2000-5000 mg daily) promotes healing, supports immunity, builds strong collagen.
- Milk thistle is hepatoprotective: 200 mg standardized extract b.i.d.
- Zinc (60 mg/d) speeds second-phase healing, localizes to healing tissues.
- B vitamins (50-100 mg) generally included in multiple vitamin formula.
- Immune support to reduce probability of infection.
- Protein powder or free-form glutamine and arginine to speed postoperative recovery and promote protein synthesis for collagen formation.
- *Arnica* and Traumeel are homeopathics traditionally used to speed recovery from injury or trauma.

## Postoperative Nutrition

Resume nutritional support as soon as patient can consume solid foods. Do not start vitamins or herbs if patient is NPO. If the patient is able to consume liquids, add herbal teas and homeopathic remedies. When solid food is allowed without restriction, resume all indicated medications. Be aware of all pharmaceuticals being used to ensure no adverse interactions with nutraceuticals. Consult *A–Z Guide to Drug-Herb-Vitamin Interactions* (Alan R Gaby, editor) or Indiana University Department of Medicine's online resource "Drug Interactions," available at http://medicine.iupui.edu/flockhart. Continue all presurgical support for at least 2 weeks after surgery or until patient is fully recovered. Particularly important at this time is modified/fractionated citrus pectin to inhibit aggregation and attachment of dislodged circulating tumor cells. Continue pectin for 3 to 6 months thereafter.

Additional postoperative nutrients include the following:

- **Vitamin E**: reduces risk of thromboses and adhesions
- **Bromelain**: reduces inflammation, pain, and risk of thrombophlebitis
- **Protein drinks and smoothies**: amino acids for tissue collagen repair

Patient must do the following:

- **Ambulate** as soon as possible to prevent blood clots, constipation, muscle atrophy
- **Return home** as soon as possible to prevent nosocomial infection, sleep disruptions, medication errors
- **Not leave hospital** if patient feels something is wrong

## Chemotherapy and Biologic Response Modifiers

Clinical uses of chemotherapy treatment include the following:

- **Neoadjuvant**: before other treatments; shrinks tumor for easier treatment by surgery or radiation; used in breast cancers, some rectal cancers, bladder cancer, esophageal cancer.
- **Adjuvant**: after control of visible tumor with surgery or radiation; destroys undetectable cancer cells; reduces likelihood of recurrence; used in breast cancer, colon cancer.
- **Second-line chemotherapy**: tumor recurrence; to put the patient into remission; agents different from first treatment (may be resistance cells).

- **Palliative**: to reduce symptoms, such as pain, by temporarily shrinking tumor pressing on vital organ or nerve; not intended to cure; may extend life for short period.
- **High-dose chemotherapy**: to kill all cancer cells; side effect is loss or complete destruction of bone marrow capacity; patient needs "rescue" therapy—bone marrow or stem cell transplant; used in hematologic malignancies (e.g., leukemia, multiple myeloma) or in aggressive cancers (e.g., advanced breast cancer).

## Actions of Chemotherapeutic Drugs

- **Cytotoxic**: kill all rapidly dividing cells
- **Cytostatic**: slow cell division but does not cause cell death
- **Secondary effects**: antiangiogenic in lower dosages

Given in combinations of agents to take advantage of differences in actions for particular tumor types. Given in cycles: specific number of infusions followed by rest period.

## Families of Chemotherapy Drugs

- **Alkylating agents and platinum compounds**: substitute alkyl group for hydrogen to produce defects in DNA. Examples: cisplatin, carboplatin, cyclophosphamide.
- **Antitumor antibiotics**: bind between DNA base pairs, interfere with normal mitosis, generate free radicals. Examples: doxorubicin, mitomycin, bleomycin.
- **Antimetabolites**: substitute structural analogues of normal metabolites, interfere with DNA replication. Examples: methotrexate, fluorouracil, hydroxyurea.
- **Microtubule and chromatin inhibitors**: interfere with normal intracellular mechanisms necessary for mitosis. Block either topoisomerase enzymes used in DNA replication or bind to tubulin and block assembly or disassembly of microtubules. Microtubule inhibitors: vinblastine, vinorelbine, paclitaxel, docetaxel. Topoisomerase inhibitors: CPT-11 and etoposide.
- **Biologic response modifiers**:
  - —**Antiangiogenic agents**: inhibit the growth of new blood vessels. Examples: thalidomide, angiostatin, endostatin, cetuximab, bevacizumab, matrix metalloproteinase inhibitors, taxane-based agents at low doses.
  - —**Immune modulators, vaccines, monoclonal antibodies**: increase immune response. Examples: interferon,

interleukins, trastuzumab. Bone marrow stimulating agents: filgrastim, epoetin alfa, sargramostim.
—**Hormones and hormone inhibitors**: manipulate signals that regulate cell growth. Estrogen inhibitor: tamoxifen. Testosterone inhibitor: leuprolide. Therapeutic hormone: prednisone. Appetite stimulant: megestrol.
—**New-breed chemotherapy agents**: work by variety of methods. Specificity of action limits effects to tumor cells. Example: imatinib mesylate. Photosensitizing agents: less toxicity than systemic agents; specific activation in areas desired by laser.

## Side Effects of Chemotherapy

Vary depending on agent, timing, dosage, and protective measures used to reduce side effects. Individual factors include general health, efficiency of liver enzymes, amount of prior treatment (bone marrow suppression). Side effects are specific to agent.

- **Short-term side effects**: nausea and vomiting, mucositis, diarrhea, fatigue, hair loss, anemia, leucopenia, thrombocytopenia, bruising, cardiac damage, neuropathy, pneumonitis, nephropathy, tinnitus, infections, "chemo brain," hand-foot syndrome, alterations of taste and smell, anorexia.
- **Long-term side effects**:
  —Development of tumor resistance to chemotherapy
  —Increased risk of secondary cancers
  —Increased risk of leukemia and lymphoma
  —Infertility and premature menopause
  —Persistent unexplained fatigue
  —Persistent bone marrow suppression or myelodysplasia
  —Persistent "chemo brain" or short-term memory dysfunction

## Chemotherapy Resistance Testing

- Testing tumor tissue for resistance to chemotherapeutic agents. Small amount of fresh, unpreserved tumor tissue is taken during biopsy or surgery. Cell cultures are grown and tested for resistance to agents. Technique is new, controversial, not yet widely available, but makes sense. Requires fresh living tumor tissue shipped by overnight express on dry ice.
- Genetic testing of tumor tissue for characteristics indicating best agents and recurrence risk.

## General Recommendations for Chemotherapy

### To Improve Effectiveness

Specific nutrients can enhance specific chemotherapy agents. Addition of appropriate nutrients increases therapeutic efficacy. Take for at least 2 weeks before chemotherapy until completion of treatment. Actions: normalize cell division, increase apoptosis, increase cancer cell uptake of chemotherapy drugs, reduce drug resistance, stimulate normal cell differentiation.

- **Melatonin**: 20 mg melatonin nightly may double response rates and rates of survival at 1 year in a variety of stage IV cancer types. Reduces toxicity: thrombocytopenia, neurotoxicity, cardiotoxicity.
- **Green tea**: enhances inhibitory effects of doxorubicin against Erlich ascites tumors 2.5 fold in mice. Effect only seen in tumor cells, not healthy cells.

### To Reduce Side Effects

Variations in mode of action and path of elimination for each chemotherapy agent cause damage to certain organs. Minimize side effects with nutritional support throughout treatment; drug damage may be irreversible. General measures for all cases: optimal hydration, healthy diet, high-potency multiple vitamin.

Know each agent being used and relevant nutrient interactions and contraindications, especially when combinations of drugs are used. Selection of appropriate nutrients and botanicals is complex and based on many factors. General recommendations are safe for all types of chemotherapy.

- **Multiple vitamin:**
  —Vitamin A: 5000 IU
  —Mixed natural carotenoids: 10,000-25,000 IU
  —B complex: 25-50 mg
  —Folic acid: 400-800 μg
  —Vitamin $B_{12}$: 200-1000 μg
  —Vitamin E succinate: 400 IU
  —Vitamin C: 500-1000 mg
  —Vitamin D 400-800 IU
  —Trace minerals: full complement
- **Melatonin**: 20 mg at bedtime
- **Vitamin C**: 3000-10,000 mg q.d. in divided doses according to bowel tolerance

- **Fish oils**: to provide 2 g total combined eicosapentaenoic acid and docosahexaenoic acid daily
- **Mushroom extracts/immune support**: use a variety of immune modulators, switching them regularly to avoid downregulation of receptors. Standard doses for *Coreolis versicolor* mushroom is 3 g of the extract daily. Suggested dosage for maitake D fraction is 0.5-1.0 mg of extract per kilogram body weight. Other botanical immune modulators may be used as desired.
- **Enzymes**: use pancreatic enzymes with meals and mixed enteric-coated enzymes between meals.
- **Green tea**: capsules and beverages to total the equivalent of 5-10 cups daily. Caffeinated form is preferred if patient tolerates caffeine.
- **Whey protein shake**: administer with fruit daily as a source of easily assimilated protein and amino acids, particularly glutamine.

### Recommendations for Specific Individual Chemotherapy Agents

Individual agents are discussed below with nutrients considered in addition to basic protocol above. Unless larger doses are indicated for agent already mentioned, it will not be discussed in this section. For more on chemotherapy agents, consult the *Physicians' Cancer Chemotherapy Drug Manual 2007* by Edward Chu and Vincent DeVita, Jr.

- **Doxorubicin (Adriamycin)**: cardiotoxicity from free radicals may be reduced with additional green tea, vitamins C and E, and coenzyme Q10.
- **Cyclophosphamide (Cytoxan)**: orally active alkylating agent rendered effective by p450 enzymes. Use fish oils, folic acid, vitamin E, ashwaganda, and mushroom extracts. Tendency to cause cystitis; keep patient well hydrated.
- **Cisplatin and carboplatin**: intravenous glutathione immediately before administration of cisplatin. Simultaneous coadministration of selenium with cisplatin allows higher doses with less toxicity and higher therapeutic index. Milk thistle extract reduces toxicity. Vitamin A: synergistic with cisplatin for head and neck cancers. Vitamins C and E improve antineoplastic activity. Spleen extracts stabilize white blood cells, body weight, and fatigue. *Coriolus* mushroom extract enhances cytotoxicity against ovarian cancer.

- **Fluorouracil (5-FU), capecitabine (Xeloda), and floxuridine (FUDR)**: Vitamin E increases colorectal antitumor activity by upregulating proapoptotic enzyme p21 and augmenting proapoptotic protein "bax." Spleen extracts enhance action of 5-FU. Vitamin $B_6$ at 100 mg q.d. reduces incidence and severity of hand-foot-mouth syndrome.
- **Methotrexate (MTX)**: blocks activation of folic acid to inhibit DNA duplication. Folic acid at multivitamin levels is not problematic. Avoid higher doses. Avoid aspirin, other nonsteroidal antiinflammatory drugs, and penicillin, which reduce renal elimination of drug. L-Glutamine may increase intratumor levels of methotrexate by decreasing intratumor glutathione. Glutamine reduces mucositis and diarrhea caused by methotrexate. Vitamin A limits gastrointestinal damage.
- **Paclitaxel (Taxol) and docetaxel (Taxotere)**: semisynthetic isolates from yew species. Bind microtubules to inhibit cell division. Radiosensitizers, making tumors more sensitive to radiation therapy. Vitamin C improves response to docetaxel. Glutamine at 10 g t.i.d. reduces myalgia and neuropathy. Essential fatty acids (gamma-linolenic acid [GLA], alpha-linolenic acid [LNA], eicosapentaenoic acid [EPA], docosahexaenoic acid [DHA]) enhance cytotoxicity against breast cancer. GLA is most active; linoleic acid is of no benefit.

## Radiation Therapy

**Effect**: damages DNA of cells, leading to apoptosis during next mitosis cycle.

### Types of Radiation Therapy

- **Machine sources**:
  —Photon radiation: no mass and no charge.
  —Particle radiation, including neutron therapy and proton therapy. Effective even in low-oxygen environments.
    - Neutrons have mass but no charge.
    - Protons have mass and positive charge.
- **Brachytherapy**: use of localized radiation sources placed within a tumor. Precise targeting spares healthy tissue.
  —Permanent placement of seeds now common for prostate cancer.
  —Temporary placement of high-intensity source within tumor.

- **Radioimmunotherapy**: radioactive moieties linked to monoclonal antibodies injected into bloodstream. Antibodies target abnormal tissue marker and deliver bulk of radiation to specific tumor tissues, sparing other tissues.

### Side Effects of Radiation Therapy

Radiation therapy is more tolerable than chemotherapy. Factors influencing side effects include:

- Location of tumor
- Size of treatment field
- Organs or tissues within treatment field
- Prior or concurrent chemotherapy (radiosensitizing)
- Presence or absence of radioprotective agents

**Early side effects**: localized superficial burning; discoloration and desquamation; fatigue; reduced blood counts; and collateral damage to localized nerves, organs, and tissues within treatment field.

**Long-term side effects**: secondary cancers, scarring or tissue fibrosis, and impaired organ function.

## Naturopathic Support During Radiation Therapy

### Goals

- Assist patient in deciding if radiation is appropriate by reviewing survival data.
- Identify most advanced equipment in region to maximize tumor kill while minimizing collateral damage to healthy tissues.
- Consider radiosensitizing support to maximize tumor kill.
- Consider and select appropriate radioprotective agents.

## Radiopotentiation

Improving radiation tumor kill by the following:

- **Pharmaceuticals**: fluorouracil (5-FU), paclitaxel, cisplatin given concurrently.
- **Increase tissue oxygenation** (radiation is less effective in hypoxic tissues): hyperthermia (increases local circulation by vasodilation), carbogen gas inhalation, hemoglobin-inducing therapies (either erythropoietin or transfusions).

- **Natural therapies**: either enhance tumoricidal action or prevent need for dose reduction because of side effects (radioprotection). Natural radiopotentiators include the following:
  —**Melatonin**
  —**Flavonoids**: genestein (most active) and quercetin
  —***Withania somnifera*** (ashwaganda): radiosensitizing
  —***Coriolus* mushroom extract**: improves survival, enhances immunity
  —**Combined vitamin $K_3$ plus vitamin C**: pretreatment for radiation therapy, reduces tumor volume

### Radioprotection

All antioxidants are helpful. Standard doses of antioxidants in a high-potency multiple vitamin will not reduce efficacy of radiation therapy but will protect normal cells. Antioxidants are crucial to apoptotic cascade; they trigger apoptosis after radiation therapy.

- **Glutamine** protects mucus membranes during radiation therapy; helps heal radiation-induced enteritis and proctitis.
- **Alkylglycerols and squalene** maintain bone marrow function and white blood cell counts during radiation therapy. Squalene prolongs survival after lethal doses of whole-body radiation.
- **Topical agents** to reduce burning of skin surface during radiation therapy: aloe vera gel (fresh leaf most effective), vitamin E, methylsulfonylmethane creams, calendula creams. Apply nightly throughout treatment, but must be completely washed off before treatment so as not to alter penetration or scattering of radiation therapy beams.

## Antioxidants, Chemotherapy, and Radiation

Use of antioxidants with chemotherapy is controversial. Most antioxidants reduce side effects and improve tumoricidal action. Antioxidants enhance cancer cell apoptosis. Common chemotherapy agents induce tumoricide without lipid or protein oxidation. Oxidative stress actually *reduces* efficacy of chemotherapy agents. Antioxidants enhance tumor-killing action of chemotherapy agents. Oxidative byproducts of chemotherapy damage organs, increase risk of secondary cancers, and increase production of vascular endothelial growth factor, which is implicated in growth and invasiveness of tumors. Benefits of appropriately chosen and dosed antioxidants outweigh theoretical concerns.

- Many patients discontinue or delay chemotherapy because of side effects that can be reduced with nutrition.
- Others refuse chemotherapy because of the fear of side effects.
- Chemotherapy and radiation therapy are implicated in secondary cancers, which are theoretically preventable with nutrition.
- Approximately 50% of tumors have abnormal p53 enzymes involved in apoptosis, thus less responsive to chemotherapy. Antioxidants can partially reverse this abnormality.
- Chemotherapy alone for common cancers does not dramatically improve survival. Antioxidants allow higher, more effective doses without dose-limiting toxicity.

Antioxidants reduce negative side effects, increase tumor responses, and increase survival times. With a few specific exceptions, consider them essential to any naturopathic cancer protocol.

### Clinical Trials

- **Phase I**: toxicity and tolerable doses
- **Phase II**: responses or shrinkage of tumors
- **Phase III**: large groups of patients with similar diagnoses and prognoses tested to compare response to new drug versus standard drugs
- **Phase I and II trials**: little gain for patient and high risk of toxicity injury
- **Phase III trials**: randomized, giving 50-50 chance patient will not receive new drug.

Unless an extremely promising, dramatically superior new drug, there is increased risk with little gain from participating in a trial unless free testing or medical care for duration of the trial is provided.

### Diet for Cancer Patients

Approximately 30% to 40% of cancers are preventable by lifestyle and diet. High-fiber, nutrient-dense whole organic foods: fruits, vegetables, beans, seeds, small wild cold-water fish. Minimize high-calorie, low-nutrient foods: junk foods, candy, soft drinks. Incorporate allium (onions, garlic) and cruciferous vegetables (e.g., broccoli). See *How to Prevent and Treat Cancer with Natural Medicine* by Michael Murray et al.

# Carpal Tunnel Syndrome

## DIAGNOSTIC SUMMARY

- Numbness, tingling, and/or burning pain on palmar surfaces of first three digits and lateral half of fourth digit of the hand.
- Positive Tinel's sign (tingling or shocklike pain on volar wrist percussion).
- Positive Phalen's sign (appearance or exacerbation of symptoms caused by flexion of wrist for 60 seconds).
- Electromyography may show decreased nerve conduction velocity across carpal tunnel.

## GENERAL CONSIDERATIONS

Carpal tunnel syndrome (CTS) is unilateral or bilateral paresthesia in the palmar aspect of first three digits and lateral half of fourth digit of hand caused by median nerve compression within the carpal tunnel. Pain may be felt in wrist, palm, and/or forearm proximal to the area of compression. Loss of strength in abduction and opposition of thumb and atrophy of opponens pollicis muscle may develop. Fine motor skills may show loss. Severity ranges from mild to severe. Mild CTS often presents with intermittent symptoms. Severe CTS may cause permanent loss of sensation and paralysis of the thumb.

### Etiology

Any condition increasing volume of structures in the carpal tunnel or causing tunnel narrowing can impinge the median nerve. Conditions decreasing tunnel volume are subluxation of carpals, separated distal radius and ulna, Colles fracture, arthritic spurs, tumor, or thickening of flexor retinaculum. Conditions increasing volume of contents of tunnel are fluid retention, fat deposition, carpal synovitis, or tenosynovitis. A large percentage of cases are idiopathic; they may involve vitamin $B_6$ deficiency or collagen dysplasia.

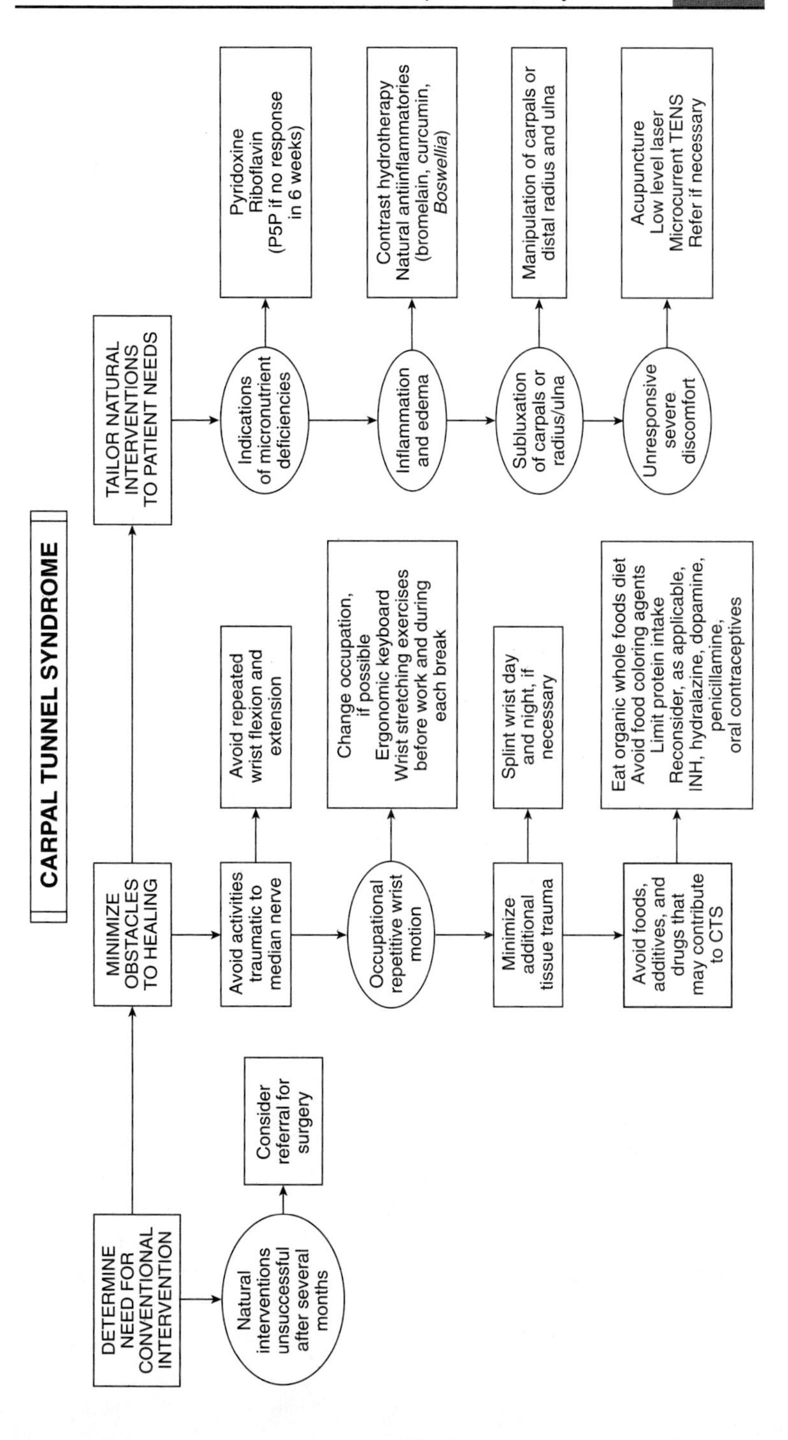
CARPAL TUNNEL SYNDROME
DETERMINE NEED FOR CONVENTIONAL INTERVENTION
Natural interventions unsuccessful after several months
Consider referral for surgery
MINIMIZE OBSTACLES TO HEALING
Avoid activities traumatic to median nerve
Avoid repeated wrist flexion and extension
Occupational repetitive wrist motion
Change occupation, if possible
Ergonomic keyboard
Wrist stretching exercises before work and during each break
Minimize additional tissue trauma
Splint wrist day and night, if necessary
Avoid foods, additives, and drugs that may contribute to CTS
Eat organic whole foods diet
Avoid food coloring agents
Limit protein intake
Reconsider, as applicable, INH, hydralazine, dopamine, penicillamine, oral contraceptives
TAILOR NATURAL INTERVENTIONS TO PATIENT NEEDS
Indications of micronutrient deficiencies
Pyridoxine
Riboflavin
(P5P if no response in 6 weeks)
Inflammation and edema
Contrast hydrotherapy
Natural antiinflammatories (bromelain, curcumin, Boswellia)
Subluxation of carpals or radius/ulna
Manipulation of carpals or distal radius and ulna
Unresponsive severe discomfort
Acupuncture
Low level laser
Microcurrent TENS
Refer if necessary

### Risk Factors and Frequency of Occurrence

Most obvious causes are traumatic injury and occupational injury through repetitive use. Other factors include repetitive activities with flexed or extended wrist, hysterectomy without oophorectomy, and last menstrual period in menopausal women 6-12 months earlier. A higher incidence is found in pregnant women, women taking oral contraceptives, menopausal women, and patients on hemodialysis. CTS is more prevalent among women and occurs frequently between ages 40 and 60 years.

## DIAGNOSTIC CONSIDERATIONS

- **Symptoms**: pain and tingling or numbness in hand; worse at night and may awaken patient; relief from shaking or rubbing hand; can be bilateral; clumsiness from inability to hold or feel an object.
- **Physical examination**: impaired sensation in distribution of median nerve. If condition is prolonged, atrophy of thenar eminence and weakness of thumb abductor may be present. Tinel's and Phalen's tests are accepted for diagnosing CTS in general practice. Tinel's sign is tingling in the distribution of the median nerve when tapping nerve in middle of palm over the transverse carpal ligament. Phalen's test is positive when symptoms are reproduced by holding the wrist in forced flexion for 60-90 seconds. Katz and Stirrat devised a self-administered hand diagram that is 80% sensitive and 90% specific for classic or probable CTS. Another in-office test is subjective assessment of swelling in the hand and palpation of the hand and wrist. Continued subjective swelling during treatment with wrist splinting correlates with poorer clinical response. Palpation of wrist and thumb in various directions of motion is a predictor of CTS. Wrist motion restriction correlates with electromyographic (EMG) diagnosis of CTS.
- **Other diagnostic tests**: EMG helps confirm median nerve compression in the carpal tunnel. Nerve conduction velocity is normal from elbow to wrist and diminished from wrist to hand and fingers. Both sensory and motor nerve conduction velocities are measured. Magnetic resonance imaging and high-definition ultrasound imaging measure median nerve size and interior dimensions of the carpal tunnel. These tests are used for preoperative assessment of CTS to choose the best approach to surgery.

- **Differential diagnosis**: CTS paresthesia is confused with paresthesia of brachial plexus in thoracic outlet syndrome or paresthesia of radial or ulnar nerves. Hand pain may be presenting feature of reflex sympathetic dystrophy (shoulder-hand syndrome). Also consider impingement of median nerve below the elbow, where the nerve passes under the pronator teres muscle. Specific dermatome pattern of CTS, without proximal dysfunction, should lead to history and tests establishing diagnosis of CTS. Left-sided CTS may be confused with angina pectoris.

## THERAPEUTIC CONSIDERATIONS

Most patients respond well to nutritional and conservative physical medicine. A few require surgical intervention. Nutritional support is needed to address underlying metabolic weakness.

### Nutrition

- **Vitamin B supplementation**: 50 mg $B_6$ initially, increased to 200-300 mg as needed, is significantly effective in treating CTS. Vitamin $B_2$ is useful, with even greater effect when given in conjunction with $B_6$. $B_2$-containing enzymes convert $B_6$ to the more active form, pyridoxal-5′-phosphate, the form of $B_6$ also used for CTS. Therapeutic response may require 3 months. Increased incidence of CTS parallels increased $B_6$ antimetabolites in environment: hydrazine dyes (FD&C yellow #5), drugs (isoniazid, hydralazine, dopamine, penicillamine, oral contraceptives), and excessive protein intake. Researchers have found no correlation between blood levels of $B_6$ and the presence of or improvement in CTS symptoms. Given safety and positive clinical studies with $B_6$ in reasonable dosages (e.g., 25-50 mg t.i.d.), a trial of $B_6$ is warranted (especially before opting for surgery).

### Medicines

Oral and locally injected steroids and nonsteroidal antiinflammatory medications provide some symptomatic relief. "Natural" antiinflammatory botanicals (bromelain, curcumin, *Boswellia*) and oils have not been studied. Natural medicines should be tried based on empirical knowledge and clinical experience. The increase in disorganized connective tissue in the carpal tunnel suggests bromelain for its antiinflammatory and proteolytic properties.

## Physical Medicine

- **Hydrotherapy**: inflammation and edema in CTS cause compression of local capillaries, decreasing nutrition to median nerve, making nerve fibers hyperexcitable. Contrast hydrotherapy increases circulation and nutrition to the area and reduces pain. Immerse in hot water for 3 minutes followed by immersion in cold water for 30 seconds; repeat 3 to 5 times.
- **Immobilization**: splinting wrist in a neutral position is required day and night for several weeks. Nighttime splinting only when symptoms appear is ineffective.
- **Manual manipulation**: manipulation of subluxation of carpals or separation of distal radius and ulna may relieve pressure in carpal tunnel, relieving impingement of median nerve. Also add manipulating cervical spine, right elbow, and right wrist three times weekly for 4 weeks. Myofascial release and frequent self-stretching techniques (three to five times daily) may offer subjective improvement, increase dimensions in the carpal tunnel, and reduce distal latencies in nerve conduction or increase motor response. Soft tissue and joint mobilization of the forearm, wrist, and hand may be helpful, but not from spinal manipulation alone.
- **Low-level laser therapy** combined with microcurrent transcutaneous electrical nerve stimulation applied to patients with mild to moderate CTS unresponsive to pharmaceuticals and surgery; may improve condition, according to McGill Pain Questionnaire, EMG sensory and motor latency, and Tinel's and Phalen's tests.
- **Stretching**: carpal tunnel pressure is twice normal in patients with CTS. After 1 minute of stretching/loading exercises, pressure drops to normal and remains so for 20 minutes. Exercise: flexing wrists and fists with arms extended for 5 minutes. This slow, sustained movement prepares nerve for repetitive actions. Do exercises before work starts and during every break. They may reduce need for surgery by 50%. Yoga therapy may also reduce pain.
- **Other nonsurgical interventions**: ultrasound therapy has produced mixed results. Therapeutic touch was found to be no more useful than placebo. Ergonomic keyboard (bent keyboard) may reduce CTS pain. Work practices (other than high-force work) have not been determined to have a direct influence on CTS.

## Surgery

**Options**: open carpal tunnel release with a long incision or a short incision; endoscopy with a single portal or a dual-portal technique;

tenosynovectomy; epineurotomy. Alternatives to open carpal tunnel release may not offer better relief. Surgery with early mobilization, surgery with oral homeopathic *Arnica* and topical *Arnica* ointment (not on unhealed, open skin), and surgery with controlled cold therapy all showed benefit over surgery alone.

## THERAPEUTIC APPROACH

Prevention is best. Avoid activities causing trauma to median nerve by repeated wrist flexion and extension as well as direct trauma to wrist. Maintain wrist posture. Apply treatment as soon as possible to avoid long-term damage to median nerve or associated muscles. Avoid all sources of hydrazine dyes. If treatment is unsuccessful after several months, consider surgery. Antiinflammatory agents may be useful.

- **Diet**: avoid foods containing yellow dyes and limit daily protein to maximum of 0.75 g /kg body weight.
- **Supplements**:
  —**Pyridoxine** (vitamin $B_6$): 50-200 mg q.d. Use pyridoxal-5′-phosphate if no response within 6 weeks.
  —**Riboflavin** (vitamin $B_2$): 10 mg q.d.
- **Physical medicine**:
  —**Contrast hydrotherapy**: immerse for 3 minutes in hot water followed by 30-second immersion in cold water three to five times daily.
  —**Manipulate carpals** and ensure proper spacing of distal radius and ulna.
- **Microcurrent**: simple noninvasive intervention to control pain.
- **Splint wrist** in neutral position night and day for unresponsive cases.
- **Regular wrist exercises**: useful intervention; key elements of prevention. Perform regular stretching of flexors and extensors of forearm several times daily to treat CTS and break up strenuous and repetitive activities that increase stress on the carpal tunnel.

# Celiac Disease

## DIAGNOSTIC SUMMARY

- Chronic intestinal malabsorption caused by intolerance to gluten
- Bulky, pale, frothy, foul-smelling, greasy stools with increased fecal fat
- Weight loss and signs of multiple vitamin and mineral deficiencies
- Increased levels of serum gliadin antibodies
- Diagnosis confirmed by jejunal biopsy

## GENERAL CONSIDERATIONS

Celiac disease (CD) is also known as nontropical sprue, gluten-sensitive enteropathy, or celiac sprue. Characteristics include malabsorption and abnormal small intestine structure that reverts to normal on removal of dietary protein gluten. Gluten and polypeptide derivative, gliadin, are found in wheat, barley, and rye. Symptoms appear in the first 3 years of life, after cereals are introduced to the diet. The second peak is the third decade. Breastfeeding has prophylactic effect; breast-fed babies have decreased risk. Early introduction of cow's milk is a major etiologic factor. Breastfeeding plus delay in introducing cow's milk and cereals are preventive steps.

- **Chemistry of grain proteins**: gluten is a major component of wheat endosperm, composed of gliadins and glutenins. Gliadin triggers CD. In rye, barley, and oats, the proteins triggering CD are secalins, hordeins, and avenins, respectively, and prolamines collectively. The cereal grain family is Gramineae; close taxonomic relation to wheat suggests ability to activate CD. Rice and corn do not activate CD and are further removed taxonomically from wheat. Gliadins are single polypeptide chains (molecular weight 30,000-75,000 mol) with high glutamine and proline. Gliadin's four electrophoretic fractions are alpha-, beta-, gamma-, and

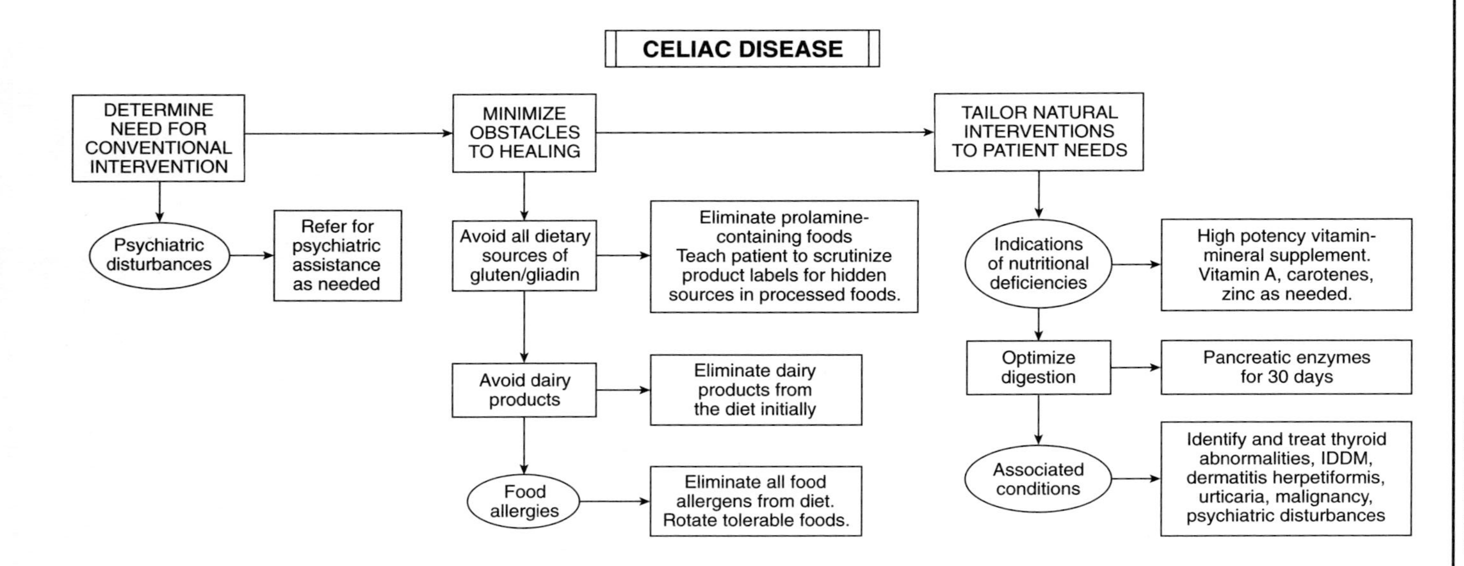
CELIAC DISEASE
DETERMINE NEED FOR CONVENTIONAL INTERVENTION
Psychiatric disturbances
Refer for psychiatric assistance as needed
MINIMIZE OBSTACLES TO HEALING
Avoid all dietary sources of gluten/gliadin
Eliminate prolamine-containing foods Teach patient to scrutinize product labels for hidden sources in processed foods.
Avoid dairy products
Eliminate dairy products from the diet initially
Food allergies
Eliminate all food allergens from diet. Rotate tolerable foods.
TAILOR NATURAL INTERVENTIONS TO PATIENT NEEDS
Indications of nutritional deficiencies
High potency vitamin-mineral supplement. Vitamin A, carotenes, zinc as needed.
Optimize digestion
Pancreatic enzymes for 30 days
Associated conditions
Identify and treat thyroid abnormalities, IDDM, dermatitis herpetiformis, urticaria, malignancy, psychiatric disturbances

omega-gliadin. Alpha-gliadin may be the fraction most capable of activating CD, but beta- and gamma-gliadin also are capable. Omega-gliadin is nonactivating but has the highest glutamine and proline. Hydrolyzed gliadin does not activate CD, suggesting deficient brush border peptidase or similar digestive defect.

- **Opioid activity**: pepsin hydrolysates of wheat gluten have opioid activity, the factor linking wheat ingestion to schizophrenia. Hypothesis: gluten is a pathogenic factor in schizophrenia (substantiated by studies).
- **Pathogenesis**: genetic etiology linked to human leukocyte antigen (HLA) DQ2 in 95% of patients and DQ8 in the remainder. These gene loci relate to immunologic recognition of antigens and specific T-cell immune responses. Hypothesis: CD may arise from abnormalities in immune response, rather than gliadin "toxicity." Gliadin sensitizing is humoral and cell mediated; T-cell dysfunction is a key factor in enteropathy. Circulating antibodies are specific for CD (antiendomysial antibody [AEA]) and are used as serum markers to screen patients and estimate CD prevalence. Tissue transglutaminase (tTG) is the autoantigen for AEA; enzyme-linked assay using recombinant tTG is highly sensitive and specific for CD. Anti-tTG antibody titers fall and can become undetectable during gluten-free diet; tTG-gliadin complexes stimulate gluten-specific T cells to induce anti-tTG antibody production. T cells may react to smaller gliadin peptides, and B cells may respond to the larger tTG enzyme. Breastfeeding has prophylactic effect; breastfed babies have decreased risk, with greater protection when breastfed after gluten is introduced. CD risk is greater when large amounts of gluten are introduced. Early introduction of cow's milk is a major etiological factor. Breastfeeding plus delayed exposure to cow's milk and cereal grains are preventive.
- **Clinical aspects:** CD lesions are often histologically indistinguishable from tropical sprue, food allergy, diffuse intestinal lymphoma, and viral gastroenteritis. CD can cause disaccharidase deficiency, leading to lactose intolerance. Increased intestinal permeability causes multiple food allergies. Cow's milk intolerance may precede CD.
- **Associated conditions**: thyroid abnormalities, insulin-dependent diabetes mellitus, psychiatric disturbances (including schizophrenia), dermatitis herpetiformis, and urticaria are linked to gluten intolerance. Increased risk of malignant neoplasms exists (e.g., non-Hodgkin's lymphoma) in celiac patients,

perhaps because of decreased micronutrient absorption of vitamin A and carotenoids (*Textbook,* "Beta-carotene and Other Carotenoids" and "Vitamin A") and gliadin-activated suppressor cell activity. Alpha-gliadin activates suppressor cells of celiac patients but not healthy control subjects or patients with Crohn's disease. Casein and beta-lactoglobulin do not activate suppressor cells. Depressed immunity increases susceptibility to infection and neoplasm.

## DIAGNOSIS

Jejunal biopsy was definitive before new biomarkers. Human antitissue tTG antibody test (immunoglobulin [Ig] A anti-tTG) is most widely used; lower cost than antiendomysium (IgA EMA) and more sensitive than antigliadin antibodies (AGA). In one study the specificity and sensitivity of IgA anti-tTG was compared with IgA EMA and AGA (IgA and IgG AGA) for the diagnosis of celiac disease. Positive predictive value of IgA anti-tTG was 90%; negative predictive value was 98%. In comparison, IgA EMA was 100% and 97%, respectively; IgA AGA was 94% and 90%, respectively; and IgG AGA was 70% and 98%, respectively.

## THERAPEUTIC CONSIDERATIONS

- **Diet**: gluten-free diet—no wheat, rye, barley, triticale, or oats. Buckwheat and millet also are excluded; they contain prolamins with antigenicity similar to alpha-gliadin. Rotate other foods. Eliminate milk and milk products until patient redevelops normal intestinal structure and function.
- **Patient response:** clinical improvement is seen within a few days or weeks (30% respond within 3 days, another 50% within 1 month, and 10% within another month). Ten percent only respond after 24-36 months of gluten avoidance. Failure to respond suggests incorrect diagnosis; patient not adhering to diet or exposed to hidden sources of gliadin; or associated disease or complication, such as zinc deficiency. Multivitamin/mineral supplements treat underlying deficiency and provide cofactors for growth and repair. CD is refractive to dietary therapy if underlying zinc deficiency is present.
- **Pancreatic enzymes**: Pancreatic insufficiency occurs in 8%-30% of celiac patients. Pancreatic enzyme supplements (2 capsules per meal, with each containing lipase 5000 IU, amylase 2900 IU, and protease 330 IU; total of six to 10 capsules daily) enhance clinical

benefit of gluten-free diet during first 30 days but with no greater benefit after 60 days. Use pancreatic enzymes during first 30 days after diagnosis (*Textbook*, "Celiac Disease").

## THERAPEUTIC APPROACH

- Eliminate all sources of gliadin.
- Initially eliminate dairy products.
- Correct underlying nutritional deficiencies.
- Treat associated conditions.
- Identify and eliminate all food allergens.
- If no response within 1 month, reconsider diagnosis and search for hidden sources of gliadin.

A strict gluten-free diet is difficult in the United States because of the ubiquitous distribution of gliadin and other activators of CD in processed foods. Read labels carefully for hidden sources of gliadin (soy sauce, modified food starch, ice cream, soup, beer, wine, vodka, whisky, malt, etc.). Patients should consult resources for patient information on gluten-free recipes.

### Patient Resources

Celiac Sprue Association
PO Box 31700
Omaha, NE 68131-0700
www.csaceliacs.org

Celiac Disease Foundation
13251 Ventura Blvd., Suite 1
Studio City, CA 91604
http://celiac.org

Gluten Intolerance Group
31214 124th Ave. SE
Auburn, WA 98092-3667
www.gluten.net

# Cellulite

## DIAGNOSTIC SUMMARY

- "Mattress phenomenon": pitting, bulging, and deformation of the skin
- Total of 90%-98% of cases occur in women
- Feeling of tightness and heaviness in areas affected (legs)
- Skin tenderness when pinched, pressed on, or vigorously massaged

## GENERAL CONSIDERATIONS

Cellulite is a cosmetic defect causing great distress among millions of European and American women. No inflammatory or infectious process is involved (as in cellulitis). Better terms would be "dermo panniculosis deformans" or "adiposis edematosa."

### Histologic Features

- Subcutaneous tissue of thighs has three layers of fat, with two planes of connective tissue (CT) (ground substance) between them. Construction of subcutaneous tissue of the thigh differs in men and women. In women, the uppermost subcutaneous layer consists of "standing fat cell chambers," separated by radial and arching dividing walls of CT anchored to overlying CT of skin (corium). The uppermost subcutaneous tissue in men is thinner, with a network of crisscrossing CT walls, and the corium (CT structure between dermis and subcutaneous tissue) is thicker than in women.
- Pinch test: pinching skin and subcutaneous tissue of woman's thighs exhibits pitting, bulging, and deformation of skin. In most men, skin folds or furrows but does not bulge or pit.
- With aging, corium, already thinner in women than men, becomes thinner and looser. Fat cells migrate into this layer. CT walls between fat cell chambers become thinner, allowing them to hypertrophy. Breakdown (thinning) of CT is a major contributor to cellulite and granular "buckshot" feel of cellulite.

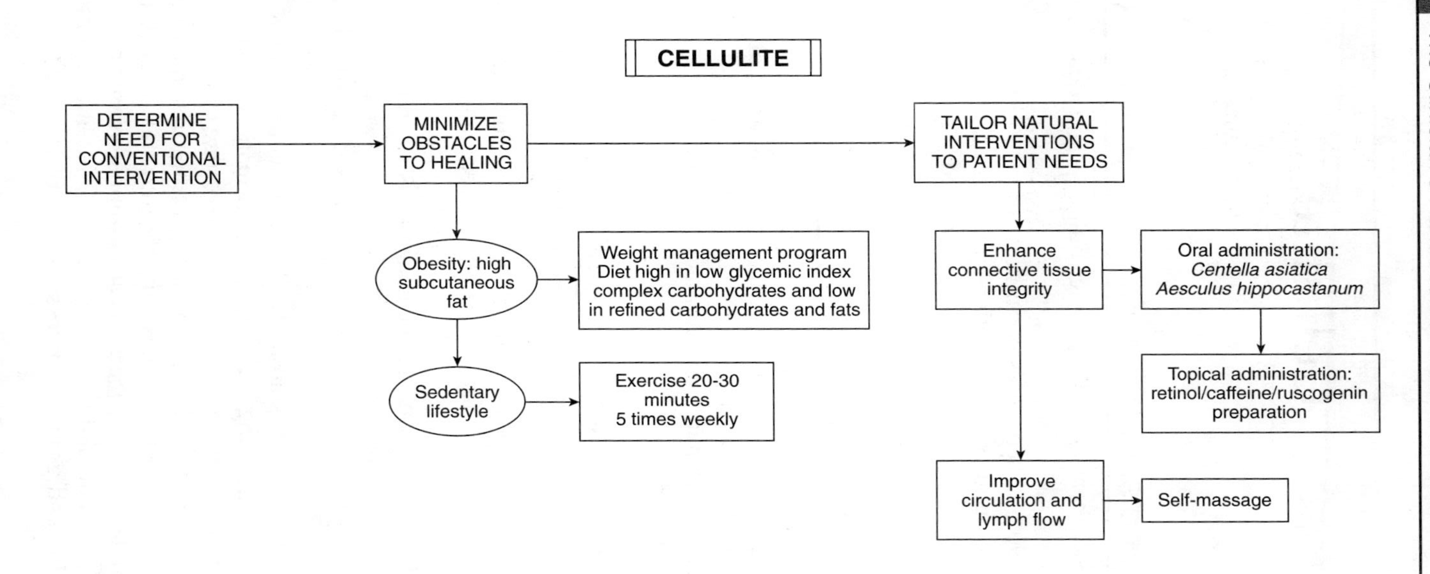
CELLULITE
DETERMINE NEED FOR CONVENTIONAL INTERVENTION
MINIMIZE OBSTACLES TO HEALING
TAILOR NATURAL INTERVENTIONS TO PATIENT NEEDS
Obesity: high subcutaneous fat
Weight management program
Diet high in low glycemic index complex carbohydrates and low in refined carbohydrates and fats
Sedentary lifestyle
Exercise 20-30 minutes 5 times weekly
Enhance connective tissue integrity
Oral administration: *Centella asiatica* *Aesculus hippocastanum*
Topical administration: retinol/caffeine/ruscogenin preparation
Improve circulation and lymph flow
Self-massage

- Condition arises from alternating depressions and protrusions in the upper compartment of fat tissue. The vertical orientation of women's fat cell compartments and weakening of tissues allows protrusion of fat cells into lower corium.
- Distension of lymphatic vessels of upper corium and decrease in number of subepidermal elastic fibers.

## CLINICAL FEATURES

Areas of body involved (gluteal and thigh regions, lower abdomen, nape of neck, and upper arms) are areas affected in gynecoid (female) obesity.

### Four Major Stages

- **Stage 0**: skin on thighs and buttocks has smooth surface when subject is standing or lying. Pinch test: skin folds and furrows but does not pit or bulge. This is the "normal" stage of most men and slim women.
- **Stage 1**: skin surface is smooth while standing or lying. The pinch test is clearly positive for pitting, bulging, deformity of affected areas, which is normal for most women. In men it may be a sign of deficiency of androgenic hormones. This is the best classification most can expect because of structural predisposition.
- **Stage 2**: skin surface is smooth while lying but when standing shows pitting, bulging, and deformity of affected skin. This is common in women who are obese or older than 35-40 years of age.
- **Stage 3**: mattress phenomenon when lying or standing. This is very common after menopause and in obesity.

Most women desire stage 0, but stage 1 is the best achievable because of structural predisposition.

## THERAPEUTIC CONSIDERATIONS

The best approach is prevention. The number and size of fat cells are largely determined by maternal prenatal nutritional status that generates significant predisposition. Maintain slim subcutaneous fat layer with exercise and maintain normal body weight throughout life. (Slim women and female athletes have little or no cellulite.)

### Lifestyle

- **Weight reduction and exercise**: primary mode of treatment. Weight reduction should be gradual, especially in women older than 40 years. Rapid weight loss may exacerbate the condition.
- **Massage**: quite beneficial, particularly self-administered with hand or brush; improves circulation of blood and lymph. The direction of massage should be from periphery to heart.

### Topical Treatments

Most cosmetic and herbal preparations have no scientific support. *Fucus vesiculosus* (bladderwrack) is a seaweed used for obesity since the seventeenth century. Its high iodine content may stimulate thyroid function. But its effects for cellulite have not been confirmed, although it does soothe, soften, and tone tissues. One formula containing retinol, caffeine, and ruscogenin (from butcher's broom [*Ruscus aculeatus*]) was proven effective based on noninvasive tests—skin macrorelief ("orange peel" effect ), dermal and hypodermal structure, skin mechanical characteristics, and cutaneous flowmetry (microcirculation). This formula has synergistic effects. Topical vitamin A (retinol) improves skin histology in women with cellulite, increasing elasticity and decreasing viscosity and improving tensile properties. Effects are more evident where "mattress phenomenon" is the only evidence of cellulite. The lumpy-bumpy look changed little, the number of factor XIIIa+ dendrocytes in the dermis and fibrous strands of the hypodermis increased twofold to fivefold. Caffeine potentiates catecholamine-induced lipolysis. *Cola* species are rich in caffeine. Ruscogenin enhances integrity of CT structures.

### Oral Botanical Medicines

- ***Centella asiatica* (gotu kola)**: oral extracts containing 70% triterpenic acids (asiatic acid and asiatoside) are clinically impressive for cellulite, venous insufficiency of the lower limbs, and varicose veins. *Centella* normalizes CT metabolism, enhancing tissue integrity by stimulating glycosaminoglycan (GAGs) synthesis without promoting excessive collagen synthesis or cell growth. GAGs comprise amorphous intercellular matrix (ground substance) surrounding collagen fibers. *Centella* enhances CT structure, reduces sclerosis, and improves blood flow through affected limbs.

- **Escin**: a compound isolated from seeds of *Aesculus hippocastanum* (horse chestnut) with antiinflammatory and antiedema properties. It decreases capillary permeability by reducing number and size of small pores of capillary walls. It is a venotonic with positive effect on varicose veins and thrombophlebitis. It is given orally or as escin/cholesterol complex applied topically. Topical application of escin is beneficial in treating bruises and decreases capillary fragility and swelling.

## THERAPEUTIC APPROACH

Cellulite is not a disease but a cosmetic disorder caused by tissue changes. Excessive subcutaneous adipose or degeneration of subcutaneous CT leads to fat chamber enlargement and the mattress phenomenon. Reduce subcutaneous fat and enhance CT integrity. Varicose veins often occur with cellulite; both conditions largely result from loss of integrity of supporting CT (*Textbook,* "Cellulite"). Mattress phenomenon in men is a sign of androgen deficiency—primary or secondary hypogonadism.

**Diet**: high in complex carbohydrates (low glycemic index/low glycemic load) and low in refined carbohydrates (high glycemic index) and fats. Promote weight loss in obese patients.

**Physical Measures:**

- **Exercise**: 20-30 minutes aerobic exercise a minimum of 5 days/week
- **Massage**: regular self-massage of affected area

### Botanical Medicines

- **Oral administration**
  —*Centella asiatica* extract (70% triterpenic acids): 30 mg t.i.d.
  —*Aesculus hippocastanum*
    - Bark of root: 500 mg t.i.d.
    - Escin: 10 mg t.i.d.
- **Topical application** of salve, ointment, and so forth twice daily
  —Cholesterol/escin complex: 0.5%-1.5%
  —*Cola vera* extract (14% caffeine): 0.5%-1.5%
  —*Fucus vesiculosus*: 0.25%-75%

# Cervical Dysplasia

## DIAGNOSTIC SUMMARY

- Abnormal Pap smears (atypical cells of undetermined significance; low-grade squamous intraepithelial lesions; high-grade squamous intraepithelial lesions)
- Colposcopy, endocervical curettage, cervical biopsies: one of following three options for managing ASC-US is acceptable:
  1. Refer to colposcopy.
  2. Repeat Pap twice at 4- to 6-month intervals with referral to colposcopy if repeat Pap is the same or worse.
  3. Human papilloma virus (HPV) testing with referral to colposcopy for high-risk subtypes.
- Management guidelines for ASC-H, LSIL, and HSIL are as follows:
  —ASC-H: direct referral to colposcopy
  —LSIL and HSIL: direct referral to colposcopy

HPV testing is not helpful in initial management of either of these cytologic reports because most will be positive for high-risk HPV.

### Terminology

**ASC-US**: atypical cells of undetermined significance
**ASC-H**: atypical cells, cannot rule out high-grade lesions
**CIN I**: condyloma (warty tissue) or mild cervical dysplasia
**CIN II**: moderate cervical dysplasia
**CIN III**: severe cervical dysplasia or carcinoma in situ
**LGSIL**: low-grade intraepithelial lesions, including CIN I
**HGSIL**: high-grade epithelial lesions, including CIN II and CIN III

## GENERAL CONSIDERATIONS

Cervical dysplasia (CD) is a precancerous lesion with risk factors similar to cervical cancer. Etiologic lifestyle factors include early age of first intercourse, multiple sexual partners, other infectious agents (chlamydia, herpes simplex), history of genital warts,

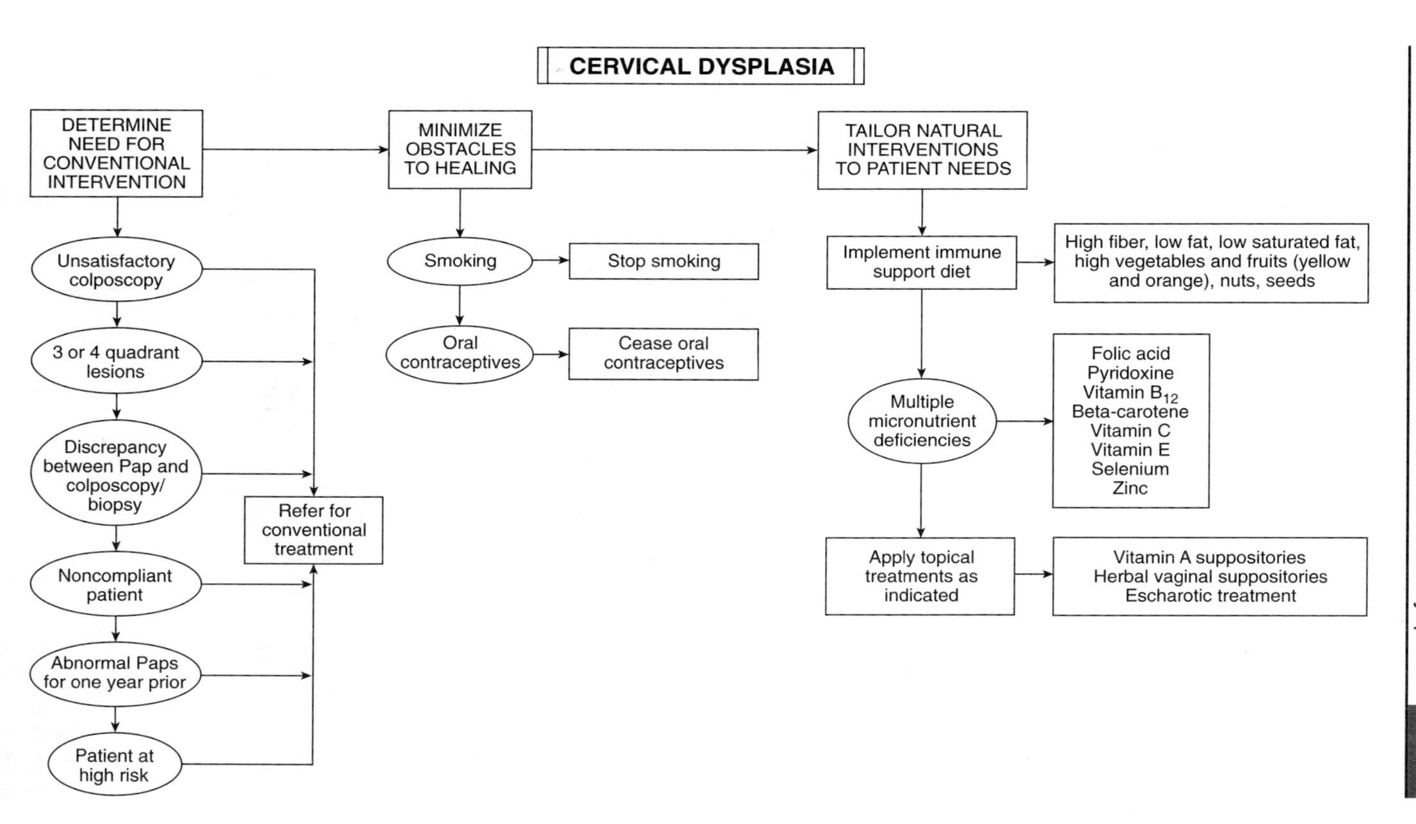
CERVICAL DYSPLASIA
DETERMINE NEED FOR CONVENTIONAL INTERVENTION
Unsatisfactory colposcopy
3 or 4 quadrant lesions
Discrepancy between Pap and colposcopy/ biopsy
Noncompliant patient
Abnormal Paps for one year prior
Patient at high risk
Refer for conventional treatment
MINIMIZE OBSTACLES TO HEALING
Smoking
Stop smoking
Oral contraceptives
Cease oral contraceptives
TAILOR NATURAL INTERVENTIONS TO PATIENT NEEDS
Implement immune support diet
High fiber, low fat, low saturated fat, high vegetables and fruits (yellow and orange), nuts, seeds
Multiple micronutrient deficiencies
Folic acid
Pyridoxine
Vitamin $B_{12}$
Beta-carotene
Vitamin C
Vitamin E
Selenium
Zinc
Apply topical treatments as indicated
Vitamin A suppositories
Herbal vaginal suppositories
Escharotic treatment

immunosuppression (HIV, organ transplant), smoking, oral contraceptive use, pregnancy, and many nutritional factors. All risk factors are closely related.

- **Epidemiology**: cervical cancer is linked to long-term persistent HPV infection, transmitted by genital-to-genital contact. Time from exposure to lesion or abnormal Pap can be a few weeks or decades. Approximately 80% of adults may be infected. Roughly 60% of young women are infected, but less than 10% develop cervical lesions. Host immunity defends against clinical disease. HPV infections often are transient, resulting only in ASC-US. Clinical disease can include flat or raised genital warts; cervical, vaginal, vulvar, or perianal dysplasias; or invasive cancers. HPV is detected in 50%-80% of vaginal, 50% of vulvar, and nearly all penile and anal cancers.
- **Total of 120 HPV varieties**: 30 HPV types infect squamous epithelium of lower anogenital tracts of men and women. HPV types 6, 11, 42, 43, and 44 result in classic genital warts of cauliflower appearance or flat lesions. Types 16, 18, 31, 33, 35, 45, 51, 52, and 56 are high-risk types found in lower genital tract cancers and intraepithelial lesions. Lesions caused by low risk and high risk HPV types can regress to normal even without treatment, but prognosis cannot be predicted. 80% of cervical cancers are linked to types 16, 18, 31 and 45; 15% are associated with types 31, 33, 35, 51, or 52. Low-grade intraepithelial lesions (LGSIL) can be caused by both low and high risk HPV types. High risk types are in 75%-85% of low grade lesions; mixed low and high risk types in 15%; low risk types exclusively in only 2%-25%.
- **Histology**: 95% of cervix cancers originate in the squamocolumnar junction of the cervical os. In adolescence, glandular epithelium covers much of exocervix, but as adolescence progresses columnar epithelium is replaced by squamous cells. This actively growing area is susceptible to multiple insults and HPV because of the metaplastic nature of the conversion process.
- **Development and progression**: HPV exposure commonly occurs during unprotected intercourse in heterosexual women. Approximately 60% of those in their teens and 20s test positive for HPV DNA by polymerase chain reaction. Three outcomes from HPV exposure: (1) permanent latency or only transient cytologic changes; (2) cytologic changes diagnostic of HPV (60% of women with atypia or LGSIL spontaneously regress and 20%-30% persist); and (3) development of HGSIL in 10%. A total of 70% of

women clear the virus within the first year. Low-grade lesions can regress, persist, or progress. Progression peaks between ages 25 and 29 years, 4 to 7 years after peak incidence of mild dysplasia. Most low-grade lesions do not progress to invasive cancer, even without treatment. Even HPV type 16, detected in 60% of cancers, tends to result in regression. Invasive cancer incidence plateaus in white American women 15 years after peak incidence of CIN III, between the ages of 40 and 45 years.

### Risk Factors

- **Sexual activity**: early age at first intercourse and/or multiple sexual contacts without condom increase risk for cervical dysplasia or carcinoma. Cervical cancer may be a sexually transmitted disease linked to HPV. The variability in time from exposure to identified lesion prevents identification of sexual partners that transmitted HPV. Oral HPV lesions are rare. Nonsexual exposure may occur from examination tables, doorknobs, tanning beds, etc. Other infectious agents (herpes simplex, Chlamydia, bacterial vaginosis) may be cofactors that alter cervical immunity, cause inflammation, facilitate HPV entry into basal cells, accelerate HPV replication in cell nuclei, and/or coexist with HPV.
- **Smoking**: smokers have three times the risk of nonsmokers and 17 times the risk in women aged 20 to 29 years. Smoking may depress immunity and induce vitamin C deficiency. Cervical cells may concentrate nicotine. Smoking may be linked to risky sexual behavior.
- **Oral contraceptives**: oral contraceptive (OC) use shows no overall change in risk of invasive cervical cancer but a modestly increased risk in long-term OC users. OCs are linked to a rare cervical cancer, adenocarcinoma, with increased incidence over the past several decades; invasive squamous cancer has declined since "the Pill" was introduced. An increased risk of invasive adenocarcinoma may occur with OC use longer than 12 years. OCs potentiate the adverse effects of smoking and decrease levels of nutrients: vitamins C, $B_6$, and $B_{12}$; folic acid; riboflavin; and zinc.

## THERAPEUTIC CONSIDERATIONS

### Nutrition

**Multiple nutrient deficiencies**: cofactors for CD. Approximately 67% of CD patients have abnormal anthropometric or biochemical parameters: height/weight ratios, triceps skin fold thickness, mid-arm muscle circumference, serum albumin, total iron-binding capacity, hemoglobin, creatinine height index, prothrombin time, and lymphocyte count. Other patients have marginal "normal" nutritional status.

**Vitamin assessment by biochemical evaluation**: plasma and red cell folate; serum beta-carotene; vitamins A, $B_{12}$, and C; erythrocyte transketolase for thiamin determination; erythrocyte glutathione reductase for riboflavin determination; and erythrocyte aspartate transaminase for pyridoxine determination. At least one abnormal vitamin level is found in 67% of cervical cancer patients. Approximately 38% display multiple abnormalities.

**General dietary factors**: High fat intake increases risk for cervical cancer. A diet rich in fruits and vegetables (with fiber, carotenes, and vitamin C) protects against carcinogenesis.

- **Vitamin A and beta-carotene**: minor association between dietary retinoids and CD risk, but a strong inverse correlation between beta-carotene intake and CD risk. Only 6% of patients with untreated cervical cancer have less-than-normal serum vitamin A, but 38% have stage-related abnormal beta-carotene. Low serum beta-carotene is linked to a three times increased risk for severe dysplasia. Serum vitamin A and beta-carotene are much lower in CD patients than in control subjects. Carotenes and retinols improve integrity and function of epithelial tissues, provide antioxidant properties, and enhance immune function (*Textbook*, "Beta-carotene and Other Carotenoids"). Beta-carotene is more advantageous than retinoids: greater antioxidant properties, immune-enhancing effects, and tendency to be concentrated in epithelial tissues.
- **Topical vitamin A**: Four consecutive 24-hour applications of retinoic acid, followed by two more applications at 3 and 6 months applied with a collagen sponge in a cervical cap may induce regression of moderate dysplasia.
- **Vitamin A suppositories**: part of multifactorial treatment using oral folic acid, vitamin C, and carotenes with topical vitamin A suppositories and herbal vitamin suppositories. For more severe disease, topical "escharotic" treatment can be used for moderate, severe dysplasia and carcinoma in situ.
- **Vitamin C**: diminished intake and plasma levels of vitamin C in CD patients. Inadequate intake is an independent risk factor for

premalignant cervical disease and carcinoma in situ. Ascorbate acts as an antioxidant, maintains normal epithelial integrity, improves wound healing, enhances immunity, and inhibits carcinogen formation.

- **Folic acid**: cervical cytological abnormalities related to folate deficiency precede hematologic abnormalities. Folate is the most commonly deficient vitamin in the world, especially among women who are pregnant or taking OCs. Folate deficiency is the probable cause of many abnormal cytologic smears rather than "true" dysplasia. OCs induce localized interference with folate metabolism—tissue levels at end-organ targets (cervix) are deficient. Red blood cell (RBC) folate is decreased (especially with CD), whereas serum levels are normal or increased. OCs induce synthesis of a macromolecule that inhibits folate uptake by cells. Low RBC folate enhances effect of other CD risk factors: HPV infection. Low RBC folate is a risk factor for cervical HPV infection. Folate supplements (10 mg q.d.) improve or normalize cytologic smears in CD patients. Regression rates for untreated CD are 1.3% for mild and 0% for moderate infection. Folate-induced regression-to-normal rates are reported to be 20%, 63.7%, and 100% in different studies. Progression rate of untreated CD is 16% at 4 months. Folate-supplemented rate is 0% (even though women remained on OCs). Progression from CD to CIN II untreated occurs in 86 months for very mild dysplasia to 12 months for severe dysplasia; regression is uncommon. Implement folate regimen (along with other considerations discussed) in mild to moderate dysplasia, with follow-up Pap and colposcopy at 3 months.
- **Vitamin $B_{12}$**: use vitamin $B_{12}$ with folate to avoid folate masking underlying $B_{12}$ deficiency.
- **Pyridoxine**: vitamin $B_6$ (RBC transaminase test) is decreased in one third of CD patients. Decreased $B_6$ status affects metabolism of estrogens and tryptophan and impairs immunity.
- **Selenium**: serum, dietary, and soil selenium are inversely correlated with all epithelial cancers and are much lower in CD patients. One anticarcinogenic effect is increased glutathione peroxidase activity. Toxic elements (lead, cadmium, mercury, gold) have selenium-antagonistic properties.
- **Copper/zinc ratio**: increased serum copper/zinc ratio (Cu/Zn) is a nonspecific reaction to inflammation or malignancy. Serum Cu/Zn may be a tool to establish extent of cancer. A ratio greater than 1.95 indicated malignancy in 90% of patients studied. Elevated ratios also are seen in OC use, pregnancy, acute and chronic

infections, chronic liver disease, and inflammatory conditions. Serum Cu/Zn should not be used to predict malignancy in these patients. Decreased available Zn may cause retinol-binding protein to be absent or undetectable in 80% of dysplastic tissue versus 23.5% of normal tissue. There is an inverse relationship between serum retinol and Zn and incidence of CD.

### Miscellaneous Considerations

- **Vaginal depletion pack (vag pack)**: has a long history of efficacy for CD. The mechanism of action is not yet elucidated. It may promote sloughing of superficial abnormal cervical cells. It is effective as part of a multifaceted approach (*Textbook*, "Vaginal Depletion Pack").

## THERAPEUTIC APPROACH

### Candidates for Natural Treatment

- ASC-US
- Cervical condylomata
- LGSIL on Pap with endocervical curettage negative and satisfactory colposcopy
- HGSIL with endocervical curettage negative and satisfactory colposcopy or at discretion of physician
- LGSIL with endocervical curettage positive, satisfactory colposcopy, and patient considered low risk or at discretion of physician
- HGSIL and endocervical curettage positive, satisfactory colposcopy, and patient at low risk or at discretion of practitioner

For ASC-US and LGSIL, nutriceuticals and topicals, either suppositories or escharotic treatment, are sufficient. For patients who undergo loop electrosurgical excision procedure, cryotherapy, or conization, nutritients and even topical suppositories 3 weeks after completion of conventional treatment may reduce recurrence risk and affect local cervical immunity.

**Refer for conventional treatment:** unsatisfactory colposcopy, three- or four-quadrant lesions, significant discrepancy between Pap smear and colposcopy or biopsy, noncompliant patient, history of abnormal Pap smears longer than 1 year prior, or patient at high risk.

Eliminate all factors linked to CD (smoking and OCs). Optimize patient's nutritional status with supplemental folic acid, beta-carotenes, and vitamin C.

- **Diet**: immune supportive diet: high fiber, low fat, low saturated fat, high vegetables and fruits (especially yellow and orange), raw organic nuts and seeds
- **Supplements**:
  - —Folic acid: 10 mg q.d. for 3 months, then 2.5 mg q.d.
  - —Pyridoxine: 50 mg t.i.d.
  - —Vitamin $B_{12}$: 1 mg q.d.
  - —Beta-carotene: 200,000 IU q.d.
  - —Vitamin C: 1 to 6 g q.d.
  - —Vitamin E: 200 IU q.i.d. (mixed tocopherols)
  - —Selenium: 400 μg q.d.
  - —Zinc: 30 mg q.d.

Typical treatment protocols include the following:

- ASC-US
  - —Topical:
    - Week 1: vitamin A suppository nightly for 6 nights
    - Week 2: herbal vaginal suppository nightly for 6 nights (myrrh, *Echinacea*, usnea, *Hydrastis canadensis* [goldenseal], *Althea*, *Geranium*, yarrow)
    - Week 3: repeat vitamin A suppository
    - Week 4: repeat herbal suppository
  - —Supplements daily for 3 months minimum:
    - Folic acid: 10 mg
    - Beta-carotene: 150,000 IU
    - Vitamin C: 3-6 g
    - Multiple vitamin/mineral supplement
- LGSIL
  - —Topical:
    - Week 1: vitamin A suppository nightly for 6 nights; vag pack suppository on night 7
    - Week 2: herbal suppository nightly for 6 nights; vag pack suppository on night 7
    - Week 3: repeat vitamin A suppository; vag pack suppository on night 7
    - Week 4: repeat herbal suppository; vag pack suppository on night 7
  - —Supplements daily for minimum of 3 months:
    - Folic acid: 10 mg
    - Beta-carotene: 150,000 IU
    - Vitamin C: 3-6 g
    - Selenium 400: μg daily
    - Multiple vitamin/mineral supplement

- HGSIL
  - —Topical:
    - Escharotic treatment twice weekly for 5 weeks
    - Follow last treatment with 1 month of suppository routine as in LGSIL
  - —Supplements:
    - Folic acid: 10 mg
    - Beta-carotene: 150,000 IU
    - Vitamin C: 3-6 g
    - Selenium: 400 μg
    - Vitamin E: 800 IU (mixed tocopherols)
- Multiple vitamin/mineral supplement

# Chronic Candidiasis

## DIAGNOSTIC SUMMARY

- Chronic fatigue and malaise
- Gastrointestinal bloating and cramps
- Vaginal yeast infection
- Allergies and/or low immune function
- Carbohydrate craving
- History of broad-spectrum antibiotic use

## GENERAL CONSIDERATIONS

*Candida* is normal in the gastrointestinal (GI) tract and vagina. Overgrowth, depleted immunity, damaged GI mucosa allow absorption of yeast cells, particles, toxins; result is "yeast syndrome," or "feeling sick all over": fatigue, allergies, immune system malfunction, depression, chemical sensitivities, and digestive disturbances. Women are eight times more likely than men to have syndrome; contributors are estrogen, birth control pills, and greater antibiotic use.

- **Causal factors**: multifactorial; correct factors predisposing overgrowth; requires more than killing yeast with antifungals, synthetic or natural; prolonged antibiotic use is the key factor in most cases—suppresses normal intestinal bacteria that control yeast, suppresses immunity, generates antibiotic-resistant microbes, may contribute to Crohn's disease.
- **Related syndromes**: small intestinal bacterial overgrowth and leaky gut associated with *Candida* overgrowth; may produce identical symptoms to the yeast syndrome.

## DIAGNOSIS

- **Screening method**: comprehensive questionnaire (see *Textbook*, "*Candida* Questionnaire").
- **Best method**: clinical evaluation—knowledge of yeast-related illness, detailed medical history, patient questionnaire.

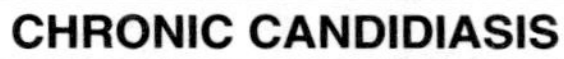
CHRONIC CANDIDIASIS

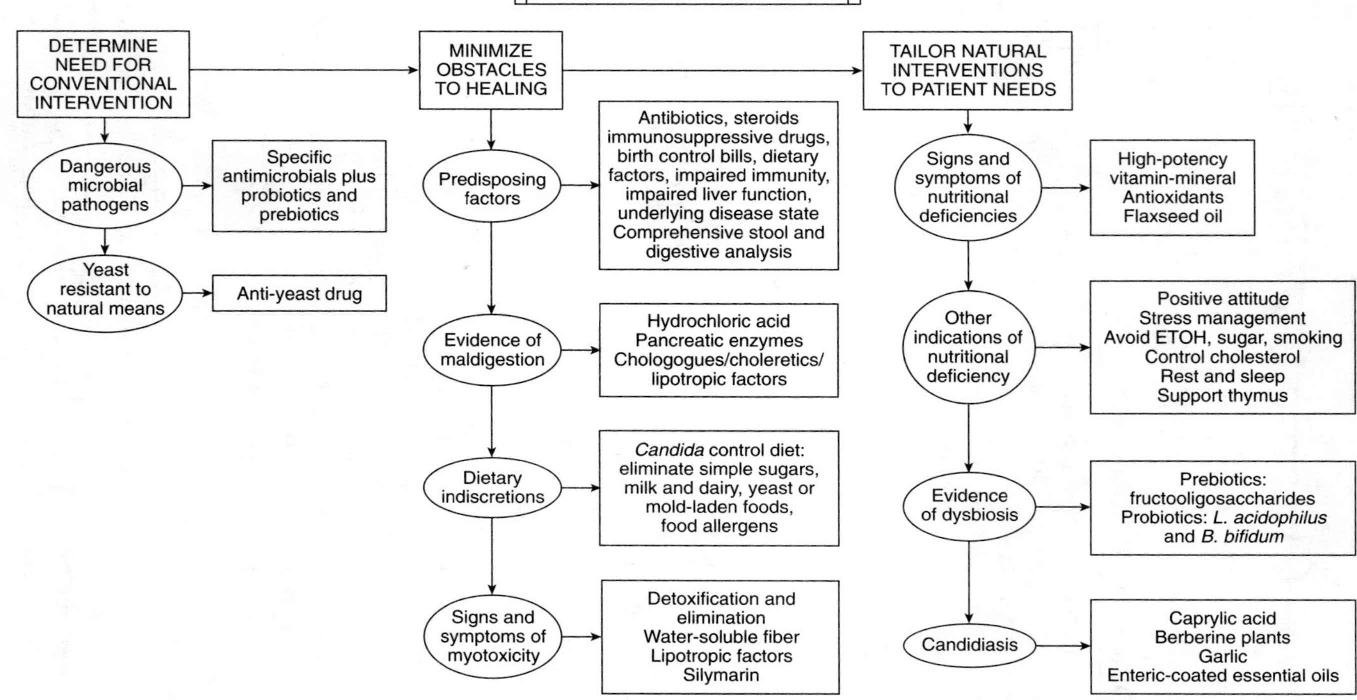
DETERMINE NEED FOR CONVENTIONAL INTERVENTION
Dangerous microbial pathogens
Specific antimicrobials plus probiotics and prebiotics
Yeast resistant to natural means
Anti-yeast drug
MINIMIZE OBSTACLES TO HEALING
Predisposing factors
Antibiotics, steroids immunosuppressive drugs, birth control bills, dietary factors, impaired immunity, impaired liver function, underlying disease state Comprehensive stool and digestive analysis
Evidence of maldigestion
Hydrochloric acid Pancreatic enzymes Chologogues/choleretics/ lipotropic factors
Dietary indiscretions
Candida control diet: eliminate simple sugars, milk and dairy, yeast or mold-laden foods, food allergens
Signs and symptoms of myotoxicity
Detoxification and elimination Water-soluble fiber Lipotropic factors Silymarin
TAILOR NATURAL INTERVENTIONS TO PATIENT NEEDS
Signs and symptoms of nutritional deficiencies
High-potency vitamin-mineral Antioxidants Flaxseed oil
Other indications of nutritional deficiency
Positive attitude Stress management Avoid ETOH, sugar, smoking Control cholesterol Rest and sleep Support thymus
Evidence of dysbiosis
Prebiotics: fructooligosaccharides Probiotics: L. acidophilus and B. bifidum
Candidiasis
Caprylic acid Berberine plants Garlic Enteric-coated essential oils

- **Comprehensive stool and digestive analysis (CSDA)**: more clinically useful; evaluates digestion, intestinal environment, and absorption; indicates underlying digestive disturbance; may pinpoint other causes (e.g., small intestinal bacterial overgrowth, leaky gut syndrome).
- **Laboratory techniques (used only to confirm)**: stool cultures for *Candida*, antibody to *Candida*, *Candida* antigens in the blood; rarely needed; confirm what history, physical examination, CDSA reveal; confirm *Candida* is factor, monitor therapy.

## THERAPEUTIC CONSIDERATIONS

Comprehensive approach more effective than simply killing yeast with drug or natural agent; address causes. Eradicate *Candida* with natural therapies; follow-up stool culture and analysis confirm *Candida* eliminated. If symptoms remain after yeast is eliminated, condition is unrelated to *Candida*; consider small intestinal bacterial overgrowth, pancreatic enzymes, and berberine-containing plants. Address predisposing factors, recommend *Candida* control diet, support organ systems as needed.

### Diet

- **Sugar**: chief nutrient of *Candida*; restrict sugar, honey, maple syrup, and fruit juice.
- **Milk and dairy products**: high lactose content promotes *Candida*; contain food allergens; may contain trace levels of antibiotics disrupting GI bacteria, promoting *Candida*.
- **Mold and yeast-containing foods**: avoid foods with high yeast or mold levels: alcohol, cheese, dried fruits, peanuts.
- **Food allergies**: common in patients with yeast syndrome; enzyme-linked immunosorbent assay (ELISA) tests for immunoglobulin (Ig) E- and IgG-mediated food allergies.

### Hypochlorhydria

Gastric HCl, pancreatic enzymes, and bile inhibit *Candida* and prevent its penetration into intestinal mucosa; decreased secretion allows yeast overgrowth; antiulcer and antacid drugs induce *Candida* overgrowth in the stomach; pancreatic enzymes: proteases keep small intestine free from parasites. Supplement as-needed HCl, pancreatic enzymes, substances promoting bile flow; use CDSA as guide.

## Enhancing Immunity

- **Immune function** essential; rule out other chronic infections caused by depressed immunity.
- **Decreased thymus function**: major factor in depressed cell-mediated immunity; history of repeated viral infections (e.g., acute rhinitis, herpes, prostatic or vaginal infections).
- **Vicious cycle**: triggering event (e.g. antibiotic, nutrient deficiency) induces immune suppression, allowing yeast overgrowth, competition for nutrients, secretion of mycotoxins and antigens that tax immune system.
- **Restore immunity**: improve thymus function; prevent thymic involution with antioxidants (carotenes, vitamins C and E, zinc, selenium), nutrients for synthesis or action of thymic hormones, and concentrates of calf thymus tissue.

## Promoting Detoxification

Liver damage is the underlying factor; nonviral liver damage reduces immunity, allowing *Candida* overgrowth; liver support: healthy lifestyle, avoidance of alcohol, regular exercise, vitamin/mineral supplement, lipotropic formula, silymarin, 3-day fast at change of each season.

- **Lipotropic factors**: promote flow of fat and bile through liver for a "decongesting" effect; increase intrahepatic levels of S-adenosylmethionine, a major lipotropic compound, and glutathione, a major detoxifying compound; daily dose: 1000 mg choline and 1000 mg of either L-methionine and/or L-cysteine.
- **Silymarin**: extract of milk thistle (*Silybum marianum*); protects liver from damage; enhances detoxification; dosage: 70-210 mg t.i.d.
- **Promote elimination**: high-fiber plant foods; fiber formulas as needed.

## Probiotics

Colon microflora affect immunity, cholesterol metabolism, carcinogenesis, aging; species: *Lactobacillus acidophilus, Bifidobacterium bifidum* (dosage of 1-10 billion viable organisms); application: to promote proper intestinal environment after antibiotic therapy, vaginal yeast infections, and urinary tract infections.

## Natural Antiyeast Agents

- **Herxheimer ("die off") reaction**: worsening symptoms; caused by rapid killing of *Candida* and absorption of yeast toxins, particles, and antigens; to minimize, follow dietary recommendations for 2 weeks before antiyeast agent; support liver; start antiyeast medication at a low dose and gradually increase over 1 month to full level.

- **Caprylic acid**: natural fatty acid antifungal; readily absorbed by intestines; use timed-release or enteric-coated formula for release throughout GI tract; dosage for delayed release: 1000-2000 mg with meals.
- **Berberine-containing plants (*Hydrastis canadensis, Berberis vulgaris, B. aquifolium, Coptis chinensis*)**: berberine alkaloids are broad-spectrum antibiotics against bacteria, protozoa, and fungi, including *Candida*; dosage based on berberine content: solid extract (4:1 or 8%-12% alkaloids), 250-500 mg t.i.d.
- ***Allium sativum* (garlic)**: significant antifungal activity and inhibition of *Candida*; dosage based on allicin content—at least 10 mg allicin or a total allicin potential of 4000 μg or one clove (4 g) fresh garlic.
- **Enteric-coated essential oils (oregano, thyme, peppermint, rosemary)**: antifungal agents; oregano oil is 100 times more potent than caprylic acid; enteric coating ensures delivery to small and large intestines; dosage: 0.2-0.4 mL b.i.d. between meals.
- **Propolis**: rich in flavonoids, phenolics, terpenes, and other compounds found to be antifungal; mechanism of action unknown; dosage depends on product.
- ***Melaleuca alternafolia*** (tea tree oil): topical application.

## THERAPEUTIC APPROACH

- **Step 1**: identify and address predisposing factors—antibiotics, steroids, immune-suppressing drugs, birth control pills (unless absolutely medically necessary); comprehensive stool and digestive analysis; dietary factors, impaired immunity, impaired liver function, or an underlying disease state.
- **Step 2**: *Candida* control diet—eliminate simple sugars, milk and dairy, yeast or mold-laden foods, food allergens.
- **Step 3**: nutritional support—high-potency multiple vitamin, antioxidants, 1 tbsp flaxseed oil daily.
- **Step 4**: support immunity—promote positive attitude and stress coping; avoid alcohol, sugar, smoking, cholesterol; get rest and sleep; support thymus (750 mg crude polypeptide fractions daily).

- **Step 5**: detoxification and elimination—3-5 g water-soluble fiber (guar, psyllium, pectin) at night; lipotropic factors, silymarin.
- **Step 6**: probiotics —1-10 billion viable *L. acidophilus* and *B. bifidum* cells daily.
- **Step 7**: antiyeast therapy—nutritional and/or herbal supplements; antiyeast drug if needed.
- Repeat stool cultures and antigen levels to monitor progress; take stronger prescription anti–yeast agents if needed.

# Chronic Fatigue Syndrome

## DIAGNOSTIC SUMMARY

- Mild fever
- Recurrent sore throat
- Painful lymph nodes
- Muscle weakness
- Muscle pain
- Prolonged fatigue after exercise
- Recurrent headache
- Migratory joint pain
- Depression
- Sleep disturbance (hypersomnia or insomnia).

Chronic fatigue syndrome (CFS) is not a new disease; medical literature references to a similar condition appeared in the 1860s. Old names for CFS: chronic mononucleosis-like syndrome, chronic Epstein-Barr virus syndrome, yuppie flu, postviral fatigue syndrome, postinfectious neuromyasthenia, chronic fatigue and immune dysfunction syndrome, Iceland disease, Royal Free Hospital disease. Centers for Disease Control and Prevention (CDC) criteria are controversial and restrictive; British and Australian criteria are less strict. CDC criteria allow a U.S. prevalence estimate of 11.5%; British criteria suggest 15%, and Australian criteria 38%.

## ETIOLOGY

- **Epstein-Barr virus**: Epstein-Barr virus (EBV) is a member of the herpes group (which includes herpes simplex 1 and 2, varicella zoster, cytomegalovirus, and pseudorabies virus) that can maintain lifelong latent infection kept in check by functional immunity. Immunocompromise permits viral replication and dissemination, as in AIDS, cancer, or drug-induced immunosuppression. Almost all human beings are exposed to EBV by early adulthood. Primary infection in childhood often is asymptomatic; but in adolescence or early adulthood mononucleosis

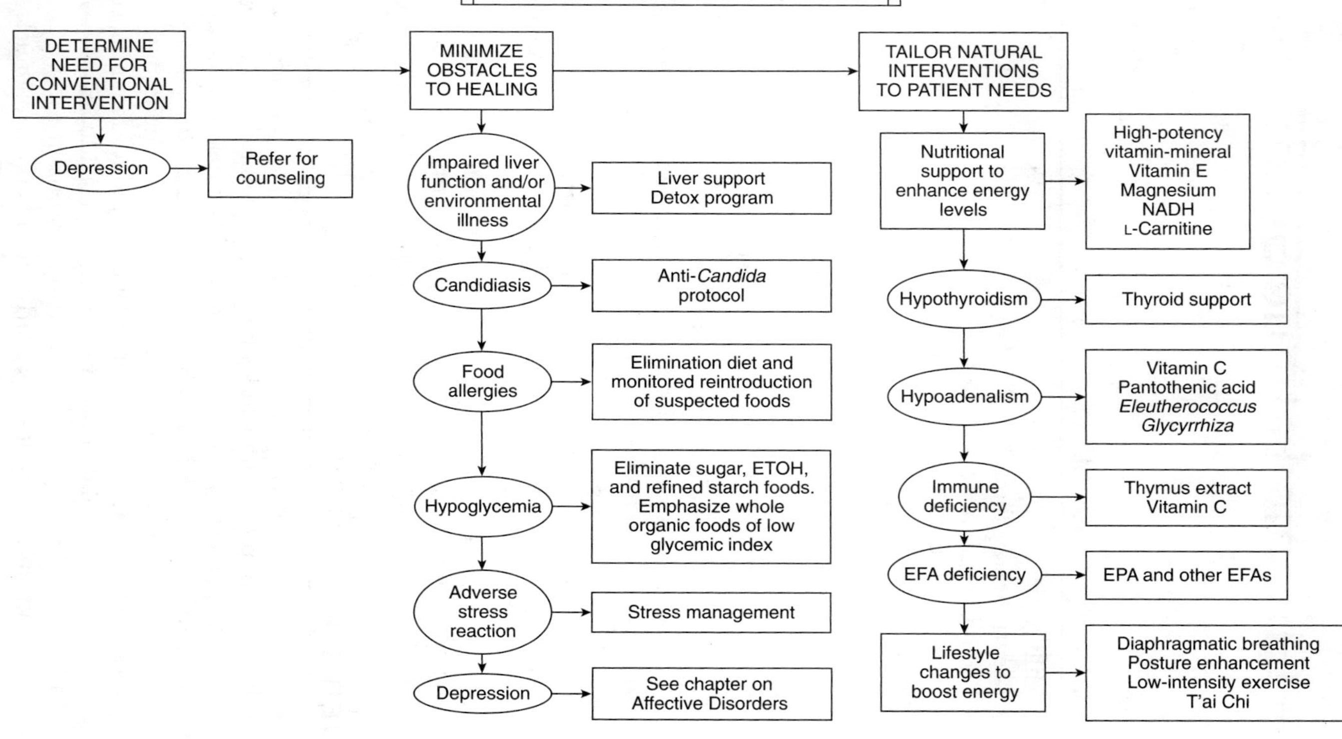
CHRONIC FATIGUE SYNDROME
DETERMINE NEED FOR CONVENTIONAL INTERVENTION
Depression
Refer for counseling
MINIMIZE OBSTACLES TO HEALING
Impaired liver function and/or environmental illness
Liver support
Detox program
Candidiasis
Anti-*Candida* protocol
Food allergies
Elimination diet and monitored reintroduction of suspected foods
Hypoglycemia
Eliminate sugar, ETOH, and refined starch foods. Emphasize whole organic foods of low glycemic index
Adverse stress reaction
Stress management
Depression
See chapter on Affective Disorders
TAILOR NATURAL INTERVENTIONS TO PATIENT NEEDS
Nutritional support to enhance energy levels
High-potency vitamin-mineral
Vitamin E
Magnesium
NADH
L-Carnitine
Hypothyroidism
Thyroid support
Hypoadenalism
Vitamin C
Pantothenic acid
*Eleutherococcus*
*Glycyrrhiza*
Immune deficiency
Thymus extract
Vitamin C
EFA deficiency
EPA and other EFAs
Lifestyle changes to boost energy
Diaphragmatic breathing
Posture enhancement
Low-intensity exercise
T'ai Chi

symptoms appear in 50% of cases. Persistently elevated serum anti-EBV capsid antibody (titers >1:80) are found in many patients with CFS symptom pattern. The infection itself can compromise and/or disrupt immunity, leading to other diseases. Elevated EBV antibody levels are observed in diseases with immunodysfunction. Elevated antibody titers to herpes group viruses, measles, and other viruses are found in CFS. Antibody testing for herpes group viruses and measles may be a useful measure of immunity and host resistance but should not be relied on for diagnosis of CFS.

- **Other infectious agents under investigation**: human herpes virus-6, Inoue-Melnick virus, *Brucella*, *Borrelia burgdorferi*, *Giardia lamblia*, cytomegalovirus, enterovirus, retrovirus.
- **Immune system abnormalities**: elevated antibodies to viral proteins; decreased natural killer (NK) cell activity; low or elevated antibody levels; increased or decreased levels of circulating immune complexes; increased cytokines (e.g., interleukin-2); increased or decreased interferon; altered helper/suppressor T-cell ratio. No specific immunodysfunction pattern has been recognized, but the most consistent abnormality is decreased number or activity of NK cells. NK cells destroy cancerous or virus-infested cells. (CFS was at one time called low natural killer cell syndrome). Reduced lymphocyte response to stimuli is perhaps caused by reduced activity or production of interferon, found in most cases. Low interferon permits reactivation of latent viruses. High interferon and interleukin-1 may cause CFS symptoms from physiologic effects, as seen during interferon therapy for cancer and viral hepatitis.
- **Fibromyalgia and multiple chemical sensitivities**: the only difference in diagnostic criteria for fibromyalgia (FM) and CFS is musculoskeletal pain in FM and fatigue in CFS. Diagnosis of FM or CFS depends on type of physician consulted. Approximately 70% of patients with FM and 30% with multiple chemical sensitivities (MCS) meet CDC criteria for CFS; 80% of both FM and MCS patients meet CFS criterion of fatigue for more than 6 months with 50% reduction in activity. More than 50% of CFS and FM patients have adverse reactions to various chemicals.
- **Other causes of CFS**: preexisting physical condition (diabetes, heart disease, lung disease, rheumatoid arthritis, chronic inflammation, chronic pain, cancer, liver disease, multiple sclerosis), prescription drugs (antihypertensives, antiinflammatory agents,

birth control pills, antihistamines, corticosteroids, tranquilizers, and sedatives), depression, stress/low adrenal function, impaired liver function and/or environmental illness, impaired immune function, chronic candidiasis, other chronic infections, food allergies, hypothyroidism, hypoglycemia, anemia and nutritional deficiencies, and sleep disturbances.

## DIAGNOSIS

- **Identify as many factors as possible** contributing to fatigue.
- **Complete physical examination**: swollen lymph nodes (chronic infection), diagonal crease in both earlobes (impaired blood flow).
- **Lab**: avoid expensive tests unless absolutely necessary. Complete blood count and chemistry panel (including serum ferritin for menstruating women). Avoid tests to confirm diagnosis that will not affect treatment. Assess thyroid function, liver detoxification function, bowel dysbiosis, and gastrointestinal permeability (*Textbook,* "Chronic Fatigue Syndrome," "Comprehensive Stool Analysis 2.0," and "Intestinal Permeability Assessment").

## THERAPEUTIC CONSIDERATIONS

- **Multifactorial conditions** require tailored multiple therapies.
- **Energy level and emotional state**: determined by internal focus and physiology. The mental focus of CFS is on fatigue. Physiology is affected by chemicals, hormones, posture, and breathing (shallow). Address mind and body.
- **Depression**: a major cause of chronic fatigue and common in CFS. Depression is the most common cause of chronic fatigue in the absence of preexisting pathosis.
- **Stress**: underlying factor in a patient with depression, low immune function, or other cause of chronic fatigue (*Textbook,* "Stress Management"). Evaluate stress effects with the Social Readjustment Rating Scale by Holmes and Rahe.
- **Impaired liver function and/or environmental illness**: exposure to toxins (food additives, solvents [cleaning materials, formaldehyde, toluene, benzene, etc.], pesticides, herbicides, heavy metals [lead, mercury, cadmium, arsenic, nickel, and aluminum]) causes "congested" or "sluggish" liver and impaired hepatic detoxification, leading to diminished bile flow (cholestasis) and decreased phase I and/or phase II enzyme detoxification activity. Causes

of cholestasis: dietary factors (saturated fat, refined sugar, low fiber intake), obesity, diabetes, gallstones, alcohol, endotoxins, hereditary disorders (Gilbert's syndrome), pregnancy, steroid hormones (anabolic steroids, estrogens, oral contraceptives), chemicals (cleaning solvents, pesticides), or drugs (antibiotics, diuretics, nonsteroidal antiinflammatory drugs, thyroid hormone), viral hepatitis.

- **Clinical judgment and lab tests**: serum bilirubin, aspartate aminotransferase, alanine aminotransferase, lactate dehydrogenase, glycoprotein 4-beta-galactosyl transferase, bile acid assay, clearance tests (*Textbook,* "Chronic Fatigue Syndrome"). Test results may be abnormal only after significant liver damage; many conditions in subclinical stages have normal lab values. Common patient symptoms: depression, general malaise, headaches, digestive disturbances, allergies and chemical sensitivities, premenstrual syndrome, constipation. Hair mineral analysis can screen for heavy metals; if inconclusive, use 8-hour lead mobilization test with chelating agent edetate calcium disodium, which measures lead excreted in urine for 8 hours after injection of EDTA.
- **Excessive gastrointestinal permeability**: common finding in CFS, measured by lactulose/mannitol absorption test (*Textbook,* "Intestinal Permeability Assessment"). Use food allergy control and nutrients to stimulate gastrointestinal regeneration. Support hepatic phase I and II detoxification and use oligoantigenic rice protein food replacement formula.
- **Impaired immune function and/or chronic infection**: fatigue is the body's response to infection; the immune system works best when the body rests. Use immune function questionnaire on page 176, and lab tests in *Textbook,* "Immune Function Assessment.
- **Chronic *Candida* infection**: impaired immunity allows *Candida* overgrowth in the intestines. Diagnosis is difficult; no single specific test exists. Stool cultures and elevated *Candida* antibody levels plus detailed history and patient questionnaire (*Textbook,* "Chronic Candidiasis").
  - **Patient profile**: female, 15-50 years old, chronic fatigue, lack of energy, malaise, decreased libido, thrush, bloating, gas, intestinal cramps, rectal itching, altered bowel function, vaginal yeast infection, frequent bladder infections, menstrual symptoms, depression, irritability, inability to concentrate, allergies, chemical sensitivities, low immunity, craving for foods rich in carbohydrates or yeast.

  - **History**: chronic vaginal yeast infections, long-term antibiotic use for infections or acne, oral birth control use, oral steroid hormone use.
  - **Associated conditions**: premenstrual syndrome; sensitivity to foods, chemicals, and other allergens; endocrine disturbances; psoriasis; irritable bowel syndrome.
  - **Predisposing factors**: impaired immunity, antiulcer drugs, broad-spectrum antibiotics, cellular immunodeficiency, corticosteroids, diabetes mellitus, excess sugar intake, intravascular catheters, intravenous drug use, lack of digestive secretions, oral contraceptives.
- **Food allergies**: chronic fatigue is a key feature of food allergies, formerly known as "allergic toxemia" or "allergic tension-fatigue syndrome." Symptoms include fatigue, muscle and joint aches, drowsiness, difficulty concentrating, nervousness, depression. From 55% to 85% of people with CFS have allergies (*Textbook,* "Food Allergy Testing").
- **Hypothyroidism**: common cause of chronic fatigue that is often overlooked. Failure to treat reduces efficacy of other interventions (*Textbook,* "Hypothyroidism").
- **Hypoglycemia**: must be ruled out because it contributes to depression. Depressed people have hypoglycemia, and depression is most common cause of chronic fatigue.
- **Hypoadrenalism**: disruption of hypothalamic-pituitary-adrenal (HPA) axis may be involved in CFS. Chronic fatigue patients have lower cortisol levels on wakening, reduced evening cortisol, and low 24-hour urinary-free cortisol, elevated basal adrenocorticotropic hormone (ACTH), and increased adrenal cortical sensitivity to ACTH but reduced maximal response and attenuated net integrated ACTH response to corticotrophin-releasing hormone (CRH). This suggests a mild, central adrenal insufficiency resulting from either a deficiency of CRH or other central stimulus to the pituitary-adrenal axis. Hyperresponsiveness to ACTH may reflect a secondary adrenal insufficiency in which adrenal ACTH receptors are hypersensitive because of inadequate exposure to ACTH. Reduced response to large doses of ACTH suggests adrenal atrophy. Mild hypocortisolism reflects a defect at or above the hypothalamus, decreasing CRH and/or other secretagogues. HPA axis dysfunction may exacerbate symptoms. Glucocorticoid deficiency causes debilitating fatigue. A stressful event can induce fever, arthralgia, myalgia, adenopathy, postexertional fatigue, exacerbation of allergies, and distur-

bances of mood and sleep—symptoms typical of CFS and seen in partial or subclinical adrenal insufficiency. Endocrine testing, such as ACTH stimulation, is needed for accurate diagnosis. Glucocorticoids suppress immune function. Adrenal insufficiency may allow allergic responses, enhanced antibody titers to viral antigens, and increased cytokines. CFS may not be a discrete disease with singular cause; it may be a clinical presentation with a variety of infectious and noninfectious antecedents and contributing factors. Pathophysiologic antecedents (acute infection, stress, preexisting or concurrent psychiatric illness) may converge in a final common clinical presentation. Reduced adrenal cortical secretion is a major feature.

- **Mind and attitude**: affect immunity and energy. Many CFS patients are depressed or have no enthusiasm for life. They often lack social support. Cognitive therapy may help. Inform CFS patients that they can get better. Positive mental attitude is critical to healing. Exercise or condition the attitude as conditioning the body. Prescribe mental exercises: visualizations, goal setting, affirmations, empowering questions.

## Diet

Energy is related to quality of foods routinely ingested. Eliminate or restrict caffeine and refined sugar. Acute caffeine intake stimulates; regular caffeine intake induces chronic fatigue. Excessive caffeine intake is quite common in psychiatric disorders. The degree of fatigue correlates to the quantity of caffeine ingested. Abrupt cessation of coffee may trigger caffeine withdrawal—fatigue, headache, intense desire for coffee—that may last a few days.

## Nutritional Supplements

- **High-potency vitamin/mineral combination**: deficiency of any nutrient can produce fatigue and susceptibility to infection.
- **Extra vitamin C**: 3000 mg/day in divided doses.
- **Magnesium**: subclinical magnesium (Mg) deficiency can result in chronic fatigue. Low RBC Mg (a more accurate measure of Mg status than routine blood analysis) is found in CFS. Cell Mg deficiency may not be caused by low intake, yet Mg supplements can alleviate fatigue. Oral Mg and K aspartate (1 g each) provide notable relief after 4-5 days; sometimes 10 days are required. Continue treatment for 4-6 weeks. Fatigue may not return. Mg is easily absorbed orally as aspartate or citrate, Krebs cycle

intermediates that support cell adenosine triphosphate (ATP) production. Dose: 500-1200 mg/day in divided doses.

- **Essential fatty acids**: supplementation (combined linoleic acid, gamma-linolenic acid [GLA], eicosapentaenoic acid [EPA], docosahexaenoic acid [DHA]) given as eight 500-mg caps q.d. for 3 months may improve clinical picture and RBC membrane phospholipid profile of patients with postviral fatigue. Brain lateral ventricular enlargement can occur in CFS. Cerebral magnetic resonance imaging at baseline and 16 weeks indicates that eicosapentaenoic acid markedly reduces lateral ventricular volume during treatment.
- **Nicotinamide adenine dinucleotide**: or NADH, the active coenzyme form of vitamin $B_3$, counters jet lag effects on cognition and wakefulness and encourages adenosine triphosphate generation. NADH may improve quality of life in CFS. Dose: stabilized oral absorbable form at 10 mg daily for 1 month. In one small study, 31% responded favorably in contrast to 8% on placebo. No severe adverse effects are noted in human beings; no toxicity noted in animals at megadoses.
- **L-Carnitine**: essential for transport of long-chain fatty acids across mitochondrial membrane. Two months of treatment gave statistically significant clinical improvement in 12 of 18 studied parameters after 8 weeks with no clinical deterioration. The greatest improvement occurs between 4 and 8 weeks. It is extremely safe, with no significant side effects. Use the L-form; avoid the D-form.

## Other Therapies

- **Breathing, posture, and bodywork**: diaphragm breathing, good posture, bodywork (massage, spinal manipulation, etc.).
- **Exercise**: moderate level improves mood, ability to handle stress. Increases (up to 100%) NK activity and stimulates immune system. Intense exercise can have opposite effect. Tai chi exercises may enhance immunity. Graded exercise begins with mild walking and weight exercises, increasing time and intensity as is comfortable. This method is superior to relaxation and flexibility exercises.

## Botanical Medicines

- *Eleutherococcus senticosus* (Siberian ginseng): supports adrenals, is a nonspecific adaptogen, increases T-helper cells and NK activity—valuable in treating CFS.

- ***Glycyrrhiza glabra*** (licorice): antiviral and glucocorticoid-potentiating properties (*Textbook, "Glycyrrhiza glabra* [Licorice]") but not well studied in CFS. Use whole root because glucocorticoid-potentiating glycyrrhizic and glycyrrhetinic acids are removed from deglycyrrhizinated licorice (DGL).

## THERAPEUTIC APPROACH

- **Comprehensive diagnostic and therapeutic approach**: identify underlying factors affecting energy or immunity. Strong correlation among CFS, FM, and MCS suggests hepatic detoxification, food allergy control, and gut restoration diet. Support the immune system (*Textbook,* "Food Reactions").
- **Diet**: identify and control food allergies. Increase water, eliminate caffeine and alcohol. Eat whole organic foods. Control hypoglycemia; eliminate sugar and refined starch foods and take regular healthy small meals and snacks. Use medical food replacement (e.g. UltraClear, Metagenics, San Clemente, Calif.) for several weeks to speed detoxification.
- **Lifestyle**: diaphragmatic breathing, proper posture, regular low-intensity exercise.
- **Supplements**:
  - —High-potency vitamin/mineral combination (*Textbook,* "Nutritional Medicine")
  - —Vitamin C: 500-1000 mg t.i.d.
  - —Vitamin E: 200-400 IU/day (mixed tocopherols)
  - —Thymus extract: 750 mg crude polypeptides q.d. or b.i.d.
  - —Mg bound to citrate or Krebs intermediates: 200-300 mg t.i.d.
  - —Pantothenic acid: 250 mg q.d.
  - —NADH: 10 mg q.d. on an empty stomach
  - —L-Carnitine: 3000-4000 mg q.d. in divided doses
  - —Fish oil: 5 g q.d. for at least 3 to 4 months
- **Botanicals**:
  - —***Eleutherococcus senticosus***: dried root, 2-4 g; tincture (1:5), 10-20 mL; fluid extract (1:1), 2.0-4.0 mL; solid (dry powdered) extract (20:1 or standardized to >1% eleutheroside E); 100-200 mg.
  - —***Glycyrrhiza glabra***: powdered root, 1-2 g; fluid extract (1:1): 2-4 mL; solid (dry powdered) extract (4:1); 250-500 mg.
- **Counseling**: directly or refer to professional counselor to reinforce pattern of mental, emotional, and spiritual affirmations.

Questionnaire for recognition of impaired immune function:

- Do you get more than two colds per year?
- When you catch a cold, does it take more than 5-7 days to get rid of the symptoms?
- Have you ever had infectious mononucleosis?
- Do you have herpes?
- Do you have chronic infections of any kind?

# Congestive Heart Failure

## DIAGNOSTIC SUMMARY

- **Left ventricular failure**: exertional dyspnea, cough, fatigue, orthropnea, cardiac enlargement, rales, gallop rhythm, and pulmonary venous congestion.
- **Right ventricular failure**: elevated venous pressure, hepatomegaly, dependent edema.
- **Left and right ventricular failure**: combinations of above.
- Diagnosis confirmed by echocardiograph.

**Stages of Congestive Heart Failure as Defined by the New York Heart Association (NYHA)**

| | |
|---|---|
| Stage I | Symptom free at rest and with treatment |
| Stage II | Impaired heart function with moderate physical effort; SOB with exertion common; no symptoms at rest |
| Stage III | Even minor physical exertion results in SOB and fatigue; no symptoms at rest |
| Stage IV | Symptoms (SOB) and signs (lower extremity edema) present when patient is at rest. |

*SOB*, Shortness of breath.

## GENERAL CONSIDERATIONS

Congestive heart failure (CHF) is the inability of the heart to pump enough blood effectively. Contractile function of the heart is governed by five factors: (1) contractile state of myocardium, (2) preload of ventricle, (3) end-diastolic volume, (4) impedance to left ventricular ejection, and (5) heart rate (HR).

- **Causes of CHF**: long-term hypertension, previous myocardial infarction, disorder of heart valve, cardiomyopathy, and chronic lung disease.

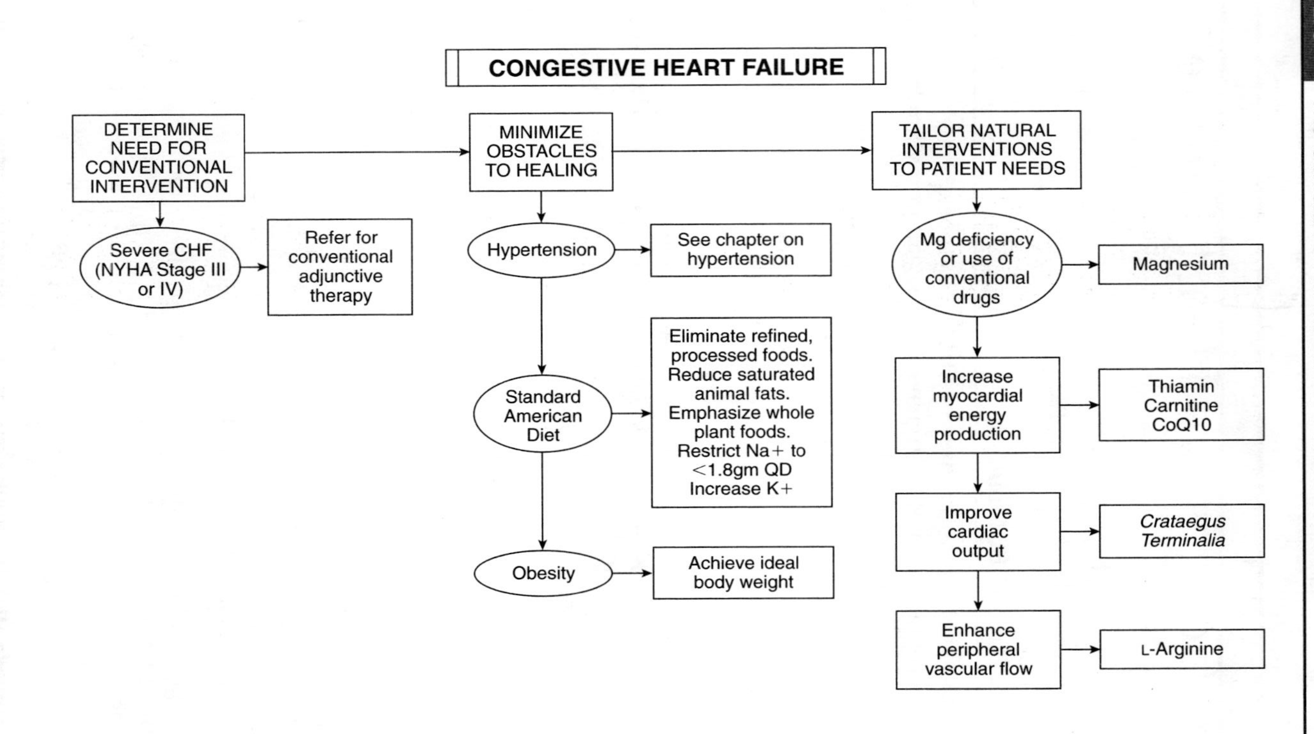
CONGESTIVE HEART FAILURE
DETERMINE NEED FOR CONVENTIONAL INTERVENTION
Severe CHF (NYHA Stage III or IV)
Refer for conventional adjunctive therapy
MINIMIZE OBSTACLES TO HEALING
Hypertension
See chapter on hypertension
Standard American Diet
Eliminate refined, processed foods. Reduce saturated animal fats. Emphasize whole plant foods. Restrict Na+ to <1.8gm QD Increase K+
Obesity
Achieve ideal body weight
TAILOR NATURAL INTERVENTIONS TO PATIENT NEEDS
Mg deficiency or use of conventional drugs
Magnesium
Increase myocardial energy production
Thiamin Carnitine CoQ10
Improve cardiac output
*Crataegus* *Terminalia*
Enhance peripheral vascular flow
L-Arginine

- **Precipitating or exacerbating factors**: increased demand (anemia, fever, infection, fluid overload, increased sodium (Na) intake, high environmental temperature, renal failure, hepatic failure, thyrotoxicosis, arteriovenous shunt, respiratory insufficiency, emotional stress, pregnancy, obesity), arrhythmias, pulmonary embolism, alcohol use, nutrient deficiency, uncontrolled hypertension, drugs (beta-adrenergic blockers, antiarrhythmic drugs, Na-retaining drugs [steroids, nonsteroidal antiinflammatories]).
- **Consequences of reduced cardiac output (CO)**: reduced renal blood flow and glomerular filtration, causing Na and fluid retention. Activation of renin-angiotensin-aldosterone (RAA) system increases peripheral vascular resistance, ventricular afterload, and levels of circulating vasopressin, a vasoconstrictor and antidiuretic.
- **Compensatory mechanisms for reduced CO**: tachycardia, increased sympathetic nervous system activation, ventricular dilation, and hypertrophy. These are a mixed blessing; increased sympathetic activity increases CO by increasing HR and force of contraction but it also increases vascular resistance.
- **Signs and symptoms of CHF**: depend on which ventricle has failed; left, pulmonary congestion and edema; right, systemic venous congestion and peripheral edema. Weakness, fatigue, and shortness of breath (SOB) are common to both as is biventricular failure.

## DIAGNOSTIC CONSIDERATIONS

CHF is most effectively treated by natural measures in early stages. Early diagnosis and prevention by addressing causative factors are imperative. First symptoms are SOB and chronic nonproductive cough. Conduct extensive cardiovascular evaluation—complete physical examination looking for characteristic signs (peripheral signs of heart failure, enlarged and sustained left ventricular impulse, diminished first heart sound, gallop rhythm, etc.), electrocardiogram, and echocardiogram.

## THERAPEUTIC CONSIDERATIONS

During initial stages of CHF, natural measures for underlying causes (e.g., hypertension) or improving myocardial metabolic function (*Textbook,* "Angina") are often quite effective. At later stages, conventional treatments—diuretics, angiotensin-converting enzyme (ACE) inhibitors, and/or digitalis glycosides—are indicated in most cases. Measures described here are used as adjuncts in more severe cases. Expect excellent clinical results in NYHA stages I and II with natural measures described later.

## Nutritional Supplements

Improve myocardial energy production because CHF is always characterized by energy depletion, often from nutrient or coenzyme deficiency (e.g., magnesium [Mg], vitamin $B_1$, coenzyme Q10 [CoQ10], carnitine). Dietary recommendations for hypertension are appropriate for most CHF patients, especially if CHF is caused by hypertension. Recommend diet low in $Na^+$ and high in potassium ($K^+$); restrict Na+ intake to <1.8 g q.d. Intake of several nutrients are deficient in CHF patients: Mg, calcium (Ca), zinc (Zn), copper (Cu), manganese (Mn), vitamins $B_1$ and $B_2$, folic acid. A high-potency multiple vitamin/mineral formula is critical, especially in diuretic therapy.

- **Mg**: critical nutrient for producing adenosine triphosphate (ATP). Low white blood cell Mg is common in CHF patients. Mg levels correlate directly with survival rates. Mg deficiency is linked to cardiac arrhythmias, reduced cardiovascular prognosis, worsened ischemia, and increased mortality rate in acute MI. Deficiency is probably caused by inadequate intake; increased wasting by overactivation of RAA system, common in patients with heart failure; and diuretics such as furosemide. Mg supplementation prevents Mg depletion caused by conventional drug therapy for CHF: digitalis, diuretics, and vasodilators (beta-blockers, Ca-channel blockers, etc.). Mg supplements produce positive effects in CHF patients taking conventional drugs, even if serum Mg is normal. Mg supplementation is not indicated in renal failure because of predisposition to hypermagnesemia—a risk factor for death. ACE inhibitors have a Mg-sparing effect in patients on furosemide. Dosage = 200 to 300 mg q.d. to t.i.d. (citrate). Monitor serum Mg to prevent hypermagnesemia in patients with renal impairment and those on digoxin. Mg reduces frequency and complexity of ventricular arrhythmias in digoxin-treated patients with CHF even without digoxin toxicity, but too much Mg may interfere with digoxin.
- **Thiamine**: vitamin $B_1$ deficiency has cardiovascular effects: "wet beri beri," $Na^+$ retention, peripheral vasodilation, and heart

failure. Furosemide (Lasix) causes $B_1$ deficiency in animals and patients with CHF. Severe $B_1$ deficiency is uncommon (except in alcoholics), but many do not get RDA (1.5 mg), especially elderly in hospitals or nursing homes. Significant percentage of geriatric population is deficient in B vitamins critical to cardiovascular and brain function. Daily doses of 80-240 mg of $B_1$ improve clinical picture; 13%–22% increase of left ventricular ejection fraction. Increased ejection fraction is linked to greater survival rate in CHF. The benefit, lack of risk, and low cost of 200-250 mg $B_1$ q.d. warrant its use in CHF, especially if the patient is taking furosemide.

- **L-Carnitine**: essential for transport of fatty acids into myocardial mitochondria for ATP production. The normal heart stores more carnitine and $CoQ_{10}$ than it needs, but heart ischemia quickly decreases both. Carnitine supplements improve cardiac function in CHF patients. The longer carnitine is used, the more dramatic the improvement. A dosage of 500 mg t.i.d. for 6 months increases maximal exercise time by 16%-25% and ventricular ejection fraction by 12%-13%.
- **$CoQ_{10}$**: Most studies used $CoQ_{10}$ as adjunct to conventional drugs. The largest study included 2664 patients in NYHA classes II and III in open study in Italy. The daily dosage was 50-150 mg orally for 90 days (majority of patients, 78%, took 100 mg q.d.). Proportions of patients with improved clinical signs and symptoms: cyanosis, 78.1%; edema, 78.6%; pulmonary edema, 77.8%; hepatomegaly, 49.3%; venous congestion, 71.81%; SOB, 52.7%; heart palpitations, 75.4%; sweating, 79.8%; subjective arrhythmia, 63.4%; insomnia, 66.2%; vertigo, 73.1%; nocturia, 53.6%. Improvement of at least three symptoms occurred in 54% of patients, with significantly improved quality of life with $CoQ_{10}$. Mild side effects were not common, only 1.5%. $CoQ_{10}$ may not achieve therapeutic benefit in more severe stages of CHF or if blood levels of $CoQ_{10}$ do not reach suggested threshold of 2.5 μg/mL.
- **L-Arginine**: amino acid of value in CHF. CHF patients are less able to achieve peripheral vasodilation during exercise. Endothelial cells make natural vasodilator nitric oxide from L-arginine. Dosage of 5.6-12.6 g q.d. oral L-arginine increases peripheral blood flow by 29%. The 6-minute walking distance increases by 8% and arterial compliance increases by 19%. L-Arginine improves endothelial cell function and renal function (improved glomerular filtration rate, natriuresis, and plasma endothelin level) in patients with CHF.

### Botanical Medicines

- ***Crataegus oxyacantha* (hawthorn)**: quite useful in early stages as sole agent and later stages in combination with digitalis cardioglycosides. *Crataegus* extract standardized to 15 mg procyanidin oligomers per 80-mg capsule b.i.d. for 8 weeks was better than placebo in improving heart function. It mildly reduces systolic and diastolic blood pressure (BP) with no adverse reactions at recommended dosage. *Crataegus* given to patients with CHF (NYHA stage II) at 600 mg standardized *Crataegus* extract q.d. for 56 days was better than placebo at increasing patient working capacity on bicycle ergometer (25 vs. 5 W). The *Crataegus* group also had a drop in systolic BP from 171 to 164 mm Hg and HR from 115 to 110 beats/min, with no change in BP or HR in the placebo group.
- ***Terminalia arjuna***: traditional Ayurvedic botanical for cardiac failure. CHF patients (class IV NYHA) received bark extract (500 mg every 8 hours) for 2 weeks or placebo. The extract group had statistically significant improvement in end-systolic volume and left ventricular ejection fraction (by echocardiogram). The uncontrolled phase of the study using combination of *T. arjuna* and conventional drugs for 2 years found nine patients showing remarkable improvement to NYHA class II and other three improving to class III.

## THERAPEUTIC APPROACH

Diet and natural agents are effective in early stages (NYHA stages I and II); in later stages, adjunct drug therapy is necessary. Treatment is designed to address underlying pathophysiology and improve myocardial function through improved energy production.

- **Diet**: Achieve ideal body weight. Restrict $Na^+$ intake (<1.8 g q.d.). Increase whole organic plant foods. Reduce saturated fat. Follow other guidelines for lowering BP (see the chapter on hypertension).
- **Nutritional supplements**:
  —Magnesium: 200-400 mg t.i.d. (citrate)
  —Thiamin: 200-250 mg q.d.
  —L-Carnitine: 500-1000 mg t.i.d.
  —Coenzyme $Q_{10}$: 100-300 mg q.d.
- **Botanical medicines**:
  —Hawthorn extract (1.8% vitexin-4′-rhamnoside or 10% procyanidin content): 200-300 mg t.i.d.
  —*Terminalia arjuna* extract: 500 mg t.i.d.

# Cystitis

## DIAGNOSTIC SUMMARY

- Burning pain on urination
- Increased urinary frequency, nocturia
- Turbid, foul-smelling, or dark urine
- Lower abdominal pain
- Urinalysis showing significant pyuria and bacteriuria

## GENERAL CONSIDERATIONS

Bladder infections in women are common: 10%-20% of all women have urinary tract discomfort at least once a year; 37.5% of women with no history of urinary tract infection (UTI) will have one within 10 years; 2%-4% of healthy women have elevated bacteria in urine, indicating unrecognized UTI. A woman with history of recurrent UTI has an episode once a year. Recurrent bladder infections are significant problems; 55% eventually involve kidneys. Recurrent kidney infection causes progressive damage: scarring and, for some, kidney failure. UTIs are much less common in males, except infants, and indicate anatomic abnormality, prostate infection, or unprotected rectal intercourse.

### Causes

Urine excreted by the kidneys is sterile until reaching the urethra. Bacteria can ascend the urethra or, much less commonly, reach the urinary system by the bloodstream. Bacteria are introduced into the urethra from fecal contamination or, in women, vaginal secretions. Factors influencing ascending infection are anatomic or functional obstructions to flow (allowing pooling of urine) and immune dysfunction. Major defenses against infection: free flow, large urine volume, complete bladder emptying, optimal immune function. Urine flow washes away bacteria. The inner surface of the bladder has antimicrobial properties. Urine pH inhibits growth of many bacteria. In men prostatic fluid has antimicrobial substances.

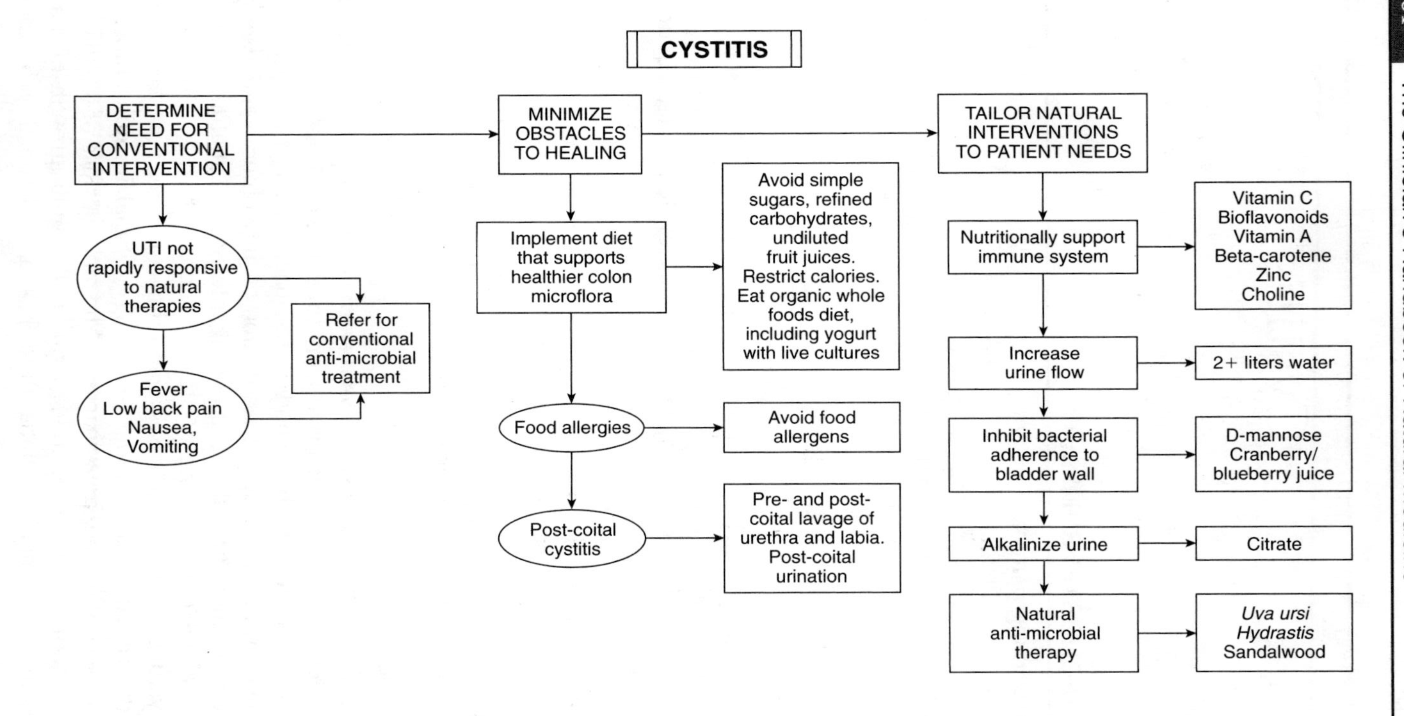
CYSTITIS
DETERMINE NEED FOR CONVENTIONAL INTERVENTION
UTI not rapidly responsive to natural therapies
Fever
Low back pain
Nausea,
Vomiting
Refer for conventional anti-microbial treatment
MINIMIZE OBSTACLES TO HEALING
Implement diet that supports healthier colon microflora
Avoid simple sugars, refined carbohydrates, undiluted fruit juices. Restrict calories. Eat organic whole foods diet, including yogurt with live cultures
Food allergies
Avoid food allergens
Post-coital cystitis
Pre- and post-coital lavage of urethra and labia. Post-coital urination
TAILOR NATURAL INTERVENTIONS TO PATIENT NEEDS
Nutritionally support immune system
Vitamin C
Bioflavonoids
Vitamin A
Beta-carotene
Zinc
Choline
Increase urine flow
2+ liters water
Inhibit bacterial adherence to bladder wall
D-mannose
Cranberry/ blueberry juice
Alkalinize urine
Citrate
Natural anti-microbial therapy
Uva ursi
Hydrastis
Sandalwood

The body quickly mobilizes white blood cells (WBCs) to control bacteria.

- **Risk factors**: pregnancy (twice as frequent); sexual intercourse (nuns have 1/10 incidence); homosexual activity (men); mechanical trauma or irritation; and, most importantly, structural abnormalities of the urinary tract blocking free urine flow.
- **Reflux of infected urine** from bladder upward infects kidneys and establishes recurrence.

## DIAGNOSIS

Bladder infection diagnosis is imprecise; clinical symptoms and presence of significant amounts of bacteria in urine do not correlate well. Only 60% of women with UTI symptoms have abundant bacteria in urine; 20% have serious kidney involvement. Diagnosis is according to signs, symptoms, and urinary findings. Pelvic examination is indicated if history suggests vaginitis or cervicitis or if any diagnostic confusion exists. Microscopic examination of infected urine reveals high WBCs and bacteria. Urine culture determines quantity and type of bacteria. *Escherichia coli* (from the colon) are most common. Fever, chills, and low back pain suggest kidney involvement. Recurrent infections warrant intravenous urogram to rule out structural abnormality.

### Collection of Urine Specimen for Culture

Optimal method is the voided midstream specimen. Clean urethral meatus and vaginal vestibule before collecting. Spread labia and cleanse area with two gauze sponges moistened with cleansing solution and a dry gauze sponge. Wash by making single front-to-back motion with each of two moist sponges and then dry sponge. While labia are still held apart, a small amount of urine is allowed to pass into toilet or bedpan. Then midstream specimen is collected in sterile container and immediately closed. Collection by catheterization is more invasive and carries 1%-2% chance of initiating UTI. Suprapubic aspiration is the most accurate method but also is the most invasive.

### Examining Collected Urine

Routine methods include dipsticks, microscope, and culture. For most accurate results, examine urine within 1 hour. If examination must be delayed, refrigerate at 5° C. Culturing requires that urine not be refrigerated for more than 8 hours.

- **Dipsticks**: reagent strips are dipped into urine and removed. Parts of dipstick are impregnated with chemicals that react with specific substances in urine to produce various colors. Careful matching of dipstick color to color standard at appropriate time is essential. Dipsticks are invaluable for qualitative and rough quantitative analysis: pH, protein, glucose, ketones, bilirubin, hemoglobin, nitrite, and urobilinogen. Some dipsticks detect WBCs and bacteria (including semiquantitative cultures). Leukocyte esterase test detects WBCs (80%-90% sensitive). Many organisms reduce urine nitrate to nitrite (*Citrobacter* spp., *E. coli, Klebsiella pneumonia, Proteus* spp., *Pseudomonas* spp., *Serratia marcescens, Shigella, Staphylococcus* spp. [most]). Measuring nitrite (50% sensitive) is inexpensive and a rapid detector of bacteriuria; confirm by culture.
- **Microscopic examination**: Perform within first hour. Place a drop of fresh urine or a drop of resuspended sediment from centrifuged fresh urine on slide, cover with cover glass, and examine with high-dry objective under reduced illumination. More than 10 bacteria per field in unstained specimen suggests bacteria count >100,000/mL. Gram stain under oil immersion objective; WBCs indicate infection. Abundant protein and/or WBC casts indicate renal involvement, commonly pyelonephritis.
- **Urine culture**: Only quantitative cultures typically are used. Diluted urine is introduced to suitable medium and incubation. Colonies counted and multiplied by dilution factor, giving bacterial count per milliliter. Bacteriuria is significant if >100,000/mL but 1000 colonies/mL is clinically significant in the presence of UTI symptoms. Semiquantitative tests using dipsticks or glass slides coated with culture media commonly are used. Colonies are counted or appearance is compared 12-24 hours later. Recurrent or chronic infection warrants sensitivity studies. Roughly 95% of UTIs involve single bacterial species. Mixed species suggest contamination. *S. epidermidis,* diphtheroids, and *Lactobacillus* are common in distal urethra but rarely cause UTI. The most common organisms are *E. coli, Proteus miribili, Klebsiella pneumonia, Enterococcus, Enterobacter aerogenes, Pseudomonas aeruginosa, Proteus* spp., *S. marcescens, S. epidermidis,* and *S. aureus.*

## THERAPEUTIC CONSIDERATIONS

Primary goal is to enhance normal host defenses—to enhance urine flow by proper hydration, promote protective urine pH, prevent bacterial adherence to bladder endothelium, and enhance immune system. Use antimicrobial botanical medicines as needed.

**Chronic interstitial cystitis**: underdiagnosed persistent form of cystitis and source of undiagnosed chronic pelvic pain not caused by infection. These patients have higher incidence of inflammatory bowel disease, lupus, irritable bowel syndrome, and fibromyalgia. Focus on enhancing integrity of bladder interstitium and endothelium. "Leaky bladder urothelium" theory: lack of integrity in glycosaminoglycan layer of bladder epithelium, increasing permeability to potassium and causing inflammation and pain. Eliminate food allergens that can produce cystitis in some patients. *Centella asiatica* extracts improve integrity of connective tissue that composes interstitium and heal bladder ulcerations (*Textbook, "Centella asiatic* [Gout Kola]").

### General Measures

- **Increase urine flow**: Increase fluid intake: pure water, herbal teas, fresh fruit and vegetable juices diluted with equal amounts of water. Drink 2+ L of liquids, at least half of that as water. Avoid soft drinks, concentrated fruit drinks, coffee, and alcohol.
- **Cranberry juice**: effective in several clinical studies. 0.5 L q.d. cranberry juice is beneficial in 73% of male and female UTI subjects. Withdrawal of cranberry juice from people who benefited resulted in recurrence in 61%. To acidify urine, 1+ L cranberry juice must be consumed at one sitting; concentration of hippuric acid in urine from drinking cranberry juice is insufficient to inhibit bacteria. Constituents in cranberry juice reduce ability of *E. coli* to adhere to bladder and urethral endothelium. Only cranberry and blueberry contain this inhibitor; blueberry juice is a suitable alternative to cranberry juice in bladder infections. Avoid immunosuppressive effects of sweetened cranberry juice. Instead use fresh cranberry (sweetened with apple or grape juice) or blueberry juice. Cranberry extracts may be more cost effective than juice; ensure that ample water is ingested if tablets are used. The theoretical concern that cranberry can induce kidney stone formation, because cranberry contains oxalate, may not be warranted. Urinary oxalate excretion does not increase after drinking cranberry juice; no cranberry studies have reported increased kidney stone incidence.
- **Acidify or alkalinize?**: Acidifying urine is difficult. Popular methods (ascorbic acid, cranberry juice) have little effect on pH at commonly prescribed doses. Alkalinizing urine is more

effective, especially in women without pathogenic bacteria in urine. The best method for alkalinizing is citrate salts (potassium citrate and sodium citrate) that are rapidly absorbed and metabolized without affecting gastric pH or producing laxative effect. They are excreted partly as carbonate, raising urine pH. Potassium citrate and/or sodium citrate are used to treat lower UTIs and are often used as "holding exercise" until urine culture is completed. Dosage of 4 g sodium citrate every 8 hours for 48 hours: 80% of 64 women had relief of symptoms, 12% had reduction of symptoms, and 91.8% rated treatment acceptable. Significant symptomatic relief experienced by 80% of another 159 women studied who were abacteriuric. Urine culture can be restricted to women who do not respond to alkalinization. Many herbs used to treat UTIs (*Hydrastis canadensis, Arctostaphylos uva ursi*) contain antibacterial components that work most effectively in alkaline environment. Enhance immune function (*Textbook*, "Immune Support").

## Nutritional Supplements

**D-Mannose**: simple sugar that helps prevent pili of *E. coli* and other bacteria from adhering to bladder wall. D-Mannose is in cranberry juice but in lower concentrations than in specific supplements. No clinical trials are available, but clinical experience supports its use. Adult dose: 0.5 to 1 tsp t.i.d. mixed in a little water. It can be used in reduced doses for pediatric UTIs.

## Botanical Medicines

- ***Arctostaphylos uva ursi* (bearberry or upland cranberry)**: Urinary antiseptic component is arbutin, composing 7%-9% of leaves. Arbutin is hydrolyzed to hydroquinone in the body. Hydroquinone is most effective in alkaline urine. Crude plant extracts are more effective medicinally than isolated arbutin. *Uva ursi* is especially active against *E. coli* and has diuretic properties. Prophylactic effect of standardized extract on recurrent cystitis continued over 1-year period of study without side-effects. Regular use may prevent bladder infections. *Uva ursi* increases susceptibility of bacteria to antibiotics such as β-lactams. Catechins, compound P, epicatechin gallate from green tea, and baicalin from *Scutellaria amoena* may have similar effects. Avoid excessive dosages of *Uva ursi*; as little as 15 g (0.5 oz) dried leaves can be toxic in susceptible individuals. Toxic signs include tinnitus, nausea and vomiting, sense of suffocation, shortness of breath, convulsions, delirium, collapse.

- ***Allium sativum*** **(garlic)**: antimicrobial activity against many disease-causing organisms, including *E. coli, Proteus* spp., *K. pneumonia, Staphylococcus* spp., *Streptococcus* spp.
- ***Hydrastis canadensis*** **(goldenseal)**: very effective antimicrobial agent against *E. coli, Proteus* spp., *Klebsiella* spp., *Staphylococcus* spp., *Enterobacter aerogenes* (requires large dosage), and *Pseudomonas* spp. Berberine constituent works better in an alkaline urine (*Textbook, "Hydrastis canadensis* [Goldenseal] and Other Berberine-Containing Botanicals").

## THERAPEUTIC APPROACH

Most cases of cystitis are relatively benign, but must be properly diagnosed, treated, and monitored. Patient must notify physician of any change in condition. If culture positive, follow up with another culture 7-14 days after treatment is started. Citrates can ameliorate symptoms. Pyelonephritis requires immediate antibiotic therapy and sometimes hospitalization. Patient must promptly inform physician of fever, low back pain, and nausea or vomiting. Occasional acute bladder infection is easily treated; chronic cystitis is a challenge. Find underlying cause: structural abnormalities, excessive sugar intake, food allergies, nutritional deficiencies, chronic vaginitis, local foci of infection (prostate, kidneys), current or childhood sexual abuse. Causative agents for cystitis have not changed, but bacterial multidrug resistance to antibiotics (trimethoprim-sulfamethoxazole, β-lactam drugs, fluoroquinolone) is an alarming trend. Natural therapeutics protect urinary tract, support immunity, and inhibit bactericidal attack as first-line therapy in nonpyelonephritic cases and as an adjunctive to efficacy of antibiotics, if needed.

- **General measures**: large amounts of fluids (2+ L q.d.), including 0.5+ L unsweetened cranberry or 0.25+ L blueberry juice q.d.. For recurrent postcoital cystitis, urinate after intercourse; wash labia and urethra with strong tea of *Hydrastis canadensis* (2 tsp/cup) before and after. If this is inadequate, use dilute solution of povidone-iodine.
- **Diet**: UTIs arise and ascend with stool bacteria. Diet alters stool bacterial composition; UTI risk can change by modifiying diet. Avoid all simple sugars, refined carbohydrates, full-strength fruit juice (diluted is acceptable), and food allergens. Restrict calories. Eat unsweetened yogurt with live probiotics and liberal amounts of garlic and onions.

**Bacteriologic Susceptibility to Nutrients and Botanical Medicines**

| Bacteria Species | Agent |
|---|---|
| Abacterial | Citrates |
| *Enterobacter aerogenes* | |
| *Enterococcus* | |
| *Escherichia coli* | *Allium sativum*<br>*Hydrastis canadensis*<br>*Uva ursi* |
| *Klebsiella pneumonia* | *Allium sativum*<br>*Hydrastis canadensis* |
| *Proteus miribili* | *Allium sativum*<br>*Hydrastis canadensis* |
| *Pseudomonas aeruginosa* | *Hydrastis canadensis* |
| *Staphylococcus saprophyticus* | *Allium sativum*<br>*Hydrastis canadensis* |

- **Nutritional supplements**:
  - —D-Mannose powder: 0.75 tsp t.i.d.
  - —Vitamin C: 500 mg every 2 hours
  - —Bioflavonoids: 1000 mg q.d.
  - —Vitamin A: 25,000 IU q.d. (<10,000 IU q.d. during pregnancy)
  - —Beta-carotene: 200,000 IU q.d.
  - —Zinc: 30 mg q.d. (e.g., picolinate)
  - —Choline: 1000 mg q.d.
- **Botanical medicines** (t.i.d.):
  - —*Uva ursi:* dried leaves or as a tea, 1.5-4.0 g (1-2 tsp); freeze-dried leaves, 500-1000 mg; tincture (1:5), 4-6 mL (1-1.5 tsp); fluid extract (1:1), 1.0 mL (0.25-0.5 tsp); powdered solid extract (10% arbutin), 250-500 mg
  - —*Hydrastis canadensis:* dried root (or as tea), 1-2 g; freeze-dried root, 500-1000 mg; tincture (1:5), 4-6 mL (1-1.5 tsp); fluid extract (1:1), 0.5-2.0 mL (0.25-0.5 tsp); powdered solid extract (8% alkaloid), 250-500 mg
  - —Sandalwood oil, 1-2 drops (natural, not artificial)

# Dermatitis Herpetiformis

## DIAGNOSTIC SUMMARY

- Pruritic, blistering rash usually on extensor surfaces.
- Most common in middle-aged white males, although may present in individuals of any age.
- Immunoglobulin (Ig) A deposits in papillary skin; confirmed by immunofluorescence.
- Asymptomatic "celiac" disease (gluten-sensitive enteropathy) in 75%-90% of patients.

## GENERAL CONSIDERATIONS

Dermatitis herpetiformis (DH), described as "celiac disease of the skin," is a dermatologic condition caused by a gastrointestinal (GI) immunologic disorder. Jejunal biopsy in DH patients reveals villous atrophy characteristic of celiac disease, but GI symptoms are rare. Absorption studies (*Textbook,* "Intestinal Permeability Assessment") are used to assess degree of enteropathy. Average age of onset of rash is 7.2 years, with a predilection for elbows, knees, and buttocks. Skin biopsy reveals granular IgA deposits. Skin lesions are itchy, grouped vesicles often located on extensor surfaces.

## THERAPEUTIC CONSIDERATIONS

- **Gluten**: most important factor in DH is to eliminate all sources of gluten. Frazer's criteria for diagnosing gluten-sensitive enteropathy (improvement on gluten-free diet and relapse after reintroduction) indicate rash and villous atrophy are largely gluten dependent. Gluten elimination improves virtually all patients, including disappearance of reticulin and gluten antibodies in DH. Gliadin polypeptide of gluten is key antigen; indirect immunofluorescence shows antibodies to gliadin in sera of 45% of DH patients. Titer and correlation increase with increasing disease severity. Approximately 81% of patients with severe jejunal abnormalities show antibodies to gliadin. Gluten connection is never

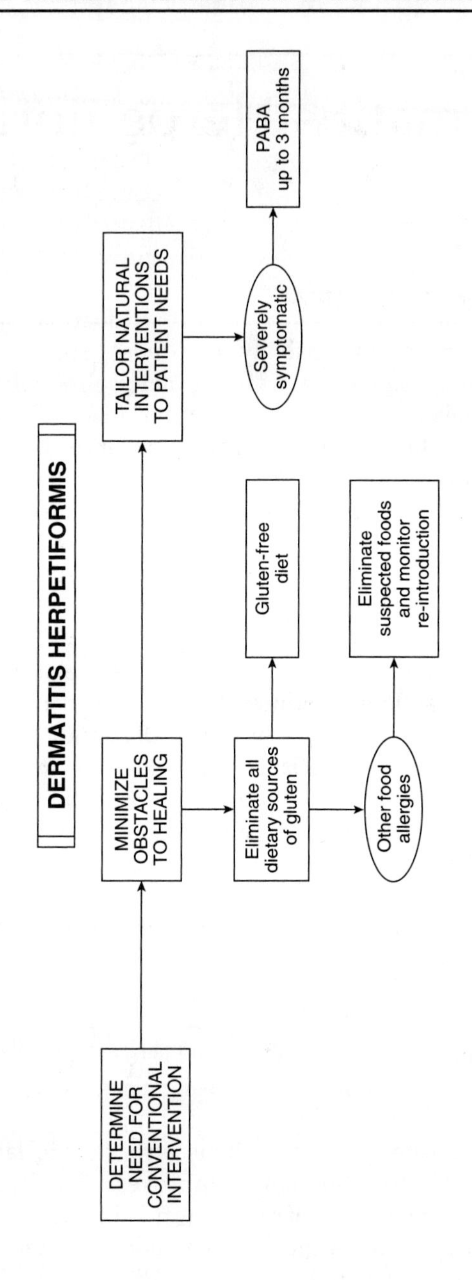
DERMATITIS HERPETIFORMIS
DETERMINE NEED FOR CONVENTIONAL INTERVENTION
MINIMIZE OBSTACLES TO HEALING
Eliminate all dietary sources of gluten
Gluten-free diet
Other food allergies
Eliminate suspected foods and monitor re-introduction
TAILOR NATURAL INTERVENTIONS TO PATIENT NEEDS
Severely symptomatic
PABA up to 3 months

mentioned in conventional medical textbooks. Gluten-free diet is superior to drugs such as dapsone and its severe side effects. Beneficial effects of gluten-free diet: at least 65% of patients have complete resolution and remainder substantially improve. DH enteropathy completely resolves; harsh medicines can be eliminated or substantially reduced; most patients experience improved sense of well-being. Those using gluten-free diet rather than drugs are protected against developing lipomas.

- **Food allergy**: 35% of patients are not adequately helped by gluten-free diet; only half of patients totally eliminate cutaneous IgA deposits and develop normal jejunal tissue. Other food allergies develop from increased leakage of macromolecules across damaged GI mucosa. Milk allergy is significant in some patients. According to enzyme-linked immunosorbent assay, 75% of DH patients have serum antibodies to gliadin, bovine milk, or ovalbumin. Thus other food sensitivities can also induce DH. Elemental diet, followed by careful food reintroduction, gives better results than gluten-free diet.
- **Para-aminobenzoic acid**: has been used successfully to control DH, even in those not controlling dietary gluten. It provides only symptom control and no repair of villous atrophy. It is not recommended as treatment of choice but as adjunct in unresponsive or severe cases.

## THERAPEUTIC APPROACH

Eliminate all gluten and gliadin sources. Identify and eliminate other food allergens (*Textbook,* "Food Allergy Testing"). Use therapeutic regimen similar to atopic dermatitis. Patience is necessary because response may take several weeks to 6 months.

- **Diet**: normal, healthy, unprocessed diet free of all grains and allergic foods.
- **Supplements**:
  —**Para-aminobenzoic acid**: 5 g q.d. until remission (maximum of 3 months).

# Diabetes Mellitus

## DIAGNOSTIC SUMMARY

- Elevated blood glucose determination
  - —Fasting (overnight): venous plasma glucose ≥126 mg/dL on at least two separate occasions
  - —After ingestion of 75 g glucose: venous plasma glucose ≥200 mg/dL at 2 hours postingestion and at least one other sample during 2-hour test
  - —Random blood glucose of 200 mg/dL or more plus presence of suggestive symptoms
- Classic symptoms: polyuria, polydipsia, polyphagia
- Presenting symptoms: fatigue, blurred vision, poor wound healing, periodontal disease, frequent infections

## GENERAL CONSIDERATIONS

Diabetes is a chronic disorder of carbohydrate, fat, and protein metabolism characterized by fasting elevations of blood glucose and greatly increased risk of heart disease, stroke, kidney disease, retinopathy, and neuropathy. Causes: the pancreas does not secrete enough insulin, or cells of body become resistant to insulin. Sugar cannot enter muscle or fat cells, causing serious complications. More than 18.5 million Americans have diabetes, but one third do not know this or ever consult a physician.

**Major complications of diabetes**: cardiovascular disease, hypertension, retinopathy, renal disease, neuropathy, amputations, periodontal disease, pain (arthritis, neuropathy, circulatory insufficiency, muscle pain [fibromyalgia]), depression (even years before diabetes diagnosis), autoimmune disorders (e.g., thyroid disease, arthritis)

### Classification

Two major categories:

- **Type 1 (insulin-dependent diabetes mellitus [IDDM])**: most often in children and adolescents (juvenile-onset diabetes).

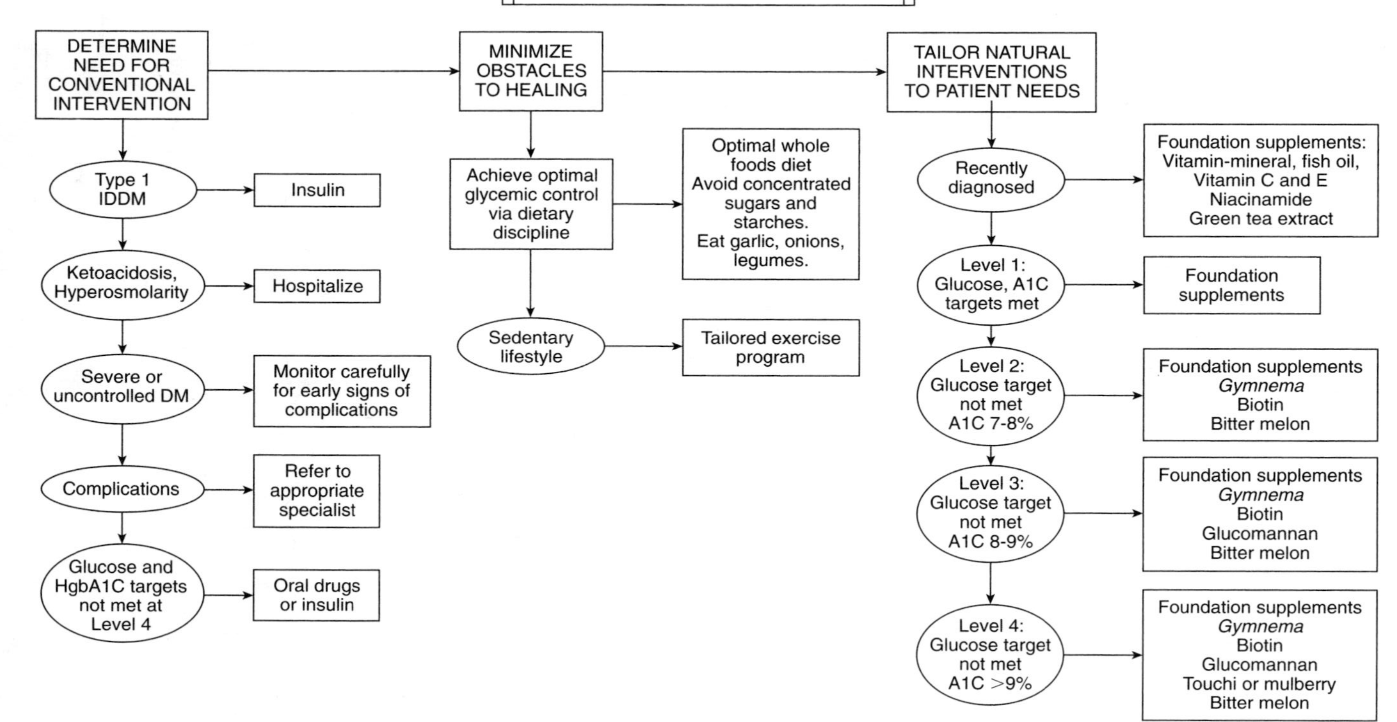
DIABETES MELLITUS TYPE 1
DETERMINE NEED FOR CONVENTIONAL INTERVENTION
Type 1 IDDM
Insulin
Ketoacidosis, Hyperosmolarity
Hospitalize
Severe or uncontrolled DM
Monitor carefully for early signs of complications
Complications
Refer to appropriate specialist
Glucose and HgbA1C targets not met at Level 4
Oral drugs or insulin
MINIMIZE OBSTACLES TO HEALING
Achieve optimal glycemic control via dietary discipline
Optimal whole foods diet Avoid concentrated sugars and starches. Eat garlic, onions, legumes.
Sedentary lifestyle
Tailored exercise program
TAILOR NATURAL INTERVENTIONS TO PATIENT NEEDS
Recently diagnosed
Foundation supplements: Vitamin-mineral, fish oil, Vitamin C and E Niacinamide Green tea extract
Level 1: Glucose, A1C targets met
Foundation supplements
Level 2: Glucose target not met A1C 7-8%
Foundation supplements Gymnema Biotin Bitter melon
Level 3: Glucose target not met A1C 8-9%
Foundation supplements Gymnema Biotin Glucomannan Bitter melon
Level 4: Glucose target not met A1C >9%
Foundation supplements Gymnema Biotin Glucomannan Touchi or mulberry Bitter melon

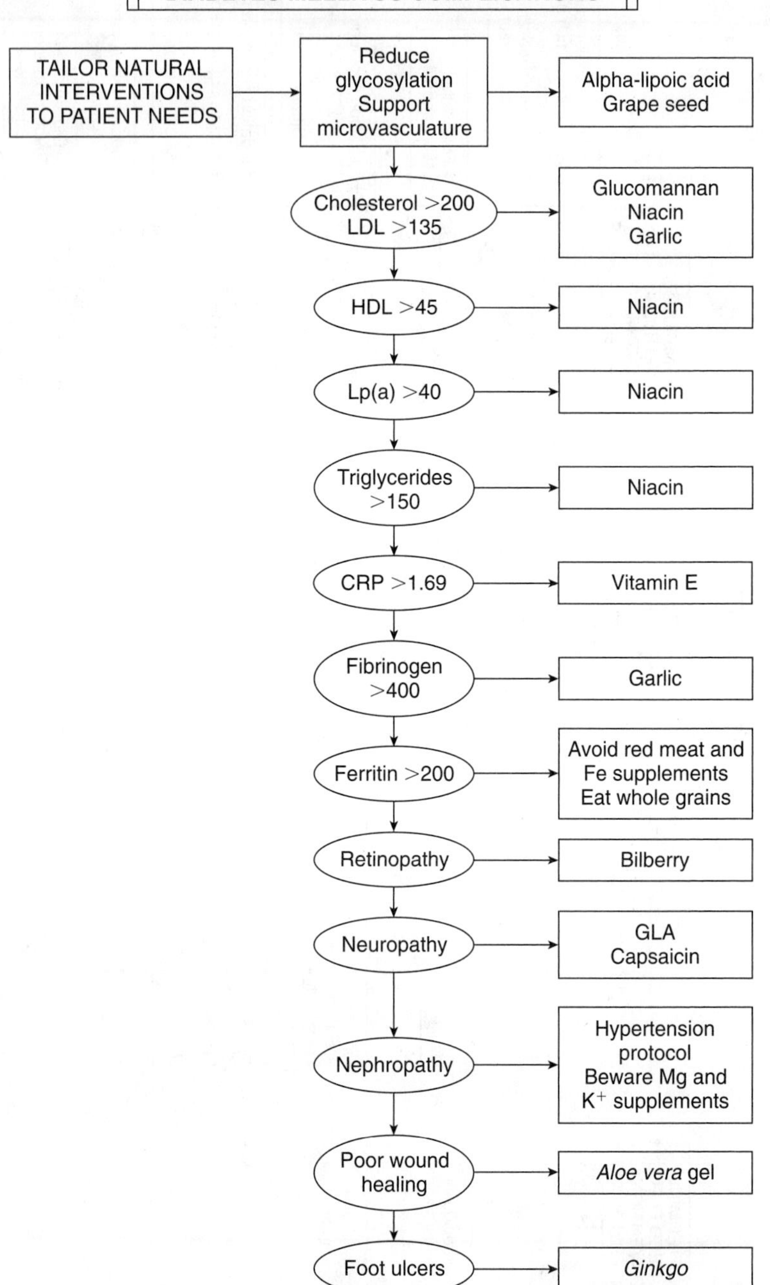
DIABETES MELLITUS COMPLICATIONS
TAILOR NATURAL INTERVENTIONS TO PATIENT NEEDS
Reduce glycosylation Support microvasculature
Alpha-lipoic acid Grape seed
Cholesterol >200 LDL >135
Glucomannan Niacin Garlic
HDL >45
Niacin
Lp(a) >40
Niacin
Triglycerides >150
Niacin
CRP >1.69
Vitamin E
Fibrinogen >400
Garlic
Ferritin >200
Avoid red meat and Fe supplements Eat whole grains
Retinopathy
Bilberry
Neuropathy
GLA Capsaicin
Nephropathy
Hypertension protocol Beware Mg and K+ supplements
Poor wound healing
Aloe vera gel
Foot ulcers
Ginkgo

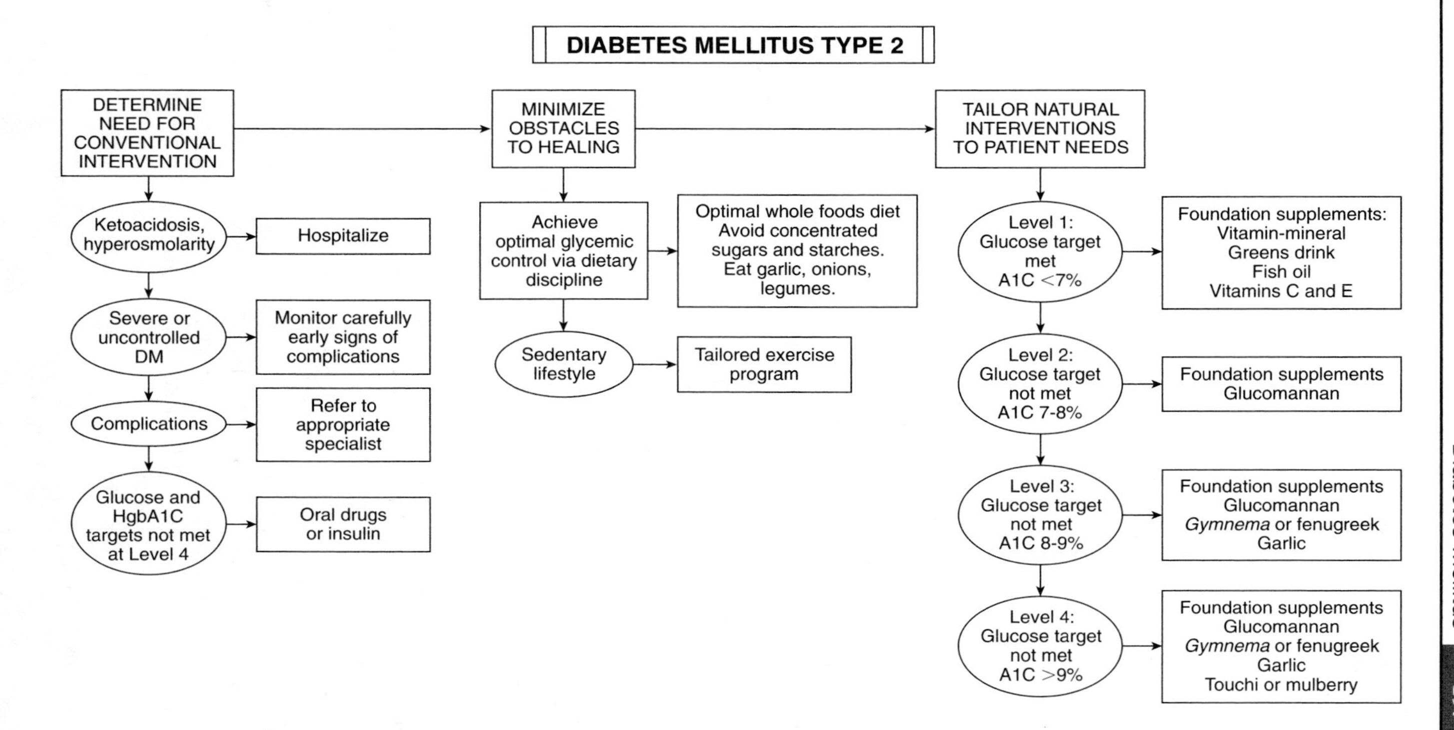

DIABETES MELLITUS TYPE 2
DETERMINE NEED FOR CONVENTIONAL INTERVENTION
Ketoacidosis, hyperosmolarity
Hospitalize
Severe or uncontrolled DM
Monitor carefully early signs of complications
Complications
Refer to appropriate specialist
Glucose and HgbA1C targets not met at Level 4
Oral drugs or insulin
MINIMIZE OBSTACLES TO HEALING
Achieve optimal glycemic control via dietary discipline
Optimal whole foods diet Avoid concentrated sugars and starches. Eat garlic, onions, legumes.
Sedentary lifestyle
Tailored exercise program
TAILOR NATURAL INTERVENTIONS TO PATIENT NEEDS
Level 1: Glucose target met A1C <7%
Foundation supplements: Vitamin-mineral Greens drink Fish oil Vitamins C and E
Level 2: Glucose target not met A1C 7-8%
Foundation supplements Glucomannan
Level 3: Glucose target not met A1C 8-9%
Foundation supplements Glucomannan Gymnema or fenugreek Garlic
Level 4: Glucose target not met A1C >9%
Foundation supplements Glucomannan Gymnema or fenugreek Garlic Touchi or mulberry

- **Type 2 (non-insulin-dependent diabetes mellitus [NIDDM])**: onset after age 40 years (adult-onset diabetes). Incidence of this type is rising in sedentary, obese children. Fifteen percent of adults diagnosed with type 2 actually have type 1.

| Features | Type 1 | Type 2 |
|---|---|---|
| Age at onset | Usually <40 years | Usually >40 years |
| Percentage of all diabetics | <10% | >90% |
| Seasonal trend | Fall and winter | None |
| Family history | Uncommon | Common |
| Appearance of symptoms | Rapid | Slow |
| Obesity at onset | Uncommon | Common |
| Insulin levels | Decreased | Variable |
| Insulin resistance | Occasional | Often |
| Treatment with insulin | Always | Not required |
| Beta-cells | Decreased | Variable |
| Ketoacidosis | Frequent | Rare |
| Complications | Frequent | Frequent |

- **IDDM (type 1)**: complete destruction of pancreas beta-cells, which manufacture insulin. Patients require lifelong insulin supplementation and must manage blood sugar daily by modifying insulin types and dosage schedules according to results of regular blood sugar testing. Ten percent of diabetics are type 1. Current causal theory focuses on injury to beta-cells plus a defect in tissue regeneration. Autoimmune component is revealed by antibodies to beta-cells present in 75% of cases compared with 0.5%-2.0% of normals. Antibodies to beta-cells may develop in response to cell destruction from other mechanisms (chemical, free radical, viral, food allergy).
- **NIDDM (type 2)**: affects 90% of diabetics. Insulin is elevated because of a loss of sensitivity to insulin by cells of body. Obesity is the major contributor; 90% of type 2 diabetics are obese. Achieving ideal body weight is linked to restoring normal blood sugar in most cases. Diet is of primary importance, implemented diligently before drug use. Most type 2 diabetics can be controlled by diet alone.

- **Other types of diabetes**:
  —Secondary diabetes: a result of conditions or syndromes (pancreatic disease, hormone disturbances, drugs, malnutrition)
  —Gestational diabetes: glucose intolerance during pregnancy
  —Impaired glucose tolerance: includes prediabetic, chemical, latent, borderline, subclinical, and asymptomatic diabetes

Individuals with impaired glucose tolerance have blood glucose and glucose tolerance test results intermediate between normal and clearly abnormal. Reactive hypoglycemia may be a prediabetic condition.

### Prediabetes and Syndrome X

Prediabetes (impaired glucose tolerance) entails abnormally high glucose. Although not high enough to fit the definition of NIDDM, it still needs to be treated. Many cases progress to type 2 DM. Impaired glucose tolerance is usually reversible, and DM is avoidable. High cholesterol, blood pressure, inflammation biomarkers, and blood clotting tendency are typical, increasing risk for cardiovascular disease, stroke, and so forth. Syndrome X is a cluster of abnormalities linked to refined carbohydrate consumption in the genetically predisposed. Syndrome X (metabolic cardiovascular risk syndrome [MCVS]), metabolic syndrome, Reaven's syndrome, insulin resistance syndrome, atherothrombogenic syndrome) includes mild to moderately impaired glucose tolerance, hyperinsulinemia from insulin resistance, hypercholesterolemia, hypertriglyceridemia, hypertension, and abdominal obesity. Key factor is hyperinsulinemia caused by refined carbohydrates coupled with insulin resistance. Prediabetes, hypoglycemia, hyperinsulinemia, syndrome X, and type 2 DM are facets of the same disease and underlying dietary, lifestyle, and genetic causes.

## DIAGNOSIS

In the patient with type 2 DM, classic symptoms are milder and often unnoticed. Fatigue, blurred vision, poor wound healing, periodontal disease, and frequent infections are presenting symptoms.

- **Fasting blood glucose**: taken after fasting at least 10 hours but not more than 16 hours. Normal fasting blood glucose is 70-99 mg/dL. Fasting blood glucose >126 mg/dL (7 mmol/L) on two separate occasions is diagnostic of diabetes. Fasting glucose ≥110 and <126 mg/dL indicates impaired glucose tolerance. Levels <50 mg/dL indicate fasting hypoglycemia.

- **Postprandial glucose**: 2 hours after meal. Level >200 mg/dL (11 mmol/L) indicates DM.
- **Random glucose**: anytime regardless of last meal. Level >200 mg/dL (11 mmol/L) indicates DM.
- **Glucose tolerance test (GTT)**: gold standard because of its long-standing use but less reliable than fasting blood glucose if combined with hemoglobin $A_1c$ ($HgbA_1c$).

### Glucose Tolerance Test Response Criteria

- **Normal**: no level >160 mg/dL (9 mmol/L) and <150 mg/dL (8.3 mmol/L) at end of first hour; <120 mg/dL (6.6 mmol/L) at end of second hour.
- **Flat**: no variation >± 20 mg/dL (1.1 mmol/L) from fasting value.
- **Prediabetic**: 140 mg/dL (7.8 mmol/L) to 180 mg/dL (10 mmol/L) at end of second hour.
- **Diabetic**: >180 mg/dL (10mmol/L) during first hour; 200 mg/dL (11.1 mmol/L) or higher at end of first hour; 150 mg/dL (8.3 mmol/L) or higher at end of second hour.
- **Glycosylated hemoglobin**: proteins with attached glucose molecules (glycosylated peptides) are elevated severalfold in DM. Normal levels are 5%-7% of Hgb. Mild glucose elevations cause $A_1c$ increase to 8%-10%; high glucose can increase $A_1c$ to 20%. $A_1c$ assay is a time-averaged indicator for preceding 2-4 months. It is simple and useful for assessing treatment efficacy and patient compliance. $A_1c$ plus fasting glucose can diagnose DM but not as only criteria. A third of diabetics diagnosed with GTT have normal $A_1c$. Couple $A_1c$ with fasting glucose and 2-hour postprandial glucose for a more accurate diagnosis. $A_1c$ assay can determine relative glucose load and monitor therapy.

## CAUSES OF DIABETES

### Risk Factors for Type 1 Diabetes Mellitus

Type 1 DM is multifactorial. Genetic factors (susceptibility genes) predispose beta-cell damage through impaired defense, immune sensitivity, or a defect in tissue regeneration. Less than 10% of genetically susceptible persons actually develop type 1 DM. Diet and environment are chief factors in the onset.

- **Environmental and dietary risk factors:** abnormalities of gut immune system: poor protein digestion induces development of antibodies by the gastrointestinal (GI) immune system that attack beta-cells. Diet can modify the development of autoimmune DM. Absorbed whole proteins can trigger formation of antibodies. Antibodies cross-react with beta-cell antigens. Incriminated food proteins are in milk (bovine serum albumin and bovine insulin) and wheat (gluten). Antibodes may attack human insulin and activate T-killer cells to attack beta-cells. Breastfeeding helps optimize intestinal immunity, reducing type 1 DM risk, food allergies, and intestinal infection risk. Ingestion of cow's milk at any age may increase risk of type 1 DM. Gluten sensitivity produces celiac disease, another autoimmune disorder. Breastfeeding may be preventive; early introduction of cow's milk may be causative. Risk of type 1 DM is higher in children with celiac disease. Celiac patients have the highest level of antibodies to cow's milk proteins.
- **Factors that set the stage for autoimmunity in type 1 diabetes**: immune system usually develops tolerance to bovine insulin. Factors affecting autoimmunity response: gut microflora, breastfeeding, GI infections, nutritional status.
- **Enteroviruses and type 1 diabetes:** type 1 DM can arise from GI viral infection. Enteroviruses (polioviruses, coxsackieviruses, echoviruses) and rotavirus are common in children, can activate immune cells, and can infect beta-cells, triggering a white blood cell attack. GI virus infections may increase intestinal permeability. Small intestinal leaky gut during and after rotavirus infections exposes gut immune cells to intact protein.
- **Vitamin D deficiency**: cod liver oil vitamin D may be protective. Supplementation during early childhood can prevent type 1 DM. Protective dosage is 2000 IU daily. Children taking vitamin D from cod liver oil have an 80% reduced risk of type 1 DM; vitamin D–deficient children have a 300% increased risk. Vitamin D from cod liver oil during pregnancy reduces type 1 DM frequency. Lack of sun exposure during childhood may explain higher type 1 DM rates in Northern countries. Vitamin D helps normalize immune system development and inhibit autoimmune reactions against beta-cells.
- **Omega-3 fatty acid deficiency**: omega-3 fatty acids in cod liver and other fish oils are also protective. Compounds that generate free radicals (e.g., nitrosamines, alloxan) destroy beta-cells. Fish oil can prevent chemically induced type 1 DM by improving cell

membrane function, enhancing antioxidant status, and suppressing formation of inflammatory cytokines.

- **Nitrates**: the increase in nitrates in diet and water is linked to an increased rate for type 1 DM. Sources of nitrates include agricultural fertilizer runoff and cured and smoked meats. Nitrates are converted in the body into nitrosamines, which can cause DM. Infants and young children are particularly vulnerable. Nitrates in water may be a key factor in the 3% annual growth in type 1 DM. High-quality water purifiers are recommended.

## Early Treatment and Possible Reversal of Type 1 Diabetes Mellitus

Early intervention resolving autoimmunity or oxidation may slow or reverse the disease process.

- **Niacinamide (nicotinamide)**: may help prevent immune-mediated destruction of beta-cells and reverse disorder. It must be given soon enough at onset of DM to restore beta-cells or retard destruction. A dosage of 3 g niacinamide daily may prolong non-insulin-requiring remission, lower insulin requirements, improve metabolic control, and increase beta-cell function as determined by C-peptide secretion. Time-released niacinamide may not provide sufficient peak concentrations to block autoimmunity (e.g., cytokine production). Complete reversal in some patients makes its use worth the effort because no reasonable alternative is available. Dosage is based on body weight: 25-50 mg niacinamide per kilo (2.2 lb) of body weight to maximal dosage of 3 g q.d. in divided doses. No side effects were reported in type 1 DM clinical trials. It can harm the liver; monitor liver enzymes every 3 months.
- **Epicatechin**: bark from the Malabar kino tree (*Pterocarpus marsupium*) is used in India for DM. Epicatechin extract prevents beta-cell damage in rats. Epicatechin and crude extract of *Pterocarpus marsupium* can regenerate beta-cell function in diabetic animals. Green tea (*Camellia sinensis*) extract has a higher epicatechin content and broader range of beneficial effects. Green tea polyphenols have antiviral activity against rotavirus and enterovirus, suspected of causing type 1 DM. Dosage for children younger than 6 years is 50-150 mg; children 6-12 years, 100-200 mg; children >12 years and adults, 150-300 mg. Decaffeinated green tea extracts with a polyphenol content of 80% are preferred.

## Risk Factors for Type 2 Diabetes Mellitus

- **Obesity (excess body fat)**: 80% to 90% of type 2 diabetics are obese (body mass index >30). Abdominal adipocytes, engorged with fat, secrete resistin, leptin, tumor necrosis factor, and free fatty acids that dampen the effect of insulin, impair glucose use in skeletal muscle, promote liver gluconeogenesis, and impair beta-cell insulin release by pancreatic beta-cells. The increasing size of adipocytes reduces secretion of compounds (adiponectin) that improve insulin sensitivity, reduce inflammation, lower triglycerides, and inhibit atherosclerosis. Adipose is part of the endocrine system. Blood levels of adiponectin/adipohormone may predict type 2 DM. Increasing insulin resistance leads to compensatory increased insulin secretion to the point of beta-cell exhaustion or burn out.
- Family history: parent or sibling with type 2 DM
- Increased waist/hip ratio
- Increasing age beginning at age 45 years
- Race/ethnicity (African American, Hispanic, Native American/First Nation, Native Australian or New Zealander, Asian American, Pacific Islander)
- Impaired fasting glucose (IFG) or impaired glucose tolerance (IGT)
- History of gestational diabetes or delivery of infant larger than 9 lb
- Hypertension (blood pressure >140/90 mm Hg)
- Triglycerides >250 mg/dL
- Low adiponectin, elevated fasting insulin
- Polycystic ovary syndrome (adult women: overweight, acne, infertile)
- **Genetics of type 2 diabetes and obesity:** even with the strongest genetic predisposition, DM can be avoided in most cases. When DM-prone ethnic groups follow the traditional diet and lifestyle of their original culture, DM incidence is extremely low. These groups are simply sensitive to the Western lifestyle.
- **Diet, exercise, lifestyle, and diabetes risk:** type 2 DM is a disease of diet and lifestyle: lack of exercise, failure to eat whole plant foods, high intake of harmful fat, and obesity. Lifestyle changes alone are associated with a 58% reduced risk of developing DM in people with impaired glucose tolerance.
- **Glycemic index and glycemic load (GL)**: glycemic index is the numeric value expressing a rise of blood glucose after eating a

particular food. The standard of 100 applies to the ingestion of glucose itself. The insulin response matches blood sugar elevation. Glycemic index reflects the quality of carbohydrates, not the quantity of sugar to be metabolized. Glycemic index is not related to portion size. GL is calculated by amount of carbohydrate in a serving multiplied by the food's glycemic index (compared with glucose), then divided by 100. The higher the GL, the greater the stress on insulin. GL has a stronger link in predicting DM than glycemic index. A high-GL diet increases risk for heart disease because of lower high-density lipoprotein (HDL) and higher triglyceride levels. Increased DM and heart risk start at daily GL of 161. GL should not exceed 150 daily.

- **Fiber and glycemic index/GL**: inadequate dietary fiber increases DM risk. Fibers most beneficial to glycemic control are water-soluble forms (hemicelluloses, mucilages, gums, and pectin, as in legumes, oat bran, nuts, seeds, psyllium seed husks, pears, apples, most vegetables). They slow down digestion and absorption, preventing rapid glycemic rises, increasing tissue insulin sensitivity, and improving uptake of glucose by muscles and liver. Recommend 35+ g fiber daily from a variety of food sources, especially vegetables. Fiber supplements can also be used.
- **The wrong type of fats**: saturated fat and trans fats (hydrogenated vegetable oils, as in margarine, vegetable shortening) with relative insufficiency of monounsaturated and omega-3 fats. Cell membrane fluidity, affected by fatty acid composition, affects insulin binding to receptors. Monounsaturated fats (olive oil, nuts, nut oils) and omega-3 oils improve insulin action and protect against onset of type 2 DM. Eating nuts reduces risk of type 2 DM. Raw or lightly roasted and unsalted fresh nuts and seeds are preferred over commercially roasted and salted.
- **Low intake of antioxidants**: Cumulative free radical damage ages cells and contributes to type 2 DM. Fruits and vegetables (even dark green salads) improve glycemic control and reduce risk. Vitamins C and E and carotenes lower risk. Antioxidant deficits and lipid peroxides increase risk.
- **Free radicals**: type 2 diabetics have higher levels of reactive oxygen species (ROS) and reactive nitrogen species (RNS), which exhaust antioxidant mechanisms while damaging DNA, proteins, and membrane fatty acids. ROS, RNS, high blood glucose, and saturated fat activate inflammatory compounds (nuclear factor kappa B), increase insulin resistance and impair insulin secretion.

- **Lifestyle vs. drugs to prevent type 2 DM**: the benefits of drugs pale compared with the efficacy of diet and lifestyle changes.

## MONITORING THE DIABETIC PATIENT

- **Urine glucose monitoring**: kidneys conserve glucose until blood glucose reaches 180 mg/dL (10 mmol/L). A negative urine glucose means blood glucose since previous voiding has been <180 mg/dL. Urine testing is crude; it gives no indication of blood glucose below 180 mg/dL. It is worthless for severe hypoglycemia or hyperglycemia.
- **Urine ketone testing**: when fat is the primary source of energy, ketones are produced. High ketone level spills over into urine. In the diabetic, ketonuria occurs with severe deficits in insulin availability or activity. Examples: a patient with IDDM accidentally or purposefully fails to take insulin; or a diabetic is ill, injured, or is given high doses of cortisone-related drugs. Loss of insulin effect impairs glucose uptake and use of glucose. The result is hyperglycemia, fat burning for energy, and toxemia from acidic ketones, with severe dehydration from water loss caused by glycosuria. This state is the deadly medical emergency termed "diabetic ketoacidosis," necessitating intravenous (IV) insulin, IV fluids, and intensive care unit monitoring. Urine ketone testing is critical, especially in IDDM. Urine ketones (with hyperglycemia) may indicate impending or established ketoacidosis, requiring immediate intervention. Advise patients to test urine for ketones during acute illness; during severe stress, when blood glucose is consistently elevated (>300 mg/dL [16.7 mmol/L]), regularly during pregnancy; or in the presence of symptoms of ketoacidosis (nausea, vomiting, abdominal pain).
- **Self-monitoring of blood glucose**: glycemic control is the most important factor in the long-term risk of serious complications in type 1 and type 2 DM. Self-monitoring of blood glucose allows the patient to modify treatment to maintain glycemic control, detect hypoglycemia, adjust care to daily circumstances (food intake, exercise, stress, illness), detect and treat severe hyperglycemia, increase therapeutic compliance, and improve motivation from immediate feedback.
- **Optimal schedule for self-monitoring of blood glucose**
  —Awakening and just before each meal. Ideal before meals is <120 mg/dL (6.7 mmol/L).

**Optimal Range for Self-Monitored Blood Glucose***

| | |
|---|---|
| Fasting or before meals | 80-110 mg/dL (4.4-6.7 mmol/L) |
| Two hours after eating (postprandial) | <140 mg/dL (7.8 mmol/L) |
| At bedtime | 100-140 mg/dL (5.6-7.8 mmol/L) |

Whole blood values typically run 10 mg/dL (0.6 mmol/L) higher than serum values. To avoid confusing numbers, some home glucose monitoring kits, even those using whole blood samples, calibrate to serum levels. Check instruction manual to find out if kit is set up to determine whole blood or serum glucose levels.

*Slightly higher values may be acceptable in elderly or young children because of the higher risk of dangerous hypoglycemia.

—Two hours after each meal. Ideal 2 hours after meals is <140 mg/dL (7.7 mmol/L).

—Bedtime. Ideal at bedtime is <140 mg/dL (7.7 mmol/L).

- **Type 1 diabetes and self-monitoring of blood glucose**: all type 1 diabetics must frequently monitor blood glucose to make ongoing adjustments to insulin injections, diet, and exercise. Until recently, type 1 diabetics often were prescribed combinations of short- and medium-action or long-action insulin one to two times per day. Many diabetics monitored glucose infrequently, some less than once daily. Diabetics are now trained to maintain ideal levels 24/7 by intensive insulin therapy (IIT) plus frequent glycemic monitoring. Using rapid-acting and short-duration insulins, IIT involves either frequent injections of insulins (Humalog [Insulin Lispro] or Novolog [Insulin Aspart]) or an insulin pump (continuous electronic injection of very-short-acting insulins with extra boluses before meals). Rapid-acting, short-duration insulin allows timing and size of doses to be adjusted to daily events. Despite multiple injections (before meals and at bedtime) and glycemic testing six or more times daily, IIT allows greater freedom, higher quality of life, and superior glycemic control.
- **Type 2 diabetes and self-monitoring of blood glucose**: every type 2 diabetic must own a monitor and be intimately familiar with its use. Even if glucose is well controlled by diet, lifestyle, and supplements, they should monitor regularly. Type 2 NIDDM patients with good glucose control according to regular lab testing, including $A_1c$, should designate a day every 1-3 weeks as intensive glycemic measuring day. Check before breakfast (fasting), just before meals, 2 hours after meals, and before bed. Record measurements, diet, exercise, and supplements in a

journal to increase awareness of the effects of factors on blood glucose. Type 2 diabetics with poor control should monitor intensively each day and seek professional help to regain control. Diabetics in advanced stages, with diminished insulin secretion, may need IIT. Blood test for C-peptide estimates insulin output. IIT requires self-monitoring of blood glucose as frequently as type 1 diabetics (before and 2 hours after each meal). Advanced type 2 diabetics with diminished insulin production have less than normal C-peptide. Common intervention trend: one injection of new, very-long-acting insulin (insulin glargine [Lantus]) for smooth, continual 24-hour release plus diet and medication. With this regimen, self-monitoring should be done before and 2 hours after each meal.

- **C-Peptide determination:** assessing insulin secretion influences treatment, especially in a diabetic hoping to avoid or stop using insulin, and the type of pharmaceuticals and nutriceuticals likely to be effective. Pancreas manufactures proinsulin first. Enzymes snip off a piece of this proinsulin (C-peptide); both C-peptide and insulin are secreted. For type 2 diabetics with poor glycemic control, high or normal C-peptide confirms their pancreatic output and directs attention to insulin resistance and sensitivity. A patient with low C-peptide may need insulin replacement.

| C-Peptide Results | Interpretation |
|---|---|
| Normal | The insulin production is at normal level |
| Less than normal | A. Newly diagnosed type 1 diabetic<br>B. Chronic, long-term type 2 diabetic |
| Greater than normal | A. Newly diagnosed type 2 diabetic<br>B. Benign tumor of the pancreas; insulinoma (rare). |
| Undetectable | A. Chronic type 1 diabetic<br>B. Status postsurgical removal of pancreas (rare) |

- **Physician monitoring**: physician monitoring of diabetics by lab testing of glycemic control has a major positive impact on long-term health. The $A_1c$ test reflects average glycemic level over the preceding 3 months. $A_1c$ correlates to risk for complications. Ideal is $A_1c \leq 6\%$. $A_1C < 7$ still indicates much lower risk. Test all diabetics, types 1 and 2, for $A_1c$ every 3 to 4 months, depending on stability of status.

## Clinical Management of the Patient With Diabetes

| | Quarterly | Annually |
|---|---|---|
| **Review Management Plan** | | |
| Blood glucose self-monitoring results | X | |
| Medication/insulin regimen | X | |
| Nutritional plan | X | |
| Exercise program | X | |
| Psychosocial support | X | |
| **Physical Examination** | | |
| Weight | X | |
| Height (for child/adolescent) | X | |
| Sexual maturation (for child/adolescent) | X | |
| Skin, including insulin injection sites | X | |
| Feet: pulses, capillary refill, color, sensation, nails, skin, ulcers | X | |
| Neurologic: reflexes, proprioception, vibratory sensation, touch (distal temperature sensation, distal pinprick or pressure sensation, standardized monofilament) | | X |
| Regular retinal exam | X | |
| Dilated retinal exam | | X |
| Electrocardiogram | | X |
| **Laboratory Tests** | | |
| Fasting or random plasma glucose: normal/ target range 80-120 mg/dL before meals | X | |
| Hgb $A_1$c: target range <7% in adults, <7.5% in children | X | |
| Urinalysis: glucose, ketones, microalbumin, protein, sediment | X | |
| Complete cardiovascular profile:<br>Cholesterol <200 mg/dL<br>Triglycerides <200 mg/dL<br>LDL <130 mg/dL<br>HDL >35 mg/dL<br>Lipoprotein(a) <40 mg/dL<br>C-reactive protein <1.69 mg/L<br>Fibrinogen <400 mg/L<br>Homocysteine <16 μmol/L<br>Ferritin 60 to 200 μg/L (if elevated—transferrin saturation, if elevated genetic testing for hemochromatosis)<br>Lipid peroxides <normal | | X |
| Serum creatinine (in adults; in children, do only if protein is present in urine) | X | |

## COMPLICATIONS OF DIABETES

Risk of complications is a reflection of glucose control; good glucose control greatly reduces risk; monitoring and controlling hyperglycemia are critical to preventing complications.

### Acute Complications

- **Hypoglycemia**: in type 1 DM from taking too much insulin, missing a meal, or overexercising; "brittle" type 1; or any diabetic on insulin or sulfonylurea who neglects monitoring. Daytime hypoglycemic symptoms: sweating, nervousness, tremor, and hunger. Nighttime hypoglycemia may be asymptomatic or display night sweats, unpleasant dreams, or early morning headache.
- **Diabetic ketoacidosis**: in poorly controlled or untreated type 1. Hypoinsulinemia allows extreme hyperglycemia and ketoacidosis, which can cause coma or death. Because ketoacidosis is a medical emergency, prompt recognition is imperative. The coma usually is preceded by a day or more of increased urination and thirst as well as marked fatigue and nausea and vomiting. A simple urine dipstick can be used at home by diabetics to measure the level of ketones in the urine. This procedure should be done during illness or severe stress. A mistake occasionally made by inexperienced medical personnel is to avoid giving insulin to a type 1 diabetic because the person is fasting before surgery. This mistake also can be made at home by a misinformed diabetic when he or she is too sick too eat. Generally the stress of illness or surgery is sufficient to drive blood glucose up even when no food is taken. This is because the stress hormones cortisol and epinephrine result in a massive release of glucose from the liver and muscles and usual insulin doses are generally required.
- **Nonketogenic hyperosmolar hyperglycemia**: in type 2 DM with some insulin production or in type 1 DM on inadequate insulin for acute situation. It evolves over days with severe dehydration and electrolyte (sodium, potassium) disturbance. If comatose, mortality rate is >50%. Cause is profound dehydration from deficient fluid intake or precipitating events (pneumonia, burns, stroke, recent surgery, certain drugs [phenytoin, diazoxide, glucocorticoids, and diuretics]). Onset is insidious over period of days or weeks; symptoms include weakness, polyuria and thirst, and worsening signs of dehydration (weight loss, loss of skin elasticity, dry mucous membranes, tachycardia, hypotension).

This condition is completely preventable by regular monitoring during illness or stress.

## Long-Term Complications

More common than acute complications are long-term ones. Contributing factors include the following:

- **Poor glucose control**: glycemic control reduces risk of complications—retinopathy (up to 76%), nephropathy (up to 56%), neuropathy (up to 60%). Keep Hgb-$A_1$c at 7.0% or less.
- **Glycosylation of proteins**: changing structure and function of proteins deactivates enzymes, inhibits regulatory molecule binding, and forms abnormal protein structures. Glucose binds to low-density lipoprotein (LDL), blocking its binding to liver receptors that signal cessation of cholesterol synthesis. Antioxidants, such as vitamins C and E, flavonoids, and alpha-lipoic acid, help reduce glycosylation.
- **Sorbitol accumulation**: sorbitol is a sugar molecule formed from glucose within cells. In nondiabetics, sorbitol is quickly converted into fructose to allow excretion from the cell. Intracellular sorbitol accumulation creates an osmotic effect that forces damaging leakage of amino acids, inositol, glutathione, niacin, vitamin C, magnesium, and potassium. These losses increase susceptibility to damage. Sorbitol buildup is a major cause of complications. Ascorbate and flavonoids (quercetin, grapeseed extract, and bilberry extract) help lower intracellular sorbitol.
- **Oxidative damage**: elevated free radicals and oxidative compounds destroy cellular compounds and increase inflammatory mediators (C-reactive protein).
- **Nutrient deficiency**: risk of complications is inversely proportional to micronutrient status. Symptoms of deficiency can mimic long-term complication of diabetes. (Vitamin $B_{12}$ deficiency or dysmetabolism causes numbness, pins and needles sensation, or a burning feeling in the hands and/or feet—virtually identical to DM neuropathy.)
- **Homocysteine**: elevation is an independent risk factor for cardiocerebrovascular disease. In DM, homocysteine is linked to retinopathy.
- **Hypertension**: more than half of all diabetics have hypertension. A single layer of endothelial cells lining all blood vessels acts as the interface between blood components and blood vessels that regulates blood flow, coagulation, and formation of compounds

controlling blood pressure. These cells are damaged by oxidized LDL and free radicals.

## Specific Complications

- **Atherosclerosis**: major feature in many chronic complications. Diabetics have a two to three times higher risk of dying prematurely of atherosclerosis than do nondiabetics; 55% of deaths in diabetics are caused by cardiovascular disease. Lesions in microvasculature reduce oxygen and nutrients supply to nerves, the eyes, kidneys.
- **Diabetic retinopathy**: leading cause of blindness in the United States between ages 20 and 64 years. The retina is damaged by microhemorrhages, scarring, and glycosylation of proteins. Within 20 years of diagnosis, 80% of type 1 and 20% of type 2 diabetics have significant retinopathy. Diabetics are prone to cataracts.
- **Diabetic neuropathy**: loss of peripheral nerve function with tingling, numbness, loss of function, and burning pain (neuropathic pain). First comes a loss of sensation in the hands and feet ("stoking glove" neuropathy). Progressing deeper to autonomic nerves disturbs stomach emptying, heart function, alternating diarrhea and constipation, and inability to empty the bladder. Impotence is a common effect caused by damage to microvasculature of penis and neuropathy of autonomic nerves controlling penile blood flow. Sixty percent of diabetics eventually develop neuropathy.
- **Diabetic nephropathy**: 40% of cases of severe nephropathosis and most common reason for hemodialysis and kidney transplant. It is a leading cause of death in DM. Monitor kidney function by lab tests: microalbuminuria, 24-hour urine protein, blood urea nitrogen (BUN), uric acid, creatinine, creatinine clearance.
- **Poor wound healing and foot ulcers**: poor wound healing and foot ulcers are common. Microvascular damage impairs circulation, causing functional deficiency of vitamin C and immune dysfunction that allows chronic foot infections. Fifty percent of lower limb amputations in the United States (70,000 yearly) are the result of DM foot ulcers.
- **Immune system dysfunction**: begins long before DM diagnosis. Recurrent vaginal or skin yeast infection is the clue. Serious infections or complications of simple infections are a risk, such as secondary pneumonia during influenza. Chronic, hidden infections induce cardiovascular disease. C-reactive protein is often elevated from oral, respiratory, or blood infections.

- **Depression and cognitive difficulties**: are common in diabetics. Depression may begin decades before onset of type 2 DM. Brain is sensitive to glycemic levels and may suffer from deprivation linked to insulin resistance. Depression is common in the overweight and obese because of insulin resistance and diminished self-esteem. Cognitive changes begin after severe hypoglycemic episodes stressful to the brain; repeated severe hypoglycemia can cause cognitive impairment. Glycemic awareness training with frequent monitoring and new insulins can optimize control.

## THERAPEUTIC CONSIDERATIONS

- **Diet therapy**: strictly avoid foods with a high glycemic load. Rigorous sugar and starch discipline is required for glycemic and $A_1c$ control. Achieve and maintain ideal body weight. Initially, GL may need to be no more than 20 per meal; space these meals 3 hours apart. High-fiber, low-GL diets are beneficial in both adults and children and in both type 1 and type 2 DM. Similar results occur in adults with type 1 DM, including pregnant women with type 1 DM. Low glycemic index/GL diet is the most scientifically proven dietary support for type 1 DM. Diet alone can be effective as the sole intervention to treat and reverse type 2 DM. Treating type 2 begins with diet. A low glycemic index/GL diet has the most scientifically proven benefit on blood sugar and DM sequelae, including cardiovascular risk and hypertension. Key goal: increase total fiber intake from foods to 50+ g daily, especially soluble type.
- **Psychological support**: help patient deal with the diagnosis, develop a sense of empowerment, and make lifestyle changes. Cognitive therapy is effective for adolescents with type 1 DM, improving mood and glycemic control.
- **Stress management**: higher stress is linked to higher blood glucose in type 1 and type 2 DM. Stress response increases adrenaline and cortisol, which elevate blood sugar and blunt insulin response. Implement stress management such as relaxation training.
- **Exercise**: exercise is essential to prevent and manage DM and pre-DM states of glucose intolerance and syndrome X. Insulin sensitivity and glycemic control improve because of increased lean muscle mass and metabolism. Cardiovascular health, HDL, anxiety, depression, sexual function, confidence, self-esteem, and

weight management improve. Types of exercises for DM: aerobic (walking, jogging, dancing, cycling, swimming), strength training (light to moderate weights three times weekly), and stretching (daily).

## Nutritional and Herbal Supplements

**Objectives**: achieve ideal glycemic control and metabolic targets; reduce risk of complications. (1) Establish optimal nutrient status, (2) reduce postprandial glucose elevations, (3) improve insulin function and sensitivity, and (4) prevent nutritional and oxidative stress. Treatment requires careful integration of diet, lifestyle, and natural medicines. All type 1 and many type 2 diabetics require conventional treatments depending on adequacy of pancreatic output (C-peptide) and response to diet and lifestyle measures. The most important factor determining need for drugs and insulin is glycemic control.

**Establish optimal nutritional status**: nutrient-dense diet plus high-potency multiple vitamin/mineral supplement to improve glycemic control, reduce complications, and boost immune function. Special supplements include:

- **Chromium (Cr)**: component of glucose tolerance factor that works closely with insulin, facilitating glucose uptake into cells. Cr deficiency is a factor in DM, hypoglycemia, and obesity. Supplementing Cr decreases fasting glucose, improves glucose tolerance, lowers insulin, and decreases total cholesterol and triglycerides while increasing HDL. Reversing Cr deficiency lowers body weight and increases lean body mass. Its effects are from increased insulin sensitivity. Cr produces meaningful improvements in glycemic control only in people who are Cr deficient. Cr has no recommended daily allowance (RDA), but at least 200 μg q.d. is necessary for optimal sugar regulation. Diabetics should take 200-400 μg q.d. Cr is depleted by refining of carbohydrates and lack of exercise. Cr polynicotinate, Cr picolinate, and Cr-enriched yeast are preferred.
- **Vitamin C**: insulin enhances transport of vitamin C into cells. Many diabetics have intracellular deficiency despite usually adequate intake. Diabetics need extra ascorbate. A major function of vitamin C is the manufacture of collagen, the main protein substance of connective tissue. Vitamin C is vital for wound repair,

healthy gums, excess bruising prevention, immune function, manufacture of certain neurotransmitters and hormones, and absorption and utilization of other nutritional factors. Chronic latent vitamin C deficiency causes increased bleeding tendency (increased capillary permeability), poor wound healing, microvascular disease, elevated cholesterol, and depressed immune function. Ascorbate reduces generation of compounds linked to DM complications, reduces hypertension, and improves arterial stiffness and blood flow. Doses ranging from 100-2000 mg q.d. reduce accumulation of sorbitol in red blood cells (RBCs) of diabetics, independent of glycemic control, by inhibiting aldose reductase, the enzyme that converts glucose to sorbitol. It also inhibits glycosylation of proteins. Encourage vitamin C–rich foods that also contain flavonoids and carotenes, which enhance effects of vitamin C. Dietary sources of vitamin C include broccoli, peppers, potatoes, Brussels sprouts, and citrus fruits.

- **Vitamin E**: antioxidant protecting cell membranes, especially nerve cells. Vitamin E improves insulin action, prevents free radical damage to LDL and vascular lining, improves the functioning of blood vessels and endothelium, increases intracellular magnesium, decreases C-reactive protein (biomarker of inflammation), increases glutathione (intracellular antioxidant), improves nerve impulse conduction, improves blood flow to eyes in diabetic retinopathy, improves kidney function, and normalizes creatinine clearance in diabetics with mild elevations. Diabetics require lifelong supplementation. Dosage: 400-800 IU daily.
- **Niacin and niacinamide (nicotinamide)**: niacin (vitamin $B_3$)-containing enzymes are important in energy production; metabolism of fat, cholesterol, and carbohydrate; and the synthesis of many body compounds (sex and adrenal hormones). Niacin is an essential component of glucose tolerance factor. Niacinamide supplements may prevent type 1 DM and help restore beta-cells or at least slow their destruction. Niacinamide prolongs non-insulin-requiring remission, lowers insulin, improves metabolic control, and increases beta-cell function. Niacinamide can induce complete resolution in some newly diagnosed type 1 diabetics. The main difference between positive and negative studies in recent-onset IDDM is older age and higher baseline fasting C-peptide in positive studies. The mechanism of action is inhibition of macrophage- and interleukin-1-mediated beta-cell damage, inhibition of nitric oxide production, and antioxidant activity.

Niacinamide (500 mg t.i.d.) improves C-peptide release and glycemic control in type 2 diabetics unresponsive to oral antihyperglycemic drugs alone. The daily dose of niacinamide is 25 mg/kg. Children use 100-200 mg q.d. Niacin lowers cholesterol safely and extends life.

- **Inositol hexaniacinate**: useful in type 1 and type 2 DM to lower hyperlipidemia. It lowers cholesterol and improves blood flow in intermittent claudication and improves sugar regulation and is much better tolerated than niacin. High-dose niacin can disrupt glucose control in diabetics; closely monitor glucose and discontinue if worsening of diabetic control.
- **Vitamin $B_6$**: supplements protect against diabetic neuropathy. Vitamin $B_6$ inhibits glycosylation of proteins. Diabetics tend to be deficient in $B_6$. Longstanding DM or signs of peripheral nerve abnormalities indicate need for $B_6$. At 100 mg q.d., it is a safe and effective treatment for gestational diabetes. Dosage in general is up to 150 mg q.d.
- **Magnesium (Mg)**: Mg deficiency is common in diabetics and lowest in those with severe retinopathy. Mg may prevent DM retinopathy and heart disease. Mg (at 400-500 mg q.d.) improves insulin response and action, glucose tolerance, and fluidity of RBC membranes. RDA is 350 mg q.d. for men and 300 mg q.d. for women. Diabetics may need twice this amount. Emphasize dietary sources: tofu, legumes, seeds, nuts, whole grains, green leafy vegetables. Add 300-500 mg of Mg q.d. as aspartate or citrate. Supplement at least 25 mg $B_6$ q.d. and vitamin E to ensure entry of Mg into cells.
- **Zinc (Zn)**: cofactor in 200 enzyme systems and involved in all aspects of insulin metabolism. Marginal deficiency is common in the elderly and diabetics, increasing susceptibility to infections, poor wound healing, diminished sense of taste or smell, skin disorders, and onset of DM. Zn is protective against beta-cell destruction and has antiviral effects. Diabetics excrete Zn excessively in urine. Supplements improve insulin levels in type 1 and type 2 DM. Sources: whole grains, legumes, nuts, and seeds. Dose for diabetics is 30 mg q.d.
- **Manganese (Mn)**: cofactor in many enzymes of glucose control, energy metabolism, thyroid hormone function, and antioxidant enzyme superoxide dismutase. Mn deficiency in lab animals results in DM and offspring with pancreatic abnormalities or no pancreas at all. Diabetics have only half the Mn of normal persons. Daily dose for diabetics is 3-5 mg.

- **Biotin**: functions in manufacture and utilization of carbohydrates, fats, and amino acids. Biotin deficiency impairs sugar metabolism. It is synthesized in intestines by gut bacteria; vegetarian diet alters intestinal flora to enhance synthesis and promote absorption of biotin. Supplements enhance insulin sensitivity and increase activity of glucokinase, the enzyme in the first step of utilization of glucose by the liver. Glucokinase is low in diabetics. Dosage of 16 mg biotin q.d. significantly lowers fasting glucose and improves glucose control in type 1 DM; in type 2 DM, similar effects occur at 9 mg biotin q.d. Biotin also helps treat diabetic neuropathy. Insulin use must be adjusted.
- **Omega-3 fatty acids from fish**: protect against heart disease in DM. At doses of 3 to 18 g/day (18% eicosapentaenoic acid [EPA]/12% docosahexaenoic acid [DHA]), fish oil has no adverse effect on glycemic control. Insist on pharmaceutical-grade products that do not elevate LDL. Take fish oil at or near beginning of meals to avoid fishy aftertaste or burping. Combined total omega-3 supplemention should be 600-1200 mg q.d.
- **Fiber supplements**: enhance glycemic control, decrease insulin, and reduce calories absorbed from food. To reduce postprandial glucose, lower cholesterol, and promote weight loss, choose water-soluble fibers: glucomannan (from konjac root), psyllium, guar gum, defatted fenugreek seed powder, seaweed fibers (alginate and carrageenan), ground flaxseed, and pectin. With water, they form a gelatinous, viscous mass, which slows absorption of glucose, reduces calorie absorption, and induces satiety. Glucomannan has greatest viscosity, which is enhanced when combined with alginate and xanthum gum. Viscosity of soluble fiber is directly related to physiologic effects and benefits: decreased postprandial gylcemia, increased insulin sensitivity, diminished appetite, weight control, improved bowel movements, and decreased cholesterol. Glucomannan lowers postprandial glucose by 20% and insulin secretion by 40% and produces whole-body insulin sensitivity index improvement of 50%, which is unequalled by any drug or natural product. Glucomannan-alginate-xanthum gum blend improves all aspects of syndrome X.
- **Natural glucosidase inhibitors**: alpha-glucosidases that line intestines to breakdown carbohydrates into absorbable glucose. Inhibiting these enzymes can diminish postprandial glucose and insulin. The drugs acarbose (Precose) and miglitol (Glyset) inhibit alpha-glucosidase but have side effects: flatulence, diarrhea, and

abdominal discomfort. Superior natural alternatives are touchi or mulberry extract.

- **Touchi**: ancient Asian fermented soy product concentrated for alpha-glucosidase inhibitors. In type 2 diabetics, 300 mg touchi extract before each meal for 6 months reduced fasting glucose by 10+ mg/dL in 80% of patients and Hgb $A_1c$ by 0.5+% in 60% of patients. It also mildly lowered triglycerides and cholesterol. No side effects have been observed and no GI complaints were noted.
- **Mulberry plant (*Morus indica*)**: food for silkworms that has an alpha-glucosidase inhibitor and other compounds that improve glycemic control. At a dose of 3 g/day versus one tablet of glyburide (5 mg/day) for 4 weeks, mulberry lowers fasting glucose 27% in diabetics; no significant differences were observed in the blood glucose between before and after glyburide. Mulberry acts as an antioxidant, reducing lipid peroxidation in RBC membranes, and decreases membrane cholesterol of type 2 diabetics. Mulberry is superior to glyburide.

## Improve Insulin Function and Sensitivity

**Achieve ideal body weight**: follow dietary and lifestyle recommendations, including high-potency vitamin/mineral supplement. As needed, add one or combination of the following:

- ***Gymnema sylvestre***: plant native to tropical forests of India that is effective in types 1 and 2 DM. It enhances production or activity of insulin and promotes regeneration of pancreas beta-cells. In type 1 DM, leaf extract reduces insulin requirements and fasting glucose and improves glycemic control. It improves glycemic control in type 2 DM, reducing hypoglycemic drug needs. Applied to the tongue, gymnemic acid blocks sensation of sweetness. Subjects who had *Gymnema* applied to the tongue ate fewer calories at meals compared with control subjects. Capsules or tablets do not produce the same effect. Dosage: 200 mg (standardized to 24% gymnemic acid) b.i.d. No side effects reported; diabetics on insulin must monitor blood glucose because insulin dosages may have to be decreased.
- ***Momordica charantia* (bitter melon, balsam pear)**: charantin is hypoglycemic constituent composed of mixed steroids more potent than the drug tolbutamide. Insulinlike constituent polypeptide, polypeptide-P, lowers blood glucose when injected subcutaneously like insulin into type 1 diabetics, with fewer side

effects than insulin. Fresh juice and extract of unripe fruit lower blood sugar in clinical trials. Dosage: 2 oz fresh juice.

- ***Panax quinquefolium* and *Panax ginseng***: American ginseng is the most evidenced-based herbal therapy for type 2 DM. Whole powdered American ginseng root at 3 g before each meal reduces postprandial glucose in type 2 DM. Panax ginseng at 200 mg elevates mood, improves psychophysiologic performance, and reduces fasting glucose and body weight. It also improves Hgb $A_1c$, serum aminoterminalpropeptide concentrations, and physical activity.
- **Fenugreek seeds (*Trigonella foenum-graecum*)**: active principles are special soluble fiber, alkaloid trigonelline, and 4-hydroxyisoleucine. It is helpful in types 1 and 2. Defatted seed powder at 50 g b.i.d. in type 1 DM reduces fasting glucose and improves glucose tolerance, with 54% reduction in 24-hour urinary glucose excretion and significant reductions in LDL, VLDL, and triglycerides. In type 2 diabetics, 15 g powdered seed soaked in water significantly reduced postprandial glucose during meal tolerance test. Type 2 diabetics on 1 g/day fenugreek seed extract for 2 months had improved blood glucose (fasting glucose dropped from 148.3 to 119.9 mg/dL) but with decreased insulin output, indicating improved insulin sensitivity. This effect is most likely attributable to 4-hydroxyleucine.
- ***Allium cepa* and *Allium sativum***: Onions and garlic have blood sugar–lowering action. The active principles are sulfur-containing compounds allyl propyl disulfide (APDS) and diallyl disulfide oxide (allicin), respectively. Flavonoids may play a role. APDS lowers glucose by competing with insulin (also a disulfide) for insulin-inactivating sites in the liver, thereby increasing free insulin. ADPS in doses of 125 mg/kg given to fasting human beings drops blood glucose and increases serum insulin. Allicin at doses of 100 mg/kg has similar effect. Graded doses of onion extracts (1 mL of extract = 1 g whole onion) at levels found in diet (1-7 oz onion) reduce glucose in dose-dependent manner. Effects are similar in raw and boiled onion extracts; they also lower cholesterol and blood pressure. Garlic improves glycemic control, lowers cholesterol and blood pressure, and inhibits increases in fibrinogen.

## Preventing Nutritional and Oxidative Stress

Diabetics have elevated damaging, proinflammatory free radicals and oxidative compounds. Flood the body with antioxidants to counteract negative effects of free radicals and pro-oxidants. Use flavonoid-rich extracts and alpha-lipoic acid.

- **Flavonoids**: Quercetin promotes insulin secretion and inhibits glycosylation and sorbitol accumulation. Bilberry and hawthorn extracts help diabetic retinopathy and microvascular abnormalities. Flavonoids increase intracellular vitamin C, decrease leakiness and breakage of small blood vessels, prevent easy bruising, promote wound healing, and provide immune system support. Sources: citrus fruits, berries, onions, parsley, legumes, green tea,

**Flavonoids for Diabetes and Diabetic Complications**

| Flavonoid-Rich Extract | Daily Dose | Indication |
|---|---|---|
| Bilberry extract (25% anthocyanidins) | 160-320 mg | Best choice in diabetic retinopathy or cataracts. |
| *Ginkgo biloba* extract (24% ginkgo flavonglycosides) | 120-240 mg | Best choice for most people older than 50 years. Protects brain and vascular lining. Very important in improving blood flow to the extremities, neuropathy, and foot ulcers. |
| Grapeseed extract or pine bark extract (95% procyanidolic oligomers) | 150-300 mg | Systemic antioxidant; best choice for most people younger than 50 years especially if retinopathy, hypertension, easy bruising, and poor wound healing are present. Also specific for the lungs, varicose veins, and protection against cardiovascular disease. |
| Green tea extract (60%-70% total polyphenols) | 150-300 mg | Best choice in the early stage of type 1 diabetes or a family history of cancer. |
| Hawthorn extract (10% procyanidins) | 150-300 mg | Best choice in cardiovascular disease or hypertension. |
| Milk thistle extract (70% silymarin) | 100-300 mg | Best choice if showing signs of impaired liver function. |
| Mixed citrus flavonoids | 1000-2000 mg | Least expensive choice but may not provide same level of benefit. Acceptable if no complication is present. |
| Quercetin | 150-300 mg | Good choice if allergies, symptoms of prostate enlargement or bladder irritation, or eczema is also present. |

red wine. Tissue affinity of flavonoids allows targeting of specific tissues. Identify most appropriate flavonoids for specific patient needs.

- **Alpha-lipoic acid**: vitamin-like substance termed "nature's perfect antioxidant." It is efficiently absorbed, easily crosses cell membranes, quenches both water- and fat-soluble free radicals within cells and in intracellular spaces, and extends biochemical life of other antioxidants. It is an approved drug in Germany for diabetic neuropathy. Dosage: 300-600 mg q.d. It improves glucose metabolism, improves blood flow to peripheral nerves, stimulates regeneration of nerve fibers, and increases insulin sensitivity.

## Recommendations for Specific Long-Term Complications

The most important method for reducing risk of complications is achieving optimal glycemic control.

- **Elevated cholesterol**: key natural products are soluble fiber, garlic, and niacin (see chapter on atherosclerosis). Niacin at higher dosages (3000+ mg q.d.) can impair glucose tolerance, but lower dosages (1000 to 2000 mg q.d.) have not adversely affected glucose regulation. Niacin addresses all of the most common blood lipid abnormalities in type 2 DM—elevated triglycerides, decreased HDL, and preponderance of smaller, denser LDL particles—better than lipid-lowering drugs. Side effects of niacin: skin flushing, gastric irritation, nausea, liver damage. To reduce flushing, use time-released formulas at bedtime or inositol hexaniacinate. Some people only respond to regular niacin. Dosage for regular niacin or inositol hexaniacinate: start with 500 mg at bedtime for 1 week; increase to 1000 mg the next week and 1500 mg the following week. Stay at 1500 mg for 2 months before checking the response. Adjust dosing up or down depending on response. Dose time-release niacin at 1500 mg at bedtime from the beginning. Check cholesterol, $A_1c$, and liver function every 3 months.
- **Retinopathy and cataracts**: Two forms: simple (bursting of blood vessels, hemorrhage, swelling) and proliferative (newly formed vessels, scarring, hemorrhage, retinal detachment). Laser photocoagulation treats proliferative retinopathy but is not indicated in milder forms. Key factor in prevention: maintaining optimal glycemic control. Monitor Hgb A1c frequently. Use flavonoid-rich extracts that have affinity for blood vessels of the eye and improve circulation to the retina (bilberry, pine bark, grapeseed).

- **Neuropathy**: Alpha-lipoic acid and Mg are important.
  —Gamma-linolenic acid (GLA) improves and prevents neuropathy. GLA bypasses disturbances in fatty acid conversion. Sources: borage, evening primrose, black currant oils. GLA at 480 mg/day for 1 year improved 16 parameters, including conduction velocities, hot and cold thresholds, sensation, tendon reflexes, and muscle strength, with better results among patients with better glucose control.
  —Capsaicin from cayenne pepper (*Capsicum frutescens*) blocks small pain nerve fibers by depleting substance P. Topical capsaicin relieves pain of neuropathy in 80% of patients. Apply over-the-counter 0.075% capsaicin cream b.i.d. to affected area. (Cover hand with plastic wrap to avoid capsaicin contacting eyes or mucous membranes.) Allow a few days to take effect. It will only continue to work with regular application.
- **Nephropathy**: high-protein diets strain kidneys forced to excrete more waste—nitrogenous byproducts of protein metabolism (ammonia and urea). A low-protein diet is required only for progressed nephropathy, but it is wise to modulate protein intake. Dietary water-soluble fibers are fermented by colon bacteria into short chain fatty acids that fuel colonic cells and increase waste removal capabilities of the colon, acting as a "third kidney" collecting and excreting nitrogenous wastes from the blood. Vitamin C (1250 mg) and vitamin E (680 IU) q.d. for 4 weeks reduces elevated urinary albumin by 20% in type 2 diabetics, indicating retardation of nephropathy progression. Normalize blood pressure with drugs (angiotensin-converting enzyme (ACE) inhibitors and ACE receptor blockers in low doses) if necessary.
- **Poor wound healing**: any nutrient deficiency can impair wound healing. Key nutrients: vitamin C and zinc. Use high-potency multiple vitamin mineral formulas. Topical: pure (100%) aloe vera gel, which contains vitamins C and E and zinc. Apply it to affected areas (not open wounds) b.i.d. or t.i.d.
- **Foot ulcers**: causative factors: lack of blood supply, poor wound healing, and peripheral neuropathy. Strategies: proper foot care—care of nails and calluses by podiatrist, regular physician exams of feet, avoiding injury, avoiding tobacco, improving local circulation. Keep feet clean, dry, warm. Wearing well-fitted shoes. Support circulation with regular exercise; avoid sitting with legs crossed or positions that compromise circulation; massage feet lightly upwards. *Ginkgo biloba* and grapeseed extract support circulation.

## THERAPEUTIC APPROACH

Although the information here has focused on type 2 DM, it is equally appropriate for type 1, with the exception that the type 1 diabetic will always require insulin.

- **Step 1:** Thorough diagnostic work-up. Investigate DM complications, diet, environment, lifestyle issues, glucose intolerance. Stay alert to early signs/symptoms of acidosis and hyperosmolar non-ketogenic coma and have patient hospitalized at the first signs.
- **Step 2:** Develop individualized diet, exercise, supplement program. Normalize weight.
- **Step 3:** Monitor carefully, especially if on insulin—symptoms, home glucose monitoring, HgbA1c. Alter drug dosing via prescribing doctor as therapies take effect,

**Note:** Under no circumstances should a patient suddenly stop taking diabetic drugs, especially insulin. According to current information, an IDDM patient will never be able to stop taking insulin.

- **Diet:** optimal health food diet. Avoid simple, processed and concentrated sugars and starches. Stress high fiber foods. Minimize fats. Encourage legumes, onions, garlic.
- **Supplementation for IDDM:** dependent on degree of glycemic control: self-monitored blood glucose and HgbA$_1$C levels.

### Recently Diagnosed Type 1 Diabetes Mellitus

- **Foundation supplements**
  —High-potency multiple vitamin/mineral
  —Fish oils: 600 mg combined EPA/DHA q.d.
  —Vitamin C: 500 to 1500 mg q.d.
  —Vitamin E: 400 to 800 IU q.d. (mixed tocopherols)
- **Niacinamide:** 25 to 50 mg per kg body weight
- **Green tea extract** (80% polyphenol, decaffeinated): children younger than 6 years: 50 to 150 mg; children aged 6 to 12 years: 100 to 200 mg; children older than 12 years and adults: 150 to 300 mg.
- **Level 1:** achieved target glucose levels, A$_1$C <7%, no lipid abnormalities, no complications.
  —Foundation supplements
  High-potency multiple vitamin/mineral
  Fish oils: 600 mg of combined EPA/DHA q.d.

Vitamin C: 500 to 1500 mg q.d.
Vitamin E: 400 to 800 IU q.d. (mixed tocopherols)

- **Level 2:** failure to achieve target glucose, $A_1C$ at 7% to 8%.
  —Foundation supplements
  —*Gymnema sylvestre* extract (24% gymnemic acid): 200 mg b.i.d.
  —Biotin: 8 mg b.i.d.
  —Optional: bitter melon juice: 2 to 4 oz. q.d.
- **Level 3:** failure to achieve target glucose levels, $A_1C$ 8% to 9%.
  —Foundation supplements.
  —*Gymnema sylvestre* extract (24% gymnemic acid): 200 mg b.i.d.
  —Biotin: 8 mg b.i.d.
  —Glucomannan (or other soluble source at equivalent dosage): 1000 mg before meals
  —Optional: bitter melon juice: 2 to 4 oz q.d.
- **Level 4:** failure to achieve target glucose levels, $A_1C > 9\%$.
  —Foundation supplements.
  —*Gymnema sylvestre* extract (24% gymnemic acid): 200 mg b.i.d.
  —Biotin: 8 mg b.i.d.
  —Glucomannan (or other soluble source at equivalent dosage): 1,000 mg before meals.
  —Glucosidase inhibitor: either touchi extract (300 mg t.i.d. with meals) or mulberry extract (equivalent to 1000 mg dried leaf t.i.d.)
  —Optional: bitter melon juice: 2 to 4 oz. q.d.

If self-monitored glucose levels do not improve after 4 weeks of following recommendations for current level, move to next higher level. If glucose and $A_1C$ do not reach targets with Level 4 support, either oral drug or insulin is required.

### Supplementation for Type 2 Diabetes Mellitus

Dependent on degree of glycemic control: self-monitored blood glucose and $A_1C$.

- **Level 1:** achieved target glucose and $A_1C$ <7%, no lipid abnormalities, no complications.
  —Foundation supplements
  High-potency multiple vitamin/mineral
  Greens drink: one serving q.d.
  Fish oils: 600 mg combined EPA/DHA q.d.

Vitamin C: 500 to 1500 mg q.d.
Vitamin E: 400 to 800 IU q.d. (mixed tocopherols)

- **Level 2:** failure to achieve target glucose, $A_1C$ 7% to 8%.
  —Foundation supplements.
  —Glucomannan (or other soluble source at equivalent dosage): 1000 mg before meals.
- **Level 3:** failure to achieve target glucose, $A_1C$ 8% to 9%.
  —Foundation supplements
  —Glucomannan (or other soluble source at equivalent dosage): 1000 mg before meals.
  —Insulin enhancer: either gymnema sylvestre extract (24% gymnemic acid) (200 mg b.i.d.) or fenugreek extract (1 g q.d.)
  —Garlic: 4000+ µg allicin q.d.
- **Level 4:** failure to achieve target glucose, $A_1C$ > 9%.
  —Foundation supplements
  —Glucomannan (or other soluble source at equivalent dosage): 1000 mg before meals
  —Insulin enhancer: either *Gymnema sylvestre* extract (24% gymnemic acid) (200 mg b.i.d.) or fenugreek extract (1 g q.d.)
  —Garlic: 4000+ µg allicin q.d.
  —Glucosidase inhibitor: either touchi extract (300 mg t.i.d. with meals) or mulberry extract (equivalent to 1000 mg dried leaf t.i.d.)

If self-monitored glucose levels do not improve after 4 weeks of following recommendations for current level, move to next higher level. If glucose and $A_1C$ do not reach targets with Level 4, oral drug or insulin is required.

## Additional Supplements for Prevention and Treatment of Complications

With any complication add:

- Alpha-lipoic acid: 300 to 600 mg q.d.
- Grape seed extract (or other flavonoid-rich extract): 150 to 300 mg q.d.

For specific complications, follow the foundation supplement program with the addition of alpha-lipoic acid and an appropriate flavonoid-rich extract and add the specified supplement(s) in the following list.

- **High cholesterol and other cardiovascular risk factors**
  —Total cholesterol >200 mg/dL or LDL >135 mg/dL (100 mg if history of myocardial infarction [MI]):

Glucomannan (or other soluble source at equivalent dosage): 1000 mg before meals
Niacin (or inositol hexaniacinate): 1000 to 1500 mg at bedtime
Garlic: 4000+ µg of allicin q.d.
—HDL <45 mg/dL niacin (or inositol hexaniacinate)—1000 to 1500 mg at bedtime
—Lipoprotein (a) >40 mg/dL: niacin (or inositol hexaniacinate)—1500 mg at bedtime
—Triglycerides >150 mg/dL: niacin (or inositol hexaniacinate)—1500 mg at bedtime
—C-reactive protein >1.69 mg/L: vitamin E—800 IU q.d. (mixed tocopherols)
—Fibrinogen > 400 mg/L garlic extract—4000 µg q.d.
—Ferritin (iron-binding protein) >200 µg/L: eliminate red meat; avoid iron supplements; increase whole grains

- **Diabetic retinopathy**
  —Bilberry extract: 160 to 320 mg q.d. or grapeseed extract: 150 to 300 mg q.d.
- **Diabetic neuropathy**
  —Gamma-linolenic acid from borage, evening primrose, or blackcurrant oil: 480 mg q.d.
  —Capsaicin (0.075%) cream: apply to affected area b.i.d.
- **Diabetic nephropathy**
  —Follow recommendations for cardiovascular risk factors as previously mentioned unless kidney function falls below 40% of normal. Be cautious when recommending magnesium and potassium supplements.
- **Poor wound healing**
  —*Aloe vera* gel: apply to affected areas b.i.d.
- **Diabetic foot ulcers**
  —*Ginkgo biloba* extract: 120 to 240 mg q.d. or grapeseed extract: 150 to 300 mg q.d.

# Endometriosis

## DIAGNOSTIC SUMMARY

- **Triad of symptoms**: dysmenorrhea, dyspareunia, infertility.
- **Physical examination**: reveals one or more of the following: tenderness of the pelvic area and/or cul-de-sac, enlarged or tender ovaries, a uterus that tips backward and lacks mobility, fixed pelvic structures, adhesions.
- **Pelvic ultrasounds**: detection and consistency of endometriomas.
- **Definitive diagnosis**: laparoscopy or laparotomy visualizing pelvic endometrial implants.

## GENERAL CONSIDERATIONS

Endometriosis affects 10%-15% of menstruating women between ages of 24 and 40 years. Main risk factor is heredity—a mother or sister with endometriosis. Other risk factors include shorter menstrual cycles; longer duration of flow; lack of exercise from an early age; high-fat diet; intrauterine device use; estrogen imbalance; natural red hair color; personal history of abuse; pelvic immune action with antibody to sperm; immune dysfunction; prenatal exposure to estrogens, xenoestrogens, or endocrine disruptors (polychlorinated biphenyls [PCBs], weed killers, plastics, detergents, household cleaners, aluminum can liners), or dioxin; liver dysmetabolism of estrogens. Endometriosis can cause infertility and miscarriage, producing excess free radicals involved in implantation. Endometriomas (ectopic endometrium on ovaries) are found in two thirds of endometriosis patients. Infertility may cause endometriosis from tubal scarring, adhesions, unruptured follicles.

## DIAGNOSTIC CONSIDERATIONS

- **Symptoms begin at onset of menstruation or later**, worsening with time. Triad of symptoms: dysmenorrhea, dyspareunia,

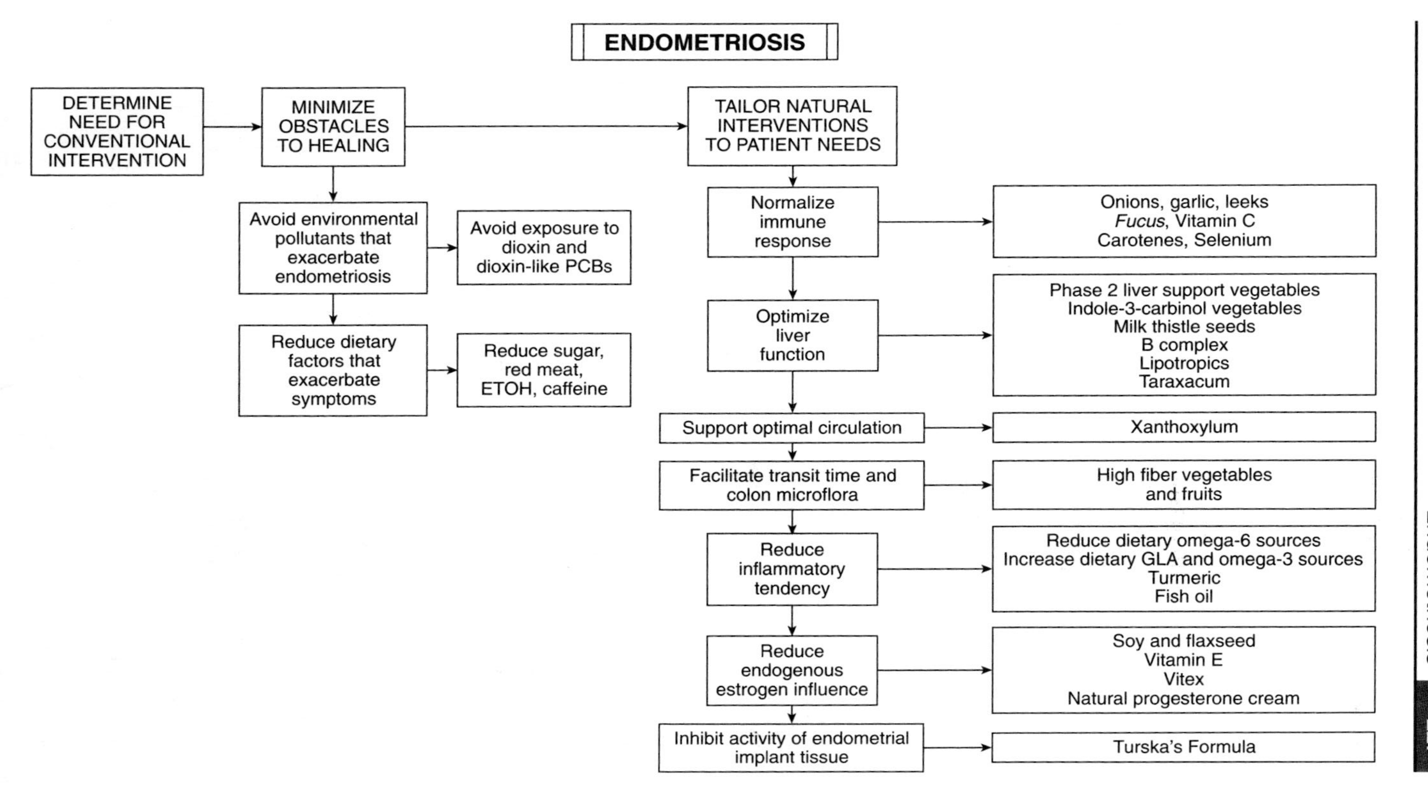
ENDOMETRIOSIS
DETERMINE NEED FOR CONVENTIONAL INTERVENTION
MINIMIZE OBSTACLES TO HEALING
TAILOR NATURAL INTERVENTIONS TO PATIENT NEEDS
Avoid environmental pollutants that exacerbate endometriosis
Avoid exposure to dioxin and dioxin-like PCBs
Reduce dietary factors that exacerbate symptoms
Reduce sugar, red meat, ETOH, caffeine
Normalize immune response
Onions, garlic, leeks
Fucus, Vitamin C
Carotenes, Selenium
Optimize liver function
Phase 2 liver support vegetables
Indole-3-carbinol vegetables
Milk thistle seeds
B complex
Lipotropics
Taraxacum
Support optimal circulation
Xanthoxylum
Facilitate transit time and colon microflora
High fiber vegetables and fruits
Reduce inflammatory tendency
Reduce dietary omega-6 sources
Increase dietary GLA and omega-3 sources
Turmeric
Fish oil
Reduce endogenous estrogen influence
Soy and flaxseed
Vitamin E
Vitex
Natural progesterone cream
Inhibit activity of endometrial implant tissue
Turska's Formula

infertility. Features include acute pain before menses, lasting a day or two during menses or throughout the month; vomiting; diarrhea; fainting concurrent with pelvic/abdominal cramping and labor-like pains; chronic bearing down pain; pressure on low back; pains radiating down legs; pain with urination or bowel movements; bleeding from nose, bladder, or bowels; fatigue.
- **Curious feature**: pain and extent of disease correlate poorly. Symptom severity correlates with depth of lesions rather than number of lesions.
- **Physical examination**: one or more of the following: tenderness in pelvic area and/or cul-de-sac; enlarged or tender ovaries; uterus tips backward and lacks mobility; fixed pelvic structure; adhesions. Other findings include endometrial tissue or surgical scar tissue in vagina or on cervix. Examination during the first or second day of menses: tender septum between rectum and vagina.
- **Pelvic ultrasound**: useful assessing pain and tumors but not definitive; detects mass on ovary; determines size, characteristics, consistency of endometriosis. Blood test CA-125 can be positive in endometriosis but cannot distinguish endometriosis, fibroids, malignancies, and even normal tissue.
- **Definitive diagnosis**: biopsy by laparoscopy or laparotomy of visualized tissue.
- **Estrogens stimulate growth of implants**: therapy manipulating endogenous hormones may be effective.

## THERAPEUTIC CONSIDERATIONS

### Diet

- **Objectives**:
  —Normalize immune response
  —Optimize liver function to metabolize hormones and detoxify toxins
  —Eliminate metabolic wastes
  —Facilitate transit time and intestinal microflora
- **High-fiber foods** optimize intestinal transit time and balance friendly gut microflora that displace undesirable strains that deconjugate estrogens, allowing them to recirculate. Less protein, high-fiber organic vegetarian diet: decreases plasma active unconjugated estrogens; reduce intake of proinflammatory arachidonic acid. Vegetable protein, soy, nut butters (almond), salmon are preferred. Emphasize phase 2 liver support vegetables: carrots,

beets, artichokes, lemons, dandelion greens, watercress, burdock root, cabbage family vegetables. Indole-3-carbinol, in broccoli, Brussels sprouts, cabbage, cauliflower, favors less-active estrogen metabolites. Onions, garlic, and leeks contain immunity-enhancing organosulfur compounds and bioflavonoids (quercetin) that protect against oxidation, block inflammation, and inhibit tumor growth.
- **Phytoestrogens**: soy isoflavones and flaxseed lignans help alleviate endometriosis symptoms.
- **Seasonings**: Turmeric (curcumin) protects against environmental carcinogens, decreases inflammation, increases bile secretion. Milk thistle seeds soaked and ground helps liver function. Fresh flaxseeds increase antiinflammatory fatty acids. *Fucus* (seaweed) stimulates T-cell production and absorbs toxins.
- **Decrease** sugar, caffeine, dairy, red meat, alcohol.

## NUTRITIONAL SUPPLEMENTS

- **Vitamin C**: increases cellular immunity, decreases autoimmunity and fatigue, decreases capillary fragility and tumor growth.
- **Beta-carotene**: enhances immunity, increases T-cell levels, protects against early stages of tumor growth. One third of beta-carotene is converted to vitamin A (retinol). Immune function is from carotenoids rather than vitamin A.
- **Vitamin E**: helps correct abnormal progesterone/estradiol ratios in patients with mammary dysplasia (increased growth of cells), which parallels abnormal growth of lesions in endometriosis. It inhibits the arachidonic lipid pathway, preventing release of inflammatory chemicals.
- **Essential fatty acids**: Gamma linolenic acid (in borage, black currant, evening primrose oil) and alpha-linolenic acid (in flaxseed, canola, pumpkin, soy, walnuts) help decrease tissue inflammatory responses by increasing noninflammatory prostaglandins. The higher the ratio of omega-6 to omega-3 fatty acids, the longer the survival time and secretion of interleukin-8 in cells from women with or without endometriosis. The cells from women with endometriosis secrete higher levels of interleukin-8, and the levels are proportionately higher at higher ratios of omega-6 to omega-3.
- **B vitamins**: help the liver inactivate estrogen. Supplementation may cause the liver to become more efficient in processing estrogen.

- **Selenium**: aids synthesis of liver detoxification antioxidant enzymes and stimulates white blood cells and thymus function. Selenium deficiency impairs cell-mediated immunity, decreases T-cells, and promotes inflammation.
- **Lipotropics**: enhance liver function and detoxification reactions. Choline, betaine, and methionine promote bile flow that facilitates excretion of estrogen metabolites.

### Botanical Medicines

Use same herbs as for menstrual cramps: valerian, cramp bark, black cohosh.

- ***Vitex agnus-castus* (chaste tree)**: treats hormone imbalances in women, acting on the pituitary to increase luteinizing hormone, which stimulates progesterone production. Uses: reducing estrogen excess linked to fibroids, premenstrual syndrome, perimenopause, symptoms of endometriosis.
- ***Taraxacum officinale* (dandelion root)**: supports liver and gallbladder detoxification efforts to expel wastes and deactivate excess estrogens. Dandelion may have antitumor activity. Dandelion leaf contains vitamins A, C, and K; calcium; and lipotropic choline.
- ***Xanthoxylum americanum* (prickly ash)**: treats capillary engorgement and sluggish circulation. It stimulates blood flow bodywide, enhancing oxygen and nutrient transport and removal of cellular wastes. It relieves pelvic congestion by enhancing pelvic circulation.
- ***Leonurus* (mother wort)**: antispasmodic that gently soothes nerves. To alleviate uterine cramps and pain, it promotes relaxation during extreme "bearing down" uterine or pelvic pain. It is a mild sedative for needed rest during menstrual cramps.
- **Turska's formula**: old naturopathic treatment for decreasing aberrant cancer cell growth, useful in endometriosis because of similarities to pelvic cell growth. Ingredients include monkshood (*Aconite napellus*), yellow jasmine (*Gelsemium sempervirens*), bryony (*Bryonia alba*), and poke root (*Phytolacca americana*). Monkshood and yellow jasmine alkaloids disrupt assembly of microtubules of undifferentiated mesenchymal cells and abnormal ectopic pelvic lesions. Bryony provides antitumor effects. Poke root glycoproteins stimulate lymphocyte transformation for immune enhancement. It also has antiinflammatory properties. Tinctures of this formula are toxic if misused.

### Other Considerations

- **Natural progesterone**: progesterone modifies the action of estradiol by decreasing retention of receptors and diminishing serum estradiol. Progesterone insufficiency causes estrogen excess imbalance. Progesterone sedates painful uterine contractions and relieves entire pelvic region. Natural progesterone is not used alone but as part of a comprehensive plan. For some women, cream preparations are applied—¼ teaspoon t.i.d. for 3 weeks on and 1 week off (week off is week of menses). Others need it only the week before menses. And others require higher doses of natural oral micronized progesterone in a cyclic dosing pattern.
- **Dioxin exposure**: increases incidence and severity of endometriosis in monkeys; promotes growth and survival of surgically implanted endometrial tissue in rodents. Dioxin is a carcinogen, influencing growth factors, cytokines, and hormones affecting endometriosis. Dioxin-like PCBs, but not non-dioxin-like PCBs, are linked to endometriosis.

## THERAPEUTIC APPROACH

### Diet

Increase high-fiber fruits and vegetables. Decrease omega-6 fatty acids (domesticated land animal products). Increase omega-3 fatty acids (wild fish, flax). Increase indole-3-carbinol (broccoli, Brussels sprouts, cabbage, cauliflower). Limit caffeine.

## SUPPLEMENTS

- **Vitamin C**: 6-10 g q.d. in divided doses
- **Beta-carotene**: 50,000-150,000 IU q.d.
- **Vitamin E**: 400-800 IU q.d. (mixed tocopherols)
- **Fish oil**: 1000 mg q.d.
- **Vitamin B complex**: 50-100 mg q.d.
- **Selenium**: 200-400 μg q.d.
- **Lipotropics**: 1000 mg choline and 1000 mg methionine or cysteine t.i.d.

### Botanical Medicines

- Chaste tree + dandelion root + prickly ash + motherwort tincture (equal parts): ½ tsp to 1 tsp. t.i.d.

- Turska's formula (*Aconite* 1½ drams + *Bryonia* 1½ drams + *Gelsemium* 1½ drams + *Phytolacca* 3 drams + ½ dram water): 5 drops q.d.
- Topical progesterone cream:
  - —Option 1
    - Day 1-7, no cream
    - Day 8-28, ¼-½ tsp b.i.d.
  - —Option 2
    - Day 1-14, no cream
    - Day 15-28, ¼-½ tsp b.i.d.
  - —Option 3
    - Day 1-21, no cream
    - Day 22-28, ¼-½ tsp b.i.d.

# Epilepsy

## DIAGNOSTIC SUMMARY

- Recurrent seizures
- Characteristic electroencephalographic (EEG) changes accompanying seizures
- Mental status abnormalities or focal neurologic symptoms may persist for hours postictally

## GENERAL CONSIDERATIONS

Epilepsy is not a disease in itself, but a symptom of disease. Epilepsy describes a group of disorders characterized by sudden, recurrent, and episodic changes in neurologic function caused by abnormalities in electrical activity of the brain. An episode of neurologic dysfunction is called a seizure. Seizures are termed *convulsive* when accompanied by motor manifestations and *nonconvulsive* when accompanied by sensory, cognitive, or emotional events. Epilepsy can result from many abnormalities: neural injuries, structural brain lesions, systemic diseases. It is termed *idiopathic* when neither history of neural insult nor other apparent neural dysfunction is present. The common denominator is the epileptic attack or seizure.

- **Epidemiology**: prevalence of chronic, recurrent epilepsy is 10 in 1000. Ten percent of the population will have seizure at some point in life. Cumulative lifetime incidence is 3%. From 2%-5% of the population will have a nonfebrile seizure at some point in life; an additional 2%-5% of children have febrile convulsions during the first several years of life. Ten percent of these children, especially with prolonged febrile seizures, have epilepsy later in life. Sixty percent of newly diagnosed patients enter remission with conventional treatment.
- **Genetic factors**: prevalence of seizures in close relatives is three times that of the overall population.

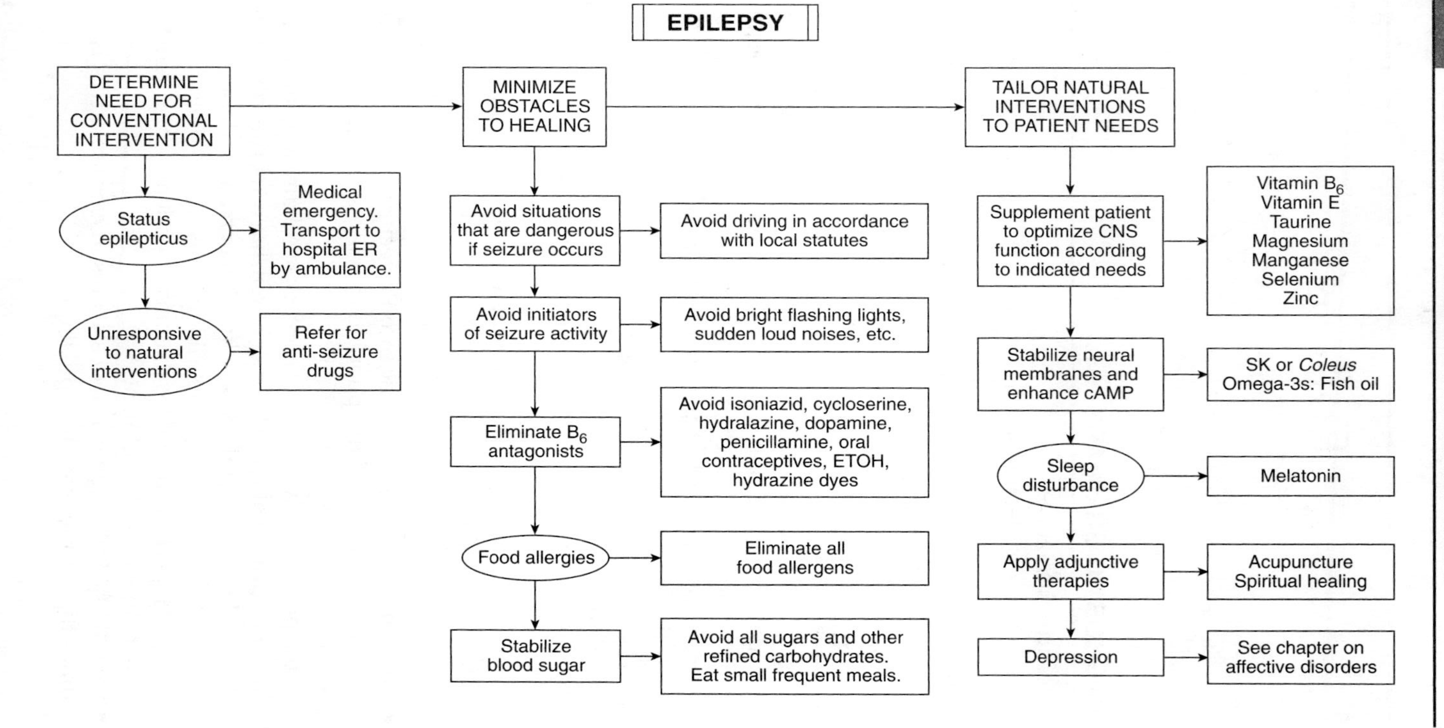
EPILEPSY
DETERMINE NEED FOR CONVENTIONAL INTERVENTION
Status epilepticus
Medical emergency. Transport to hospital ER by ambulance.
Unresponsive to natural interventions
Refer for anti-seizure drugs
MINIMIZE OBSTACLES TO HEALING
Avoid situations that are dangerous if seizure occurs
Avoid driving in accordance with local statutes
Avoid initiators of seizure activity
Avoid bright flashing lights, sudden loud noises, etc.
Eliminate B6 antagonists
Avoid isoniazid, cycloserine, hydralazine, dopamine, penicillamine, oral contraceptives, ETOH, hydrazine dyes
Food allergies
Eliminate all food allergens
Stabilize blood sugar
Avoid all sugars and other refined carbohydrates. Eat small frequent meals.
TAILOR NATURAL INTERVENTIONS TO PATIENT NEEDS
Supplement patient to optimize CNS function according to indicated needs
Vitamin B6
Vitamin E
Taurine
Magnesium
Manganese
Selenium
Zinc
Stabilize neural membranes and enhance cAMP
SK or Coleus
Omega-3s: Fish oil
Sleep disturbance
Melatonin
Apply adjunctive therapies
Acupuncture
Spiritual healing
Depression
See chapter on affective disorders

- **Etiology**: classified as symptomatic or idiopathic. Symptomatic means a probable cause can be identified. From 70%-80% of cases are idiopathic.

**Probable Causes Determined by Age of Onset**

| Age of Onset | Presumptive Causes |
|---|---|
| Birth to 2 years | Birth injury, degenerative brain disease |
| 2-19 years | Congenital birth injury, febrile thrombosis, head trauma, infection (meningitis or encephalitis) |
| 20-34 years | Head trauma, brain neoplasm |
| 35-54 years | Brain neoplasm, head trauma, stroke |
| 55 years and older | Stroke, brain neoplasm |

## Common Causes of Seizures

- Brain damage before or at birth (congenital malformations, anemia, fetal infection)
- Head trauma injuring brain and gliosis
- Central nervous system infections (meningitis, encephalitis, brain abscess, neurosyphilis, rabies, tetanus, falciparum malaria, toxoplasmosis, cysticercosis of brain)
- Metabolic disorders (hypocalcemia, hypoglycemia, hypoparathyroidism, phenylketonuria, withdrawal from alcohol and drugs)
- Brain tumors and other space-occupying lesions
- Stroke and other vascular disorders
- Degenerative brain disease
- Genetic disease
- Toxic conditions
- Idiopathic

## Classification

Classification is based on clinical and EEG criteria (International League Against Epilepsy).

### Partial (Focal, Local) Seizures

- Simple partial seizures (consciousness not impaired)
  —Motor signs
  —Somatosensory or special sensory symptoms

—Autonomic symptoms or signs
—Psychic symptoms
- Complex partial (consciousness impaired)
  —Simple partial onset followed by impaired consciousness
  —Consciousness impaired at onset
- Partial seizures evolving to generalized seizures (tonic, clonic, or tonic-clonic)
  —Simple partial seizures evolving to generalized seizures
  —Complex partial seizures evolving to generalized seizures
  —Simple partial seizures evolving to partial seizures evolving to generalized seizures

### Generalized Seizures (Convulsive or Nonconvulsive)

- Absence seizures
  —Typical (brief stare, eye flickering, no emotion)
  —Atypical (associated with movement)
- Myoclonic seizures
- Clonic seizures
- Tonic seizures
- Tonic-clonic seizures
- Atonic seizures
- Unclassified seizures

## DIAGNOSIS

Differentiating between partial or focal seizures and generalized seizures is of great clinical significance. Partial seizures begin focally as a specific sensory, motor, or psychic aberration reflecting the affected part of the cerebrum. These seizures may remain localized. Generalized seizures affect consciousness and motor function. Partial seizures are indicative of focal brain disorders (e.g., tumors, gliosis). Generalized seizures rarely have a definable etiology (perhaps metabolic disorders). Eyewitness account of the onset is valuable in classifying the seizure. Explore past trauma, infections, drugs, alcohol use, and family history. A complete neurologic examination is a preliminary screen for neoplasms. Epilepsy is not diagnosed from a solitary seizure; the recurrence rate after a single seizure is 27% over a 3-year period.

- **Diagnosis workup**: serum glucose and calcium, complete blood count, liver and kidney function tests, syphilis serology, skull radiographs, EEG, computed tomographic scan (all adult-onset seizures), magnetic resonance imaging (MRI). Cerebrospinal fluid exam is indicated if infection or meningeal neoplasm is suspected. MRI is the gold standard to investigate epilepsy; resolution is superior to computed tomographic scan. EEG during functional MRI maps normal and pathologic brain function.

## PATHOPHYSIOLOGY

Hallmark of altered physiologic state of epilepsy is rhythmic and repetitive, synchronous discharge of many neurons in a localized brain area. Discharge pattern is recorded on EEG during attack. The cause of abnormal discharges is unknown. Synchronous depolarization of masses of neurons results from the combination of increased excitation and decreased inhibition. Gamma-aminobutyric acid (GABA) blockers are potent convulsants. Antiepileptic drugs (phenobarbital, benzodiazepines) enhance GABA. In some forms of chronic focal epilepsy, inhibitory terminals on neurons in areas around cortical gliotic lesions are diminished. Nerve cell membranes in epileptics are unstable; during seizures, stored intracellular $Ca^{2+}$ is released and moves toward inner cell membranes, binding to $Ca^{2+}$-receptive proteins, causing protein conformational changes. These changes trigger transmembranal $Ca^{2+}$, $K^+$, and $Na^+$ channels to remain open, potentiating excitation. Earliest symptoms (aura) generated by focal discharge are the best clue to localization and characterization of the responsible lesion.

## THERAPEUTIC CONSIDERATIONS

### Environmental Toxins

- **Heavy metals**: lead, mercury, cadmium, and aluminum induce seizures by disrupting neural function. Rule out heavy metal toxicity; hair mineral analysis is the most cost-effective screening method (*Textbook,* "Environmental Medicine" and "Metal Toxicity: Assessment of Exposure and Retention").
- **Neurotoxic chemicals**: many neuron-, axon-, and myelin-toxic chemicals are released into the ecosystem. Explore possible exposure during detailed history taking (*Textbook,* "Environmental Medicine").

### Dietary Considerations

- **Hypoglycemia**: important metabolic cause of seizures. Serum glucose is unusually low before a seizure. From 50%-90% of epileptics have constant or periodic hypoglycemia. Seventy percent of epileptics have abnormal glucose tolerance test results. The correlation of glucose abnormalities and epilepsy is well documented, but the mechanism is unknown. Hypoglycemia may impair adenosine triphosphate (ATP) production in neurons, reducing efficacy of sodium–adenosine triphosphatase pump. Defective sodium (Na) pump increases intracellular Na, depolarizing the cell membrane and lowering the firing threshold. Single measurements of serum glucose are inadequate to determine glycemic status; extended glucose tolerance test is required.

- **Ketogenic diet**: has a long history of use to reduce seizure activity. Components are large amounts of fat and minimal proteins and carbohydrates. Low carbohydrates inhibit fat metabolism, causing production of excess ketone bodies (acetone, acetoacetic acid, beta-hydroxybutyric acid), which are intermediary oxidation products. Beneficial effects are caused by metabolic acidosis, which corrects underlying tendency of epileptics toward spontaneous alkalosis. Acidification may normalize nerve conductivity, irritability, and membrane permeability. Two types of ketogenic diets: classic ketogenic diet (CKD) and medium-chain triglyceride ketogenic diet (MCTKD). CKD limits carbohydrates and protein to <10% of calories combined. MCTKD diet uses medium-chain triglycerides to produce ketosis, allowing a larger intake of carbohydrates and protein. Forty percent of 27 children aged 1-16 years had a seizure reduction of >50%, with 25% becoming seizure free; 35% discontinued diet because of the difficulty following the rigorous guidelines. A ketogenic diet is effective in one third to one half of cases in children and partially effective in another third. Success rate of the ketogenic diet exceeds that of medications, is cheaper, and has fewer side effects. Linear growth may be maintained or retarded, but body weight decreases in children on both diets because of inadequate energy intake. Protein intake is adequate. MCTKD resulted in a 0.7 decrease in ratio of total cholesterol to high-density lipoprotein cholesterol at 4 months. Biochemical indexes, including albumin, were normal, but long-term studies are needed. MCTKD may be more nutritionally adequate. Long-term risks are associated with a high-fat diet, and it is unhealthy for a growing child. For children, recommend adequate calories and protein, a higher proportion of unsaturated to saturated fats; consider vitamin/mineral supplements. Do not allow children to eat very large meals, which predispose to seizures. Small, frequent meals may decrease hypoglycemia. The Atkins diet also is ketogenic and less restrictive on protein. The Atkins diet reduced intractable focal and multifocal epilepic seizures in a small pilot study.

- **Food allergy**: little research has explored the correlation between food allergy and epilepsy. Epileptic patients may have allergic reactions in the brain similar to swelling, anoxia, and inflammatory chemical reactions of local allergic reactions. Suspect allergy in epileptics with multiple other symptoms of food allergy (*Textbook*, "Epilepsy" and "Food Allergy Testing"). Folic acid deficiency is a common side effect of most antiepileptic drugs. Link between celiac disease, epilepsy, and cerebral calcifications indicates celiac disease be ruled out (even in the absence of gastrointestinal symptoms) in all cases of epilepsy and cerebral calcifications of unexplained origin, especially when epilepsy is characterized by occipital seizures and calcification located bilaterally in posterior regions. Epileptic children have higher rates of eczema in mothers, rhinitis in siblings, allergic states in both of these groups, allergy to cow's milk, and asthma compared with control subjects.

## Nutritional Considerations

- **Pyridoxine**: two types of vitamin $B_6$–related seizures in newborns and infants <18 months old—$B_6$ deficient and $B_6$ dependent with similar neurologic symptoms, EEG abnormalities, and prognosis of mental retardation if untreated. $B_6$-dependent type is an autosomal, recessive inherited error of metabolism with recurrent long-lasting seizures, with onset in infancy and up to age 3 years. Seizures resist anticonvulsants. It is fatal if diagnosis and pharmacologic dosing of $B_6$ is delayed too long. Suspect $B_6$ dependency if convulsions in the first 18 months of life have the following clinical features:
  —Seizures of unknown origin in previously normal infant without abnormal gestational or perinatal history
  —History of severe convulsive disorders
  —Long-lasting focal or unilateral seizures, often with partial preservation of consciousness
  —Irritability, restlessness, crying, and vomiting preceding actual seizure

  MRI with spectroscopy can assess parenchymal changes despite normal-appearing brain MRI in patients with $B_6$-dependent seizures. Atypical presentations of $B_6$-responsive seizures suggest empiric trial of parenteral $B_6$ for neonate or infant with long-lasting convulsions, especially with no clear-cut etiology. Dose is 100-200 mg IV or 20 mg every 5 minutes to a total of 200 mg. If seizures stop, child has $B_6$-responsive seizures. Diagnosis of $B_6$ responsiveness is lost if $B_6$ is given together with, or after, anticonvulsant drugs. $B_6$ deficiency responds to dietary amounts, but $B_6$ dependency requires continuous high-dose supplementing at 25-50 mg q.d. The mechanism is not fully understood, but it is related to $B_6$ as a cofactor in synthesis of neurotransmitters dependent on amino acid decarboxylation. Absorbed $B_6$ is phosphorylated to pyridoxal-5-phosphate (P5P), a coenzyme in converting glutamic acid to GABA, an inhibitory neurotransmitter. Proposed mechanism: pyridoxal phosphate does not bind with usual affinity to glutamic acid decarboxylase, reducing GABA production; thus higher levels of $B_6$ are required for activity of this enzyme. Uncontrollable infantile spasms or sequelae improve in 2-14 days with oral P5P (20-50 mg/kg). Adverse reactions include elevated transaminase levels, nausea, and vomiting. Administering $B_6$ to epileptics must be strictly monitored and improvements noted; daily doses of 80-400 mg interfere with anticonvulsants.

- **Folic acid**: low serum and red blood cell folic acid occurs in 90% of patients using barbiturates or the anticonvulsants phenytoin or carbamazepine; these drugs interfere with intestinal uptake of folate by mucosa. Lamotrigine and zonisamide do not seem to cause this problem; valproate has mixed reports. Supplementing folic acid appears safe even up to 15 mg/day, protecting against birth defects for women of childbearing potential and elevated homocysteine, a cardiac risk factor for antiepileptic medicines.
- **Thiamin**: deficiency may promote epileptic episodes in those with subclinical predisposition for seizures. Vitamin $B_1$ may play a significant role in nerve conduction. Vitamin $B_1$ deficiency may accompany low concentrations of GABA. In patients with late-onset epilepsy, thiamin deficiency may be a cause.
- **Taurine**: one of the most abundant amino acids in the brain, taurine is involved in hyperpolarizing neurons by changing ion permeability. It may mimic effects of GABA and glycine. Taurine's anticonvulsive mode of action is a membrane-stabilizing effect (normalizes flow of $Na^+$, $K^+$, and $Ca^{2+}$ into and out of the cell). Taurine acts as a GABA-like neurotransmitter and may increase GABA levels by enhancing action of glutamic acid decarboxylase. Epileptics have much lower taurine levels in platelets than do control subjects. Anticonvulsant effects have been demonstrated, but the rate of efficacy is far below the level warranting recommendation as standard treatment. No consensus exists on amenable seizure types, dosage, or whether taurine traverses the blood-brain barrier. Daily dose was 0.05-0.3 g/kg

in one study and 750 mg in another—effective in some cases of intractable epilepsy, decreasing seizures by >30% in one third of subjects unresponsive to any other anticonvulsant. Partial epilepsy showed best results, with those achieving highest taurine concentrations showing the best response. Monitoring platelet or plasma taurine levels is useful.

- **Magnesium (Mg)**: epileptics have much lower serum Mg compared with normal control subjects. Seizure severity correlates with level of hypomagnesemia. The mechanism is not fully understood. Mg may be lowered by antiepileptic drugs. Mg is beneficial in control of some seizures. Mg deficiency induces muscle tremors and convulsive seizures; dose = 450 mg q.d.
- **Manganese (Mn)**: low whole blood and hair Mn levels are common in epileptics; those with lowest levels have the highest seizure activity. Mn is a critical cofactor for glucose utilization within neurons, adenylate cyclase activity, and neurotransmitter control. Optimal central nervous system function requires sufficient Mn. Supplements may help control seizure activity in some patients.
- **Zinc (Zn)**: children with epilepsy have much lower serum Zn levels, especially in West or Lennox syndromes. Epileptics may have elevated copper (Cu)/Zn ratio. Seizures may be triggered when Zn levels fall, as in the absence of adequate taurine. The exact role of Zn or Cu/Zn ratio is unclear; it may involve storage or binding of GABA. Supplementing is warranted because anticonvulsants may cause Zn deficiency.
- **Choline, betaine (N,N,N,-trimethylglycine), dimethylglycine (DMG), and sarcosine**: produce anticonvulsant activity in human and animal studies. Choline is converted to betaine when acting as a methyl donor; betaine is converted to DMG when donating a methyl group to homocysteine to produce methionine. Supplemental betaine is quite effective in alleviating seizures in human beings with homocystinuria. DMG blocks seizures induced in lab animals. DMG strikingly decreased seizure frequency in a patient with longstanding mental retardation at dose of 90 mg b.i.d. Glycine and betaine may act indirectly on glycine metabolism and glycine-mediated neuronal inhibition, enhance GABA activity, or simply have a nonspecific effect on biologic membranes.
- **Vitamin D**: anticonvulsant drugs are linked to disorders of mineral metabolism (hypocalcemia, rickets, osteomalacia). Studies of serum levels of vitamin D in epilepsy are conflicting. Supplemental vitamin D is recommended when the climate or

lifestyle does not allow adequate exposure to sunlight (particularly important for people with dark skin pigmentation). Supplementing epileptics with 4000-16,000 IU vitamin D has significantly decreased the number of seizures, but that large dosage can be quite toxic, requiring careful monitoring.

- **Vitamin E and selenium (Se)**: function synergistically. Vitamin E deficiency produces seizures; antiepileptic drugs decrease vitamin E and beta-carotene levels. Vitamin E and Se levels are low in epileptics. Phosphate diesters of vitamins E and C prevent epileptogenic focus formation or attenuate seizure activities in animal models. Vitamin E and Se supplements may improve control of seizures. Se is helpful in children with reduced glutathione peroxidase activity, intractable seizures, multiple infections, and resistance to anticonvulsants. Other antioxidants (green tea (-)-epigallocatechin and (-)-epigallocatechin-3-O-gallate; alpha lipoic acid) scavenge radical oxygen species and may be prophylactic for epileptic discharges induced in animal models.
- **Essential fatty acids (EFAs)**: long-chain polyunsaturated EFAs may alleviate or prevent cerebrovascular pathology and reinforce blood-brain barrier competency. Dosage of 5 g q.d. 65% omega-3 fatty acid spread reduced frequency and strength of seizures. Yet gamma-linolenic acid and linoleic acid (omega-6) as evening primrose oil (EPO) induced temporal lobe epilepsy in three hospitalized schizophrenics. Monitor closely when using EFAs for epilepsy. Omega 3 EFAs are best choice; use EPO (as well as borage and black currant oils) with caution.
- **Melatonin (5-methoxy-*N*-acetyltryptamine)**: powerful antioxidant that treats abnormalities in sleep-wake cycle, jet lag, cancer, and Parkinson's disease. Epileptic children have a higher incidence of sleep problems; epilepsy is exacerbated by sleep deprivation. Melatonin has antiepileptic activity. Mechanism may be antiexcitotoxic neuroprotection by lowering lipid peroxidation and raising coenzyme $Q_{10}$ within the central nervous system. In children aged 3 to 12 years seizure free on sodium valproate (10 mg/kg/day) for 6 months, fast-release 3-mg melatonin tablet 1 hour before bedtime improved attention, memory, language, anxiety, behavior, and other cognitive processes. Very high dosages (up to 300 mg/day) are well tolerated in adults; slowly increasing dose beyond 3 mg gives better results.

## Botanical Medicines

- **Chinese herbal medicine**: Chinese herbal combination Saiko-Keishi-To (SK) demonstrated dramatic therapeutic effects on

some difficult cases unresponsive to anticonvulsants. SK is a combination of nine botanicals:
—*Bupleuri radix*: 5.0 g
—*Scutellaria radix*: 3.0 g
—*Pinelliae tuber*: 5.0g
—*Paeoniae radix*: 6.0 g
—*Cinnamon cortex*: 2.0 g
—*Zizyphi fructus*: 4.0 g
—*Ginseng radix*: 30.0 g
—*Glycyrrhizae radix*: 1.5 g
—*Zingiber rhizoma*: 2.0 g

SK inhibits intracellular shift of $Ca^{2+}$ toward cell membrane; inhibits binding of $Ca^{2+}$ to $Ca^{2+}$-receptive membrane proteins and $Ca^{2+}$-calmodulin complex; inhibits conformational changes of $Ca^{2+}$-receptive membrane proteins; inhibits pathologic transmembrane current of $Na^+$, $K^+$, and $Ca^{2+}$. Attempts to isolate purified chemicals from component herbs failed to match crude drug's efficacy, revealing synergistic effect among herbal agents.

- ***Coleus forskohlii***: cyclic nucleotides are involved in the pathophysiology of seizures—possible mechanism of action of several botanicals. Cyclic adenosine monophosphate (cAMP) depresses electrical activity in animal models. Cyclic guanosine monophosphate (cGMP) can produce seizurelike discharge in the same tissues. cAMP inhibits $Ca^{2+}$ binding to intracellular proteins (calmodulin), decreasing extrusion of neurotransmitters into synapse. *Coleus* is an Ayurvedic herb that activates adenylate cyclase, increasing cAMP. The constituent forskolin, a diterpine, increases adenylate cyclase activity by 530%. Seven of the nine botanicals in SK (*Bupleuri radix,* Cinnamon cortex, *Glycyrrhizae radix, Paeoniae radix, Ginseng radix, Scutellaria radix,* and *Zingiber rhizoma*) also increase cAMP by enhancing adenylate cyclase or inhibiting cAMP phosphodiesterase.
- ***Ginkgo biloba***: antioxidant that improves memory and cerebral insufficiency. It may precipitate seizures in some people. *Gingko* flavonoids exert GABAergic activity as partial agonists at benzodiazepine receptors. Avoid *Ginkgo* in patients with seizure history.

## Spiritual Healing

A connection between epileptic seizures and mystical states (transcendent experiences) has been hypothesized. Mohammad, Moses, and Saint Paul are thought to have suffered from recurrent epileptic seizures. Spiritual work may reciprocally influence biologic and energetic mechanisms of epilepsy. Many epileptic patients in diverse cultures worldwide perceive some continuing benefit. Little research has evaluated its efficacy, but low risk and possible benefit warrant future study.

## THERAPEUTIC APPROACH

Avoid situations that could be dangerous if seizures occur. Be aware of state laws regarding epilepsy and driving. Avoid known initiators of seizure activity (e.g., bright flashing lights, sudden loud sounds). Continue therapy at full dosages until patient is seizure free for 2+ years. Reduce dosage gradually over several months. Epileptics not controlled with natural therapies require drug therapy. Eliminate pyridoxine antagonists (isoniazid, cycloserine, hydralazine, dopamine, penicillamine, oral contraceptives, alcohol, and hydrazine dyes [FD&C yellow #5]).

Note: Status epilepticus is a medical emergency causing serious neurologic damage or death if untreated. Immediate hospitalization is mandatory, preferably with emergency medical services transport to maintain airway, assist ventilation, and administer intravenous glucose and anticonvulsants.

Monitor for depression. Endogenous depression is more prevalent in epileptics than in the general population.

- **Diet**: eliminate all sugar and refined carbohydrates. Moderate protein intake. Identify and eliminate food allergens. Eat small, frequent meals. If ketotic effect is desired, strictly limit all carbohydrates and increase fat. Ensure adequate calories, protein, and omega-3 fatty acids. Use vitamin/mineral supplements with carefully supervised ketotic diets.
- **Lifestyle**: regular sleep patterns should be encouraged.
- **Nutritional supplements** (adult doses; reduce proportionately for children):
  —Vitamin $B_6$: 50 mg t.i.d.
  —Folic acid: 0.4 to 4 mg q.d.
  —Vitamin E: 400 IU q.d. (mixed tocopherols)
  —Taurine: 500 mg t.i.d.
  —Mg: 300 mg t.i.d.
  —Mn: 10 mg t.i.d.
  —Se: 100 μg q.d.
  —Zn: 25 mg q.d.

—Melatonin: 3 mg in children, increase up to 20 mg or more in adults.

- **Botanical medicine**:
  —Saiko-Keishi-To: 300 mL before bedtime.

Caution:

—*Gingko biloba*: contraindicated at this time.

# Erythema Multiforme

## DIAGNOSTIC SUMMARY

- Sudden onset of symmetric, erythematous, edematous, macular, papular, urticarial, bullous, or purpuric skin lesions.
- Evolves into "target lesions" ("bull's eye" lesions with clear centers and concentric erythematous rings).
- Characteristic first site: dorsum of hand.
- Characteristic distribution: extensor surfaces of extremities with relative sparing of head and trunk.
- Rare oral manifestations: range from tender superficial erythematous and hyperkeratotic plaques to painful, deep, hemorrhagic bullae and erosions.
- Tendency to recur in spring and fall.

## GENERAL CONSIDERATIONS

Erythema multiforme (EM) includes a wide range of expressions, from exclusive oral erosions (oral EM) to mucocutaneous lesions ranging from mild (EM minor) to severe multiple mucosal membranes (EM major, Stevens-Johnson syndrome [SJS]) or large area of total body surface (toxic epidermal necrolysis [TEN]). But the term EM is not accepted worldwide; various clinical categories have overlapping features. EM minor, EM major, SJS, and TEN differ in severity and expression. All variants share two common features: cutaneous target lesions and satellite cell or more widespread necrosis of epithelium. Suspected etiologic factors: herpes simplex or *Mycoplasma* are linked to 90% of cases of EM minor; SJS and TEN (80% of cases) arise from drugs: anticonvulsants, sulfonamides, nonsteroidal antiinflammatories, and antibiotics. Vaccines (e.g., *Vaccinia*, bacille Calmette-Guérin, polio), food allergy, and other infectious organisms have all induced EM minor. Common factor: highly reactive, polymorphonuclear leukocyte oxygen intermediates trigger hypersensitivity and immune system–mediated tissue damage.

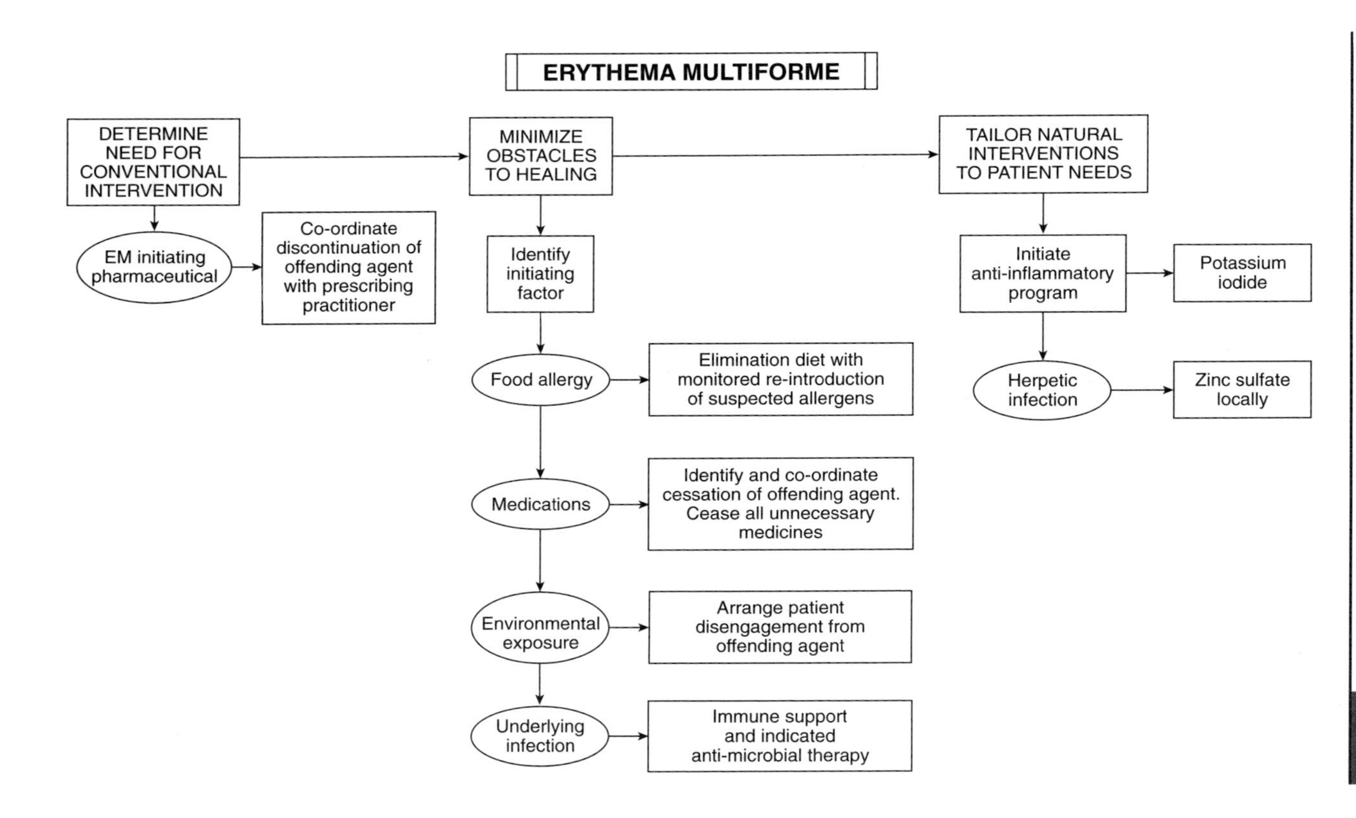
ERYTHEMA MULTIFORME
DETERMINE NEED FOR CONVENTIONAL INTERVENTION
EM initiating pharmaceutical
Co-ordinate discontinuation of offending agent with prescribing practitioner
MINIMIZE OBSTACLES TO HEALING
Identify initiating factor
Food allergy
Elimination diet with monitored re-introduction of suspected allergens
Medications
Identify and co-ordinate cessation of offending agent. Cease all unnecessary medicines
Environmental exposure
Arrange patient disengagement from offending agent
Underlying infection
Immune support and indicated anti-microbial therapy
TAILOR NATURAL INTERVENTIONS TO PATIENT NEEDS
Initiate anti-inflammatory program
Potassium iodide
Herpetic infection
Zinc sulfate locally

## THERAPEUTIC CONSIDERATIONS

- **Potassium iodide**: historically used to treat a variety of erythematous disorders, including erythema multiforme, erythema nodosum, nodular vasculitis, acute febrile neutrophilic dermatosis, and subacute nodular migratory panniculitis. Potassium iodide has documented dramatic success. Mechanism: suppression of generation of oxygen intermediates (hydrogen peroxide, hydroxyl radical) by stimulated polymorphonuclear antibodies. Iodine therapy is occasionally associated with adverse skin reactions and gastrointestinal discomfort. Never use in pregnant women in last trimester because of suppression of fetal thyroid.
- **Zinc**: zinc sulfate (0.025%-0.05%) is used locally at site of herpetic infection to prevent relapse of postherpetic erythema multiforme.

## THERAPEUTIC APPROACH

Carefully search to determine initiating factor; treat underlying infections; cease all unnecessary medicines; initiate antiinflammatory program.

- **Supplements**:
  —**Potassium iodide**: 100 mg t.i.d. for 4-6 weeks. Discontinue if adverse reactions occur.
  —**Zinc sulfate**: 0.025%-0.05% solution locally if postherpetic.

# Fibrocystic Breast Disease

## DIAGNOSTIC SUMMARY

- Very common: 20%-40% of premenopausal women.
- Pain or premenstrual breast pain and tenderness common, although the condition is often asymptomatic.
- Cyclic and bilateral with multiple cysts of varying sizes giving breasts nodular consistency.

## GENERAL CONSIDERATIONS

- **Benign breast discomfort**: conditions present in most women of reproductive age should never be labeled pathologic. Misconception: women with painful or lumpy breasts have increased breast cancer risk. Premenstrual pain and sensitivity is common; more prominent estrogen than progesterone effect at this time, when effect of progesterone is normally greater in luteal phase. This does not mean lower or higher levels of any particular hormone, but increased tissue sensitivity to estrogen with related fluid retention. This discomfort is tolerable in most women. Others need lifestyle changes or supplements. Oral contraceptives or hormone replacement therapy may cause breast discomfort: physiological, cyclical pain and swelling.
- **Mastalgia**: breast pain of severity interfering with daily life and prompting medical attention. Cyclical mastalgia is this severe 15% of the time. Noncyclical is rarer, caused by infection, old trauma, musculoskeletal conditions of chest wall.
- **Diffuse lumpiness**: cyclic or noncyclic and may or may not include pain. Normal breasts can have diffuse lumpiness—glands, fat, connective tissue. Prominent lumpiness and numerous lumps distinguish this from normal. Diffuse lumpiness is symmetric, distinguishing a normal from suspicious lump.
- **Unilateral densities**: most are benign. If mass edge merges in one or more places with surrounding tissue, it is nondominant. Evaluate masses carefully to distinguish dominant mass or mass

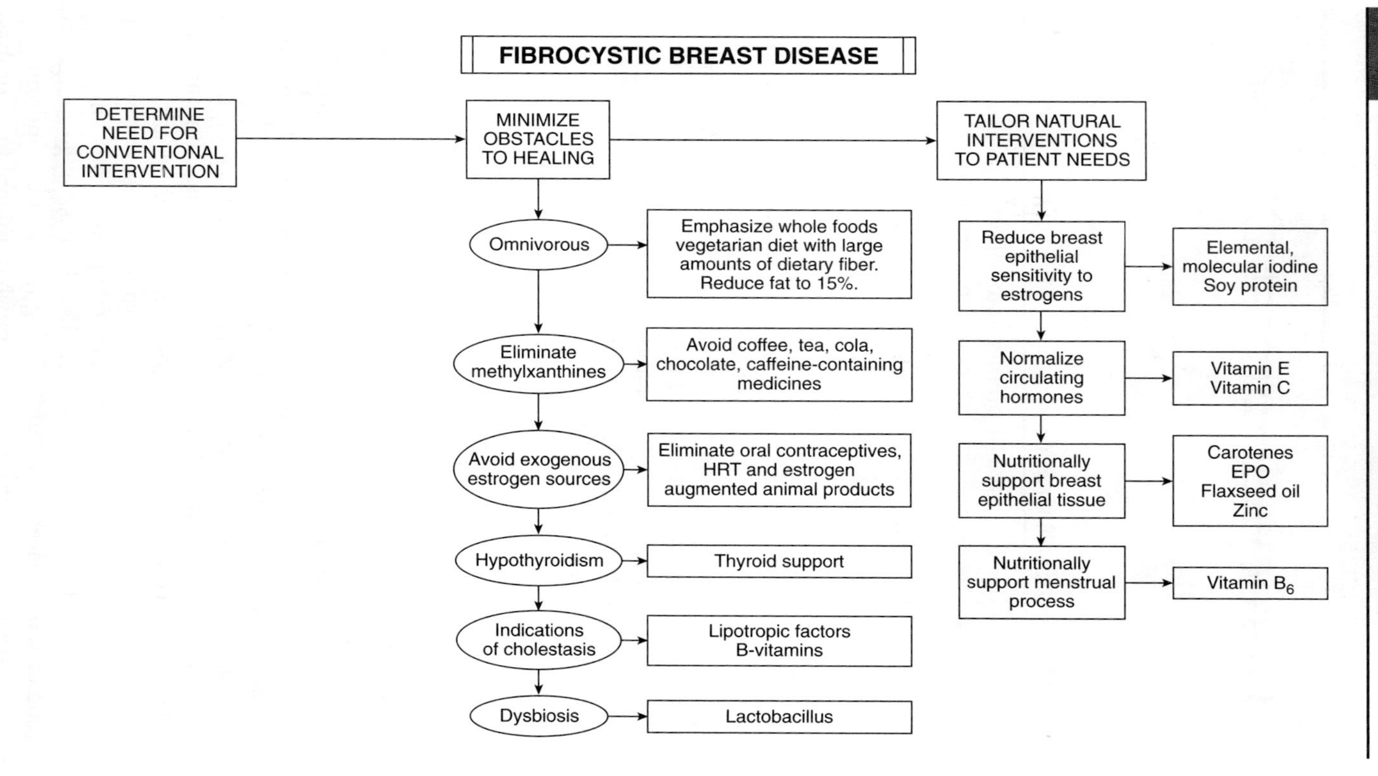
FIBROCYSTIC BREAST DISEASE
DETERMINE NEED FOR CONVENTIONAL INTERVENTION
MINIMIZE OBSTACLES TO HEALING
TAILOR NATURAL INTERVENTIONS TO PATIENT NEEDS
Omnivorous
Emphasize whole foods vegetarian diet with large amounts of dietary fiber. Reduce fat to 15%.
Eliminate methylxanthines
Avoid coffee, tea, cola, chocolate, caffeine-containing medicines
Avoid exogenous estrogen sources
Eliminate oral contraceptives, HRT and estrogen augmented animal products
Hypothyroidism
Thyroid support
Indications of cholestasis
Lipotropic factors B-vitamins
Dysbiosis
Lactobacillus
Reduce breast epithelial sensitivity to estrogens
Elemental, molecular iodine Soy protein
Normalize circulating hormones
Vitamin E Vitamin C
Nutritionally support breast epithelial tissue
Carotenes EPO Flaxseed oil Zinc
Nutritionally support menstrual process
Vitamin $B_6$

of concern. Fine-needle biopsy may be needed. Most show non-proliferative changes; 20% show proliferative changes without atypical hyperplasia with no increased breast cancer risk. Approximately 5% show atypical hyperplasia with increased risk, especially if first-degree relative has or had breast cancer.

- **Dominant masses**: noncyclical, unilateral, distinct on all sides from surrounding tissue. They persist over time and require thorough assessment, except in the very young. They are either fibroadenomas or obvious cysts. Fibroadenomas are rubbery, smooth, benign, fibrous tumors that usually do not grow bigger. Cysts are softer and disappear by draining with needle aspiration. Fibroadenomas and cysts do not increase risk but must be distinguished from malignancy.

## DIFFERENTIAL DIAGNOSIS

Fibrocystic breast disease (FBD) (cystic mastitis) cannot be definitively differentiated from breast cancer or breast fibroadenoma on clinical criteria alone. Pain, cyclic variations in size, high mobility, and multiplicity of nodules are indicative of FBD. Noninvasive procedures (mammography, ultrasonography) are helpful, but definitive procedures are needle aspiration, fine-needle biopsy or excisional biopsy.

## THERAPEUTIC CONSIDERATIONS

See the *Textbook*, "Premenstrual Syndrome," for additional factors that can influence FBD.

### Dietary Considerations

- **Methylxanthines**: caffeine, theophylline, and theobromine inhibit action of cyclic adenosine monophosphate (cAMP) and cyclic guanosine monophosphate (cGMP) phosphodiesterase and elevate their levels in breast tissue. Increased cyclic nucleotides excessively stimulate protein kinase, causing overproduction of cellular products (fibrous tissue, cyst fluid). Excess cyclic nucleotides in breast are one of the biochemical findings in breast cancer; caffeine promotes carcinogenesis in mammary gland of rats. Limiting dietary methylxanthines (coffee, tea, cola, chocolate, caffeinated medicines) improved 97.5% of 45 women who completely abstained and 75% of 28 who limited consumption. Women may have varying thresholds of response to methylxanthines. Stress plays a role; fibrocystic breasts are more responsive to epinephrine, which increases adenylate cyclase activity (cAMP).

- **Fiber**: an inverse association exists between dietary fiber and risk of benign, proliferative, epithelial breast disorders. Fiber may reduce risk of benign breast disease and cancer.
- **Soy**: in premenopausal women consuming soy protein daily for 1 year, their physicians reported subjective reduction in breast tenderness and FBD by using breast-enhanced scintigraphy test imaging. Average and maximal count breast activity and variability of tissue activity declined.

## Nutritional Supplements

- **Evening primsrose oil (EPO)**: only essential fatty acid source studied for FBD. Dosage of 3000 mg EPO for 6 months improved half of women's cyclic breast pain compared with one fifth on placebo. Approximately 27% of 33 women with breast pain throughout the month improved compared with 9% on placebo. EPO reduces cyclic and noncyclic pain. Consider other seed oils with gamma-linolenic acid (GLA): flaxseed, black currant oil, borage.
- **Vitamin E**: d-alpha-tocopherol can relieve premenstrual syndrome (PMS), including FBD and cyclical and noncyclical pain, in some patients. Results of early studies have not been duplicated. Mode of action is obscure—normalizes circulating hormones in PMS and FBD patients; 600 IU q.d. normalizes elevated follicle-stimulating hormone (FSH) and luteinizing hormone (LH) in FBD.
- **Vitamin A**: 150,000 IU q.d. for 3 months caused complete or partial remission of FBD in five of the nine patients who completed the study. Some developed mild side-effects, causing two of the original 12 to withdraw for headache, and one patient had dosage reduced. Beta-carotene may be a better source of retinol; it is much less toxic and triggers similar activity in ovarian and inflammatory disorders (*Textbook,* "Vitamin A" and "Vitamin Toxicities and Therapeutic Monitoring").
- **Thyroid and iodine**: iodine deficiency in rats induces mammary dysplasia histologically similar to human FBD. Hypothyroidism and/or iodine deficiency are linked to higher incidence of breast cancer. Thyroid hormone replacement in hypothyroid (and some euthyroid) patients may give improvement. Thyroid supplement (0.1 mg q.d. Synthroid) decreases mastodynia, serum prolactin, and breast nodules in euthyroid patients; subclinical hypothy-

roidism and/or iodine deficiency may be etiologic factors in FBD. Iodine caseinate may be an effective treatment for FBD. The theory is that absence of iodine renders epithelium more sensitive to estrogen stimulation. Hypersensitivity produces excess secretions, distending ducts and producing cysts and later fibrosis. In animal models, iodides correct cystic spaces and partially correct excess cellular reproduction; elemental iodine corrects entire disease process. Elemental iodine is preferred form for breast metabolism. Oral iodine has acute and long-term antiinflammatory and antifibrotic effects. Human studies: iodides effective in 70% of subjects but with high rate of side effects (altered thyroid function in 4%, iodinism in 3%, and acne in 15%). Elemental iodine gives same benefits but no significant side effects: short-term increased breast pain corresponding to softening of breast and disappearance of fibrous tissue plaques. Dosage of molecular iodine is 70-90 µg/kg body weight (iodine caseinate or liquid iodine).

## Other Considerations

- **Liver function**: liver is primary site for estrogen clearance. Any factor (cholestasis, "toxic liver syndrome," environmental pollution) compromising the liver can cause estrogen excess. Lipotropic factors and B vitamins are necessary for estrogen conjugation.
- **Colon function**: breast disease is linked to a Western diet and bowel function. Epithelial dysplasia in nipple aspirates of breast fluid and frequency of bowel movements (BMs) are also linked. Women having fewer than three BMs per week have 4.5-fold greater risk of FBD compared with women having one or more BMs every day. Colon bacteria transform endogenous and exogenous sterols and fatty acids into toxic metabolites (polycyclic carcinogens and mutagens). Fecal microbes can synthesize estrogens and metabolize estrogen sulfate and glucuronate conjugates. The result is absorption of bacteria-derived and previously conjugated estrogens. Diet influences microflora, transit time, and concentration of absorbable metabolites. Vegetarian women excrete two to three times more conjugated estrogens than omnivores. Omnivorous women have 50% higher unconjugated estrogens. *Lactobacillus* supplements lower fecal beta-glucuronidase.
- **Fiber**: an inverse correlation exists between dietary fiber and risk of benign, proliferative, epithelial breast disorders. Increasing dietary fiber may reduce risk for benign disease and breast cancer.

## THERAPEUTIC APPROACH

Some women have noncyclic FBD; others have cyclic premenstrual breast tenderness and lumpiness. Therapy given in the *Textbook*, "Premenstrual Syndrome," may be more appropriate for individual needs. Recommendations here include key factors in that chapter and this one.

- **Diet**: primarily vegetarian with large amounts of dietary fiber. Eliminate all methylxanthines until symptoms are alleviated, then reintroduce in small amounts. Reducing fat to 15% of total calories, while increasing complex carbohydrates, reduces premenstrual breast tenderness and swelling as well as actual breast swelling and nodularity in some women. Reducing fat intake decreases circulating estrogens. Avoid exogenous estrogens (oral contraceptives, hormone replacement therapy, estrogen-augmented animal products). Emphasize whole, unprocessed foods (whole grains, legumes, vegetables, fruits, nuts, and seeds). Drink 48+ oz pure water daily.
- **Supplements**:
  —Vitamin B complex: 10 times the recommended daily allowance.
  —Lipotropic factors:
    - Choline: 500-1000 mg q.d.
    - Methionine: 500-1000 mg q.d.

  —Vitamin $B_6$: 25-50 mg t.i.d.
  —Vitamin C: 500 mg t.i.d.
  —Vitamin E: 400-800 IU q.d. D-alpha tocopherol
  —Beta-carotene: 50,000-300,000 IU q.d.
  —Iodine (molecular iodine): 3 to 6 mg q.d. (prescription item)
  —Zinc: 15 mg q.d.
  —EPO: 1500 mg b.i.d.
  —Flaxseed oil: 1 tbsp q.d.
  —*Lactobacillus acidophilus*: 1-2 billion live organisms q.d.

# Fibromyalgia Syndrome

## DIAGNOSTIC SUMMARY

- Affects 2%-13% of population, 80%-90% of which are female.
- Chronic widespread pain involving axial pain; pain on left, right, upper, and lower parts of body.
- Abnormal tenderness at 11 or more of 18 specific anatomic tender point (TnP) sites.
- Associated symptoms include fatigue, stiffness, headache, sleep disturbance, irritable bowel, depression, cognitive dysfunction, anxiety, coldness, paresthesias, sicca symptoms, exercise intolerance, dysmenorrhea.

## DIFFERENTIAL DIAGNOSIS

- Two major criteria for fibromyalgia syndrome (FMS) are chronic (>3 months) widespread pain and tenderness.
- Hypothyroidism and cellular resistance to thyroid hormone may present with symptoms of FMS. Thyroid testing and a trial of thyroid hormone therapy can determine whether FMS is related to these disorders.
- Main disorders for differentiation are arthritis, myopathy, polymyalgia rheumatica, diabetic polyneuropathy, ankylosing spondylitis, discopathy, cardiac or pleural pain, multiple muscle myofascial pain syndromes, and lupus erythematosus.
- Distinguish FMS (except for hypothyroidism or cellular resistance to thyroid hormone) by careful pathognomy. Symptoms and signs of most FMS patients are indistinguishable from the subclass of hypothyroid or thyroid hormone–resistant patients for whom pain is the predominant symptom.

## GENERAL CONSIDERATIONS

- **Serotonin deficiency hypothesis**: central nervous system (CNS) serotonin deficiency reduces efficiency of brainstem-spinal cord descending antinociceptive system, resulting in heightened pain

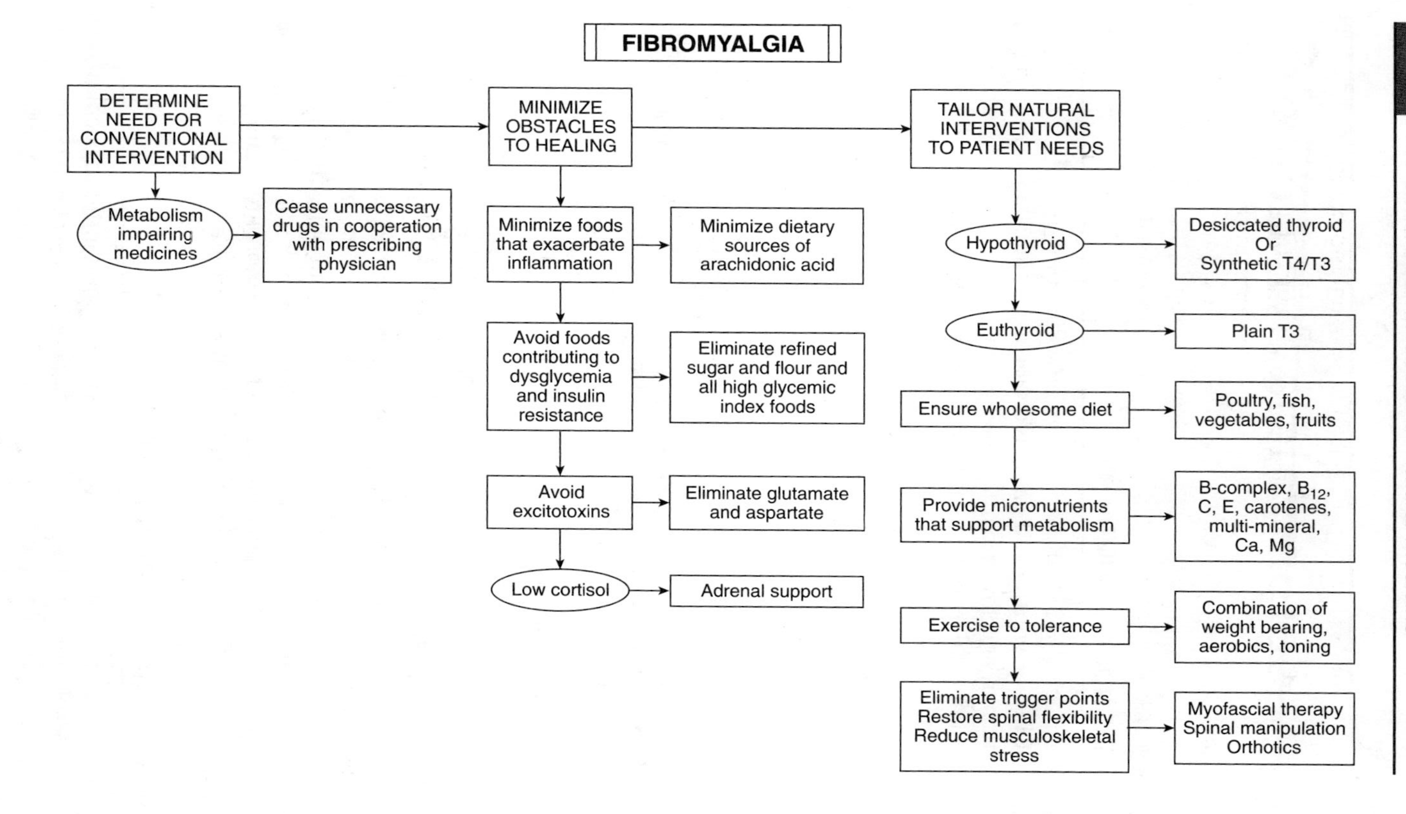
FIBROMYALGIA
DETERMINE NEED FOR CONVENTIONAL INTERVENTION
Metabolism impairing medicines
Cease unnecessary drugs in cooperation with prescribing physician
MINIMIZE OBSTACLES TO HEALING
Minimize foods that exacerbate inflammation
Minimize dietary sources of arachidonic acid
Avoid foods contributing to dysglycemia and insulin resistance
Eliminate refined sugar and flour and all high glycemic index foods
Avoid excitotoxins
Eliminate glutamate and aspartate
Low cortisol
Adrenal support
TAILOR NATURAL INTERVENTIONS TO PATIENT NEEDS
Hypothyroid
Desiccated thyroid Or Synthetic T4/T3
Euthyroid
Plain T3
Ensure wholesome diet
Poultry, fish, vegetables, fruits
Provide micronutrients that support metabolism
B-complex, $B_{12}$, C, E, carotenes, multi-mineral, Ca, Mg
Exercise to tolerance
Combination of weight bearing, aerobics, toning
Eliminate trigger points Restore spinal flexibility Reduce musculoskeletal stress
Myofascial therapy Spinal manipulation Orthotics

perception in response to normal afferent input. This theory has been refuted.

- **Hypometabolism hypothesis**: contributing factors are hypothyroidism and/or partial cellular resistance to thyroid hormone, pernicious diet, nutritional deficiencies, low physical fitness level, and metabolism-impeding drugs. Inadequate thyroid hormone regulation (ITHR) may be underlying mechanism of two main features of FMS: chronic widespread pain and abnormal tenderness. ITHR of metabolic processes in brainstem-spinal cord descending antinociceptive system can cause the following:
  —Spontaneous or ongoing pain
  —Tenderness (lowering pain threshold to mechanical stimuli)
  —Hyperalgesia (increased responsiveness to noxious stimuli)

Following are two mechanisms of the syndrome:

- ITHR increases substance P, which is released from nociceptor neurons, is high in CSF of FMS patients, and facilitates summation of slow nociceptive signals, amplifying nociceptive signals in spinal cord. Thyroid hormone inhibits substance P synthesis and secretion in many CNS cells by repressing transcription of the gene for preprotachykinin-A, a precursor of substance P, and its cognate substance P receptor. Thyroid hormone treatment lowers substance P level in the anterior pituitary, brain nuclei, and dorsal horns of the spinal cord. Excess thyroid hormone reduces substance P to subnormal levels.
- ITHR reduces synthesis and secretion of norepinephrine (NE) in the brainstem locus ceruleus cells, which are essential to the normal function of the descending antinociceptive system.

Antinociception pathways contain neurons that secrete serotonin or NE. Serotonin secretion is tonically augmented by NE secretion; normal serotonin secretion depends on NE secretion. Serotonin stimulates interneurons to secrete opiates that inhibit transmission by blocking release of the neurotransmitters glutamate and substance P from afferent neurons and block $Ca^{++}$ influx into and $K^{+}$ efflux from afferent terminals (type C and A delta fibers), inhibiting nociceptive signals to spinothalamic neurons transmitting signals to the brain. Low NE from descending neurons may reduce serotonin selectively at dorsal horn interneurons, reducing opiates. Transmission of nociceptive signals heightens pain perception.

FMS patients have decreased NE (low dopamine and NE metabolites in CSF). The locus ceruleus has the brain's heaviest concentration of triiodothyronine ($T_3$). $T_3$ regulates two rate-limiting enzymes: (1) tyrosine hydroxylase, which converts tyrosine to dihydroxyphenylalanine, which is converted to dopamine. Tyrosine hydroxylase activity in the locus ceruleus noradrenergic neurons is low in patients with hypothyroidism. Thyroid hormone therapy increases activity of tyrosine hydroxylase. (2) Dopamine-β-hydroxylase converts dopamine to NE. NE in the antinociceptive system and other tissues in thyroid disorders has not been studied extensively.

**Other factors**: Most FMS patients are physically inactive because of pain; low motor drive from low dopamine contributes to inactivity. Low physical activity contributes to inefficiency of antinociceptive system.

ITHR can account for muscle and joint pain, paresthesias, cognitive dysfunction, depression, cold intolerance, exercise intolerance, weakness and fatigue, dry skin and mucous membranes, constipation, dysmenorrhea, menorrhagia, increased platelet $\alpha_2$-adrenergic receptor density, reduced brain blood flow, reduced peripheral blood flow, sleep disturbance, deficient slow-wave sleep, hypotension, blunted sympathetic response to stress, stiffness and swelling, irritable bowel syndrome, excessive urination, high serum hyaluronic acid, low procollagen III, high ground substance proteoglycans, low pyridinoline and hydroxyproline, glycolysis abnormalities, low cell levels of high-energy phosphates, and low human growth hormone (HGH) and somatomedin C. Thyroid hormone's effect on the adrenergic system suggests that FMS is a condition of alpha-adrenergic dominance.

Virtually identical presentations occur with FMS, hypothyroidism, and peripheral cellular resistance to thyroid hormone. Ninety percent of FMS patients have some form of thyroid disease or cellular resistance. The only clinical trials fully relieving FMS used oral thyroid hormone plus other metabolism-regulating therapies.

### Other Metabolism-Regulating Therapies

Thyroid hormone is necessary but not sufficient for full recovery. Other therapies—wholesome diet, nutritional supplements, exercise to tolerance—provide some improvement but not full recovery. Additional intervention requires physical treatment.

- **Wholesome diet**: vegetarian diets; eliminate excitotoxins monosodium L-glutamate and aspartame; ingest *Chlorella pyrenoidosa*; uncooked vegan diet of berries, fruits, vegetables and roots, nuts, germinated seeds, sprouts; strict, low-salt, uncooked vegan diet rich in lactobacteria.

- **Nutritional supplements**: vitamins $B_1$, $B_6$, $B_{12}$, C, E, and beta-carotene have antinociceptive properties. Myers' cocktail (intravenous B vitamins, vitamin C, calcium, magnesium [Mg]); 5-hydroxy-L-tryptophan (5HT); S-adenosyl-L-methionine (SAM); Mg; malic acid; combined aloe vera extracts, plant saccharides, freeze-dried fruits and vegetables; *Dioscorea*; vitamin/mineral supplement; collagen hydrolysate; blend of ascorbigen and broccoli powder.
- **Exercise to tolerance**: results of exercise treatment for FMS are mixed. Cardiovascular exercise provides the most improvement, especially low-intensity endurance training. Endurance exercise reduces physical limitations of FMS. Low metabolic efficiency from ITHR renders some patients susceptible to FMS. Vigorous exercise exacerbates symptoms; high density of $\alpha_2$-adrenergic receptors on FMS patients' platelets indicates receptor density in CNS. Binding catecholamines to high density of membrane receptors inhibits energy metabolism, worsening symptoms. During early phase of treatment, use mild exercise to minimize catecholamine secretion. Thyroid hormone therapy decreases density of $\alpha_2$-adrenergic receptors and increases $\alpha_2$-adrenergic receptors, enabling cells to respond appropriately to high catecholamines. Shifting from $\alpha_2$-adrenergic receptor dominance explains the ability to engage in vigorous activity after thyroid hormone therapy.
- **Physical medicine**: necessary to eliminate FMS pain. Spinal manipulation, soft tissue manipulation, and trigger point therapy relieve pain. Lesions exacerbating FMS: myofascial trigger points and spinal joint fixations. Any nociception-generating neuromusculoskeletal lesion can exacerbate pain because of the impaired antinociceptive system. Neuromusculoskeletal lesions can disturb sleep, increasing symptoms in hypometabolic patients.

## THERAPEUTIC CONSIDERATIONS

### Laboratory Testing for Thyroid Status

#### Thyroid Function Tests

- Primary hypothyroidism (hormone deficiency from subnormal function of thyroid gland) is detected by two standard thyroid batteries:
  - —Thyroxine ($T_4$), $T_3$ uptake, free $T_4$ index, thyroid-stimulating hormone (TSH)
  - —Free $T_3$, free $T_4$, TSH

In untreated primary hypothyroidism TSH is elevated; revised upper limit of serum TSH reference range is 2.5 μU/mL.

- Thyroid-releasing hormone (TRH) stimulation test distinguishes two conditions:
  —Euthyroidism (normal function of hypothalamic-pituitary-thyroid axis)
  —Central hypothyroidism (hormone deficiency caused by pituitary or hypothalamic dysfunction)
  Basal blood TSH level is measured. TRH is then injected. Thirty minutes later TSH is measured again. Subtract baseline TSH from 30-minute level to derive TSH response to injected TRH. Normal = 8.5 to 20.0 μU/mL. Below 8.5 μU/mL suggests pituitary hypothyroidism; above 20.0 μU/mL suggests central hypothyroidism. (Exaggerated TSH response to TRH does not distinguish pituitary and hypothalamic hypothyroidism.) Diagnosis is tentative without evidence of other pituitary or hypothalamic hormone abnormalities (assays), pituitary or hypothalamic structural abnormalities (imaging), or mutations of TRH or TSH gene (nucleotide sequencing).

### Thyroid Antibodies

The most common cause of primary hypothyroidism is autoimmune thyroiditis. Test is titer of thyroglobulin and thyroid microsomal (peroxidase) antibodies, which are important in FMS. Patients with elevated thyroid antibodies may also have thyroid function test results within reference ranges for years, but high thyroid microsomal antibodies occur in those with musculoskeletal symptoms. Prevalence of antibodies is higher in women than in men. In autoimmune thyroiditis, thyroid hormone levels too low to regulate the CNS antinociceptive system can escape detection by thyroid function tests, including TSH.

### Thyroid Hormone Therapy Based on Initial Thyroid Status

- FMS with primary or central hypothyroidism: use preparation with both $T_4$ and $T_3$ in a $T_4/T_3$ 4:1 ratio. Dosage: 2 to 4 grains (76 μg $T_4$ and 18 μg $T_3$ to 152 μg $T_4$ and 36 μg $T_3$). Hypothyroid and euthyroid FMS patients tend not to recover with conventional

$T_4$ replacement. $T_4/T_3$ preparations and $T_3$ alone have been effective, in violation of conventional mandates for $T_4$ replacement:
—Hormone therapy applied despite test results indicating euthyroid.
—Dosages not titrated according to TSH levels but by clinical responses to particular dosages.

- Effective dosages suppressed TSH levels, yet no symptoms of thyrotoxicosis arose or evidence of thyrotoxicosis by electrocardiogram, bone densitometry, or serum and urine biochemical tests.
- FMS with tests indicating euthyroidism: begin with plain $T_3$. Seventy-five percent of patients testing as euthyroid have partial peripheral cellular resistance to thyroid hormone according to four criteria:
  1. Euthyroid (thyroid function tests including TRH stimulation) before beginning $T_3$
  2. Recover from hypothyroid-like FMS symptoms and signs with supraphysiologic dosages of $T_3$
  3. Extremely high serum free $T_3$ after beginning $T_3$ therapy
  4. No evidence of tissue thyrotoxicosis: serial electrocardiograms, serum and urine biochemical tests, bone densitometry

  These patients benefit only from plain $T_3$ (not sustained-release $T_3$) in a single daily dose, responding only to supraphysiologic dosages of $T_3$. $T_3$ dosage = 75 to 125 μg. For some patients safe, effective dosages are far higher. Some FMS patients have both hypothyroidism and cellular resistance to thyroid hormone. Determine over time which form of hormone works best for an individual patient.

## Dosage Adjustments

Titrate dosage changes according to tissue responses, not thyroid function tests, which have no value in finding the safest, most effective dosage for any particular patient. Inference in the metabolic status of cells (other than thyrotrophs of anterior pituitary) from thyroid function tests is not justified. Levels of $T_3$ and $T_4$ in cells of different tissues cannot be accurately predicted from plasma TSH, $T_3$, or $T_4$. TSH levels correlate poorly with tissue metabolic status, such as speed of relaxation of the Achilles reflex. Symptoms and signs are more accurate and reliable indicators of tissue metabolic status than are thyroid function tests.

### Rehabilitation Model: Data-Driven Clinical Decisions

Distinguish all factors impairing metabolism. Individualize treatment to correct, eliminate, or compensate for factors. A data-driven rehabilitation model requires baseline and repeated monitoring of clinical status by objective assessment methods.

### Objective Assessment of Patient Status

Recovery gradually occurs over a 2- to 6-month period. Quantify patient's clinical status by objective measures weekly or biweekly. Post measurement scores as data points on line graphs after each evaluation, with baseline score before therapy as initial data point on each graph. Draw a line connecting data points to create a trend line to assess regimen efficacy. Typically, all measures change together in a direction of improvement, no improvement, or worse. Patient subjective status usually closely corresponds to trend lines. False conclusions that no progress has occurred, despite minor setbacks, are quickly corrected by reviewing graphs objectively displaying real progress. Following are five objective assessments (in addition to physical examination at each evaluation):

- **Pain distribution body form**: the most sensitive indicator for changes in FMS status is pain distribution as percentage of body in pain. (Chronic widespread pain is one major criterion for assessing FMS.) Small changes in pain distribution are applied to drawings of body. Patient shades in location of aching, pain, soreness, or tenderness since last evaluation. Place a template over the patient's shaded form. The template divides the body into 36 areas, each with a percentage value. Total values of the shaded divisions. Place percentage number on a graph as a data point. Connect data points with a line to show trend of pain distribution over time.
- **Mean pressure and pain threshold of TnPs**: modified TnP examination measures pressure and pain threshold of TnPs with algometry (numerical values in kilograms per square centimeter), a more precise quantification than the 1990 American College of Rheumatology method, enabling more evidence-based decisions. Calculate mean of threshold values and post to a line graph.
- **FibroQuest Symptoms Survey**: 13 100-mm visual analog scales (VASs), one for each of 13 most common FMS symptoms also characteristic of hypothyroidism and peripheral cellular resis-

tance to thyroid hormone. Patient estimates intensity of each symptom by marking appropriate point on scale (1 to 10). Total values for each marked symptom; divide total symptom intensity by number of symptoms marked at intake (baseline). Post mean score on a line graph.

- **Fibromyalgia Impact Questionnaire (FIQ)**: measure of patient functional status. Post total score as a data point to a line graph.
- **Zing's Self-Rating Depression Scale**: depression is common in FMS. Use this scale in addition to VAS scale for depression. Post score on a line graph.
- **Physical examination**: when FMS treatment includes thyroid hormone, use the five FMS measures plus physical tests that assess tissue responses to hormone: Achilles reflex (relaxation phase), pulse rate, basal body temperature. A combination of these is more reliable than thyroid function tests.

### Integrated Metabolic Therapies Essential for All FMS Patients

Control or eliminate the following metabolism-impeding factors:

- **Thyroid hormone**: 90% of FMS patients have some form of thyroid disease.
- **Modify diet**: minimize arachidonic acid, which increases proinflammatory prostaglandin $E_2$ and leukotriene $B_4$ that contribute to chronic pain. Reduce refined carbohydrates. ITHR of glycolysis, citric acid cycle, and electron transport impedes production of adenosine triphosphate (ATP) and creatine phosphate. Dysglycemia and insulin resistance from refined carbohydrates worsen low production of high-energy phosphates from ITHR.
- **Wide array of nutritional supplements**: synergistic to thyroid hormone by optimal intracellular metabolism.
- **Exercise to tolerance**: sufficiently vigorous physical activity optimizes tissue metabolism and primes CNS descending nociceptive inhibitory system.

### Additional Factors Needed for Some Patients

- **Adrenocortical hypofunction**: low cortisol can produce some symptoms similar to FMS (weakness, fatigue, inability to handle stress, exercise intolerance, hypotension, low nociception threshold). Low cortisol can create patient intolerant of dosage of thyroid hormone high enough to be therapeutic. Yet ITHR alone can cause adrenocortical hypofunction. If low cortisol stems from ITHR, thyroid hormone therapy may correct the deficiency.

- **Neuromusculoskeletal lesion**: provide physical treatment for nociception-generating neuromusculoskeletal lesions (myofascial trigger points and spinal joint lesions) perpetuated by self-sustaining skeletal muscle contractures that may stem from low intramuscular, high-energy phosphate from ITHR.
- **Metabolism-impairing medicines**: some patients must cease some metabolism-impairing medicines and convert from maintenance to as-needed use of others.
  - —Beta-blockers: impair metabolism directly by reducing beta-adrenergic receptor density on cell membranes and increasing alpha$_2$-adrenergic receptor density, exactly as hypothyroidism does. The isoform shift may impair CNS descending antinociceptive system, with pain and tenderness characteristic of FMS.
  - —Narcotics, tranquilizers, muscle relaxants are prescribed as FMS treatments but disincline patients from vigorous physical activity, increasing anergia and heightened pain perception.
  - —Some antidepressants (commonly prescribed for FMS) and decongestants can cause tachycardia when used concurrently with exogenous thyroid hormone. Wean patients off these drugs to increase hormone dosage high enough to be therapeutic.

## THERAPEUTIC APPROACH

### Assess FMS Status

Determine FMS status before treatment is begun and at intervals throughout treatment. Reevaluate weekly to biweekly and before each increase in hormone dosage. Conduct physical examination and review five FMS measures at each evaluation:

- Pain distribution as percentage of 36 body divisions containing pain, according to body drawing
- Mean TnP score in kilograms per square centimeter—algometry
- Symptom intensity estimate—visual analog scales (FibroQuest Symptoms Survey)
- Functional status—Fibromyalgia Impact Questionnaire
- Depression—Zung's Self-Rating Depression Scale

Generate line graphs by using scores for each assessment instrument. Base changes in individualized regimen on trend of scores on line graphs combined with physical examination and clinician's and patient's subjective assessments. Continue process (2 to 6 months) until scores and line graphs normalize, patient no longer meets criteria for FMS, and patient is symptom free and fully functional.

### Patient Safety

- Conduct electrocardiogram before metabolic rehabilitation and, if indicated, at intervals throughout treatment. Arrhythmias usually are not obstacles to metabolic treatment, but identify them before thyroid hormone intervention.
- Educate patients extensively on signs and symptoms of thyrotoxicosis and its management. As indicated by history, test for adrenocortical hypofunction. If cortisol production is diminished, treat with physiologic doses of cortisol at least temporarily before thyroid hormone therapy.

### Thyroid Hormone Therapy

- **Hypothyroid**: begin with 1 grain (60 mg) of desiccated thyroid or synthetic $T_4/T_3$ preparation with a 4:1 ratio. Increase dosage by 2-to-1 grain at 1-month intervals.
- **Euthyroid**: plain $T_3$ at start. Continue dosage of 50-75 μg. Increase dosage at weekly to biweekly intervals by 6.25-12.5 μg. Continue dosage increases until patient is symptom free, no longer meets criteria for FMS, and is fully functional.

Serum and salivary thyroid hormone levels and TSH levels have no value in finding a safe and effective dosage. Titrate according to tissue responses.

### Wholesome Diet

**Components**: Lean meats (poultry and fish), fruits, vegetables; minimize whole grains and arachidonic acid, and additive excitotoxins (glutamate and aspartate). Use organic foods and filtered drinking water.

### Nutritional Supplements

- **Vitamin B complex**: at least 50 mg $B_1$ per tablet, 1 b.i.d.
- **Vitamin $B_{12}$**: 5000-10,000 μg q.d. (try for pain control)
- **Vitamin C**: 1-3 g t.i.d.
- **Vitamin E**: 800-1600 IU q.d. (mixed tocopherols)

- **Carotenoids**: 15 mg q.d.
- **Multimineral formulation**: twice daily
- **Calcium**: 2000 mg q.d.
- **Magnesium**: 1000 mg q.d.
- **Exercise to tolerance**: choose form patient enjoys and gradually increase intensity as symptoms diminish. Use combinations: weight-bearing exercise to support bone health; aerobics to strengthen cardiovascular and pulmonary systems; toning to build lean muscle mass, improving metabolism. Warm water exercise is an ideal way to begin.
- **Physical medicine**: myofascial therapy to eliminate trigger points in muscles and spinal manipulation to regain flexibility of spine and other joints also can raise nociceptive threshold and increase mobility. If an examination indicates, prepare weight-bearing castings for flexible orthotics. For some patients, orthotics reduce musculoskeletal stress and consequent nociceptive input to CNS.

### Abstention from Metabolism-Impairing Medicines

Cease beta-blockers, antidepressants, maintenance dosing of narcotics, tranquilizers, and muscle relaxing drugs.

# Gallstones

## DIAGNOSTIC SUMMARY

- May be asymptomatic or cause biliary colic with irregular pain-free intervals of days or months.
- Real-time ultrasonography provides definitive diagnosis.

## GENERAL CONSIDERATIONS

Gallstones are a "Western diet"–induced disease affecting 20% of women and 8% of men over age 40 years. Twenty million Americans have gallstones. Each year 1 million more develop gallstones. More than 300,000 cholecystectomies are performed each year for gallstones. Gallstones are risk factor for gallbladder (GB) cancer. Bile components are bile salts, bilirubin, cholesterol, phospholipids, fatty acids, water, electrolytes, other organic and inorganic substances. Gallstones arise when solubilized bile components become supersaturated and precipitate.

- **Four categories**: (1) pure cholesterol; (2) pure pigment (calcium bilirubinate); (3) mixed, containing cholesterol and derivatives plus bile salts, pigments, and inorganic calcium salts; (4) mineral.
- **Pure stones** (cholesterol or calcium bilirubinate) are rare in the United States, where 80% are mixed and 20% are exclusively minerals (calcium salts, oxides of silicon and aluminum).

## PATHOGENESIS

Three steps: (1) bile supersaturation, (2) nucleation and initiation of stone formation, and (3) enlargement of gallstone by accretion.

Cholesterol and mixed stones require cholesterol supersaturation of bile within the GB. Bile solubility and supersaturation are based on relative molar concentrations of cholesterol, bile acids, phosphatidylcholine (lecithin), and water. Free cholesterol is water-insoluble—it must be in lecithin-bile salt micelle. Increased

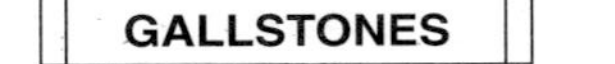
GALLSTONES

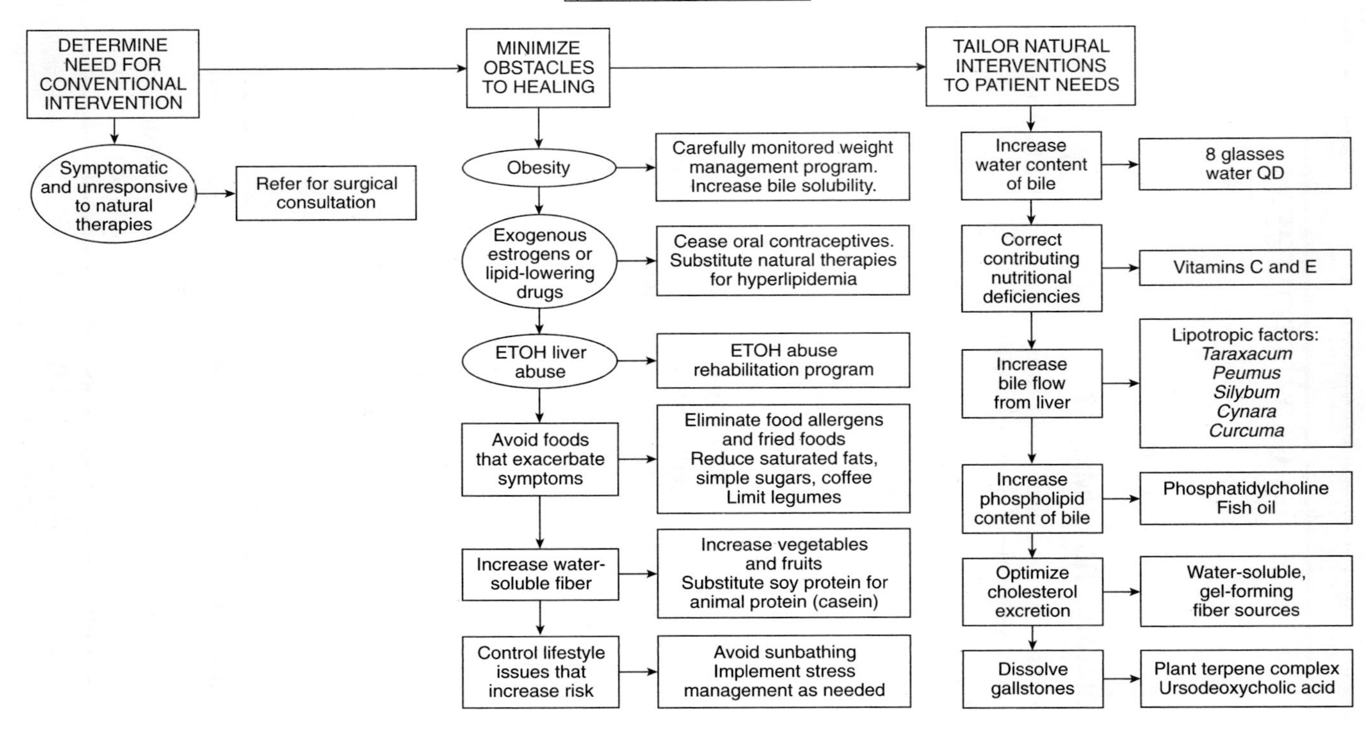
DETERMINE NEED FOR CONVENTIONAL INTERVENTION
Symptomatic and unresponsive to natural therapies
Refer for surgical consultation
MINIMIZE OBSTACLES TO HEALING
Obesity
Carefully monitored weight management program. Increase bile solubility.
Exogenous estrogens or lipid-lowering drugs
Cease oral contraceptives. Substitute natural therapies for hyperlipidemia
ETOH liver abuse
ETOH abuse rehabilitation program
Avoid foods that exacerbate symptoms
Eliminate food allergens and fried foods
Reduce saturated fats, simple sugars, coffee
Limit legumes
Increase water-soluble fiber
Increase vegetables and fruits
Substitute soy protein for animal protein (casein)
Control lifestyle issues that increase risk
Avoid sunbathing
Implement stress management as needed
TAILOR NATURAL INTERVENTIONS TO PATIENT NEEDS
Increase water content of bile
8 glasses water QD
Correct contributing nutritional deficiencies
Vitamins C and E
Increase bile flow from liver
Lipotropic factors: *Taraxacum* *Peumus* *Silybum* *Cynara* *Curcuma*
Increase phospholipid content of bile
Phosphatidylcholine
Fish oil
Optimize cholesterol excretion
Water-soluble, gel-forming fiber sources
Dissolve gallstones
Plant terpene complex
Ursodeoxycholic acid

cholesterol secretion or decreased bile acid or lecithin secretion induces supersaturation. Stone formation is initiated by biliary stasis, infection, or mucin. Radius increases at 2.6 mm/year, eventually reaching size of a few millimeters to more than a centimeter. Stone is symptomatic 8 years after formation begins. Cholelithiasis occurs in 95% of patients with cholecystitis.

Risk factors for cholesterol and mixed stones are diet, sex, race, obesity, high caloric intake, estrogens, gastrointestinal diseases (Crohn's disease, cystic fibrosis), drugs, and age.

- **Gender**: frequency is two to four times greater in women than in men. Women are predisposed because of either increased cholesterol synthesis or suppression of bile acids by estrogens. Pregnancy, oral contraceptives, or other causes of elevated estrogen increase incidence.
- **Genetic and ethnic**: gallstones are most common in Native American women older than 30 years (70% have gallstones). Only 10% of black women older than 30 years have gallstones. Differences reflect extent of cholesterol saturation of bile. Dietary factors outweigh genetic factors.
- **Obesity**: increases activity of 3-hydroxy-3-methylglutaryl coenzyme A (HMG CoA) reductase and secretion of cholesterol in bile from increased cholesterol synthesis. Obesity is linked to much increased incidence because of biliary cholesterol saturation. During active weight reduction, biliary cholesterol saturation initially increases. Secretion of biliary lipids is reduced during weight loss, but secretion of bile acids decreases more than cholesterol. When weight is stabilized, bile acid output returns to normal and cholesterol output remains low. Net effect is a significant reduction in cholesterol saturation. Prolonged dietary fat reduction can promote biliary stasis, causing cholesterol saturation. 10+ g of fat daily are needed for proper GB emptying.
- **Gastrointestinal tract diseases**: Crohn's disease and cystic fibrosis involve malabsorption of bile acids from the terminal ileum that disturbs enterohepatic circulation by reducing bile acid pool and rate of bile secretion.
- **Drugs**: tamoxifen increases gallstones. Over 5 years, incidence of stones in tamoxifen-treated patients was 37.4% versus 2.0% in those not taking drug. Other problematic agents are oral contraceptives, other estrogens, cephalosporin ceftriaxone, octreotide, HMG CoA reductase inhibitors, and possibly other lipid-lowering drugs.

- **Age**: average gallstone patient is 40-50 years old. Incidence increases with age because of inactivity of cholesterol 7-alpha-hydroxylase with increased biliary cholesterol hypersecretion, cholesterol saturation, and accelerated stone formation.
- **Risk factors for pigmented gallstones**: geography, sun exposure, severe diseases. They are more common in Asia because of liver and GB parasites (liver fluke *Clonorchis sinensis*). Bacteria and protozoa cause stasis or act as nucleating agents. In the United States, pigmented stones are caused by chronic hemolysis or alcohol liver cirrhosis.

## THERAPEUTIC CONSIDERATIONS

Gallstones are easier to prevent than reverse. Primary treatment is to reduce controllable risk factors. Therapeutic intervention is to avoid aggravating foods and increase solubility of cholesterol in bile. If symptoms persist or worsen, cholecystectomy is indicated. Eliminate foods producing symptoms. Increase dietary fiber. Eliminate food allergens. Reduce refined carbohydrates and animal protein. Gallstones increase risk for GB cancer. Vegetables and fruits protect against GB cancer; red meat (beef, mutton) increase risk of gallbladder carcinogenesis. Use nutritional lipotropic compounds and herbal choleretics to increase solubility of bile. Biliary cholesterol concentration and serum cholesterol do not correlate, but increased serum triglycerides are linked to bile saturation.

**Asymptomatic gallstones**: natural history of silent or asymptomatic gallstones suggests elective cholecystectomy is not warranted. Cumulative chance for developing symptoms is 10% at 5 years, 15% at 10 years, and 18% at 15 years. If controllable risk factors are eliminated or reduced, the patient remains asymptomatic.

### Diet

- **Dietary fiber**: diet high in refined carbohydrates and fat and low in fiber reduces liver synthesis of bile acids and lowers bile acids in the GB. Fiber reduces absorption of deoxycholic acid, produced from bile acids by gut bacteria, which lessens solubility of cholesterol in bile. Fiber decreases formation of deoxycholic acid and binds deoxycholic acid for fecal excretion. Prefer water-soluble fibers: vegetables, fruits, pectin, oat bran, and guar gum. Diets rich in legumes with water-soluble fiber (Native Americans) are linked to increased risk for cholesterol gallstones.

Legumes increase biliary cholesterol saturation because of saponin content; restrict legume intake with gallstones.

- **Vegetarian diet**: protective against gallstones because of fiber content. Animal proteins (casein from dairy) increase formation of gallstones; vegetable proteins (soy) are preventive against gallstones.
- **Food allergies**: food allergies may cause GB pain. One study demonstrated 100% of patients to be symptom free while on elimination diet (beef, rye, soybeans, rice, cherries, peaches, apricots, beets, spinach). Foods inducing symptoms, in decreasing order of occurrence, are: egg, pork, onion, fowl, milk, coffee, citrus, corn, beans, nuts. Ingestion of allergy-causing substances may cause swelling of bile ducts, impairing bile flow from GB.
- **Buckwheat**: decreases gallstone formation and reduces concentration of cholesterol in GB, plasma, and liver of animals compared with casein. Buckwheat is far more protective than soy. Buckwheat can enhance bile acid synthesis and fecal excretion of steroids. It may treat both hypercholesterolemia and gallstones and reduce colon cancer cell proliferation. Higher levels of arginine and glycine may help in buckwheat's protective function.
- **Sugars**: increase risk of biliary tract cancer based on relation between sugars, blood lipids, and gallstone formation. Sugar increases cholesterol saturation of bile. Gallstones are linked to monosaccharides and disaccharides, independent of other energy sources.
- **Caloric restriction**: total calorie and carbohydrate intake and serum triglycerides are higher in gallstone patients than in control subjects. Refined carbohydrate intake is higher in female gallstone patients; fat intake is higher in male gallstone patients. Caloric intake of more than 2500 kcal/day and diets rich in carbohydrates and saturated fats increased gallstone risk. Alcohol intake at 20-40 g/day was protective. Caloric restriction must be instituted carefully because rapid weight loss and fasting increase risk of gallstones. Those who develop gallstones have higher baseline triglyceride and total cholesterol and greater rate of weight loss than those who did not.
- **Coffee**: can promote symptoms of gallstones but may also inhibit their formation. Avoid coffee until stones are resolved: coffee (regular and decaffeinated) induces GB contractions by cholecystokinin secretion. In women, 4 cups of caffeinated coffee daily induce 28% lower risk of developing symptoms of gallstones. Drinking coffee regularly before or during early stone formation

may inhibit development or clear small stones by enhanced GB contractions from multiple daily coffee doses. Large existing stones may exacerbate symptoms if contractions are induced by coffee.

## Nutritional Factors

- **Lecithin (phosphatidylcholine)**: main cholesterol solubilizer in bile. Low lecithin in bile may be a causative factor. A pure bile salt micelle requires 50 molecules to enclose a single molecule of cholesterol; a mixed bile salt/phospholipid micelle requires only seven molecules. Taking only 100 mg lecithin t.i.d. increases lecithin in bile, and larger doses (up to 10 g) provide greater increases. Increased lecithin content of bile usually increases solubility of cholesterol. No significant effects on gallstone dissolution are obtained by using lecithin alone.
- **Nutrient deficiencies**: deficiencies of either vitamins E or C cause gallstones in animal studies.
- **Olive oil**: olive oil "liver flush" is undesirable for patients with gallstones; consuming large quantities of any oil induces contraction of GB, increasing risk of stone blocking bile duct and causing a surgical emergency. Oleic acid increases development of gallstones in lab animals by increasing cholesterol in the GB.
- **Fish oils**: in animal studies fish oil increases biliary phospholipid secretion and reduces cholesterol concentration in the GB and rate of gallstone formation. Omega-3 eicosapentaenoic acid (EPA) and docosahexaenoic acid (DHA) inhibit gallstone formation and decrease biliary calcium and total protein. Omega-3 fatty acids enhance stability of biliary phospholipid-cholesterol vesicles.
- **Lipotropic factors and botanical choleretics**: lipotropic factors are substances that hasten removal or decrease deposit of fat in the liver by interaction with fat metabolism. Lipotropic agents—choline, methionine, betaine, folic acid, and vitamin $B_{12}$—are used with herbal cholagogues and choleretics. Cholagogues stimulate GB contraction, whereas choleretics increase bile secretion by liver. Herbal choleretics have favorable effect on solubility of bile. Choleretics appropriate to gallstones are *Taraxacum officinale* (dandelion root), silymarin from *Silybum marianum* (milk thistle), *Cynara scolymus* (artichoke), *Curcuma longa* (turmeric), and *Peumus boldo* (alkaloid boldine helps treat gallstones).

## Chemical Dissolution of Gallstones

Use complex of plant terpenes alone or, preferably, in combination with oral bile acids. Decreasing GB cholesterol and/or increasing bile acids or lecithin should result in dissolution of stone. Chemical dissolution is especially indicated for gallstones in the elderly who cannot withstand stress of surgery and in others for whom surgery is contraindicated.

- **Bile acids**: increase cholesterol solubility. Oral chenodeoxycholic acid alone (750 mg q.d.) has completely dissolved gallstones in 13.5% and partially dissolved in 27% of patients in one study but often takes several years with mild diarrhea and possible liver damage. Ursodeoxycholic acid is more effective with fewer side-effects.
- **Terpenes**: natural terpene combination (menthol, menthone, pinene, borneol, cineol, camphene) is an effective alternative to surgery. It is safe even when consumed up to 4 years.
- **Combined therapy**: terpenes are effective alone but best results come from combining plant terpenes and bile acids. Lower doses of bile acids can be used, reducing risk of side effects and cost of bile acid therapy. Menthol is a major component of formula; peppermint oil, especially enteric coated, may offer similar results.

### Lifestyle

- **Sunbathing**: almost all cholesterol gallstones contain a central, pigmented nucleus with radial or lamellar pigmented bands, alternating with layers of crystalline cholesterol. Activation of the pigmentary system by ultraviolet light may increase concentrations of indole metabolites in bile, triggering their polymerization. Positive attitude toward sunbathing is linked to twice the risk of cholelithiasis compared with those with negative attitude. The association is almost entirely restricted to those who always burn after long sunbathing.
- **Social stress**: chronic social stress can increase bile retention, increase GB hypertrophy, and inhibit GB emptying. Chronic stress may be predictor of GB dysfunction and eventual gallstone formation.

## THERAPEUTIC APPROACH

Healthy diet rich in dietary fiber, with controlled caloric intake and limited saturated fats, gives adequate prevention. After development of stones, implement measures to avoid GB attacks and increase bile solubility. Limit incidence of symptoms; intolerant or allergic foods and fatty foods must be avoided. Increase solubility of bile; follow dietary guidelines plus nutritional and herbal supplementation on the following page.

- **Diet**: increase vegetables, fruits, and dietary fiber, especially gel-forming or mucilaginous fibers (ground flaxseed, oat bran, guar gum, pectin). Increase intake of buckwheat. Reduce saturated fats, cholesterol, sugar, animal proteins. Avoid all fried foods. Allergy elimination diet reduces GB attacks (*Textbook*, "Food Reactions").
- **Water**: six to eight glasses water daily to optimize water content of bile.
- **Nutritional supplements**:
  —Vitamin C: 1–3 g q.d.
  —Vitamin E: 200–400 IU q.d. (mixed tocopherols)
  —Phosphatidylcholine: 500 mg q.d.
  —Choline: 1 g q.d.
  —L-Methionine: 1 g q.d.
  —Fiber supplement (guar gum, pectin, psyllium, or oat bran): minimum of 5 g q.d.
- **Botanical medicines**:
  —*Taraxacum officinale* (t.i.d.): dried dandelion root, 4 g; fluid extract (1:1), 4-8 mL; solid extract (4:1), 250-500 mg
  —*Peumus boldo* (t.i.d.): dried leaves (or by infusion), 250-500 mg; tincture (1:10), 2-4 mL; fluid extract (1:1), 0.5-1.0 mL
  —*Silybum marianum* (milk thistle): sufficient dosage according to form to yield 70-210 mg of silymarin t.i.d.
  —*Cynara scolymus* (artichoke): extract (15% cynarin), 500 mg t.i.d.
  —*Curcuma longa* (turmeric): use liberally as a spice; curcumin, 300 mg t.i.d.

Gallstone-dissolving formula: menthol, 30 mg; menthone, 5 mg; pinene, 15 mg; borneol, 5 mg; camphene, 5 mg; cineol, 2 mg; citral, 5 mg; phosphatidylcholine, 50 mg; medium-chain triglycerides, 125 mg; chenodeoxycholic acid, 750 mg. Dosage: t.i.d. if used in combination with meals. Note: peppermint oil in enteric-coated capsule can substitute at dosage of 1-2 capsules (0.2 mL/capsule) t.i.d. between meals.

# Glaucoma: Acute (Angle Closure) and Chronic (Open-Angle)

## DIAGNOSTIC SUMMARY

### Acute Glaucoma

- Increased intraocular pressure, usually unilateral.
- Severe throbbing pain in eye with markedly blurred vision.
- Pupil moderately dilated and fixed.
- Absence of pupillary light response.
- Nausea and vomiting common.

### Chronic Glaucoma

- Persistent elevation of intraocular pressure is associated with pathologic cupping of optic discs.
- Asymptomatic in early stages.
- Gradual loss of peripheral vision resulting in tunnel vision.
- Insidious onset in older individuals.

## GENERAL CONSIDERATIONS

Glaucoma is increased intraocular pressure (IOP) from imbalance between production and outflow of aqueous humor. Obstruction to outflow is the main factor in closed-angle glaucoma. Acute glaucoma occurs only with closure of preexisting narrow anterior chamber angle. In chronic open-angle glaucoma, anterior chamber appears normal.

- **Three million cases in the United States**: 25% undetected; 90% are chronic open-angle type (no consistent anatomic basis for condition). Content and composition of collagen and glaucomatous eye are strongly correlated.
- **Collagen**: most abundant protein in the body, including eye. It provides tissue strength and integrity of cornea, sclera, lamina cribosa, trabecular meshwork, and vitreous. Inborn errors of collagen metabolism (osteogenesis imperfecta, Ehlers-Danlos

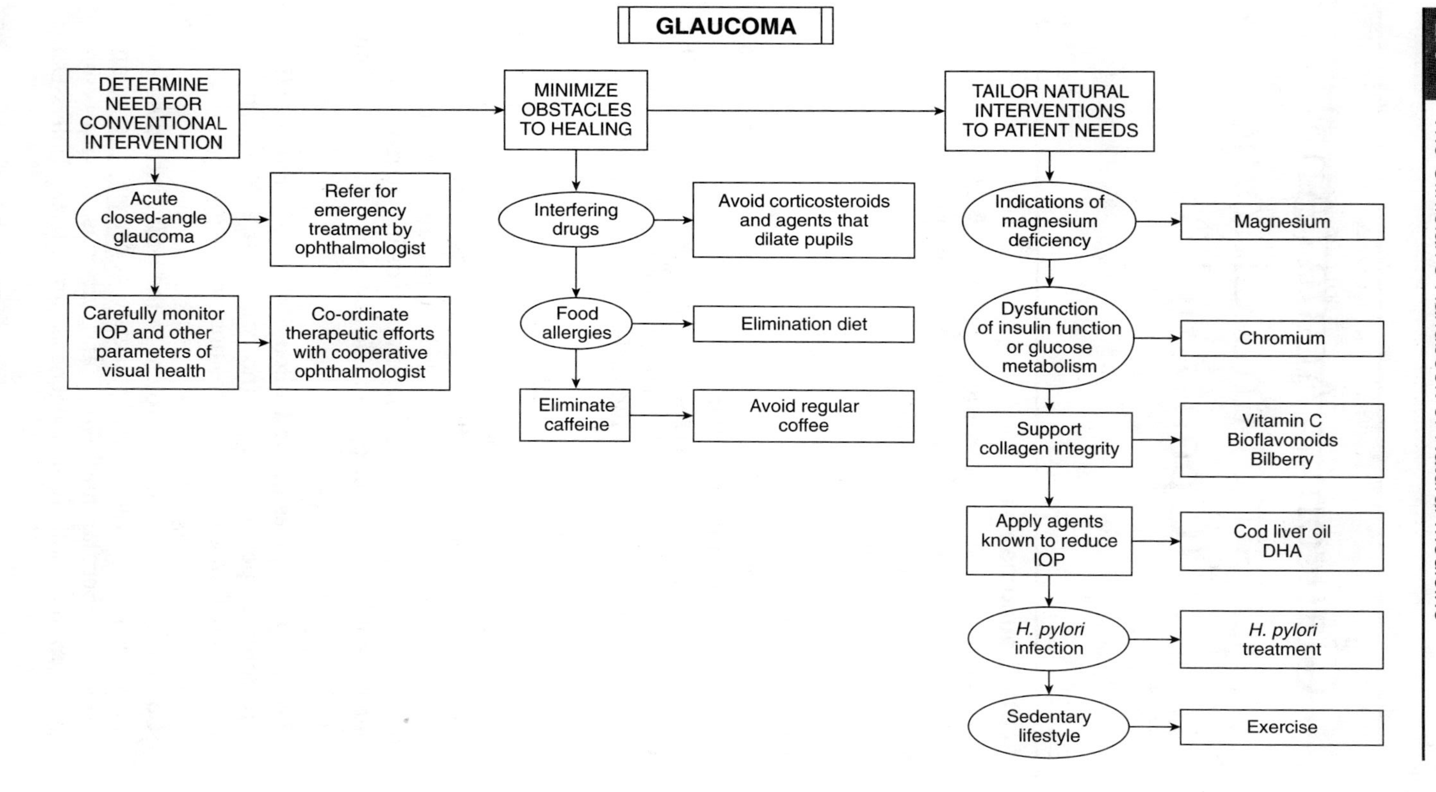
GLAUCOMA
DETERMINE NEED FOR CONVENTIONAL INTERVENTION
Acute closed-angle glaucoma
Refer for emergency treatment by ophthalmologist
Carefully monitor IOP and other parameters of visual health
Co-ordinate therapeutic efforts with cooperative ophthalmologist
MINIMIZE OBSTACLES TO HEALING
Interfering drugs
Avoid corticosteroids and agents that dilate pupils
Food allergies
Elimination diet
Eliminate caffeine
Avoid regular coffee
TAILOR NATURAL INTERVENTIONS TO PATIENT NEEDS
Indications of magnesium deficiency
Magnesium
Dysfunction of insulin function or glucose metabolism
Chromium
Support collagen integrity
Vitamin C Bioflavonoids Bilberry
Apply agents known to reduce IOP
Cod liver oil DHA
H. pylori infection
H. pylori treatment
Sedentary lifestyle
Exercise

syndrome, Marfan's syndrome) have ocular complications: glaucoma, myopia, retinal detachment, ectopia lentis, and blue sclera. Morphologic changes in lamina cribosa (scleral area pierced by optic nerve and blood vessels), trabecular meshwork (connective tissue network the aqueous humor must traverse to reach canal of Schlemm), and papillary blood vessels are found in glaucomatous eyes. Changes may elevate IOP or lead to progressive loss of peripheral vision.

- **Collagen structure changes**: may explain similar peripheral vision loss in patients with normal and elevated IOP, cupping of optic disc even at low IOP, and no apparent anatomic reason for decreased aqueous outflow.

## DIAGNOSIS

There may be slight cupping of optic disc and narrowing of visual fields. Tonometry is the key to confirming diagnosis. Early recognition is critical; delayed surgical intervention increases risk of blindness.

## THERAPEUTIC CONSIDERATIONS

- Treatment and prevention depend on reducing IOP and improving collagen metabolism in optic disc and trabecular meshwork.
- Optic disc is composed of lamina cribosa, optic nerve fibers, and blood vessels. The lamina cribosa is a meshlike network rich in collagen traversed by optic nerves and blood vessels. Collagen changes in lamina cribosa, papillary vessels, and trabecular meshwork precede pressure changes. Intervention must prevent breakdown of ground substance and collagen.
- Corticosteroid use should be discouraged in glaucoma because of inhibition of biosynthesis of collagen and glycosaminoglycans (GAGs), causing glaucoma to develop.

### Nutrition

- **Vitamin C**: achieving collagen integrity requires optimal tissue ascorbic acid (AA); AA lowers IOP in clinical studies. Daily dose of 0.5g/kg body weight (single or divided doses) reduces IOP by 16 mm Hg. Near-normal tension was achieved in some patients unresponsive to acetazolamide (a carbonic anhydrase inhibitor) and 2% pilocarpine (a miotic agent). Hypotonic action of AA on eye is long lasting if supplement continued; intravenous administration gives greater initial reduction in IOP. Patient monitoring is necessary to determine required individual dose (2-35 g q.d.). Abdominal discomfort with high doses is common but resolves after 3-4 days. Proposed mechanisms: increased blood osmolarity, diminished production of aqueous fluid by ciliary epithelium, and improved aqueous fluid outflow; AA role in collagen formation may be key.

- **Bioflavonoids**: anthocyanosides (blue-red pigments in berries) elicit AA-sparing effect, improve capillary integrity, and stabilize collagen matrix by preventing free radical damage, inhibiting enzymatic cleavage of collagen matrix, and by cross-linking with collagen fibers directly to form more stable collagen matrix. *Vaccinium myrtillus* (European bilberry) is rich in these compounds and is used in Europe to reduce myopia, improve nocturnal vision, and reverse diabetic retinopathy. Rutin lowers IOP when used as an adjunct in patients unresponsive to miotics alone.
- **Allergy**: chronic glaucoma has been successfully treated by anti-allergy measures. Immediate rise in IOP of up to 20 mm (plus other allergic symptoms) occurred in patients challenged with appropriate allergen. Allergic responses (altered vascular permeability and vasospasm) may cause congestion and edema characteristic of glaucoma.
- **Magnesium**: Channel-blocking drugs benefit some glaucoma patients. Magnesium (Mg) is "nature's physiologic calcium-channel blocker." Mg dosed at 121.5 mg b.i.d. for 1 month improved visual fields and peripheral circulation in patients with glaucoma.
- **Chromium**: primary open-angle glaucoma is strongly linked to deficiency of red blood cells, chromium (Cr), and AA and elevated red blood cell vanadium (chromium's principal antagonist). AA and Cr potentiate insulin receptors that help sustain strong ciliary muscle eye-focusing activity. AA or Cr deficiency is linked with elevated IOP, which stretches normal eye, reducing capacity for focusing power.
- **Fish oil**: cod liver oil reduces IOP dramatically in lab animals in a dose-dependent fashion. Preliminary human trials with docosahexaenoic acid (DHA) are encouraging
- **Caffeine**: Consumption of regular (180 mg caffeine in 200 ml of coffee) by normotensive glaucoma or ocular hypertensive patients elevates IOP. This elevation may be clinically significant.

## Other Recommendations

- **Exercise**: induces immediate and prolonged reduction in IOP. Within 5 minutes of starting exercise, IOP increases, then gradually decreases to lowest level 60 minutes after completion of exercise. Reduction: Walking/jogging and running—7.2% and 12.7%, respectively, more than decrease in IOP in normal eyes. Duration of IOP reduction: 84 minutes in glaucoma and 63 minutes in normal eyes. Mechanism is independent of

**Differential Diagnosis of the Inflamed Eye**

| | Acute Conjunctivitis | Acute Iritis | Acute Glaucoma | Corneal Trauma or Infection |
|---|---|---|---|---|
| Incidence | Very common | Common | Uncommon | Common |
| Discharge | Moderate to copious | None | None | Watery or purulent |
| Vision | No effect | Slightly blurred | Markedly blurred | Usually blurred |
| Pain | None | Moderate | Severe | Moderate to severe |
| Conjunctival injection | Diffuse, mostly fornices | Circumcorneal | Diffuse | Diffuse |
| Cornea | Clear | Usually clear | Steamy | Clarity may change |
| Pupil size | Normal | Small | Dilated and fixed | Normal |
| Pupil light response | Normal | Poor | None | Normal |
| Intraocular pressure | Normal | Normal | Elevated | Normal |
| Anterior chamber | Normal depth | Normal depth | Very shallow | Normal depth |
| Iris | Normal | Dull, swollen | Congested and bulging | Normal unless infected |
| Smear | Causative organisms | No organisms | No organisms | Causative organisms if there is infection |

systemic BP and sympathetic stimulation but may be influenced by increased serum osmolarity. Moderate to heavy exercise is effective in sedentary subjects, but less effective in physically fit subjects. Physically fit persons tend to have lower IOP. But if one stops exercising, effect wears off in 3 weeks. Yet, many can benefit from exercise.

- ***H. pylori***: Infection is linked to open angle glaucoma. Eradication of *H. pylori* can decrease IOP. See chapter gastric ulcer for a discussion of *H. pylori* treatment.

## THERAPEUTIC APPROACH

Acute closed-angle glaucoma is an ocular emergency; refer immediately to ophthalmologist. Unless treated within 12–48 h, patient will be permanently blinded within 2–5 days. An asymptomatic eye with narrow anterior chamber angle may convert spontaneously to angle-closure glaucoma. The process can be precipitated by anything dilating pupil (atropine, epinephrine-like drugs). Signs / symptoms: extreme pain, blurring of vision, conjunctivitis, fixed and dilated pupil. Agents which dilate pupils must be strictly avoided if glaucoma is suspected.

- Supplements:
  —vitamin C: 0.1–0.5 g/kg q.d. in divided doses
  —bioflavonoids (mixed): 1000 mg q.d.
  —magnesium: 200 mg q.d.
  —chromium: 100 μg q.d.
- Botanical medicines:
  —*Vaccinium myrtillus* extract (25% anthocyanidins): 80 mg t.i.d.

# Gout

## DIAGNOSTIC SUMMARY

- Acute onset, frequently nocturnal, of typically monarticular joint pain involving metatarsophalangeal joint of big toe in approximately 50% of cases.
- Elevated serum uric acid level.
- Asymptomatic periods between acute attacks.
- Identification of urate crystals in joint fluid.
- Aggregated deposits of monosodium urate monohydrate (tophi) chiefly in and around the joints of extremities but also in subcutaneous tissue, bone, cartilage, and other tissues.
- Uric acid kidney stones.
- Familial disease with 95% affected being male.

## GENERAL CONSIDERATIONS

Gout is a common arthritis condition caused by increased uric acid (final breakdown product of purine metabolism) in biologic fluid. Uric acid crystals (monosodium urate) deposit in joints, tendons, kidneys, and other tissues, causing inflammation and damage.

- Characterized biochemically by increased serum uric acid, leukotrienes, and neutrophil accumulation. It may debilitate from tophaceous deposits around joints and tendons. Renal involvement may cause kidney failure by parenchymal disease or urinary tract obstruction.
- Associated with affluence ("rich man's disease"). Meats (organ meats) are high in purines. Alcohol inhibits uric acid excretion by kidneys. Gout is primarily a disease of adult men (95% of cases are men older than 30 years). Incidence rate is three adults in 1000; 10%-20% of adults have hyperuricemia.

### Causes of Gout

- Two major categories:
  1. **Primary gout**: affecting 90% of all cases; usually idiopathic, but several known genetic defects cause elevated uric acid levels.

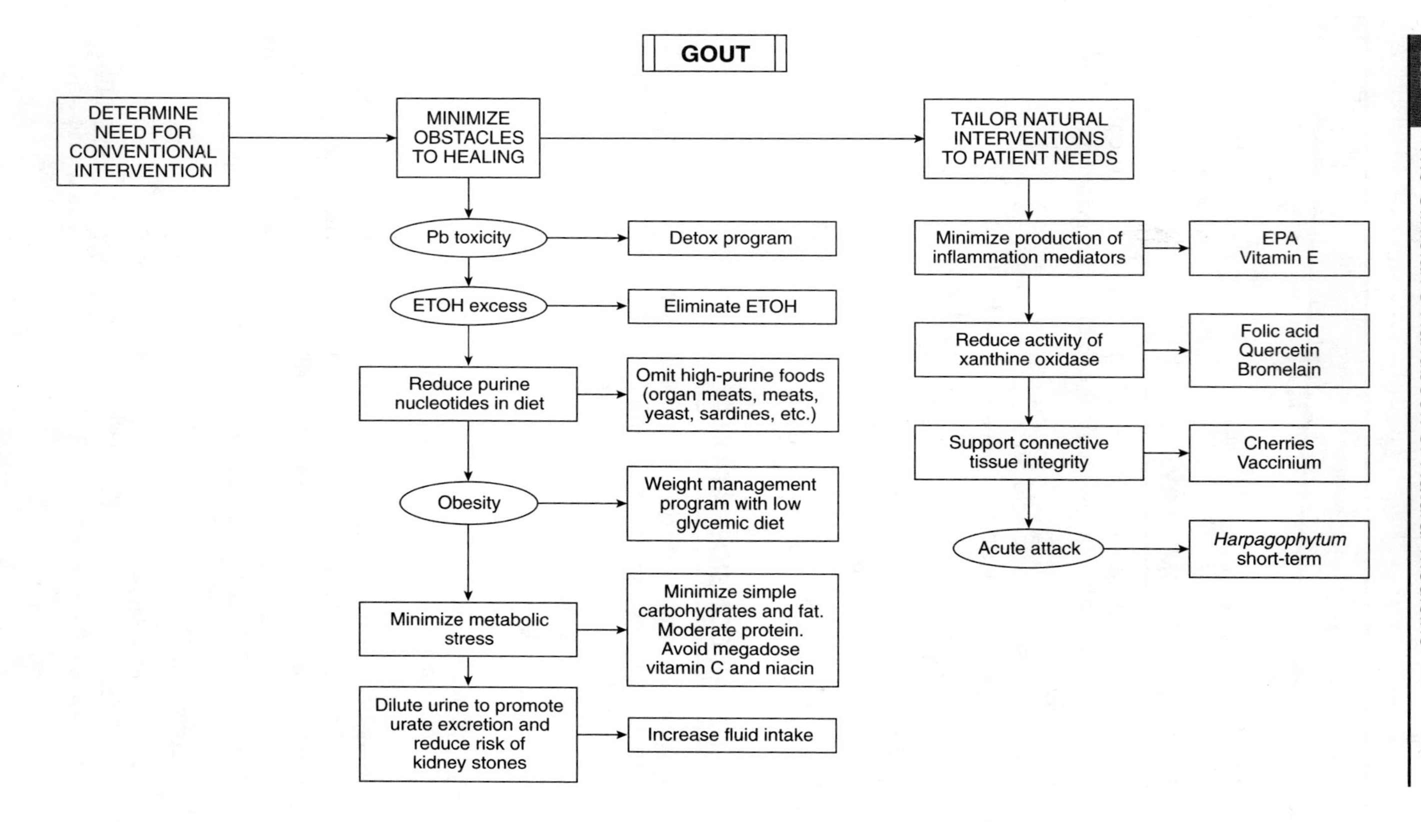
GOUT
DETERMINE NEED FOR CONVENTIONAL INTERVENTION
MINIMIZE OBSTACLES TO HEALING
TAILOR NATURAL INTERVENTIONS TO PATIENT NEEDS
Pb toxicity
Detox program
ETOH excess
Eliminate ETOH
Reduce purine nucleotides in diet
Omit high-purine foods (organ meats, meats, yeast, sardines, etc.)
Obesity
Weight management program with low glycemic diet
Minimize metabolic stress
Minimize simple carbohydrates and fat. Moderate protein. Avoid megadose vitamin C and niacin
Dilute urine to promote urate excretion and reduce risk of kidney stones
Increase fluid intake
Minimize production of inflammation mediators
EPA Vitamin E
Reduce activity of xanthine oxidase
Folic acid Quercetin Bromelain
Support connective tissue integrity
Cherries Vaccinium
Acute attack
Harpagophytum short-term

2. **Secondary gout**: affecting 10% of cases; elevated uric acid is attributable to some other disorder (e.g., excessive breakdown of cells or renal disease). Diuretics for hypertension and low-dose aspirin are causes because they decrease uric acid excretion.

- Hyperuricemia of primary idiopathic gout has three causes:
  1. **Increased synthesis of uric acid** (majority of cases)
  2. **Reduced ability to excrete uric acid** (30% of cases)
  3. **Overproduction of uric acid and underexcretion of uric acid** (minority of cases)
- Exact metabolic defect unknown in most cases but the disease is controllable.
- From 200-600 mg uric acid are excreted daily in urine of adult male, two thirds of the amount produced. The remainder is excreted in bile and other gastrointestinal secretions. Dietary component of uric acid is 10%-20%; in hyperuricemia, 1 mg/100 mL added to serum, enough to precipitate into tissues if individual is near saturation threshold.
- Almost all plasma urate is filtered at glomerulus; only a small amount bound to protein is not filtered. Renal excretion is peculiar; 80% of filtered uric acid is reabsorbed in proximal tubule of nephron. Distal tubule secretes most uric acid in urine. Distal to this site, postsecondary reabsorption occurs. Uric acid is highly insoluble. At a pH of 7.4 and at body temperature, serum is saturated at 6.4-7.0 mg/100 mL. An unknown factor in serum inhibits urate precipitation. The chance of acute attack is 90% when level >9 mg/100 mL. Lower temperatures decrease saturation point; urate deposits form in areas where temperature is lower than mean body temperature (e.g., pinna of ear). Uric acid is insoluble below pH 6.0 and can precipitate as urine is concentrated in collecting ducts and passes to renal pelvis.

## Signs and Symptoms

First attack includes intense pain, usually involving only one joint; first joint of big toe affected in 50% of first attacks and involved in 90% of cases. If attack progresses, fever and chills appear. First attacks usually occur at night, preceded by specific event (dietary excess, alcohol consumption, trauma, certain drugs, or surgery). Subsequent attacks are common, usually within 1 year; but 7% never have a second attack. Chronic gout is extremely rare; dietary therapy and drugs lower urate levels. Some kidney dysfunction occurs in 90% of subjects with gout, who have a higher risk of kidney stones.

## THERAPEUTIC CONSIDERATIONS

- **Colchicine**: conventional acute treatment; an antiinflammatory drug originally isolated from the plant *Colchicum autumnale* (autumn crocus, meadow saffron). Colchicine has no effect on uric acid levels; it stops inflammation by inhibiting neutrophil migration into areas of inflammation. Approximately 75% of patients improve within the first 12 hours of taking colchicine, but 80% of patients are unable to tolerate the optimal dose because of gastrointestinal side effects preceding or coinciding with improvement. Colchicine may cause bone marrow depression, hair loss, liver damage, depression, seizures, respiratory depression, and even death. Other antiinflammatory agents also are used (indomethacin, phenylbutazone, naproxen, fenoprofen).
- **Postacute episode measures to reduce risk of recurrence**: drugs to normalize urate levels, controlled weight loss in obese patients, avoidance of known precipitating factors (alcohol excess or diet rich in purines), low-dose colchicine to prevent attacks.
- **Dietary factors exacerbating gout**: alcohol, high-purine foods (organ meats, meat, yeast, poultry), fats, refined carbohydrates, caloric excess. Gout patients typically are obese, hypertensive, prone to diabetes, and at greater risk for cardiovascular disease. Obesity is the most important dietary factor.
- **Naturopathic approach**: similar to conventional approach—dietary and herbal measures instead of drugs to maintain normal urate levels, weight management to reduce obesity, control of known precipitating factors, nutritional substances to prevent acute attacks.
- **Lead toxicity**: a secondary type of gout ("saturine gout") results from lead (Pb) toxicity. The source is leaded crystal (port wine elutes Pb when stored in crystal decanters). Pb level increases with storage time, becoming toxic after several months. Even a few minutes in crystal glass produces measurable increases of Pb in wine. Mechanism of action is a decrease in renal urate excretion.

### Dietary Guidelines

Eliminate alcohol; achieve ideal body weight; begin diet low in purines, high in complex carbohydrates, low in fat and protein, abundant in fluids, especially pure water.

- **Alcohol**: increases urate production by accelerating purine nucleotide degradation, which reduces urate excretion by increasing lactate (from alcohol oxidation) and impairing kidney function. Net effect is increased serum uric acid. Alcohol intake often initiates acute attack. Abstinence is the only change needed to prevent attacks in some patients.
- **Weight reduction**: obesity is linked to increased rate of gout. Weight reduction in obese persons reduces serum urate. Use low-glycemic, high-fiber, low-fat diet to improve insulin sensitivity and manage elevated cholesterol and triglycerides common in obesity. This diet is an alkaline ash diet; alkaline pH increases urate solubility.
- **Low-purine diet**: reduces metabolic stress. Omit high-purine foods (organ meats, meats, shellfish, yeast [brewer's and baker's], herring, sardines, mackerel, anchovies). Curtail foods with moderate protein (dried legumes, spinach, asparagus, fish, poultry, mushrooms).
- **Carbohydrates, fats, and protein**: refined carbohydrates increase urate production; saturated fats increase urate retention. Enhance insulin sensitivity. Avoid excess protein (>0.8 g/kg body weight); high protein intake may accelerate urate synthesis in normal and gouty patients. Adequate protein (0.8 g/kg body weight) is necessary; amino acids decrease resorption of urate in renal tubules, increasing urate excretion and reducing serum urate.
- **Fluid intake**: liberal fluid (pure water) intake keeps urine dilute to promote urate excretion and reduce risk of kidney stones.

## Nutritional Supplements

- **Eicosapentaenoic acid (EPA)**: quite useful for gout; limits production of proinflammatory leukotrienes, mediators of inflammation and tissue damage in gout.
- **Vitamin E**: mildly inhibits production of leukotrienes and acts as an antioxidant. Selenium functions synergistically with vitamin E.
- **Folic acid**: inhibits xanthine oxidase, the enzyme that produces uric acid. The drug allopurinol is a potent inhibitor of this enzyme. A derivative of folic acid is an even greater inhibitor of xanthine oxidase than allopurinol. Folic acid at pharmacologic doses may be effective treatment. Positive results have been reported but data are incomplete and uncontrolled.
- **Bromelain**: proteolytic enzyme of pineapple is an effective anti-inflammatory and suitable alternative to stronger prescription

antiinflammatory agents. Take between meals (*Textbook*, "Bromelain").

- **Quercetin**: bioflavonoid that may offer significant protection by inhibiting xanthine oxidase in similar fashion to allopurinol, leukotriene synthesis and release, neutrophil accumulation and enzyme release. Take with bromelain between meals. (Bromelain may enhance absorption of quercetin and other medications.)
- **Alanine, aspartic acid, glutamic acid, and glycine**: these amino acids lower serum uric acid, presumably by decreasing uric acid resorption in renal tubule, increasing uric acid excretion.
- **Vitamin C**: megadoses of vitamin C are contraindicated in gout; vitamin C may increase urate in a small number of individuals.
- **Niacin**: high-dose niacin (>50 mg q.d.) is contraindicated in gout; niacin competes with urate for excretion.

### Botanical Medicines

- **Cherries**: Consuming 0.25 kg fresh or canned cherries daily is effective in lowering uric acid and preventing gout attacks. Cherries decrease plasma urate within 5 hours by 30 μmol/L, correlating with increased urine urate excretion. Plasma C-reactive protein and nitric oxide decline slightly after 3 hours. Cherries, hawthorn berries, blueberries, and other dark red-blue berries are rich sources of anthocyanidins and proanthocyanidins. These flavonoids give fruits deep red-blue color and prevent collagen destruction. Effects of anthocyanidins and other flavonoids are to cross-link collagen fibers, reinforcing natural cross-linking of collagen matrix of connective tissue; prevent free radical damage by potent antioxidant and free radical scavenging action; inhibit cleavage of collagen by enzymes secreted by leukocytes during inflammation; prevent synthesis and release of compounds promoting inflammation (histamine, serine proteases, prostaglandins, leukotrienes).
- ***Harpagophytum procumbens* (Devil's claw)**: relieves joint pain, reduces serum cholesterol and uric acid levels. Equivocal research results exist concerning antiinflammatory and analgesic effects. It may be useful in short-term management of gout. Long-term use is probably unnecessary because of efficacy of dietary regimen.

## THERAPEUTIC APPROACH

- **Basic approach**:
  —Dietary and herbal measures that maintain normal uric acid levels

—Controlled weight loss for obesity
—Avoidance of known precipitating factors (alcohol abuse, high-purine diet)
—Nutritional substances to prevent acute attacks
—Herbal and nutritional substances to inhibit inflammation

- **Diet**: Eliminate alcohol; maintain low-purine diet; increase complex carbohydrates; decrease simple carbohydrates; lower fat intake; optimize protein (0.8 g/kg body weight); drink liberal quantities of fluid (pure water); monitor dietary compliance with urinary 24-hour uric acid (maintain below 0.8 g/day); eat liberal amounts (250-500 g q.d.) cherries, blueberries, other anthocyanoside-rich red-blue berries (or extracts).
- **Nutritional supplements**:
  —EPA: 1.8 g q.d.
  —Vitamin E: 400-800 IU q.d. (mixed tocopherols)
  —Folic acid: 10-40 mg q.d.
  —Bromelain: 125-250 mg (1800-2000 MCU) t.i.d. between meals
  —Quercetin: 125-250 mg t.i.d. between meals with bromelain

## Botanical Medicine

- ***Harpagophytum procumbens***: dried powdered root, 1-2 g t.i.d.; tincture (1:5), 4-5 mL t.i.d.; dry solid extract (3:1), 400 mg t.i.d.
- **Anthocyanoside extracts** (e.g., *Vaccinium myrtillus*): equivalent to 80 mg anthocyanoside content q.d.

## Causes of Hyperuricemia

### Metabolic

- Increased production of purine (primary)
- Idiopathic
- Specific enzyme defects (e.g., Lesch-Nyhan syndrome, glycogen storage disease)
- Decreased enzyme activity (e.g., hypoxanthine-guanine phosphoribosyltransferase is decreased in 1%-2% of adults with gout)
- Increased enzyme activity (e.g., phosphoribosylpyrophosphate synthetase)
- Increased production of purine (secondary)
  —Increased turnover of purines
  —Myeloproliferative disorders
  —Lymphoproliferative disorders
  —Carcinoma and sarcoma (disseminated)
  —Chronic hemolytic anemia

—Cytotoxic drugs
—Psoriasis
- Increased de novo synthesis (e.g., glucose-6-phosphatase deficiency)
- Increased catabolism of purines
  —Fructose ingestion or infusion
  —Exercise

**Renal**

- Decreased renal clearance of uric acid (primary)
  —Intrinsic kidney disease
- Decreased renal clearance of uric acid (secondary)
- Functional impairment of tubular secretion
  —Drug-induced (e.g., thiazides, probenecid, salicylates, ethambutol, pyrazinamide)
- Hyperlacticemia (e.g., lactic acidosis, alcoholism, toxemia of pregnancy, chronic beryllium disease)
- Hyperketoacidemia (e.g., diabetic ketoacidosis, fasting, starvation)
- Diabetes insipidus
- Bartter's syndrome
- Lead poisoning
- Glucose-6-phosphatase deficiency

# Hair Loss in Women

## DIAGNOSTIC SUMMARY

- Increased hair loss not diagnosed as alopecia.

## GENERAL CONSIDERATIONS

### Physiology of the Hair Cycle

There are 100,000 to 350,000 hair follicles on the human scalp that go through cyclical phases of growth and rest:

- **Growth (anagen) phase**: active genetic expression of protein synthesis
- **Resting stage**
- **Migratory phase**: hair bulb migrates outward and is sloughed. Stage is set for new hair to fill remaining papilla after old hair is lost.

Age, pathology, and nutritional and hormonal factors influence duration of hair cycle. Hair loss is a normal part of aging. Hair growth slows by age 40 years. Speed of replacing old hairs declines. The issue is more apparent in men because of the effects of androgens.

## THERAPEUTIC CONSIDERATIONS

### Causes of Hair Loss in Women

- Androgenic female pattern hair loss
- Side effect of drug
- Nutritional deficiencies
- Hypothyroidism
- Antigliadin antibodies

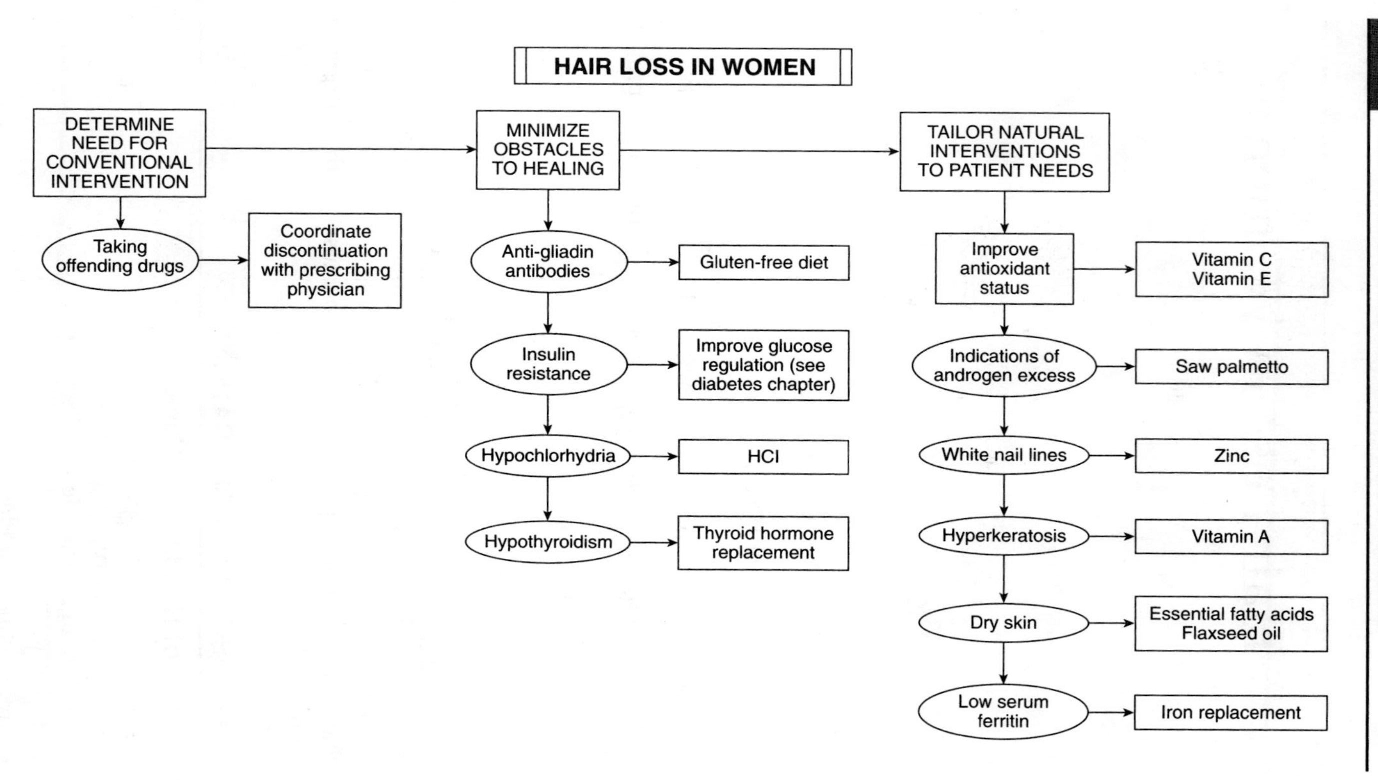
HAIR LOSS IN WOMEN
DETERMINE NEED FOR CONVENTIONAL INTERVENTION
Taking offending drugs
Coordinate discontinuation with prescribing physician
MINIMIZE OBSTACLES TO HEALING
Anti-gliadin antibodies
Gluten-free diet
Insulin resistance
Improve glucose regulation (see diabetes chapter)
Hypochlorhydria
HCl
Hypothyroidism
Thyroid hormone replacement
TAILOR NATURAL INTERVENTIONS TO PATIENT NEEDS
Improve antioxidant status
Vitamin C
Vitamin E
Indications of androgen excess
Saw palmetto
White nail lines
Zinc
Hyperkeratosis
Vitamin A
Dry skin
Essential fatty acids
Flaxseed oil
Low serum ferritin
Iron replacement

## Androgenic Female Pattern Hair Loss

Female pattern hair loss (diffuse androgen-dependent alopecia) is more diffuse than male pattern, affecting 30% of women before age 50 years. Factors include genetics, androgen excess, insulin resistance, polycystic ovarian syndrome, low antioxidant status (i.e., reduced glutathione).

Recommendations:

- Improve blood glucose regulation through dietary, lifestyle, and supplementary measures (see the chapter on diabetes mellitus)
- Increase antioxidant intake
- Saw palmetto extract
- Hormone replacement therapy

Reactive oxygen species (and testosterone) contribute to male pattern baldness and are found at higher levels in hair follicles of men (and presumably women) with this condition as a result of lower glutathione. Vitamins C and E help preserve glutathione.

Recommendations:

- **Vitamin C**: 1000 to 1500 mg q.d. in divided doses
- **Vitamin E**: 400 IU q.d. (mixed tocopherols)

Saw palmetto extract, useful in benign prostatic hypertrophy, inhibits formation of dihydrotestosterone (DHT) by enzyme 5-alpha-reductase, also increased in male and female pattern baldness (the same mechanism as finasteride [Propecia] used in female pattern hair loss). Saw palmetto extract also inhibits transport of DHT to nuclear receptors.

- Dosage: 320 mg q.d. of extract standardized to 85%-95% fatty acids and sterols.

## Side Effect of Drug

Hair loss concurrent with taking one of the following drugs does not indicate that the drug is the sole cause of hair loss. For chemotherapy agents (e.g., fluorouracil), the link is obvious. When medically appropriate, natural alternatives to suspected culprits should be used.

**Classes of Drugs That Can Cause Hair Loss**

| Class | Examples |
|---|---|
| Nonsteroidal antiinflammatory drugs (NSAIDs) | Ibuprofen, indomethacin, naproxen |
| Antibiotics | Gentamycin, chloramphenicol |
| Anticoagulants | Coumadin, heparin |
| Antidepressants | Fluoxetine, desipramine, lithium |
| Antiepileptics | Valproic acid, phenytoin |
| Cardiovascular drugs | Angiotensin-converting enzyme inhibitors, beta-blockers |
| Chemotherapy drugs | Adriamycin, vincristine, etoposide, fluorouracil |
| Endocrine drugs | Bromocriptine, clomiphene citrate, danazol |
| Gout medications | Colchicine, allopurinol |
| Lipid-lowering drugs | Gemfibrozil, fenofibrate |
| Ulcer medications | Cimetidine, ranitidine |

## Nutritional Deficiency

Zinc, vitamin A, essential fatty acids (EFAs), and iron should be considered first.

- **Zinc**: examine nails for white lines indicating poor wound healing of nail bed even with minor trauma—sign of zinc deficit.
- **Vitamin A**: examine backs of arms for hyperkeratosis—sign of vitamin A deficiency.
- **EFAs**: examine elbows and skin generally for dry skin of EFA deficiency.
- **Iron**: use serum ferritin test. Beware: many labs report low ferritin (10-30 μg/L) within normal range. If serum ferritin is <30 μg/L, iron replacement is indicated. Low serum ferritin impairs hair growth and regeneration as the body seeks to conserve iron.

Women with noticeable generalized hair loss tend to have deficiencies in all these nutrients. Increase intake of these nutrients; supplement appropriately. Caveat: many may have hydrochlorhydria. Use hydrochloric acid supplements at meals. Use a high-potency vitamin/mineral supplement containing ferrous iron and 1 tbsp of flaxseed oil daily. If serum ferritin <30 μg/L, supplement with additional iron: 30 mg iron bound to succinate, fumarate, or other chelate b.i.d. between meals. If abdominal discomfort ensues, recommend 30 mg with meals t.i.d. After 2 months, retest serum ferritin. Improved serum ferritin often correlates with improved hair health and reduced hair loss.

### Hypothyroidism

Hair loss is a cardinal sign of hypothyroidism. Use blood thyroid hormone tests as criteria. From 1% to 4% of adults have moderate to severe hypothyroidism; another 10% to 12% have mild hypothyroidism. Prevalence among American women is 20%.

### Antigliadin Antibodies

Gluten and its polypeptide derivative, gliadin, are found in wheat, barley, and rye grains. Antibodies to gliadin can cross react and attack hair follicles, leading to alopecia areata—an autoimmune disease characterized by areas of virtually complete hair loss.

Celiac disease (nontropical sprue, gluten-sensitive enteropathy, or celiac sprue) entails malabsorption and abnormal small intestine structure that reverts to normal on removal of dietary gluten. Many people with gluten intolerance do not have overt gastrointestinal symptoms; instead, gluten intolerance may appear insidiously as hair loss. Instead of antigliadin antibody test, in cases of general hair loss or alopecia areata test for human antitissue transglutaminase antibodies for greater sensitivity compared with antigliadin antibodies (see the chapter on celiac disease). This test is especially indicated with gastrointestinal symptoms suggestive of celiac disease.

### Key Diagnostic Features of Celiac Disease

- Bulky, pale, frothy, foul-smelling, greasy stools with increased fecal fat
- Weight loss and signs of multiple vitamin and mineral deficiencies
- Increased levels of serum gliadin antibodies
- Diagnosis confirmed by jejunal biopsy

# Hepatitis

## DIAGNOSTIC SUMMARY

- Prodrome of anorexia, nausea, vomiting, fatigue, flulike symptoms 2 weeks to 1 month before liver involvement depending on incubation period of virus.
- Symptoms may occur abruptly or insidiously.
- Fever, headaches, abdominal discomfort, light stools, diarrhea, myalgia, arthralgia, drowsiness, enlarged and tender liver, jaundice, itching.
- Dark urine.
- Normal to low white blood cell count, markedly elevated aminotransaminases, elevated bilirubin.

## GENERAL CONSIDERATIONS

Causes: drugs, toxic chemicals, bacterial or fungal infections, immune disorders, metabolic diseases, hepatic perfusion and oxygenation problems. Most common cause: virus types A, B, and C.

- **Hepatitis A**: caused by virus from Picornaviridiae family. It occurs sporadically or in epidemics and is transmitted primarily by fecal contamination from poor hygiene and sanitation.
- **Hepatitis B**: linked to 50% of viral cases in the United States; transmitted by infected blood or blood products or sexual contact (virus shed in saliva, semen, vaginal secretions).
- **Hepatitis C (hepatitis non-A, non-B)**: linked to hepacivirus and a member of Flaviviridae family. Transmitted by blood contamination and responsible for 90% of all cases of hepatitis through blood transfusions (10% of people receiving blood transfusions in the past developed hepatitis C). However, only 4% of cases of hepatitis C result from transfusions. Most cases are attributable to intravenous drug use; in other cases the source is unclear. The mortality rate (1%-12%) is much higher than for other forms.
- **Other viral causes**: hepatitis viruses D, E, and G; herpes simplex; cytomegalovirus; and Epstein-Barr virus.

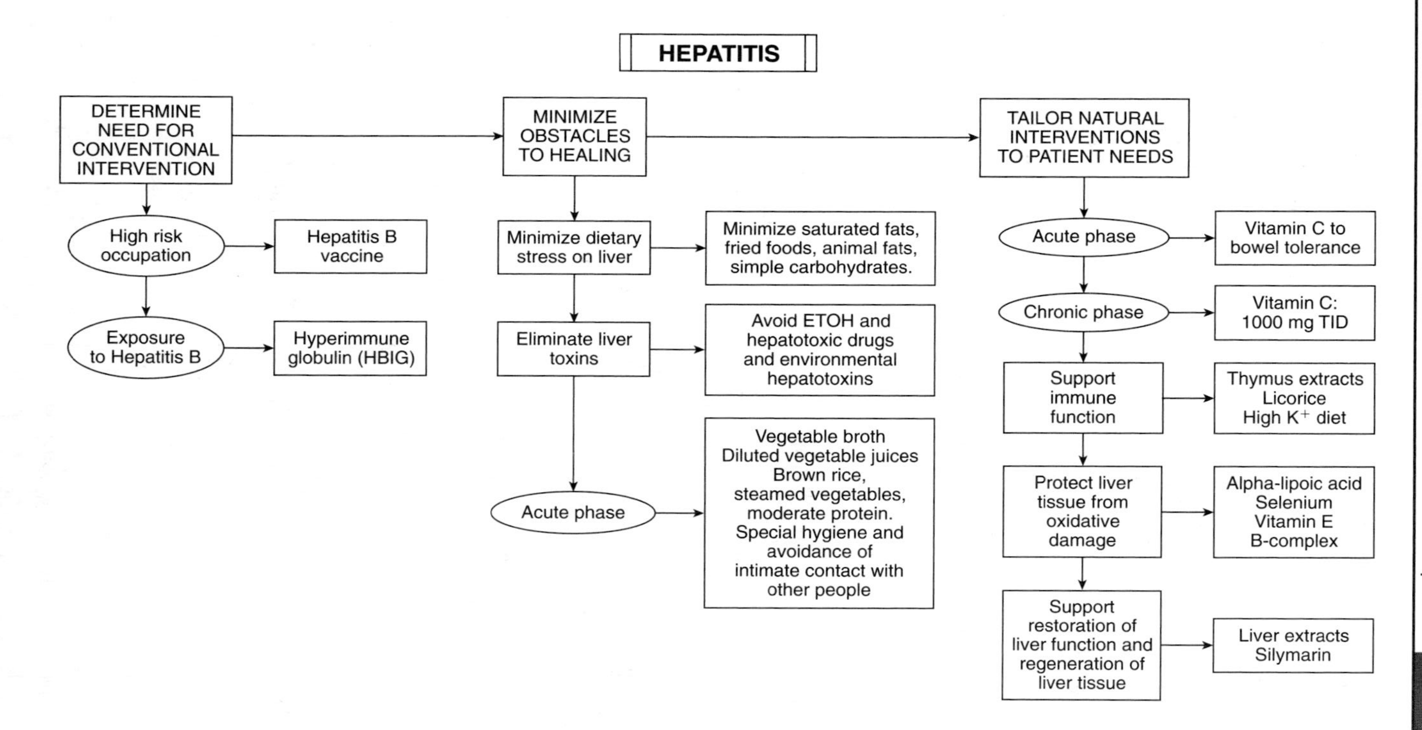
HEPATITIS
DETERMINE NEED FOR CONVENTIONAL INTERVENTION
High risk occupation
Hepatitis B vaccine
Exposure to Hepatitis B
Hyperimmune globulin (HBIG)
MINIMIZE OBSTACLES TO HEALING
Minimize dietary stress on liver
Minimize saturated fats, fried foods, animal fats, simple carbohydrates.
Eliminate liver toxins
Avoid ETOH and hepatotoxic drugs and environmental hepatotoxins
Acute phase
Vegetable broth
Diluted vegetable juices
Brown rice, steamed vegetables, moderate protein.
Special hygiene and avoidance of intimate contact with other people
TAILOR NATURAL INTERVENTIONS TO PATIENT NEEDS
Acute phase
Vitamin C to bowel tolerance
Chronic phase
Vitamin C: 1000 mg TID
Support immune function
Thymus extracts
Licorice
High K+ diet
Protect liver tissue from oxidative damage
Alpha-lipoic acid
Selenium
Vitamin E
B-complex
Support restoration of liver function and regeneration of liver tissue
Liver extracts
Silymarin

- **Acute viral hepatitis**: extremely debilitating form requiring bed rest and 2-16 weeks of recovery. Most patients completely recover (9 weeks for type A and 16 weeks for B, C, D, and G). One in 100 will die. Ten percent of hepatitis B and 10%-40% of hepatitis C cases become chronic. Hepatitis C contracted by blood transfusion has a 70%-80% rate of chronicity.
- **Symptoms of chronic hepatitis**: vary from nonexistent to chronic fatigue, serious liver damage, and even death.

## DIAGNOSTIC CONSIDERATIONS

In addition to liver enzymes, hepatitis C is monitored by the presence of hepatitis C viral RNA by polymerase chain reaction (HCV-RNA[PCR]). Hepatitis B serologic findings and their interpretation are listed in the following table.

Suspect hepatitis when typical signs and symptoms are present. Confirm by blood tests for elevated liver enzymes and presence of viral antigens or virus-specific antibodies. The type of virus is determined by identifying specific viral antigens or antibodies. In chronic hepatitis B or C, use serology to monitor progression or clearance. Hepatitis C is monitored by liver enzymes plus HCV-RNA[PCR].

**Hepatitis B Serologic Patterns and Interpretations**

| HBsAg | Anti-HBs | Anti-HBc | HBeAg | Anti-HBe | Interpretation |
|---|---|---|---|---|---|
| + | – | IgM | + | – | Acute hepatitis B |
| + | – | IgG | + | – | Chronic active hepatitis B |
| + | – | IgG | – | + | Chronic nonactive hepatitis B |
| + | + | IgG | +/– | +/– | Chronic hepatitis B |
| – | – | IgM | +/– | +/– | Acute hepatitis B |
| – | + | IgG | – | +/– | Recovery from hepatitis B |
| – | + | – | – | – | Vaccinated against hepatitis B |
| – | – | IgG | – | – | False-positive or infection in remote past |

*HBsAg*, Hepatitis B surface antigen; *HBc*, hepatitis B core antigen; *HBeAg*, hepatitis B secretory antigen; *IgG*, immunoglobulin G; *IgM*, immunoglobulin M.

## THERAPEUTIC CONSIDERATIONS

Hepatitis is greatly benefited by natural therapies—nutrients and herbs to inhibit viral reproduction, improve immune function, and stimulate regeneration of damaged liver cells (*Textbook*, "Functional Toxicology"). In chronic hepatitis, treat aggressively to reduce increased risk for hepatocellular carcinoma and cirrhosis. (If cirrhosis is present in chronic hepatitis B, 5-year survival rate is only 50%-60%.)

### Prevention

- **Hepatitis A**: vaccination for (1) children in areas with high rates of hepatitis A; (2) people at increased risk (travelers to endemic regions, homosexual men, illegal drug users, employees in research labs working with hepatitis A, persons with clotting factor disorders); (3) persons with chronic liver disease, especially chronic hepatitis B or C; and (4) outbreak communities with higher intermediate rates of hepatitis A. The vaccine curbs outbreaks when administered in a timely fashion. Administer postexposure prophylaxis (specific hepatitis A immunoglobulins) intramuscularly during first 2 weeks after exposure.
- **Hepatitis B (HBV)**: vaccination for high-risk occupations (health care professionals exposed to body fluids). For acute exposure to HBV, hyperimmune globulin (HBIG) is administered intramuscularly; it confers immediate, but short-lived, passive immunity lasting 3 months. Two doses of HBIG given within 2 weeks of exposure provide adequate protective immunity in 75% of exposed individuals. HBIG is recommended for persons exposed to HBV surface antigen–contaminated material by mucous secretions or through breaks in skin. Newborns with HBV surface antigen–positive mothers should receive vaccine (0.5 mL shortly after birth and at ages 3 and 6 months).
- **Hepatitis C**: no vaccine for hepatitis C currently exists. Minimize routes of infection. Drug abuse is the most important risk factor. Prevention includes ceasing intravenous drugs or using only unused, clean, sterile needles; cease intranasal cocaine; accept transfusions only from known, uncontaminated blood sources. Practice strict occupational safety and health standards for blood products. Never recap used needles. Sexual transmission risk is highest in male homosexuals, patients with multiple sexual partners, and those with a sexually transmitted disease. Someone in a monogamous heterosexual relationship with a hepatitis C

patient has low risk unless patient is coinfected with hepatitis C and HIV.

## Nutritional Considerations

- **Diet**: during acute phase focus on replacing fluids: vegetable broths, vegetable juices (diluted with 50% water), and herbal teas. Restrict solid foods to brown rice, steamed vegetables, and moderate lean protein. For chronic cases keep diet low in saturated fats, simple carbohydrates (sugar, white flour, fruit juice, honey), oxidized fatty acids (fried oils), and animal products. Plant foods (high-fiber diet) increase elimination of bile acids, drugs, and toxic bile substances. Avoid alcohol.
- **Vitamin C**: high dosages of vitamin C (40-100 g PO or IV) may greatly improve acute viral hepatitis in 2-4 days and clear jaundice within 6 days. Dosage of 2 g q.d. or more vitamin C dramatically prevents hepatitis B in hospitalized patients.
- **Selenium (Se)**: cofactor for enzyme glutathione peroxidase, an oxidant mediator. Deficiency consequences include immune dysfunction, cancer, and liver necrosis. Whole blood and plasma Se in patients with chronic liver disease (alcoholism and viral liver cirrhosis) are lower than in control subjects. Liver cancer cells acquire selective survival advantage under Se deficiency and oxidative stress (a feature of cirrhosis).
- **Alpha-lipoic acid (ALA) (thioctic acid)**: disulfide antioxidant that lowers liver enzymes and helps treat diabetes, AIDS, heavy metal toxicity (chelator), and age-related cardiac myopathies. ALA, produced in small quantities in cells, is a coenzyme in pyruvate dehydrogenase and alpha-ketoglutarate dehydrogenase mitochondrial enzyme complexes. It is hepatoprotective in chemical- or alcohol-induced damage, metal intoxification, carbon tetrachloride ($CCl_4$), and amanita mushroom poisoning. Administer with vitamin B complex to prevent depletion. Dosage: 600 mg q.d. R form of ALA may be more effective than R/S racemic mixture.
- **Liver extracts**: promote hepatic regeneration; effective in treating chronic liver disease, including chronic active hepatitis. Placebo-controlled study showed 70 mg liver extract for 3 months greatly lowered liver enzymes (aminotransaminases) in chronic hepatitis. Blood liver enzymes reflect damage to liver. Liver extract is effective in chronic hepatitis by its ability to improve function of damaged liver cells and prevent further liver damage.
- **Thymus extracts**: oral bovine thymus extracts are effective in acute and chronic viral hepatitis (*Textbook,* "Immune Support").

They provide broad-spectrum immune enhancement mediated by improved thymus function. Double-blind studies showed therapeutic effect noted by accelerated decreases of liver enzymes (transaminases), elimination of virus, and higher rate of seroconversion to anti–hepatitis B secretory antigen, signifying clinical remission.

## Botanical Medicines

Licorice (*Glycyrrhiza glabra*) and silymarin (flavonoid complex from milk thistle [*Silybum marianum*]) are best documented treatments. Catechin (from *Uncaria gambir*) is effective but associated with potentially serious side effects in rare cases (*Textbook,* "Catechin [+-cyanidanol-3]"). Some botanicals appropriate for other conditions may not be suitable for acute and chronic liver diseases.

- ***Glycyrrhiza glabra***: effects of licorice beneficial in hepatitis: antihepatotoxic effects, immune-enhancing actions, potentiation of interferon, antiviral effects, actions as choleretic. Glycyrrhizin reduces serum alanine transaminase and aspartate transaminase; inhibits immune-mediated cytotoxicity against hepatocytes; and antagonizes nuclear factor kappa B, a transcription factor that activates genes encoding inflammatory cytokines. A Japanese glycyrrhizin-containing product (stronger neominophagen C [SNMC]), consisting of 200 mg glycyrrhizin, 100 mg cysteine, and 2000 mg glycine in 100 mL of physiologic saline solution, is given intravenously (oral may be as effective). SNMC effectively treats chronic hepatitis B and C. Approximately 40% of patients get complete resolution (compared with 40%-50% for alpha-interferon). SNMC reduces risk for hepatocellular carcinoma. Dosage: 100 mL/day for 8 weeks followed by treatments of two to seven times weekly for periods up to 16 years. SNMC studies used intravenous glycyrrhizin, but that route may not be necessary; glycyrrhizin is readily absorbed. Goal is to achieve a high level of glycyrrhizin in blood without producing side effects. Main hazard of licorice is its aldosterone-like effects (at doses >3 g q.d. for 6+ weeks), and glycyrrhizin acid (>100 mg q.d.) may cause sodium and water retention, hypertension, hypokalemia, and suppression of the renin-aldosterone system. Monitor blood pressure and electrolytes and increase dietary potassium. Great individual variation occurs in susceptibility to symptom-producing effects of glycyrrhizin. Adverse effects are rare with doses less than 100 mg q.d. but are common above 400 mg q.d. Preventing side effects of glycyrrhizin is possible with a high-potassium, low-sodium diet. No formal trial has been performed, but patients consuming high-potassium foods and restricting sodium, even with hypertension and angina, are free from aldosterone-like side effects. Nonetheless, avoid in patients with history of hypertension or renal failure or those currently using digitalis.

- ***Silybum marianum* (milk thistle)**: contains silymarin, a mixture of flavanolignans (silybin, silydianin, silychristin), which are potent liver-protecting substances. It inhibits hepatic damage by acting as a direct antioxidant and free radical scavenger, increasing intracellular glutathione and superoxide dismutase, inhibiting formation of leukotrienes, and stimulating hepatocyte regeneration. Silymarin is effective in acute and chronic viral hepatitis. It shows no antifibrotic effect in human beings but prevents alcoholic cirrhosis in baboons. It may be of benefit before cirrhosis develops. It reverses liver cell damage (confirmed by biopsy), increases protein level in blood, and lowers liver enzymes while improving symptoms in chronic cases. Binding silymarin to phosphatidylcholine (silymarin phytosome) improves absorption and clinical results. It has very low toxicity and is well tolerated. Choleretic activity may produce looser stool; it increases bile flow and secretion at higher doses. Bile-sequestering fiber (guar gum, pectin, psyllium, oat bran) prevents mucosal irritation and loose stools. Lack of toxicity allows long-term use (*Textbook, "Silybum marianum* [Milk Thistle]").
- ***Phyllanthus amarus***: Asian herb with long tradition of use in liver disorders. An initial report indicated that 59% of hepatitis B patients lost hepatitis B secretory antigen when tested 15-20 days after treatment with *P. amarus* (200 mg dried, powdered, sterilized plant in capsules t.i.d.). Follow-up studies failed to confirm initial reports. Given benefits of thymus, licorice, and silymarin, use of *P. amarus* seems unwarranted at this time.

## Combination Antioxidant and Botanical Therapy

**Dr. Burton Berkson program** (based on three successful cases): oral supplements of alpha-lipoic acid (600 mg q.d. in two divided doses), Se (selenomethionine at 400 μg q.d. in two divided doses), silymarin (900 mg q.d. in three divided doses), vitamin B complex (50 mg), vitamin C (1000-6000 mg q.d.), and vitamin E (400 IU q.d.); diet high in fruits and vegetables: 4 oz or less of meat per meal, eight glasses of water daily. Encourage patients to walk 1 mile three times a week.

### Hepatotoxic Botanicals

The following botanicals must be avoided by patients with hepatitis:

- ***Symphytum officinale* (comfrey)**: hepatotoxic pyrrolizidine alkaloids (lasiocarpine, symphytine, and their N-oxides).
- **Chinese herbs**: Jin Bu Huan, Ma-Huang (Ephedra), *Dictamnus dasycarpus,* Sho-saiko-to, *Teucrium chamaedrys* (wild germander), *Larrea tridentata* (chaparral), *Atractylis gummifera, Callilepis laureola,* and other pyrrolizidine alkaloid–containing plants.
- ***Piper methysticum* (kava kava)**: safe at normal doses for people without liver disease; avoid during hepatic conditions.

## THERAPEUTIC APPROACH

Advise bed rest during acute phase of viral hepatitis, with slow resumption of activities as health improves. Avoid strenuous exertion, alcohol, and other liver-toxic substances. Ensure careful hygiene and avoidance of close contact with others during contagious phase (2-3 weeks before symptoms appear to 3 weeks after). Once diagnosis is made, employment in daycare centers, restaurants, or other service occupations is not recommended.

- **Diet**: natural diet low in natural and synthetically saturated fats, simple carbohydrates (sugar, white flour, fruit juice, honey), oxidized fatty acids (fried oils), and animal fat; high in fiber. Abstain from all alcohol.
- **Nutritional supplements**:
  —Vitamin C: to bowel tolerance (10-50 g q.d.) in acute cases; 1000 mg t.i.d. in chronic cases
  —Liver extracts: 500-1000 mg q.d. crude polypeptides
  —Thymus extracts: equivalent to 120 mg pure polypeptides with molecular weights <10,000 or roughly 750 mg crude polypeptide fractions
- **Botanical medicines**:
  —*Glycyrrhiza glabra* (licorice): powdered root, 1-2 g t.i.d.; fluid extract (1:1), 2-4 mL (1-2 g) t.i.d.; solid (dry powdered) extract (5% glycyrrhetinic acid content), 250-500 mg t.i.d. (Note: If licorice is to be used over a long period, increase intake of potassium-rich foods and carefully monitor for signs of hypertension.)
  —*Silybum marianum* (milk thistle): standard dose based on silymarin content (70-210 mg t.i.d.); prefer standardized

extracts; best results at higher dosages: 140-210 mg silymarin t.i.d.; dosage for silybin bound to phosphatidylcholine = 120 mg b.i.d. or t.i.d. between meals.

- **Berkson combination antioxidant approach**: See p. 300 for specific protocol.

# Herpes Simplex

## DIAGNOSTIC SUMMARY

- Recurrent viral infection of skin or mucous membranes characterized by single or multiple clusters of small vesicles on erythematous base, frequently occurring about the mouth (herpes gingivostomatitis), lips (herpes labialis), genitals (herpes genitalis), and conjunctiva and cornea (herpes keratoconjunctivitis).
- Incubation period 2-12 days, averaging 6-7 days.
- Vesicle scraping stained with Giemsa's stain gives positive Tzanck's test result.
- Regional lymph nodes may be tender and swollen.
- Outbreak may follow minor infections, trauma, stress (emotional, dietary, environmental), and sun exposure.

## GENERAL CONSIDERATIONS

More than 70 viruses compose herpes viradae. Of these, four are linked to human disease: herpes simplex (HSV), varicella zoster (VZV), Epstein-Barr (EBV), and cytomegalovirus (CMV). Serology distinguishes two types of HSV: HSV-1 and HSV-2. From 20%-40% of the U.S. population have recurrent HSV infections. From 30%-100% of adults have been infected with one or both HSV types. The greatest incidence is among lower socioeconomic groups; HSV-1 has replaced HSV-2 as the primary cause of genital lesions.

- **Recurrence rate**: genital HSV-1 lesions have a recurrence rate of 14%; HSV-2 recurrence rate is 60%. Men are more susceptible to recurrences. After primary infection resolves, HSV is a dormant inhabitant in sensory and/or autonomic ganglia. Recurrences develop at or near site of primary infection, precipitated by sunburn, sexual activity, menses, stress, food allergy, drugs, certain foods. Risk of infection after sexual contact with partner with active lesions is 75%.
- **Immunologic aspects**: host defense is paramount in protecting against HSV infection. Persistent genital infections are seen in

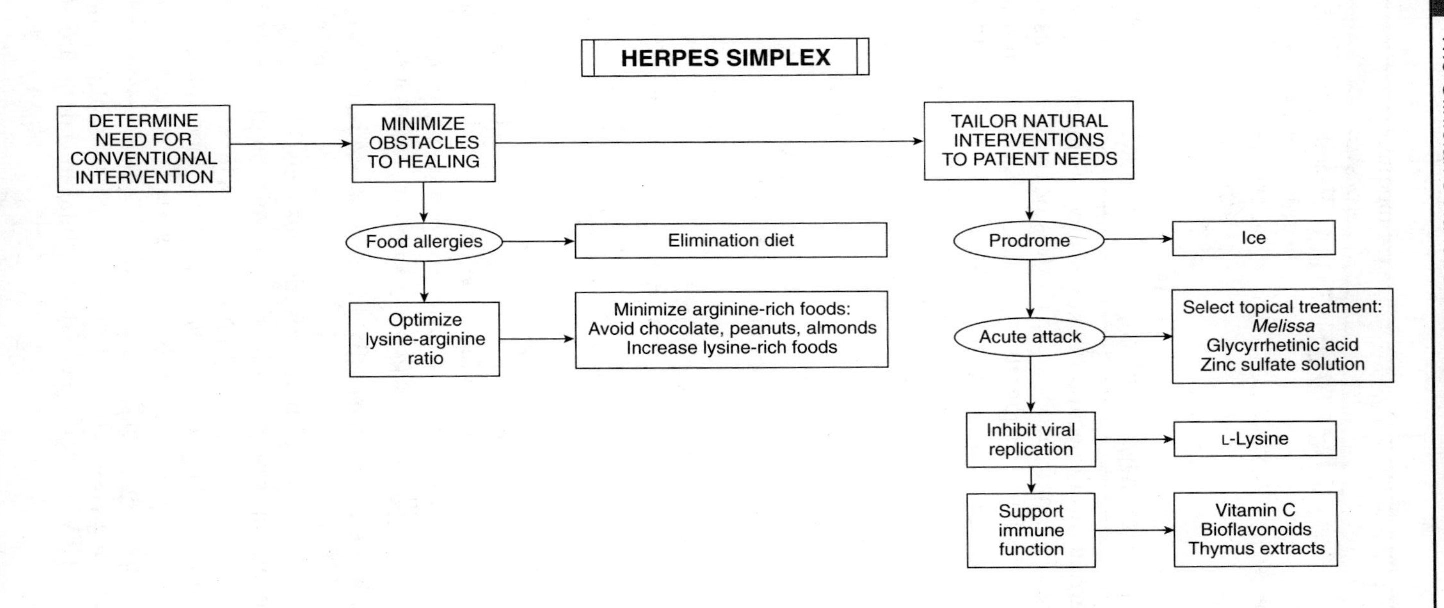
HERPES SIMPLEX
DETERMINE NEED FOR CONVENTIONAL INTERVENTION
MINIMIZE OBSTACLES TO HEALING
Food allergies
Elimination diet
Optimize lysine-arginine ratio
Minimize arginine-rich foods: Avoid chocolate, peanuts, almonds Increase lysine-rich foods
TAILOR NATURAL INTERVENTIONS TO PATIENT NEEDS
Prodrome
Ice
Acute attack
Select topical treatment: Melissa Glycyrrhetinic acid Zinc sulfate solution
Inhibit viral replication
L-Lysine
Support immune function
Vitamin C Bioflavonoids Thymus extracts

immunosuppressed individuals. Cell-mediated immunity is the major factor determining outcome of herpes exposure: resistance, latent infection, or clinical disease. HSV-neutralizing antibody found in saliva is decreased during active recurrence and is in immunoglobulin G (IgG) form, which is significant because immunoglobulin A (IgA) is the major immunoglobulin in saliva.

### Diagnosis

Gold standard is isolation of HSV from tissue scrapings. Cytopathic effects are seen within 2-7 days. Direct staining of skin scrapings is a more rapid test for mucocutaneous lesions. Type-specific serologic tests diagnose unrecognized infections or confirm suspected cases.

## THERAPEUTIC CONSIDERATIONS

Enhancing host immune status is the key to controlling herpes infection. A key natural measure to strengthen cell-mediated immunity is bovine thymus extracts. Thymus extracts reduce number and severity of recurrent infections in immune-suppressed persons and increase lymphoproliferative response to HSV, natural killer cell activity, and interferon production.

- **Zinc**: oral zinc (50 mg q.d.) is effective in clinical studies. Zn is an inhibitor of HSV replication in vitro; its effect in vivo is to enhance cell-mediated immunity. Topical 0.01%-0.025% zinc sulfate solution ameliorates symptoms and inhibits recurrence.
- **Vitamin C**: oral and topical application of vitamin C increases rate of healing of herpes ulcers. Ascorbic acid–containing pharmaceutical (Ascoxal) applied with soaked cotton wool pad t.i.d. for 2 minutes reduces number of days with scabs, number of cases of worsening of symptoms, and frequency of culturing HSV from lesions. In herpes labialis, oral ascorbate–bioflavonoid complex (1000 mg water-soluble bioflavonoids and 1000 mg vitamin C in equal increments five times daily at first onset and continued 3 days) reduces outbreak of vesiculation and prevents disruption of vesicular membranes. This therapy is most beneficial when initiated at the beginning of disease.
- **Lysine and arginine**: lysine has antiviral activity in vitro from antagonism of arginine metabolism. HSV replication requires synthesis of arginine-rich proteins. Arginine may be an operon coordinate inducer. Preponderance of lysine over arginine may

act as either allosteric enzyme inhibitor or operon coordinate repressor. Lysine at 1g t.i.d. with dietary restriction of nuts, chocolate, and gelatin for 6 months was rated much better than placebo. Lysine and arginine are dibasic amino acids that compete with each other for intestinal transport. Rats fed lysine-rich diet show 60% decrease in brain arginine, although no change in serum levels. HSV resides in ganglia during latency. Supplemental lysine and arginine avoidance is warranted but not curative; this intervention only inhibits recurrences. In some patients withdrawal from lysine is followed by relapse within 1-4 weeks.

### Topical Preparations

- ***Melissa officinalis*** **(lemon balm)**: concentrated extract (70:1) contains several components that work together to prevent virus from infecting human cells. It dramatically reduces recurrence; many patients never again have a recurrence. It rapidly interrupts infection and reduces healing time from 10 to 5 days. *Melissa* either stops recurrences of cold sores or tremendously reduces frequency of recurrences (outbreak-free period >3.5 months). Apply it fairly thickly (1-2 mm) to lesions q.i.d. during active recurrence. Extremely safe and suitable for long-term use. *Glycyrrhiza glabra* (licorice root): Preparations containing glycyrrhetinic acid (triterpenoid) inhibit growth and cytopathic effects of herpes simplex, vaccinia, Newcastle's disease, and vesicular stomatitis viruses. Topical glycyrrhetinic acid is quite helpful in reducing healing time and pain of cold sores and genital herpes.
- **Resveratrol (3,5,4′-trihydroxystilbene)**: natural component of grapes that has anti-HSV activity in vitro. Topical application of resveratrol cream (12.5%-25%) effectively blocks HSV replication and stops lesion eruption if applied early and frequently. No human studies have been reported.

## THERAPEUTIC APPROACH

- **Goals**: shorten current attack and prevent recurrences. Support the immune system; control food allergens and optimize nutrients necessary for cell-mediated immunity. Inhibit HSV replication by manipulating dietary lysine/arginine ratio. No cure is known, but strengthening the immune system is quite effective in reducing frequency, duration, and severity of recurrences.

- **Diet**: develop diet that avoids food allergens and arginine-rich foods while promoting lysine-rich foods (*Textbook*, "The Optimal Health Food Pyramid"). Foods with worst arginine/lysine ratio are chocolate, peanuts, and almonds.
- **Supplements**:
  —Vitamin C: 2000 mg q.d.
  —Bioflavonoids: 1000 mg q.d.
  —Zinc: 25 mg q.d.
  —Lysine: 1000 mg t.i.d.
  —Thymus extract: equivalent to 120 mg pure polypeptides with molecular weights <10,000 or roughly 500 mg crude polypeptide fraction.
- **Topical treatment**:
  —Ice: 10 minutes on, 5 minutes off during prodrome
  —Zinc sulfate solution: 0.025% solution t.i.d.
  —*Melissa* cream: apply b.i.d.
  —Glycyrrhetinic acid: apply b.i.d.

# HIV/AIDS

## DIAGNOSTIC SUMMARY

- **Positive test for antibody** against human immunodeficiency virus (HIV) by enzyme-linked immunosorbent assay (ELISA) and confirmed by Western blot.
- **Acute onset (acute antiretroviral syndrome)**: resembles influenza 2-6 weeks after initial infection and often goes undiagnosed as HIV because of the similarity to flu.
- **Signs and symptoms**: fever; fatigue; lymphadenopathy; pharyngitis; maculopapular rash on the face, head, and trunk; mucocutaneous ulceration of mouth, esophagus, genitals; myalgia; night sweats; diarrhea; headache; nausea and vomiting; hepatosplenomegaly; weight loss; thrush; neurologic symptoms (aseptic meningitis, encephalitis, peripheral neuropathy, facial palsy, Guillain-Barré syndrome, brachial neuritis, cognitive impairment, or psychosis); thrombocytopenia; leucopenia; transaminase elevation.
- **Insidious onset**: acquired immunodeficiency syndrome (AIDS)-associated opportunistic infection (OI) or unexplained progressive fatigue, weight loss, fever, diarrhea, and/or generalized lymphadenopathy.
- AIDS is diagnosed after positive serology and CD4+ T-cell count ≤200 cells/mm$^3$ and/or presence of designated AIDS indicator condition (1993/1997 Centers for Disease Control and Prevention [CDC] guidelines).
- The lower the CD4+ count and the higher the viral load, the higher the risk of OIs, neoplasms, or neurologic abnormalities and the higher the mortality rate.
- **Groups at high risk for contracting HIV**: intravenous drug users, gay and bisexual men, hemophiliacs and others receiving transfused blood or blood products (highest risk to recipients before May 1985), sexual partners of people in these groups, heterosexuals with more than one sex partner in the past 12 months, sexual relations without condom use in past 6 months.

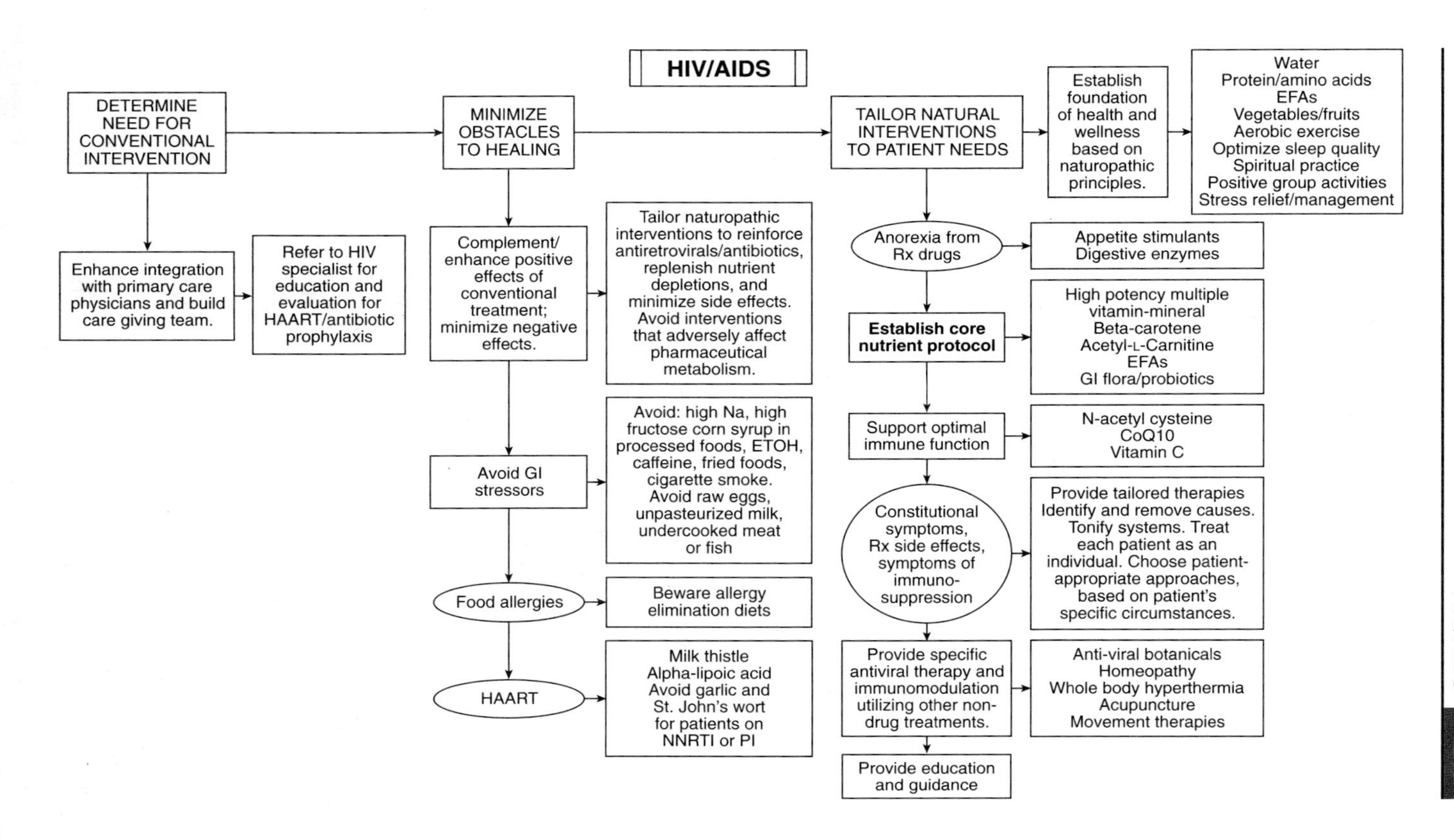
HIV/AIDS
DETERMINE NEED FOR CONVENTIONAL INTERVENTION
Enhance integration with primary care physicians and build care giving team.
Refer to HIV specialist for education and evaluation for HAART/antibiotic prophylaxis
MINIMIZE OBSTACLES TO HEALING
Complement/enhance positive effects of conventional treatment; minimize negative effects.
Tailor naturopathic interventions to reinforce antiretrovirals/antibiotics, replenish nutrient depletions, and minimize side effects. Avoid interventions that adversely affect pharmaceutical metabolism.
Avoid GI stressors
Avoid: high Na, high fructose corn syrup in processed foods, ETOH, caffeine, fried foods, cigarette smoke. Avoid raw eggs, unpasteurized milk, undercooked meat or fish
Food allergies
Beware allergy elimination diets
HAART
Milk thistle
Alpha-lipoic acid
Avoid garlic and St. John's wort for patients on NNRTI or PI
TAILOR NATURAL INTERVENTIONS TO PATIENT NEEDS
Establish foundation of health and wellness based on naturopathic principles.
Water
Protein/amino acids
EFAs
Vegetables/fruits
Aerobic exercise
Optimize sleep quality
Spiritual practice
Positive group activities
Stress relief/management
Anorexia from Rx drugs
Appetite stimulants
Digestive enzymes
Establish core nutrient protocol
High potency multiple vitamin-mineral
Beta-carotene
Acetyl-L-Carnitine
EFAs
GI flora/probiotics
Support optimal immune function
N-acetyl cysteine
CoQ10
Vitamin C
Constitutional symptoms, Rx side effects, symptoms of immuno-suppression
Provide tailored therapies
Identify and remove causes. Tonify systems. Treat each patient as an individual. Choose patient-appropriate approaches, based on patient's specific circumstances.
Provide specific antiviral therapy and immunomodulation utilizing other non-drug treatments.
Anti-viral botanicals
Homeopathy
Whole body hyperthermia
Acupuncture
Movement therapies
Provide education and guidance

## GENERAL CONSIDERATIONS

### Pathogenesis

#### Clnical Progression From Infection to AIDS

Within 2-3 weeks of infection, acute retroviral syndrome occurs. Recovery and seroconversion follow in 2-3 weeks. HIV plasma concentrations decline to viral "set point"—equilibrium between production and destruction of CD4+ cells. Viral replication plus CD4+ count are predictive of prognosis. Lower replication with higher CD4+ indicates longer asymptomatic course. Higher replication with lower CD4+ indicates shorter asymptomatic course. Gradual decline in T-cell numbers is concurrent with gradual increase in virus load, lasting 5-15 years. Eventually, T-cell depletion impairs immunity, increasing risk of OIs and ultimately leading to death.

Primary CDC criteria for AIDS in adults and children aged 13 years and older: positive serology (antibodies to HIV via ELISA and Western blot plus HIV antigen by polymerase chain reaction [PCR] or other specific HIV antigen test) and CD4+ counts <200/mm$^3$ (<14%) and/or any of the category C conditions occurs.

### CDC 1993 Surveillance Case Definition of AIDS

#### CD4+ Cell Categories

1. >500/mm$^3$ (>29%)
2. 200-499/mm$^3$ (14%-28%)
3. <200/mm$^3$ (<14%)

#### Clinical Categories

1. Asymptomatic HIV infection, persistent generalized lymphadenopathy (PGL), or acute or primary HIV infection (history or symptoms).
2. Conditions attributable to HIV or having a clinical course or requiring management complicated by HIV. Examples: bacillary angiomatosis (from *Bartonella*; erythematous papules or nodules on skin; can involve organs such as liver, bone), oral candidiasis or thrush, vulvovaginal candidiasis (persistent, frequent, or poorly responsive to therapy), cervical dysplasia (moderate or severe), cervical carcinoma in situ, constitutional symptoms such as fever or diarrhea lasting >1 month, oral hairy leukoplakia, herpes zoster (two episodes or more than one dermatome),

idiopathic thrombocytopenic purpura (ITP), listeriosis, pelvic inflammatory disease (PID), or peripheral neuropathy.

3. Specific AIDS indicator conditions (updated in 1997). Once one of the following has occurred, the person remains classified as having AIDS:
   - Candidiasis of esophagus, trachea, bronchi, or lungs
   - Cervical cancer, invasive
   - Coccidioidomycosis, extrapulmonary
   - Cryptococcosis, extrapulmonary
   - Cryptosporidiosis with diarrhea >1 month
   - Cytomegalovirus (CMV) of any organ other than liver, spleen, or lymph nodes
   - CMV retinitis
   - Herpes simplex with mucocutaneous ulcer >1 month or bronchitis, pneumonitis, esophagitis
   - Histoplasmosis, extrapulmonary
   - HIV-associated dementia: disabling cognitive and/or other dysfunction interfering with occupation or activities of daily living
   - Isosporiasis with diarrhea >1 month
   - Kaposi's sarcoma
   - Lymphoma: Burkitt's, immunoblastic, primary (brain/central nervous system)
   - *Mycobacterium avium,* disseminated
   - *Mycobacterium tuberculosis,* pulmonary or extrapulmonary
   - *Pneumocystis carinii* pneumonia
   - Pneumonia, recurrent bacterial (≥2 episodes in 12 months)
   - Progressive multifocal leukoencephalopathy
   - *Salmonella septicemia* (nontyphoid), recurrent
   - Toxoplasmosis of internal organ
   - Wasting syndrome from HIV: involuntary weight loss >10% of baseline plus chronic diarrhea (two or more loose stools/day ≥30 days) or chronic weakness and documented enigmatic fever ≥30 days

Susceptibility to complications (infectious and noninfectious) is based on CD4+ count (higher viral load is greater risk for complications):

- CD4+ of >500/$mm^3$: acute retroviral syndrome, candidal vaginitis, PGL, myopathy, or aseptic meningitis.
- CD4+ of 200-500/$mm^3$: Pneumococcal and other bacterial pneumonia, pulmonary tuberculosis, herpes zoster, oropharyngeal

candidiasis/thrush, cryptosporidiosis (self-limited), Kaposi's sarcoma, oral hairy leukoplakia, cervical intraepithelial neoplasia, cervical cancer, B-cell lymphoma, anemia, mononeuronal multiplex, idiopathic thrombocytopenic purpura, Hodgkin's lymphoma, or lymphocytic interstitial pneumonitis.
- CD4+ of 100-200/$mm^3$: *Pneumocystis carinii* pneumonia, disseminated histoplasmosis and coccidioidomycosis, miliary/extrapulmonary tuberculosis, progressive multifocal leukoencephalopathy (PML), wasting, peripheral neuropathy, HIV-associated dementia, cardiomyopathy, vacuolar myelopathy, progressive polyradiculopathy, or non-Hodgkin's lymphoma.
- CD4+ of 50-100/$mm^3$: disseminated herpes simplex, toxoplasmosis, cryptococcosis, chronic cryptosporidiosis, microsporidiosis, or candidal esophagitis.
- CD4+ of <50/$mm^3$: disseminated CMV, disseminated *Mycobacterium avium* complex, central nervous system lymphoma.

## DIAGNOSIS

### Diagnostic Testing

Risk groups needing HIV testing:

- People with sexually transmitted diseases (STDs)
- High-risk categories: intravenous drug users, gay and bisexual men, hemophiliacs, sexual partners of people in these groups, heterosexuals with more than one sex partner in past year, sexually active people not using condoms in past 6 months
- People who consider themselves at risk
- Pregnant women
- Patients with active tuberculosis
- Recipient and source of occupational exposure
- Hospital in-patients aged 15-54 years in areas of high prevalence
- Health care workers performing exposure-prone invasive procedures (consider institutional policies)
- Donors of blood, semen, and organs

Standard serologic testing for HIV begins with electroimmunoassay/ELISA using recombinant antigens to measure blood antibodies to HIV. If result is positive, test is repeated on same blood sample. If a second positive result, a Western blot test (electrophoresis to detect antibodies to specific HIV proteins) is used to confirm. Combined ELISA and Western blot have sensitivity and specificity near 100%. Newer, more rapid tests include OraQuick ADVANCE

Rapid HIV-1/2 Antibody Test (Abbott Diagnostics), the OraSure Oral Mucosal Transudate test (OraSure Technologies), the Calypte HIV-1 Urine test (Calypte Biomedical Corp.), and the Wellcozyme HIV-1&2 vaginal secretion test (Gracelisa Murex Diagnostics Ltd.). Test kits approved for home use: Confide (Johnson & Johnson), Home Access, and Home Access Express (Home Access Health Corp.) (sample taken at home and sent to lab for processing). All these tests detect antibodies to HIV. False-negative results can arise in newly infected HIV-positive patient (window period for seroconversion discussed earlier). If ELISA is negative and risk factors suggest likely infection, repeat test at 6-week, 3-month, and 6-month intervals. Counsel patients properly before testing. Ascertain risks and discuss nature and meaning of potential results. Give positive results in a face-to-face meeting. Provide education on prognosis, treatment options, and social services available. Encourage patients to and/or provide assistance to notify sexual and/or needle-sharing partners.

**Clinical history for HIV-positive patient**: standard medical history including diet history, exercise patterns, complete review of systems, plus additional information (create a table). Historical data recommended for HIV-positive patients include the following:

- Date of infection and subsequent diagnosis; probable source of infection (IV drug use, sexual contact, transfusion). If date of infection is unknown, determine any history of acute retroviral syndrome. Determine past and current HIV exposure risk factors. (Helps estimate overall heartiness and long-term prognosis.)
- Vaccinations and adverse reactions to past vaccines.
- Other STDs: date and duration of infection, therapies (efficacy, adverse reactions, duration of treatment). Screen for syphilis, gonorrhea, chlamydia, herpes simplex (all types), hepatitis (A, B, and C or E), and human papillomavirus (HPV) (skin, genital, or anal).
- Chronologic history of HIV-related problems, history of OIs or cofactor viruses/infections (mononucleosis, Epstein-Barr virus, *Molluscum contagiosum*, CMV, or yeast infections [vaginal, gastrointestinal, skin]), skin rashes or other lesions, oral lesions or tongue coating, lymphadenopathy, fevers, night sweats, weight loss, diarrhea, anorexia, fatigue, malaise, shortness of breath, or cough.
- Female specifics: abnormal Pap smears, frequency of gynecologic examinations.

- HIV viral load and CD4 count trend: indicate susceptibility to OI, need for and efficacy of highly active antiretroviral therapy (HAART) and long-term prognosis.
- HAART; other prophylactic antibiotics with duration, response, side effects, intolerance, allergies.
- Family history of chronic disease: cardiovascular disease (including dyslipidemia), diabetes mellitus, cancer.
- Psychological or emotional trauma and issues (abuse history, anxiety, depression).
- Spiritual life and support system(s), life goals, meaning of HIV in life.
- Identities of complete medical care team, reasons for seeking naturopathic care.
- Initial physical examination: must be both comprehensive and appropriately directed by history. Thoroughly examine mouth, throat, skin, genitalia. If a full pelvic examination and Pap smear cannot be done on new female patient at initial evaluation, scheduled these for shortly thereafter.

HIV-specific testing includes the following:

- **Basic initial screening tests for all HIV-positive patients**: complete blood count, serum chemistry panel (to monitor liver, kidney, and pancreas function; electrolytes; blood proteins; glucose; lipids). Baseline serum albumin serves as independent predictor of prognosis in HIV-positive women. Additional tests: STD screening (VDRL or rapid plasmin reagent [RPR] for syphilis, chlamydia, gonorrhea, herpes simplex); hepatitis (A, B, and C); purified protein derivative and baseline chest radiograph (tuberculosis screening); CMV. Female patients: regular Pap smears with initial HPV testing (increased risk of cervical cancer in HIV-positive women).
- Quarterly viral load and T-cell counts: Viral load detects viral RNA in plasma, tested by PCR, sensitive to $<50$ copies/$mm^3$ of plasma. Below this threshold, viral load is deemed undetectable. This test does not reflect HIV in compartments beyond blood (e.g., tissues or cerebrospinal fluid). Patients still can infect others even if virus is undetectable.
- **T-cell counts**: CD4+ helper cells and CD8+ suppressor cells are quantified plus CD4/CD8 ratio. Less than 200 CD4+ cells/$mm^3$, risk of OIs increases and management of HIV is modified (antimicrobial prophylaxis is initiated).

A patient on antiretrovirals with CD4+ count falling or viral load rising may be developing resistance to current HAART. Consider genetic or resistance testing to ascertain susceptibility of specific viral strain to available medicines and help formulate more effective regimen.

## THERAPEUTIC CONSIDERATIONS

### Medical Management of HIV/AIDS

AIDS is complex, multifactorial disease—both immunodeficiency and autoimmune inflammatory aspects involve every body system. HIV infects CD4+ expressing immune cells, inserts itself into cellular DNA, and lies dormant indefinitely. Those cells are activated for multiplication and reproduction of HIV virons by antigens, oxidative stress, proinflammatory cytokines, and overstressed liver detoxification and immune function.

Principles of conventional medical management of HIV/AIDS:

- Frequent monitoring: lab and physical examination
- Vaccination for OIs: e.g., pneumococcal pneumonia, hepatitis B (HBV), influenza
- HAART to slow HIV and increase CD4+ counts
- Antibiotic prophylaxis for abnormally low CD4+ counts
- Antimicrobial treatment of OIs
- Symptomatic care of HIV or HAART-induced adverse drug reactions
- Radiation and/or chemotherapy for HIV-related neoplasms
- Psychosocial support with counseling, clinical social work, medication

Conventional information resources:

- AIDSInfo Web site (www.aidsinfo.nih.gov), administered by U.S. Department of Health & Human Services, and its merger of HIV/AIDS Clinical Trials Information Service (ACTIS) and HIV/AIDS Treatment Information Service (HIVATIS).
- Johns Hopkins AIDS Service (hopkins-aids.edu) and HIV Guide (www.hopkins-hivguide.org): diagnosis and management of HIV and OIs, medications, resistance.
- *Medical Management of HIV Infection*, by John G. Bartlett and Joel E. Gallant, Johns Hopkins University, 2004, ISBN 0-9716241-1-9; phone orders: 800-537-5487.

- Best resource for patient education: www.thebody.com/index.html. This site contains valuable information on signs, symptoms, treatments, and future possibilities.

## Naturopathic Medical Management of HIV/AIDS

**Seven specific goals of naturopathic treatment:**

1. Enhance integration with primary care physicians and build caregiving team.
2. Complement and/or enhance positive effects of conventional treatment; minimize negative effects.
3. Establish foundation of health and wellness based on the naturopathic principles.
4. Establish core nutrient protocol.
   - Replace nutrient deficiencies known to exist with HIV.
   - Provide other nutrients to support optimal immune function.
5. Provide therapies for constitutional symptoms, medication side effects, symptoms of immunosuppression.
6. Provide specific antiviral therapy and immunomodulation using other nondrug treatments.
7. Provide education and guidance to patients seeking alternatives to conventional treatment.

Resource for complementary practitioners: *AIDS and Complementary & Alternative Medicine, Current Science and Practice,* by L.J. Standish, C. Calabrese, and M.L. Galantino, Churchill Livingstone, 2002, ISBN #0-443-05831-8.

1. *Enhance integration with primary care physicians and build caregiving team.*

A naturopathic physician optimizes integrated care; she may be the first and only physician coordinating or formulating a complete health care team for the patient. Identifying advantages of all available treatments and encouraging positive relationships among all providers creates unique and trusting relationships with patients who have often experienced lifetimes of fear, discrimination, victimization, and abuse. Naturopathy empowers HIV-positive patients. Ensure each HIV-positive patient has a complete care team beginning with conventional HIV specialist for HAART and familiarity with HIV signs and symptoms. HIV-positive patients have better indexes of health (low viral load and high CD4), better compliance with medicines, and better long-term survival rates when working with HIV specialists. Even though naturopaths are legally able to prescribe prophylactic antimicrobial therapy and HAART in a growing number of states, the greater need is nondrug holistic care.

2. *Complement and/or enhance positive effects of conventional treatment; minimize negative effects.*

Paradigms of natural medicine state to avoid or minimize the use of higher force (drug, surgery, radiation) interventions. Yet no therapies currently are as effective as HAART in suppressing viral load or increasing CD4 numbers. The current standard of care delays HAART in asymptomatic patients while CD4 count is consistently between or above 200-350 cells/μL and/or plasma viral load is <50,000-100,000 copies/mL. HAART must be considered and not discouraged. Regardless of HAART, HIV-positive patients benefit from nondrug therapies. Naturopaths must apply the entire therapeutic order to maximize quality of life and longevity. Stay current with arising possibilities. Ensure patient safety from adverse drug-nutrient interactions. Understand mechanisms of HAART and common nutrients used by HIV-positive patients. Four main classes of HAART currently are being used for HIV-positive patients:

- NRTI/nucleoside and nucleotide reverse transcriptase inhibitors ("nukes")
- NNRTI/NON-nucleoside reverse transcriptase inhibitors ("non-nukes")
- Protease inhibitors (PIs)
- Fusion inhibitors

These drugs have been fast-tracked through the Food and Drug Administration (FDA) and are not subjected to rigorous efficacy and safety trials. Little is known about adverse drug reactions. Naturopaths may see an HIV-positive patient more frequently than do conventional providers and may recognize adverse reactions and initiate communication with prescribing physician.

**NRTIs ("Nukes")**

NRTIs work during the transcription phase of the HIV lifecycle by competitive inhibition of HIV reverse transcriptase (RT) and DNA chain termination. Nucleoside (or nucleotide) analogues are created, which act as substrates binding to the active site of RT enzyme and are added to new DNA chain. Once inserted, normal links between chain pieces will not occur and the viral chain will be terminated without insertion into the cell's DNA.

NRTIs (given in the following list as three-character abbreviation/generic name(s)/brand name) are all nucleoside analogs except tenofovir, which is the only FDA approved nucleotide analogue:

- AZT/azidothymidine/Zidovudine/Retrovir
- 3TC/lamivudine/Epivir
- DDC/zalcitibine/Hivid
- DDI/didanosine/Videx
- D4T/stavudine/Zerit
- ABC/abacavir/Ziagen
- FTC/emtricitabine/Emtriva
- TEN/tenofovir/Viread (nucleotide)

NRTIs are fairly well tolerated (initial mild to severe nausea usually resolves), with minimal long-term adverse effects. Exceptions: AZT and the "D drugs" (DDC, DDI, D4T). AZT suppresses bone marrow, causing macrocytic anemia. D drugs are less commonly used today except in the case of multidrug resistance. D drugs cause mild to severe peripheral neuropathy and pancreatitis, linked to neural inhibition of mitochondrial DNA polymerase and reduced mitochondrial DNA content. Provide mitochondrial support with high-dose acetyl-L-carnitine, coenzyme $Q_{10}$ ($CoQ_{10}$), essential fatty acids, alpha-lipoic acid, and B vitamins, which decrease side effects.

AZT may deplete cellular carnitine, copper, zinc, and vitamin $B_{12}$ levels. Carnitine deficiency exists in HIV-positive patients not on HAART. Carnitine has high priority for supplementation. HIV patients have greatly increased animal protein requirements.

Nutrients that enhance efficacy of NRTIs: vitamin E, zinc, folate from whole grains, colorful vegetables and fruits, and high-potency vitamin/mineral supplements. Red Korean ginseng at large doses reduces AZT resistance and increases CD4 counts but is cost prohibitive and energetically "overheating" for many patients, aggravating anxiety, insomnia, heart palpitations, or sweating.

A few NRTIs are active against HBV (3TC, FTC, TEN) as well. Patient compliance is critical when taking NRTIs so as not lose this option when HAART is indicated.

### NNRTIs ("Non-nukes")

NNRTIs (given as generic name/brand name) include the following:

- efavirenz/Sustiva
- nevirapine/Viramune
- delavirdine/Rescriptor (rarely used)

NNRTIs also are fairly well tolerated (mild transient to severe rash, sleep disturbances) and may be the most important class of HAART. Without NNRTIs, patients require PIs, which cause adverse drug reactions. Patients must understand the significance of NNRTIs when initiating therapy. Side effects (depending on specific drug) include transient rash, insomnia, abnormal dreams, elevated liver enzymes, and gynecomastia (all manageable with naturopathy). NNRTIs affect transcription process, allosterically binding to HIV-1 reverse transcriptase and inhibiting both RNA- and DNA-directed DNA polymerase functions of RT enzyme. Neither nutrient depletions nor nutrient enhancement of efficacy are known for NNRTIs.

NRTIs used with NNRTIs sustain reduced plasma viral loads and improvements in immunologic responses in large, randomized, double-blind, placebo-controlled studies. Two NRTIs (zidovudine and lamivudine) were most efficacious when used in combination with one NNRTI (efavirenz). This same regimen was found to be superior to one using three NRTIs (zidovudine, lamivudine, abacavir). In another study, nevirapine and efavirenz showed similar efficacy in combination with two NRTIs. Advantages of this type of protocol are fewest side effects, excellent long-term viral suppression, and ease of dosing (fewer pills).

### Protease Inhibitors

PIs (given as generic name/brand name) include the following:

- ritonavir/Norvir
- saquinavir/Invirase
- saquinavir/Fortovase
- indinavir/Crixivan
- nelfinavir/Viracept
- lopinavir + ritonavir/Kaletra
- amprenavir/Agenerase
- atazanavir/Reyataz
- fosamprenavir/Lexiva: a calcium phosphate ester prodrug of amprenavir

PIs are effective at viral suppression but have the greatest number and most significant adverse reactions: chronic, persistent gastrointestinal (GI) abnormalities; lipodystrophy; lipoatrophy; and liver, kidney, and musculoskeletal complaints. PIs bind competitively to substrate site of viral protease (responsible for posttranslational processing), thereby inhibiting enzyme and producing immature virus particles.

NNRTIs and PIs also inhibit liver cytochrome P450 3A4 enzyme metabolism, retarding breakdown of drugs and prolonging higher blood drug levels and viral suppression. Many foods, nutrients, and botanicals upregulate this enzyme function: garlic and St. John's wort decrease NNRTI and PI levels. Avoid them in HIV patients on HAART. Be intimately aware of the mechanism of action when adding new nondrug therapies for patients on multidrug treatments. Use a multitude of low-force interventions (e.g., diet, lifestyle, homeopathy, physical medicine, counseling) for conditions otherwise treated by garlic and St. John's wort.

Milk thistle decreases trough levels of some drugs by 25% in some patients. More studies are needed on milk thistle. No nutrient depletions are linked to PIs; no nutrients are known to enhance efficacy.

### Fusion Inhibitors

Fusion inhibitors are the most recent class of drugs for HIV/AIDS. Enfuvirtide (Fuzeon) is the only HAART drug requiring injection (two subcutaneous injections daily into the upper arm, upper leg, or stomach). Enfuvirtide is salvage therapy; it enhances the effect of other HAART drugs, but it is not designed to be used alone. It is fairly well tolerated, except for injection site irritation, allergic reactions, and increased risk of bacterial pneumonia. Mechanism: it binds with cell receptor proteins gp41 necessary for HIV to identify and enter selective cell membranes. There are no known drug-nutrient interactions, nutrients known to be depleted, or nutrients known to enhance efficacy of fusion inhibitors.

3. *Establish a foundation of health and wellness based on naturopathic principles.*

A healthy diet and lifestyle cannot be overemphasized. Ensure optimal GI health and nutritional intake.

- High intake of filtered water to decrease oxidative stress and reduce toxic load of HIV and medicines.

- Optimal intake of protein. Requirements: up to 100-150 g q.d., particularly for malabsorption and/or diarrhea. Supplement if necessary to prevent weight loss. Large doses of whey protein and/or amino acids (L-glutamine, L-arginine) can reverse or prevent wasting.
- Essential fatty acids (EFAs) are deficient in HIV-positive patients. EFA supplements increase body cell mass and decrease risk of progression to AIDS.
- Fruit juices or fruit-vegetable concentrates optimize micronutrients and antioxidants. Include colorful vegetables and fruits for micronutrients, fiber, and digestive and liver support.
- Appetite stimulation and/or digestive enzyme support to combat adverse effects of HIV, HAART, and prophylactic antibiotics on the GI system. Avoid additional GI stressors, such as high sodium levels, high fructose corn syrup in processed foods, alcohol, caffeine, fried foods, and cigarette smoke. Avoid raw eggs, unpasteurized milk, undercooked meat or fish, and potentially contaminated foods to decrease risk of GI OIs and parasites.
- Beware of allergy elimination diets in HIV-positive patients because of nutrient deficiencies, maldigestion, and malabsorption caused by HIV itself and HAART medicines. Recommend replacement of food allergens one food at a time to ensure patients can maintain replacement diets without decreasing caloric and nutrient intake over time. Removing food vices and irritating foods is challenging; many other challenges and a vital need to maintain body mass are higher priorities.
- Aerobic exercise alleviates stress; enhances mood; increases CD4, CD8, and natural killer (NK) cells; and increases immune parameters. Mind-body exercises, such as Tai Chi and yoga, increase perception of health and self-confidence and allow quicker return to athletic activities after medical interventions.
- Improve sleep quality. Encourage patients to create an optimal sleeping environment and sleep 8-10 hours each night. Sleep supports tissue repair and increases circulating NK cells and lymphocytes.
- Activities that improve odds for long-term survival: group activities, positive attitude about illness, health-promoting behaviors, spiritual activities, activities that support HIV-positive community. Structured brief group intervention for bereavement decreases plasma cortisol and improves immune markers.
- Stress relief and management: cognitive behavioral stress management is guided relaxation training that improves quality of

life in HIV-positive women, decreases herpes simplex 2 antibody titers in HIV-positive men, and decreases markers of stress and improves HIV lab values. Prayer and distance healing reduce new AIDS-defining illnesses, illness severity, physician visits, and hospitalizations while improving mood. Prayer and meditation improve mental health. Laughter improves white blood cell values and decreases stress.

4. *Establish core nutrient protocol.*

- Replace known nutrient deficiencies caused by HIV.

Vitamin and mineral replenishment delays progression to AIDS and the need for antiretrovirals. Numerous deficiencies are linked to HIV disease progression. Causes of deficiencies: loss, poor absorption, or rapid use and consumption. Nutrients deficient in HIV patients, with corrective daily doses (taken in divided doses throughout day) are noted in parentheses followed by reasons for the deficiencies and/or benefits.

- **Vitamin A** (15,000-30,000 IU taken with food): slows progression to AIDS and decreases mortality rate, improves growth in infants and decreases stunting from chronic diarrhea, and prevents GI deterioration in mothers and infants. May increase risk of HIV transmission by breastfeeding but has no effect on mortality rate by 24 months. Causes of deficiency: decreased dietary intake, poor GI absorption, high urinary loss, impaired hepatic protein synthesis, increased needs from chronic infection.
- **Beta-carotene** (60-120 mg/150,000 IU taken with food): increases CD4+ count, CD4/CD8 ratios, and total lymphocyte count and decreases mortality rate. Deficiency is found in all HIV-positive patients because of poor digestion, decreased free radical elimination, and high lipid peroxidation.
- **Folate** (400 μg): normalizes cell differentiation. Deficiency due to malabsorption; AZT-induced deficiency may increase risk of bone marrow toxicity.
- **Vitamin $B_1$** (50 mg) increases survival in HIV-positive patients and decreases progression to AIDS.
- **Vitamin $B_6$** (50 mg): is essential in nucleic acid and protein metabolism and cellular and humoral immune responses. $B_6$ repletion alone and in conjunction with $CoQ_{10}$ increases circulating immunoglobulin G, CD4+ cells, and CD4/CD8 ratios.
- **Vitamin $B_{12}$** (1000 μg hydroxocobalamin, methylcobalamin, or cyanocobalamin by intramuscular injections three times per week or daily 1000 μg sublingual): benefits parameters of immune

function, cell differentiation, and nerve function and decreases homocysteine. $B_{12}$ improves lymphocyte counts, CD4/CD8 ratios, and NK cell activity. It also reverses AIDS dementia associated with $B_{12}$ deficit. Deficiency increases risk of progression to AIDS and HIV disease.

- **Vitamin E** (800 IU d-mixed tocopherols taken with food): decreases lipid peroxidation, protects against AZT oxidative damage to cardiac mitochondria, normalizes immune function, and slows progression to AIDS. Deficiency in most HIV-positive patients causes wasting in progression to AIDS.
- **Copper** (2 mg): inhibits HIV protease and viral replication. Deficiency is linked to AZT and AIDS.
- **Magnesium** (300 mg): deficient in AIDS patients.
- **Selenium** (400 μg): slows HIV proliferation, decreases HIV mortality rate, decreases anxiety in HIV-positive recreational drug users, and decreases hospitalization and medical costs. Deficiency during progression to AIDS is caused by decreased food intake, malabsorption, and infections.
- **Zinc** (15 mg; optimal intake is undetermined): decreases frequency of OIs. Deficiency in all HIV-positive patients progressing to AIDS.
- **Acetyl-L-carnitine** (2-6 g best not taken with other protein to optimize absorption): supports energy and metabolism. Deficiency is common and increases risk for alterations in fatty acid metabolism. Repletion reduces serum triglycerides, decreases risk of wasting, increases CD4 cells and reduces apoptosis, increases serum insulinlike growth factor, and reduces mitochondrial neurotoxicity and peripheral neuropathy. It treats NRTI-induced lactic acidosis.
- **Dehydroepiandrosterone (DHEA)** (15-50 mg taken with food): increases CD4 count and stimulates immune function.
- **Testosterone** (intramuscular injection weekly): if serum levels are low to maintain lean body muscle mass.
- **Glutathione/GSH** (increased through selenium and N-acetyl-cysteine or whey protein powder): decreases disease progression and mortality rate. Deficient in symptom-free HIV-positive and AIDS patients.

Many of these nutrients can be replenished by a highly nutritious diet and high-potency vitamin/mineral supplement. Multiples specifically developed for HIV-positive patients include high doses of carotenoids, B vitamins, and antioxidants and may include digestive enzymes. Multiples designed specifically for HIV reduce pill burden and enhance compliance. However, it is more cost effective to use basic multiples and supplement individual additional nutrients.

Nutrients (high doses of beta-carotene, acetyl-L-carnitine, DHEA, testosterone, GSH, catalase) not found in a multiple form must be replaced by specific dietary regimens or additional supplements. Use only natural forms of beta-carotene. Acetyl-L-carnitine is a high priority despite its high cost. Measure baseline hormone levels before supplementing to guide dosing and minimize risk of these higher force interventions.

### Support Optimal Immune Function

- ***Silybum marianum*** (milk thistle; 300 mg standardized silymarin extract taken separately from HAART): all HAART patients—improves liver function, decreases liver damage, increases antioxidant activity of blood cells.
- N-**acetyl-cysteine (NAC)** (2-8 g taken separately from other nutrients but with food to decrease GI distress): prevents loss of sulfur-containing amino acids, increases GSH, decreases TNF-alpha activity, and increases CD4 cell count.
- **$CoQ_{10}$** (100-300 mg): optimizes mitochondrial function; replaces deficiency; increases circulating immunoglobulin G, CD4+ cells, and CD4/CD8 ratios.
- **Vitamin C** (2-6 g): when combined with vitamin E, lowers oxidative stress and viral load.
- **Alpha-lipoic acid** (600 mg): protects liver, inhibits viral replication, increases intracellular GSH, increases CD4/CD8 ratios, decreases peripheral neuropathy pain by antioxidant effect.
- **L-Arginine** (7.4 g taken separately from food): improves lean body mass and increases NK cell activity. (Consider sustained-release form.) High doses can aggravate herpes simplex outbreaks. Prophylactic L-lysine may prevent or reduce aggravation.
- **EFAs** (5 g with food; preferably fish oil): improve lean body mass, increase NK cell activity, and an adjuvant therapy for tuberculosis.

These nutrients have benefits but increase cost and pill burden. Give priority to the most essential (EFAs) and lower cost (vitamin C) or to address specific symptoms.

5. *Provide therapies to address constitutional symptoms, medication side effects, and symptoms of immunosuppression.*

Naturopathic principles apply. Identify and remove causes, tone systems, treat each patient as an individual. Choose patient-appropriate approaches based on the patient's specific circumstances.

### *Candida albicans*/Oral Thrush

Occurs from HIV itself (low CD4+ reduces immunity) or from prophylactic antibiotics. Oral thrush: pain makes eating difficult, reducing intake. Intestines: inflammation and compromised nutrient absorption. Esophagus: pain; must be dealt with swiftly with antifungal drugs. Avoid foods that feed and promote yeast: sugars, baked goods, starchy vegetables (see the chapter on chronic candidiasis). Consider the following treatments:

- **Probiotics**: support healthy flora. Dose: 8 billion CFU with food. Species: *Lactobacillus acidophilus, Lactobacillus bifidus, Lactobacillus casei* ssp. *Lactobacillus rhamnosus* (LGG), *Saccharomyces boulardii* (for antibiotic-induced colitis to displace pathogenic flora).
- **Garlic** (1-2 g before meals): antifungal that spares nonpathogenic flora. Avoid in HAART patients.
- **Oregano oil** (300 mg taken separately from food): potent antifungal.
- **Nystatin and fluconazole**: pharmaceutical antifungals.

### Cardiovascular Disease

**Cause**: HAART (PIs and D-type NRTIs) adversely affects serum lipids and glucose, promoting cardiovascular disease, especially in patients already at high risk (with predisposing factors such as family history). HAART patients need preventive diet, healthy lifestyle, nutritional interventions (see the chapter on atherosclerosis). Avoid garlic because of adverse interaction with HAART. Consider the following (daily):

- **Acetyl-L-carnitine** (2-6 g away from other protein to optimize absorption) repletion reduces serum triglycerides.
- **$CoQ_{10}$** (100-300 mg) may enhance cardiovascular function.
- **Arginine** (7.4 g taken separately from food) decreases atherosclerosis. (Consider sustained-release form.)
- **EFAs** (5 g with food) may lower lipids. (Emphasize omega-3s EPA/DHA.)

### Diarrhea

Etiology guides choice of treatment. Causes include HIV-linked enteropathy, HAART side effects (especially with PIs), antibiotic side effects, GI infections, food allergies. Osmotic-type diarrhea can result from too many indigestible gel caps (medicines and supplements). First priority: remove cause if possible. Gluten intolerance is more common in HIV-positive patients. Explore lactose intolerance and irritable bowel syndrome. Rule out food allergies. Ensure sufficient patient strength to undergo food elimination; give clear alternatives for eliminated foods. Use stool cultures and ova and parasites testing to screen for infectious causes; treat as indicated. Consider stopping all nutrient supplements temporarily to see effect on diarrhea. Reintroduce supplements one at a time to determine which one is the cause.

- **Prevention**: avoid unfiltered tap water, unpasteurized milk and dairy products, ice made from unfiltered tap water, raw food unless peeled personally or washed with antimicrobial agents, raw or rare meat and fish, meat or shellfish that is not hot when served, food from street vendors.
- **Prevent dehydration**: replace electrolytes; consume broths, soups, fruit and vegetable juices, high-nutrient drinks.
- **Prevent malnutrition from malabsorption**: multiple supplements, adequate protein (requirements may increase to 100-150 g q.d.). Simplify diet (BRAT diet: bananas, rice, applesauce, toast) or use 1 tbsp tomato juice plus 1 tbsp sauerkraut juice (Dr. Bastyr's electrolyte replacement) and increase glutamine intake. Carob powder (astringent) helps relieve symptoms. Use 1 tsp in applesauce and increase up to 6 tsp q.d. as needed.

Consider the following supplements:

- **Probiotics**: for healthy flora.
- **L-Glutamine** (10-40 g taken separately from other proteins): amino acid fuel for small intestine enterocytes. Use powder (efficient and cost effective). Dose: 3 g t.i.d. Increase up to 40 g q.d. if necessary. High doses can create psychoses; monitor patient closely.
- **Pharmaceutical interventions**: Lomotil, loperamide (Imodium), psyllium husk (Metamucil).

### Herpes Simplex Virus, Herpes Zoster, Shingles

Treatment approaches for all herpes-type viruses are similar. Sequelae of herpes viruses tend to be dermatomal pattern, attributable to stress, hormonal fluctuations, and/or poor immune status. Identify and remove causes of stress (dietary, emotional, sunlight).

Support immune function. Address symptoms (pain). Consider the following:

- **Diet**: eliminate high-arginine (promotes herpes replication)—chocolate, nuts, peanuts. Increase high lysine (antagonizes L-arginine)—whole grains, dairy, fish, lima beans, soy.
- **L-Lysine**: 1000 mg t.i.d. taken separately from food during outbreak; 500 mg b.i.d. taken separately from food prophylactically.
- **Olive leaf extract** (2000 mg): effective antiviral.
- **Monolaurin**: antiviral effective against encapsulated DNA viruses; 300-600 mg t.i.d.
- ***Melissa officinalis***: antiviral topical botanical.
- ***Glycyrrhiza glabra***: antiviral oral and topical botanical.
- **Herbal tincture** (as parts): *Hydrastis* (1), *Taraxacum* root (2), *Lomatium* (2), *Passiflora* (1), *Astragalus* (1), *Gelsemium* (15 drops/oz); dose: 60 drops every 2 hours during prodrome; q.d. during outbreak; b.i.d. for prevention.
- **Acyclovir/valcyclovir**: pharmaceutical antiviral.

### Kaposi's Sarcoma

Kaposi's sarcoma (KS) is an HIV-linked vascular neoplasm occuring when CD4+ counts fall <500/mm$^3$. KS is rare outside the HIV-positive population. Etiology of AIDS-linked KS is poorly understood. Contributing factors: human herpes virus type 8, compromised immunity, hormones (KS is quite rare in women; androgen therapy increases tumor proliferation), iron-rich geographic areas. Ninety percent of AIDS KS cases in the United States occur in homosexual men.

**Progression**: from macules or elevated papules to large plaques or nodules. Color: from pink to purple or brownish-black. Shape: round or oval; do not blanche when pressed (contrast with ecchymoses). Location: first on skin of upper body or mucosal surfaces; aggressive form is widely disseminated—skin, mucous membranes, lymph nodes, viscera (GI tract from mouth to anus, lungs, liver, spleen, pancreas). Tumor secretions: angiogenic growth factors, tumor necrosis factor (TNF)-alpha, interleukin-6, basic fibroblast growth factor, platelet derived growth factor, oncostatin-M. Level of immunosuppression determines clinical course of KS in AIDS. No known cures; local and systemic approaches are aimed at palliation.

**Treatment**: chemotherapy (doxorubicin) and HAART. Surgical excision removes lesion but recurrence rate at affected site is high. Other options: radiation, liquid nitrogen cryotherapy, DC current electrical stimulation. Consider the following treatments:

- Topical and systemic retinoids.
- Topical vitamin D (1, 25-dihydroxyvitamin $D_3$).
- Iron: stimulates growth of KS cells in vitro; iron chelators reduce growth. Llimit iron intake; ensure serum iron and ferritin are at low end of normal.
- Cytokine inhibitors and antiangiogenesis compounds may reduce proliferation of vascular tumors.

Association of KS with human herpes virus type 8 suggests antiherpetic therapies if patient has herpes simplex. Topical medicinal peat preparation has triggered remission of skin KS lesions in several patients. Glutathione (N-acetylcysteine as precursor) may help KS lesions.

### Lipodystrophy

Lipodystrophy is redistribution of adipose tissue from extremities to trunk—a Cushing-like "buffalo hump" over upper thoracic region of back or trunkal obesity—impairing self-image. Cause is alterations in lipid metabolism caused by HAART or chronic (>15 years) HIV infection. Buffalo hump suggests adrenal abnormalities. Increased serum cortisol leads to increased insulin, driving blood glucose into storage in adipose cells and increasing trunkal obesity. Lipodystrophy also increases with lack of exercise. Increase exercise.

- Ensure regulation of blood glucose.
- L-Glutamine (10 g in divided doses taken separately from food).
- Acetyl-L-carnitine (2-6 g taken separately from food) optimizes mitochondria function.
- Dimethyl sulfoxide (DMSO)/bromelain (5% bromelain compounded in DMSO gel applied b.i.d. or t.i.d.). Topical applications can reduce Cushingoid adipose deposits.
- Conventional treatment: surgical removal of trunkal adipose. Invasive, but patients tend to be quite happy afterwards because of a more positive self-image.
- Buccal injections of polylactic acid (NuFill) reduces cosmetic signs of lipodystrophy and wasting.

### Macrocytic Anemia

**Cause**: malabsorption of nutrients or HAART (AZT causes bone marrow toxicity; PIs cause malabsorption). Consider the following treatments for proper cell division and differentiation:

- **Vitamin $B_{12}$** (hydroxycobalamin, methylcobalamin, cyanocobalamin 1000 μg IM each week). If intramuscular administration not available, use sublingual tablets at 1000 μg q.d. to bypass intestinal absorption.
- **Folic acid** (400 μg/day found in most good multiples) with vitamin $B_{12}$.
- **Vitamin B complex** (3 mL IM each week).

### Neuropathy

Location: periphery, particularly feet; moves proximally as severity increases. Cause is long-term HIV infection or D-type NRTIs and their toxic effect on mitochondria in neurons; diabetes mellitus (type 2); overdoses of vitamin $B_6$ (>200 mg q.d.). Consider the following treatments:

- **Acetyl-L-carnitine** (2-6 g taken separately from other protein to optimize absorption) reinforces fatty acid oxidation, energy supply, and critical metabolic functions.
- **EFAs** (5 g q.d. with food): antiinflammatory and component of neuronal membranes. (Emphasize omega-3 EPA.)
- **Vitamin $B_{12}$** (1000 μg/mL IM three times each week) for proper cell division and differentiation.
- **Vitamin B complex** (1 mL IM three times each week) for proper cell division and differentiation.
- **$CoQ_{10}$** (100-300 mg q.d.) optimizes mitochondrial function.
- **Alpha lipoic acid** (600 mg q.d.) may decrease pain.

### Pregnancy

Multiple vitamin/mineral supplements improve pregnancy outcomes in HIV-positive women, including fetal loss, low birth weight, prematurity, longer gestational length, birth weight, and head circumference. Multivitamins delay HIV disease progression and death. Supplements induce higher CD4+ counts and lower risk of diarrhea in children of nursing HIV-positive mothers. One study reported increased risk of transmission from mother to child with vitamin A and beta-carotene. Another showed that vitamin A and beta-carotene helped decrease GI deterioration in HIV-positive mothers and their children. Use vitamin A and beta-carotene with caution in pregnant or lactating women. Exclusive breastfeeding is associated with lower rate of mother-to-child transmission than breastfeeding along with other foods.

- High-potency hypoallergenic multiple vitamin/mineral; use as directed.
- Vitamin A for newborn; 200,000 IU at birth.
- Replenish HIV-induced deficiencies of folate (400 μg q.d.) and selenium (400 μg q.d.).

## Psychological Conditions

Depression, anxiety, posttraumatic stress disorder, sexual dysfunction, and substance abuse are common in HIV-positive people but are undertreated by conventional institutions. Treat each patient as a unique individual. Suicidal ideations or attempts arise as quality of life deteriorates, burden of treatment increases, and close friends die. Be vigilant for signs of suicide or loss of hope. Take these signs seriously; consult experienced professional help. Key consideration in treating psychological issues in these patients: polypharmacy and drug-nutrient interactions. Research, identify, and consider all potential interactions before initiating treatment with extreme caution. Example: St. John's wort induces liver cytochrome P-450 detoxification enzyme 3A4, reducing serum levels of HAART medicines. Avoid St. John's wort in HAART patients. Use counseling and homeopathy. Consider the following:

- **Amino acids** (if levels are low by lab analysis) in combinations tailored to replenish deficiencies.
- **Zinc** (25 mg) to normalize levels and improve efficacy of antidepressants.
- **EFAs** (5 g EPA q.d. with food): useful adjunct in depressive disorders.
- **S-adenosyl-L-methionine** (1600 mg): as effective as imipramine (150 mg) in treating major depression and better tolerated.

See the chapter on affective disorders.

## Wasting

HIV-associated wasting syndrome: involuntary weight loss of >10% of baseline body weight accompanied by chronic fever, weakness, or diarrhea. AIDS wasting syndrome must meet one of following criteria:

- Unintentional weight loss of ≥10% over 12 months
- Unintentional weight loss of ≥7.5% over 6 months
- Body cell mass (BCM) loss of ≥5% over 6 months

- Men: BCM <35% of total body weight (TBW) and body mass index (BMI) <27 kg/m$^2$
- Women: BCM <23% of TBW and BMI <27 kg/m$^2$
- BMI <20 kg/m$^2$

BCM can be measured by bioimpedance assay, a better predictor of survival than CD4 counts. Key issues are perceived weight loss, changes in appetite, diarrhea, energy level, and difficulties in performing activities of daily living.

The etiology of wasting is multifactorial:

- **Decreased food intake**: anorexia and/or nausea from medicines, systemic illness, GI pathosis; finances; dependence on others; poor choices.
- **Malabsorption/chronic diarrhea**: influenced by pathologic dysfunctions affecting any part of GI tract: infections, drug side effects, enzyme deficiencies, and malignancies.
- **Alterations of metabolism**: Resting energy expenditure is higher in HIV/AIDS patients than in control subjects. Resting energy expenditure does not downregulate if anorexia or malabsorption is present.
- **Cytokine abnormalities**: not well understood; TNF, interleukin-1 may induce anorexia and affect lipid, protein, and carbohydrate utilization; example of cachexia in cancer.
- **Endocrine abnormalities**: thyroid abnormalities, adrenal insufficiency (cortisol, DHEA), hypogonadism (testosterone), growth hormone deficiency.
- **Alcohol abuse**: accelerates progression from HIV to AIDS. Alcohol stimulates HIV production, suppresses immune defenses (lower CD4 counts), and depletes tissue antioxidants.

Remove identifiable causes, if feasible. Identify and remove possible food allergens (gluten, dairy). Ensure adequate and appropriate nutritional intake by dietary counseling. Help patient access social services as needed. Superdose nutrients. Increase protein intake to 100-150 g q.d. Encourage daily exercise. Consider the following therapies:

- **EFAs** (5 g q.d. with food). (Emphasize omega-3s.)
- **Acetyl-L-carnitine** (2-6 g q.d.): optimizes fatty acid metabolism.
- **L-Glutamine** (10-40 g): essential amino acid for enterocytes.
- **DHEA** (45 mg): promotes lean body mass.
- **Melatonin** (20 mg at bedtime): decreases cachexia and TNF.
- **Progesterone** (800 mg Megace): decreases cachexia.

- **Testosterone**: in hypogonadal men increases lean body mass and muscle strength.
- **Anabolic steroids** (nandrolone decanoate, oxandrolone, oxymetholone): increase lean body mass.
- **Thalidomide**: a cytokine modulator; increases BCM and extracellular fluid.

6. *Provide specific antiviral therapy and immunomodulation with other nondrug treatments.*

**Botanical Medicines**

- ***Glycyrrhiza glabra* (licorice)** (1500 mg): inhibits HIV fusion and viral transcription. Do not use in patients with history of hypertension or renal or cardiac problems, or in those taking digitalis or steroid medicines.
- ***Buxus sempervirens* (European boxwood)** (990 mg extract; larger doses less effective): increases CD4 + and decreases viral load after 6 months.
- ***Curcuma longa* (turmeric)** (1200 mg): inhibits HIV integrase and proteases, viral transcription; decreases nuclear factor kappa B.
- ***Olea sp.*** (olive leaf) (2-6 g extract ): increases NK cell function; effective against HIV, herpes viruses.
- ***Phyllanthus amarus*** (1200 mg): inhibits in vitro and ex vivo HIV-1 reverse transcriptase, receptors, and proteases; effective against HBV.
- ***Lentinus edodes* (shiitake mushrooms)** (1-5 mg IV twice/week): inhibits reverse transcriptase and increases CD4 and decreases p24 (surface marker).
- ***Andrographis paniculata*** (1500 mg): inhibits fusion, viral replication, and HIV-1 cell-to-cell transmission; stimulates objective measures of immune function, increases efficacy of AZT, protects against liver damage, and decreases diarrhea. Toxicity questions remain; further study needed.
- ***Silybum marianum* (milk thistle)** (300 mg extract): improves liver function and antioxidant activity of blood cells.
- ***Hyssopus officinalis* (hyssop)** (1-4 mL tincture): anti-HIV activity; inhibits integration of proviral genome into host genome.
- ***Prunella vulgaris* (self-heal)** (10 μg/mL IV): inhibits HIV replication, binding; prevents cell-to-cell infection.
- ***Rosmarinus officinalis* (rosemary)** (liberally in food): decreases HIV replication and protease activity.
- ***Momordica charantia* (bitter melon)** (6 oz fresh juice): normalizes CD4+/CD8+ ratios; inactivates viral DNA.

- ***Spirulina platensis*** **(blue-green algae)** (liberally in food): reduces fusion and viral production.
- ***Scutellaria baicalensis*** **(skullcap)** (6-15 g whole root): inhibits HIV-1 reverse transcriptase.
- **Podophyllum resin** (25% solution single topical application): helps resolve hairy leukoplakia.
- ***Melaleuca leucadendron*** **(tea tree)** (topical): effective for fluconazole-refractory oropharyngeal candidiasis in AIDS patients.
- ***Hypericum perforatum*** **(St. John's wort)** (900 mg): inhibits protein kinase C and viral uncoating, fusion, and assembly. Do not use in patients on an NNRTI or PI.
- ***Allium sativum*** **(garlic)** (4 g fresh): selectively kills HIV-1 infected cells in vitro. Do not use in patients on an NNRTI or PI.

### Physical Medicine and Acupuncture

- Whole-body hyperthermia (twice per week at 108°F for 20 minutes) may elevate CD4 count; use extreme caution in heat-intolerant patients.
- Ozone (rectal and aural insufflations) may inactivate HIV-1.
- Acupuncture and moxibustion (three treatments weekly) decrease diarrhea and illicit drug (cocaine, heroin) cravings.
- Electroacupuncture (continually stimulating acupuncture/conductance skin points associated with nervous and immune systems) ameliorates complications of HIV-related peripheral neuropathy, raises CD4+ counts, and raises other lymphocyte counts.
- Massage therapy increases NK cells, CD3 and CD4 cell counts, and CD4/CD8 ratios; improves quality of life; decreases health care costs. It increases growth, development, and overall behavior in HIV-exposed newborns; decreases anxiety; increases relaxation; increases several measures of immune function in HIV+ adults. It has no measurable effects on disease progression.
- Therapeutic touch reduces anxiety in children.
- Cranioelectrical stimulation (microcurrent 0.1 mA at 100 Hz to alligator clips attached to earlobes 20 minutes b.i.d.) decreases anxiety, insomnia, and depression.

### Movement Therapies

- **Aerobic exercise**: alleviates stress, elevates mood; improves both CD8 and NK cells in HIV-positive people.
- **Tai Chi**: improves perception of health, all functional measures compared with controls.

- **Yoga**: improves self-confidence and return to athletic activities after intervention.

7. *Provide education and guidance to patients seeking alternatives to conventional treatment.*

No known therapies currently are as effective as HAART in suppressing viral load or increasing CD4 lymphocyte cells. Avoid the temptation to allow patients to believe otherwise. If the patient is aware of the risk of high HIV viral load and/or low CD4 count yet still does not desire to initiate HAART or antibiotic prophylaxis, ensure patient access to conventional HIV specialist to provide clear education on conventional approaches and help diagnose and treat OIs. Concurrently, initiate foundation of care: healthy diet and lifestyle, nutrient support, additional therapies. Ensure patient is scheduled for frequent follow-up with health care providers to screen for and monitor OIs. If operating as a sole practitioner with a patient who refuses conventional medical and pharmaceutical intervention, consider the following therapies to decrease viral load and increase CD4 cell count:

- ***Buxus sempervirens* (European boxwood)** (990 mg extract; larger doses less effective): increases CD4 + and decreases viral load after 6 months.
- ***Curcuma longa* (turmeric)** (1200 mg): inhibits HIV integrase and proteases, viral transcription.
- ***Olea sp.* (olive leaf)** (2-6 g extract): increases NK cell function; effective against HIV and herpes viruses.
- ***Phyllanthus amarus*** (1200 mg): demonstrated in vitro and ex vivo HIV-1 inhibition of reverse transcriptase, receptors, and proteases.
- ***Lentinus edodes* (shiitake mushrooms)** (1-5 mg IV twice per week): increases CD4 and decreases p24 (surface marker).
- **Ozone** (rectal and aural insufflations): may inactivate HIV-1.

For patients seeking advice on HAART structured treatment interruptions (STI) ("drug holiday"), ensure patient clearly communicates this desire to primary care physician and HIV specialist. STI may be indicated in the following situations:

- Relieve inconvenience and toxicity of unsuccessful antiretrovirals.
- Improve response to salvage therapy (treatments for patients not responding to other HAART regimens) by allowing reemergence

of wild-type virus (predominant type in a region or population of untreated patients).

- "Reimmunize" patient to HIV and stimulate immune system to regenerate specific response to HIV. Studied in patients with optimal response to HAART (no plasma RNA for 1-3 years); associated with virologic rebound of HIV species found before HAART; associated with accelerated decrease in CD4 cell counts. Some patients respond well to reintroduction of HAART in this circumstance.
- Decrease cumulative exposure to antiretrovirals to reduce toxicity and cost and improve quality of life.
- During first trimester of pregnancy, some recommend discontinuing antiretrovirals when GI tolerance is poor and fetal organs are being formed.

STIs are controversial; financial support is lacking for reducing drug therapy and probability of increased HAART resistance. Conventional consensus is to avoid STI. If patient decides on STI knowing risks, communicate the following information:

- Patients usually revert to original set points (pre-HAART CD4 count and viral load).
- Wild-type virus returns at 6 weeks based on time needed to return to drug susceptibility in patients on discontinued HAART and is associated with increases in plasma HIV-1.
- HIV plasma RNA rebounds within days of STI and overshoots set point. Educate patient; provide supportive therapies. Measure viral load after 2 months of STI, then in 3-month intervals after stable set point.
- Consider genotyping (test to determine HAART resistance) before beginning STI (viral load must be 1000+ copies/mL for accurate genotyping).
- All resistant (mutant) and wild HIV strains are archived in all cells of body (65% of patients had HIV RNA detected in gut mucosal biopsies while undetectable in plasma).
- Hydroxyurea may lower treatment peak HIV viral load rebound during STI; viral load remained <5000 copies/mL in eight of nine patients on hydroxyurea.

The most appropriate schedule for staying off and reintroducing HAART remains unknown. The best results are in patients with a low viral load at beginning. More studies are needed to demonstrate the efficacy of STIs, but with the possibility of HAART resistance and lack of profit incentive for taking patients off a medication, additional research in this area is likely to remain sparse.

## THERAPEUTIC SUMMARY

**Diet:** natural, whole foods diet; high caloric intake; low in sugar, white flour, fruit juice, honey, processed foods; low in natural and synthetically saturated fats; low in oxidized or trans-fatty acids (fried oils); high in protein, fiber, and filtered water; abstain from alcohol, nicotine, caffeine; digestive stimulation, if appropriate; avoid broad-spectrum allergy elimination diets.

**Lifestyle:** aerobic or mind-body exercise (Tai Chi, yoga); 8-10 hours of sleep. Prayer, spiritual practice, activities that support HIV-positive community, guided forms of stress relief, and relaxation training.

### Nutritional Supplements

- High-potency, hypoallergenic multiple vitamin/mineral specifically designed to replace known nutrient deficiencies of HIV
- Beta-carotene (150,000 IU/day), best taken as food
- Acetyl-L-carnitine (2-6 g in divided doses taken separately from other protein)
- EFAs (5 g with food) (emphasize omega-3s)
- GI flora/probiotics (8 billion CFU/day with meals) (*Lactobacillus acidophilus* or *casei, Bifidobacteria bifida*)

### Botanical Medicines

- *Silybum marianum* (milk thistle) (300 mg silymarin extract): all patients on HAART.
- *Buxus sempervirens* (European boxwood) (990 mg extract; larger doses less effective): for patients resistant to or avoiding HAART.

### Physical Medicine and Acupuncture

- Whole-body hyperthermia: use extreme caution in patients with heat intolerance or peripheral neuropathies.
- Movement therapies: as indicated.
- Acupuncture and electroacupuncture: as indicated.

# Hypertension

## DIAGNOSTIC SUMMARY

- Borderline high blood pressure (BP): 130-139/85-89 mm Hg
- Mild high BP (stage 1): 140-159/90-99 mm Hg
- Moderate high BP (stage 2): 160-179/100-109 mm Hg
- Severe high BP (stage 3): 180+/110+ mm Hg

## GENERAL CONSIDERATIONS

Hypertension is a major risk factor for myocardial infarction (MI) or stroke and is the most significant risk factor for stroke. More than 60 million Americans have hypertension, including 54.3% of all Americans aged 65-74 years and 71.8% of all black Americans in the same age group.

### Classification of Hypertension by Blood Pressure

- **Optimal**
  —Systolic: <120 mm Hg
  —Diastolic: <80 mm Hg
- **Normal**
  —Systolic: <130 mm Hg
  —Diastolic: <85 mm Hg
- **Borderline (high-normal)**
  —Systolic: 130-139 mm Hg
  —Diastolic: 85-89 mm Hg
- **High BP (hypertension)**
  —**Stage 1** (mild) high BP:
    - Systolic: 140-159 mm Hg
    - Diastolic: 90-99 mm Hg

  —**Stage 2** (moderate) high BP:
    - Systolic: 160-179 mm Hg
    - Diastolic: 100-109 mm Hg

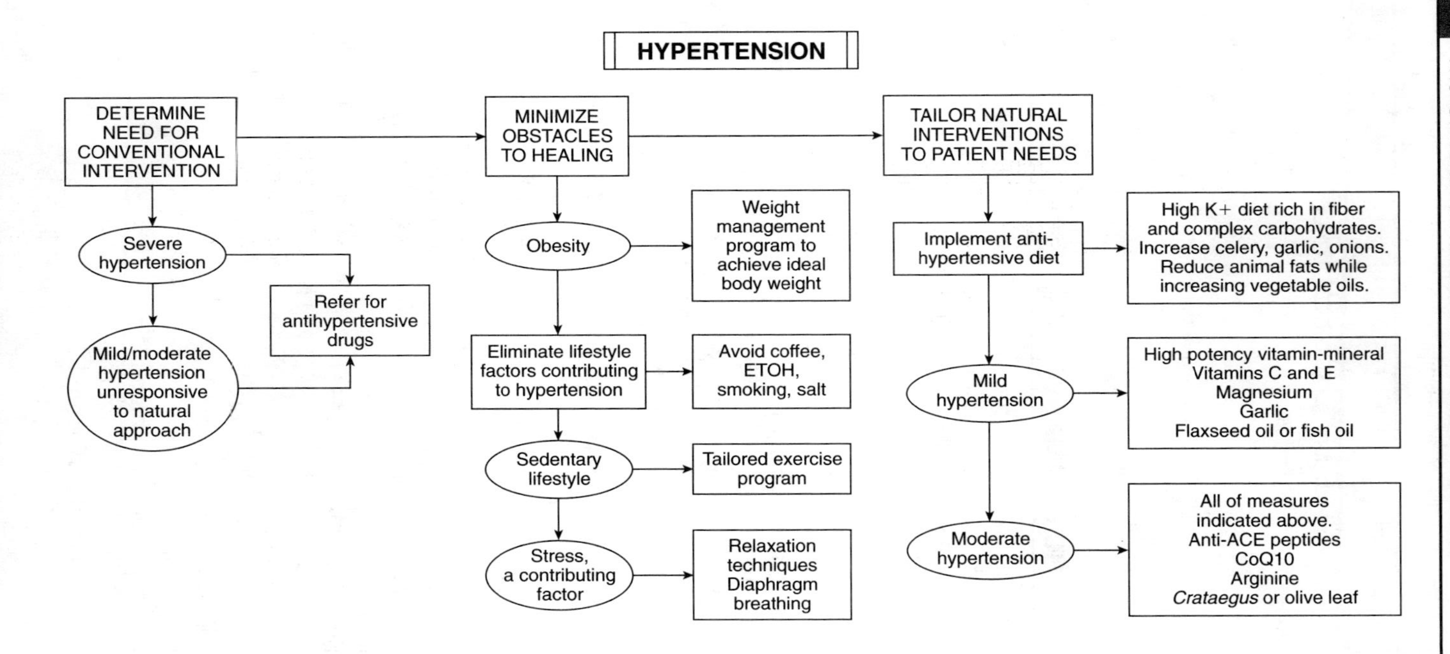
HYPERTENSION
DETERMINE NEED FOR CONVENTIONAL INTERVENTION
Severe hypertension
Mild/moderate hypertension unresponsive to natural approach
Refer for antihypertensive drugs
MINIMIZE OBSTACLES TO HEALING
Obesity
Weight management program to achieve ideal body weight
Eliminate lifestyle factors contributing to hypertension
Avoid coffee, ETOH, smoking, salt
Sedentary lifestyle
Tailored exercise program
Stress, a contributing factor
Relaxation techniques Diaphragm breathing
TAILOR NATURAL INTERVENTIONS TO PATIENT NEEDS
Implement anti-hypertensive diet
High K+ diet rich in fiber and complex carbohydrates. Increase celery, garlic, onions. Reduce animal fats while increasing vegetable oils.
Mild hypertension
High potency vitamin-mineral
Vitamins C and E
Magnesium
Garlic
Flaxseed oil or fish oil
Moderate hypertension
All of measures indicated above.
Anti-ACE peptides
CoQ10
Arginine
Crataegus or olive leaf

—**Stage 3** (severe) high BP:
  - Systolic: ≥180 mm Hg
  - Diastolic: ≥110 mm Hg

- Normal diastolic (<82 mm Hg) but elevated systolic pressure (>158 mm Hg) (increased pulse pressure) suggests decreased compliance of aorta (arteriosclerosis) and twofold increase in cardiovascular death rates. Other causes of increased pulse pressure are increased stroke volume from aortic regurgitation, thyrotoxicosis, fever.
- Classification of hypertension by cause: >90% of cases are classified as essential hypertension—no discernable cause. Essential hypertension groups are based on level of renin (enzyme secreted by kidney juxtaglomerular cells, linked to aldosterone in negative feedback loop). Renin helps generate vasoconstricting peptide angiotensin II. Renin secretion is influenced by fluid volume and sodium (Na) intake.
- Low-renin essential hypertension involves low renin activity. Aldosterone production is not being suppressed, leading to mild hyperaldosteronism with Na retention, increased fluid volume, and increased BP. This also occurs with normal-renin hypertension; low-renin hypertension may be at the end of the continuum with essential hypertension. Patients with low renin levels have increased sensitivity to angiotensin II.
- Normal-renin essential hypertensives typically are insulin resistant with abdominal obesity. Hyperinsulinemia and insulin resistance are present even in lean hypertensives without non-insulin-dependent diabetes mellitus, suggesting a strong relation between insulin sensitivity and BP. Because insulin modifies ion transport across cell membranes, insulin insensitivity decreases cytosolic magnesium (Mg) and increases cytosolic calcium (Ca) in vascular smooth muscle, increasing vascular reactivity. Normal-renin essential hypertensives typically do not respond to Na restriction.
- High-renin essential hypertensives comprise 15% of essential hypertension patients. Renin elevation (and high BP) may arise from increased adrenergic system activity.
- Categories based on renin can identify therapeutic interventions, but renin levels do not remain constant in a given patient. In low-renin essential hypertension caused by insulin resistance secondary to obesity, weight loss regains insulin sensitivity but BP may not normalize. The patient would then have normal- or high-renin essential hypertension.

## Classifications of Hypertension

I. Essential hypertension (>90% of all cases of hypertension)
   A. Low-renin
   B. Normal-renin
   C. High-renin
II. Renal etiology
   A. Chronic pyelonephritis
   B. Acute and chronic glomerulonephritis
   C. Polycystic renal disease
   D. Renovascular stenosis or renal infarction
   E. Most other severe renal diseases (e.g., arteriolar nephrosclerosis, diabetic nephropathy)
   F. Renin-producing tumors
III. Endocrine etiology
   A. Adrenocortical hyperfunction
   B. Cushing's disease and syndrome
   C. Primary hyperaldosteronism
   D. Congenital or hereditary adrenogenital syndromes (17-hydroxylase and 11-hydroxylase defects)
   E. Pheochromocytoma
   F. Myxedema
   G. Acromegaly
IV. Neurogenic etiology
   A. Psychogenic
   B. Diencephalic syndrome
   C. Familial dysautonomia (Riley-Day)
   D. Polyneuritis (acute porphyria, lead poisoning)
   E. Increased intracranial pressure (acute)
   F. Spinal cord section (acute)
V. Miscellaneous
   A. Toxemia of pregnancy
   B. Acute intermittent porphyria
   C. Coarctation of aorta
   D. Increased intravascular volume (excessive transfusion, polycythemia vera)
   E. Polyarteritis nodosa
   F. Hypercalcemia
   G. Medications (e.g., glucocorticoids, cyclosporine, oral contraceptives)

- **"White coat" hypertension**: persistent elevation of BP only at clinic or physician's office. Prevalence may be 20%-45% of diagnosed hypertensives; is more frequent in women, older patients, and persons with mild hypertension. This should not be confused with "white coat effect"—the difference in BP between office and daytime ambulatory BP that occurs in patients with white coat hypertension and other causes. Treat white coat hypertension as if it were essential hypertension; it mirrors real-life reactions to stress. It is not an innocent phenomenon because it is linked to higher mortality and twice the risk of developing sustained hypertension as normotensives.

- **Ambulatory BP monitoring**: clinically useful for assessing suspected white coat hypertension and cardiovascular risk. If white coat hypertension is confirmed, drug treatment is not indicated; treat with lifestyle and dietary modification, weight reduction, exercise, smoking cessation, and correction of glucose and lipid abnormalities. Follow-up with semiannual or annual ambulatory BP monitoring.
- **Etiology**: vascular, hormonal, renal, and neurologic factors function in complex interrelations to maintain normal BP. Disruption of any single facet creates a cascading effect on regulatory mechanisms. Genetic factors play a role, but dietary, lifestyle, psychological, and environmental factors are underlying causes. Dietary factors: obesity; high Na/potassium (K) ratio; low-fiber, high-sugar diet; high saturated fat and low omega-3 fatty acid intake; low calcium, magnesium, and vitamin C intake. Lifestyle factors: stress, lack of exercise, smoking. From 40% to 60% of hypertensives are Na sensitive. The heavy metals lead (Pb), mercury, cadmium, and arsenic target kidneys as end organs. Bone lead studies indicate that exposure to heavy metals is linked to increased risk for hypertension.

## THERAPEUTIC CONSIDERATIONS

Eighty percent of patients with hypertension are in the borderline to moderate range; thus most cases can be brought under control by diet and lifestyle. Many nondrug therapies (diet, exercise, relaxation therapies) are superior to drugs in cases of borderline to mild hypertension. Patients on diuretics and/or beta-blockers have unnecessary side effects and an increased risk for heart disease. Calcium channel blockers and angiotensin-converting enzyme (ACE) inhibitors may be safer, with fewer side effects, but not without problems.

## Conventional Antihypertensive Drugs

Conventional drug treatment may be doing more harm than good; antihypertensive drugs (diuretics and/or beta-blockers) have side effects, including increased risk for heart disease; virtually every medical authority recommends nondrug therapies for borderline to mild hypertension.

- **Antihypertensive drugs**: diuretics, beta-blockers, ACE inhibitors, calcium channel blockers.
- **Diuretics**: lower BP by reducing fluid volume in blood and tissues by promoting elimination of salt and water by increased urination. They relax smaller arteries, allowing them to expand and increase fluid capacity of arterial system. Types of diuretics: thiazides, loop diuretics, and potassium-sparing diuretics. Thiazides are more effective in lowering BP than are loop and potassium-sparing diuretics, allowing lower, safer dosing. Side effects: lightheadedness; increased blood sugar and uric acid (aggravation of gout); muscle weakness and cramps caused by low K; decreased libido; impotence; allergic reactions, headache, blurred vision, nausea and vomiting, diarrhea. Loss of K, Mg, and Ca help lower BP and prevent MI. The drugs also increase cholesterol and triglycerides, increase blood viscosity, raise uric acid, and increase platelet stickiness. Thiazides may increase risk of MI or stroke and worsen blood sugar control (difficult for diabetics).
- **Beta-blockers**: block binding of catecholamines on beta-receptors, reducing rate and force of heart contraction and relaxing arteries; treat angina and certain heart rhythm disturbances. Long-term inhibition of heart function can lead to heart failure. They fail to reduce cardiovascular mortality rate and increase risk of developing diabetes. Side effects: reduced cardiac output in relaxed arteries causes cold hands and feet, nerve tingling, impaired mental function, fatigue, dizziness, depression, lethargy, reduced libido, and impotence. They raise cholesterol and triglycerides. Beta-blocker treatment must not be discontinued suddenly because of withdrawal syndrome—headache, increased heart rate, greatly increased BP.
- **Calcium channel blockers and ACE inhibitors**: better tolerated than diuretics and beta-blockers. Calcium channel blockers lower risk for strokes and increase risk for MI.
  - **Calcium channel blockers**: block normal passage of Ca through channels in cell membranes, slowing nerve conduction and inhibiting muscle contraction. They reduce rate and force of

heart contraction, relax arteries, and slow heart nerve impulses. Side effects: constipation, allergic reactions, fluid retention, dizziness, headache, fatigue, impotence, disturbances of heart rate or function, heart failure, angina.
- **ACE inhibitors**: prevent formation of angiotensin II, which increases fluid volume and constriction of blood vessels. ACE inhibitors relax arterial walls and reduce fluid volume. They improve heart function and increase blood and oxygen flow to the heart, liver, and kidneys. They reduce risk of MI but not strokes. Side effects: dizziness, light-headedness, headache, dry nighttime cough, K buildup, and kidney problems. Monitor K levels and kidney function.

- **Most common current use**: diuretics used alone or in combination with calcium channel blockers and ACE inhibitors.
- **"Step 1" drug**: used alone (thiazides, calcium channel blockers, ACE inhibitors); step 2: two drugs; step 3: three drugs; step 4: four drugs.
- **Other types of BP-lowering drugs (steps 3 or 4)**: those acting on the central nervous system (clonidine, methyldopa, reserpine), vasodilators (nitroprusside sodium, hydralazine, prazosin, minoxidil, hydralazine), newer calcium channel blockers, and ACE inhibitors.

## Lifestyle and Dietary Factors

See the chapter on atherosclerosis.

- **Lifestyle factors**: coffee, alcohol, lack of exercise, stress, smoking.
- **Dietary factors**: obesity; high Na/K ratio; low-fiber, high-sugar diet; high saturated fat and low essential fatty acids; low calcium, magnesium and vitamin C.
- **Stress**: causative factor of hypertension in many patients; key issue is response and processing of stress rather than stress itself. Relaxation techniques (deep breathing exercises, biofeedback, autogenics, transcendental meditation, yoga, progressive muscle relaxation, hypnosis) are useful in lowering BP. Effect is modest, but stress reduction is a necessary component in natural BP-lowering protocol. Diaphragmatic breathing significantly reduces stress and increases energy. Regular short exercise sessions of slow and regular diaphragmatic breathing lower BP in hypertensives. Shallow breathing induces Na retention. Slow breathing (6 breaths/min) improves oxygen saturation, exercise tolerance,

and baroreflex sensitivity. Emphasize slow, deep diaphragmatic breathing.

- **Exercise**: Physical activity (or fitness) and hypertension are inversely related. Regular exercise is effective treatment for high BP. Even mild to moderate aerobic exercise three times weekly of 20 minutes' duration has a hypotensive effect. BP reductions: 5-10 mm Hg for systolic and diastolic. Exercise can normalize borderline or mild hypertension.
- **Diet**: obesity is the major dietary cause of hypertension. Attain ideal body weight. Increase proportion of whole organic plant foods in diet. Vegetarians have lower BP and lower incidence of hypertension and other cardiovascular diseases than do nonvegetarians. Dietary levels of sodium do not differ between these two groups, but vegetarian diet contains more K, complex carbohydrates, essential fatty acids, fiber, Ca, Mg, and vitamin C, and less saturated fat and refined carbohydrates. Increasing fruit and vegetable intake lowers BP, perhaps from the antioxidants. Hypertensives have increased oxidative stress; antioxidants block angiotensin II–induced increases in BP and promote proper nitric oxide synthesis. Most useful foods for hypertensives are celery, garlic and onions, nuts and seeds or their oils (essential fatty acids), cold-water ocean fish (e.g., salmon, mackerel), green leafy vegetables (Ca and Mg), whole grains and legumes (fiber), foods rich in vitamin C (broccoli and citrus fruits). Celery contains 3-n-butyl phthalide, which lowers BP and cholesterol. Dose: 4 to 6 ribs of celery. Garlic and onions lower BP in hypertension. Garlic's BP reductions are 8-11 mm Hg for systolic and 5-8 mm Hg for diastolic.

### DASH Diet (Dietary Approaches to Stop Hypertension)

The National Heart, Lung, and Blood Institute studied the efficacy of a system of dietary recommendations for hypertension—a diet rich in fruits and vegetables; low in dairy, saturated and total fat, and cholesterol; high in fiber, K, Ca, and Mg; and moderately high in protein. The DASH diet with lower Na lowered systolic BP by 7.1 mm Hg in nonhypertensives and by 11.5 mm Hg in hypertensives. Na intake less than 2400 mg q.d. can significantly and quickly lower BP. DASH components include those in the table on the following page.

- **Potassium (K) and sodium (Na)**: A diet low in K and high in Na is linked to hypertension. Total K content of food plus Na/K

| Food Group | Daily Servings | Serving Sizes | Examples | Significance of Each Food Group to the DASH Diet Pattern |
|---|---|---|---|---|
| Grains and grain products | 7-8 | 1 slice bread<br>½ cup dry cereal<br>½ cup cooked rice, pasta, or cereal | Whole wheat bread, English muffin, pita bread, bagel, cereals, grits, oatmeal | Major sources of energy and fiber |
| Vegetables | 4-5 | 1 cup raw leafy vegetable<br>½ cup cooked vegetable<br>6 oz vegetable juice | Tomatoes, potatoes, carrots, peas, squash, broccoli, turnip greens, collards, kale, spinach, artichokes, sweet potatoes, beans | Rich sources of potassium, magnesium, and fiber |
| Fruits | 4-5 | 6 oz fruit juice<br>1 medium fruit<br>¼ cup dried fruit<br>½ cup fresh, frozen, or canned fruit | Apricots, bananas, dates, oranges, orange juice, grapefruit, grapefruit juice, mangoes, melons, peaches, pineapple, prunes, raisins, strawberries, tangerines | Important sources of potassium, magnesium, and fiber |
| Low-fat or nonfat dairy foods | 2-3 | 8 oz milk<br>1 cup yogurt<br>1.5 oz cheese | Skim or 1% milk, skim or low-fat buttermilk, nonfat or low-fat yogurt, part-skim mozzarella cheese, nonfat cheese | Major sources of calcium and protein |
| Meats, poultry, and fish | ≤2 or less | 3 oz cooked meats, poultry, or fish | Select only lean; trim away visible fats; broil, roast, or boil instead of frying; remove skin from poultry | Rich sources of protein and magnesium |
| Nuts, seeds, and legumes | 4-5 per week | 1.5 oz or 1/3 cup nuts<br>½ oz or 2 tbsp seeds<br>½ cup cooked legumes | Almonds, filberts, mixed nuts, peanuts, walnuts, sunflower seeds, kidney beans, lentils | Rich sources of energy, magnesium, potassium, protein, and fiber |

ratio; a low-K, high-Na diet is linked to cancer and cardiovascular disease; a diet high in K and low in Na is protective against these diseases and therapeutic for hypertension. Excess sodium chloride intake, with diminished K, causes high BP in salt-sensitive persons. Na restriction alone is insufficient without high K intake. Typical Western diet: only 5% of Na is a natural constituent in food; 45% is added to prepared foods, 45% is added during cooking, and 5% is added as a condiment. Most Americans have K/Na ratio <1:2. Studies indicate a K/Na ratio >5:1 is necessary to maintain health. A natural diet rich in fruits and vegetables provides K/Na ratio >100:1 (most fruits and vegetables have K/Na ratio of 50:1). Increasing dietary potassium can lower BP. K supplements alone can reduce BP in hypertensives at a dosage of 2.5-5.0 g q.d. of potassium. Supplements are quite useful in persons older than 65 years. The Food and Drug Administration restricts the amount of K in over-the-counter supplements to a mere 99 mg/dose because of problems with high-dosage prescription K salts; yet salt substitutes (NoSalt, Nu-Salt) are potassium chloride, providing 530 mg K per 1/6 tsp. Supplement forms: salts (chloride, bicarbonate) bound to mineral chelates (aspartate, citrate, etc.) or food-based sources. High-dose salts in pills can cause nausea and vomiting, diarrhea, and ulcers. These effects are not seen when K is increased with diet only. Foods or food-based supplements are preferred. They are relatively safe except for patients with kidney disease; their inability to maintain K homeostasis may cause heart arrhythmias and other consequences of K toxicity. K supplements also are contraindicated when using some drugs (digitalis, K-sparing diuretics, and ACE inhibitor antihypertensive drugs).

- **Magnesium (Mg)**: K interacts in many body systems with Mg. Low intracellular K may result from low Mg intake. Supplement Mg (400-1200 mg q.d. in divided doses) with K. This may lower BP. Mg lowers BP in a dose-dependent way; a drop of 4.3 mm Hg systolic and 2.3 mm Hg diastolic occurs for each 10 mmol/day increase in Mg dose. Mg lowers BP by activating cellular membrane Na/K pump, which pumps Na out of, and K into, cells. High intake of Mg is linked to lower BP. Water high in minerals such as Mg is called hard water. Water hardness is inversely coordinated with high BP. Hypertensive patients who respond to Mg supplements are those taking diuretics, with high level of renin, with low red blood cell Mg, and/or with elevated intracellular Na or decreased intracellular K. Recommended daily intake for hypertensives is 6-10 mg/kg body weight. Mg bound to aspartate or Krebs cycle intermediates (malate, succinate, fumarate, citrate) are preferred. Mg supplements are well tolerated but sometimes cause looser stool (Mg sulfate [Epsom salts], hydroxide, or chloride). Use with great care in kidney disease or severe heart disease (high-grade atrioventricular block).

- **Calcium**: hypertension is linked to low intake of Ca, but the association is not as strong as for Mg and K. Ca supplements can lower BP in hypertension, but results are inconsistent. Ca supplements reduce BP in blacks and salt-sensitive patients but not patients with salt-resistant hypertension. Better results occur with Ca citrate compared with Ca carbonate. Elderly patients with mild to moderate hypertension respond to Ca.
- **Vitamin C**: The higher the intake of vitamin C, the lower the BP. A modest BP-lowering effect (drop of 5 mm Hg) occurs in people with mild hypertension. Daily dosing at 500 mg produces the same benefit as higher dosing (1000 or 2000 mg q.d.). It promotes excretion of Pb, which is linked to hypertension and increased cardiovascular mortality. Soft water supplies have increased Pb in drinking water because of the increased acidity of the water (soft water also is low in Ca and Mg, minerals protective against hypertension). Enhance efficacy by using ascorbate with other antioxidants. Combination 500 mg vitamin C, 600 mg alpha-tocopherol, 200 mg zinc sulphate, 30 mg beta-carotene q.d. has mildly reduced systolic BP.
- **Folic acid and Vitamin $B_6$**: reduce plasma homocysteine, a contributor to atherosclerosis. $B_6$ alone lowers BP. $B_6$ oral dosage of 5 mg/kg body weight for 4 weeks reduced systolic and diastolic BP and serum norepinephrine. Mean systolic pressure dropped from 167 to 153 mm Hg and diastolic pressure dropped from 108 to 98 mm Hg.
- **Omega-3 oils**: increased intake can lower BP. Fish oil and flaxseed oil are quite effective. Dosage of fish oils used: 3000 mg omega-3 EPA/DHA q.d. Prefer products with higher content of docosahexaenoic acid (DHA). In one double-blind trial comparing 4 g q.d. of purified eicosapentaenoic acid (EPA), DHA, or olive oil (placebo), only DHA reduced 24-hour and daytime ambulatory BP. Fish oil lab certified as purified against pollutants and peroxides is preferred. Flaxseed oil may be a better cost-effective choice, requiring reduced intake of saturated fat and omega-6 fatty acids. One tablespoon daily of flaxseed oil reduces systolic and diastolic BP by up to 9 mm Hg. For every absolute

1% increase in body alpha-linolenic acid content, systolic, diastolic, and mean BPs decrease by 5 mm Hg.

- **Arginine**: amino acid precursor to nitric oxide (NO) that relaxes arteries, improving blood flow, renal plasma flow, and glomerular filtration rate. Even in mild hypertension cases endothelial NO production may be disordered, especially in the kidneys. By increasing NO, arginine improves blood flow, reduces blood clot formation, and improves blood fluidity. Arginine may be most beneficial in younger subjects with essential hypertension; aging hypertensives have disturbed NO-dependent renal mechanisms. Intravenous infusion of arginine induces a significant increase in renal plasma flow, glomerular filtration rate, natriuresis, and kaliuresis without changes in filtration fraction in younger essential hypertensives but not in older subjects.
- **Anti-ACE peptides**: naturally occurring peptides in milk, chicken, and fish can inhibit ACE. Purified mixture of 9 small peptides from muscle of the fish bonito (tuna family) do not produce the side effects of ACE inhibitor drugs and do not lower BP in normotensive people, even at dosage 20 times greater than therapetic dosage for hypertensives. ACE converts angiotensin I to angiotensin II by cleaving off a small peptide. Drugs indiscriminately block this action. Anti-ACE peptides work as a decoy, causing ACE to react with the peptides instead of angiotensin. Anti-ACE peptides are transformed into even more potent inhibitors of ACE. Bonito anti-ACE peptides are prodrugs that exert an 800% greater activity. Bonito peptides and sardine dipeptide reduce systolic by 10+ mm Hg and diastolic by 7 mm Hg in borderline and mild hypertensives. Greater reductions occur in people with higher initial BP.
- **Coenzyme $Q_{10}$ ($CoQ_{10}$) (ubiquinone)**: essential mitochondrial component synthesized within the body but deficient in 39% of hypertensive patients. $CoQ_{10}$ lowers BP in hypertensives, but the effect is not seen until after 4-12 weeks of therapy. $CoQ_{10}$ is not a typical BP-lowering drug; it corrects metabolic abnormality, favorably influencing BP. It induces 10% reductions in systolic and diastolic BP. Mechanism of action causes no changes in renin, Na, or aldosterone levels. It improves cholesterol levels and peripheral vascular resistance in arteries of the arms and legs.
- **Caffeine**: coffee and tea can produce short-lived immediate increases in BP. Regular coffee drinking slightly increases BP. Coffee drinking ranging from 14 to 79 days at an average dose of 5 cups of coffee per day is linked to persistent increase in sys-

tolic and diastolic BP. Long-term avoidance of caffeine (coffee, tea, chocolate, cola drinks, some medications) is indicated because some patients respond quite favorably. Recent research suggests that caffeine is only a problem for those with low liver CYP1A2 activity.

### Botanical Medicines

- ***Crataegus* sp.**: extracts of hawthorn berries and flowering tops lower BP and improve heart function. BP-lowering effect of hawthorn is quite mild and requires at least 2-4 weeks before effect is apparent.
- ***Allium sativum* (garlic) and *Allium cepa* (onion)**: antihypertensive additions to diet along with garlic extracts. Meta-analysis conclusions: dried garlic powder standardized to contain 1.3% alliin at dosage of 600 to 900 mg q.d. (corresponding to 7.8 to 11.7 mg of alliin or 1.8-2.7 g fresh garlic q.d.) can lower systolic BP by 11 mm Hg and diastolic BP by 5.0 mm Hg over a 1- to 3-month period.
- ***Olea europaea* (olive)**: aqueous extract of olive leaf at a dosage of 400 mg q.d. for 3 months produces a modest significant decrease of BP with no side effects.
- ***Viscum album* (mistletoe)**: hypotensive action in animal studies. Mechanism of action is not fully understood. It inhibits excitability of vasomotor center in medulla oblongata. It possesses cholinomimetic activity. Hypotensive activity may depend on form in which mistletoe is administered and host tree from which it was collected. Aqueous extracts are more effective; the highest hypotensive activity is derived from macerate of leaves of mistletoe parasitizing on willow and gathered in January (*Textbook, "Viscum album* [European Mistletoe]").

## THERAPEUTIC APPROACH

**Borderline** (120-160/90-94 mm Hg) **or white coat hypertension or mild hypertension** (140-160/90-104 mg):

- Reduce excessive weight.
- Eliminate salt (sodium chloride) intake.
- Lead healthy lifestyle. Avoid alcohol, caffeine, smoking. Exercise and use stress-reduction techniques.
- Follow high-potassium diet rich in fiber and complex carbohydrates.

- Increase consumption of celery, garlic, and onions.
- Reduce or eliminate animal fats while increasing vegetable oils.
- Supplement diet with the following:
  —High-potency multiple vitamin/mineral formula
  —Vitamin C: 500-1000 mg t.i.d.
  —Vitamin E: 400-800 IU q.d. (mixed tocopherols)
  —Magnesium: 800-1200mg q.d. in divided doses
  —Garlic: equivalent of 4000 mg q.d. of fresh garlic
  —Flaxseed oil: 1tbsp q.d. or fish oils at 3 g total EPA/DHA content q.d.

Treatment period is 3-6 months. If BP has not normalized, antihypertensive medications are indicated. When a prescription drug is necessary, calcium-channel blockers or ACE inhibitors appear to be the safest.

- **Moderate hypertension** (140-180/105-114 mm Hg): Use all measures above with the addition of the following.
  Anti-ACE peptides from bonito: 1500 mg q.d.
- Coenzyme $Q_{10}$: 50 mg b.i.d. to t.i.d.
- L-Arginine: 0.5 g/10 kg body weight in divided doses throughout the day
- Take either:
  —Hawthorn extract (10% procyanidins or 1.8% vitexin-4′-rhamnoside): 100-250 mg t.i.d. *or*
  —Olive leaf extract (17%-23% oleuropein content): 250-500 mg t.i.d.

Treatment period is 1-3 months. If BP has not dropped below 140/105 mm Hg, antihypertensive medications are indicated.

**Severe hypertension** (160+/115+ mm Hg): drug intervention is required. Use all measures above. When satisfactory BP control is achieved, taper off medication gradually.

# Hyperthyroidism

## DIAGNOSTIC SUMMARY

- Weakness, sweating, weight loss, nervousness, loose stools, heat intolerance, irritability, fatigue
- Tachycardia; warm, thin, moist skin; stare; tremor
- Diffuse, nonpainful goiter
- Increased thyroxine ($T_4$), free $T_4$, and free $T_4$ index
- Failure of thyroid suppression with triiodothyronine ($T_3$) administration
- In Graves' disease: goiter (often with bruit), ophthalmopathy

## GENERAL CONSIDERATIONS

Hyperthyroidism (thyrotoxicosis) is a group of disorders characterized by increased free $T_4$ and/or $T_3$. The autoimmune disorder Graves' disease comprises 85% of all cases of hyperthyroidism. The disease is much more common in women than in men (8:1 ratio) and begins between ages 20 and 40 years. Diffuse, nonpainful goiter with hyperthyroidism is the most common presentation of Graves' disease. Less-common signs and symptoms are exophthalmos, pretibial myxedema and other skin changes, nail changes (acropachy), and paralysis in some groups. The common denominator is the antibodies against thyroid-stimulating hormone (TSH) receptors. Exophthalmos and skin changes can progress independently from thyroid dysfunction (euthyroid Graves' disease); predicting the course of disease in a given patient is difficult.

### Disease Risk

Following are patterns of susceptibility in autoimmune disease (especially Graves' disease):

- **Gender**: female/male ratio is 7:1 to 10:1; the ratio in those with ophthalmic complications is 1:1.
- **Stress**: recent stress is a precipitating factor. The most common precipitating event is "actual or threatened separation from person on whom patient is emotionally dependent." The onset

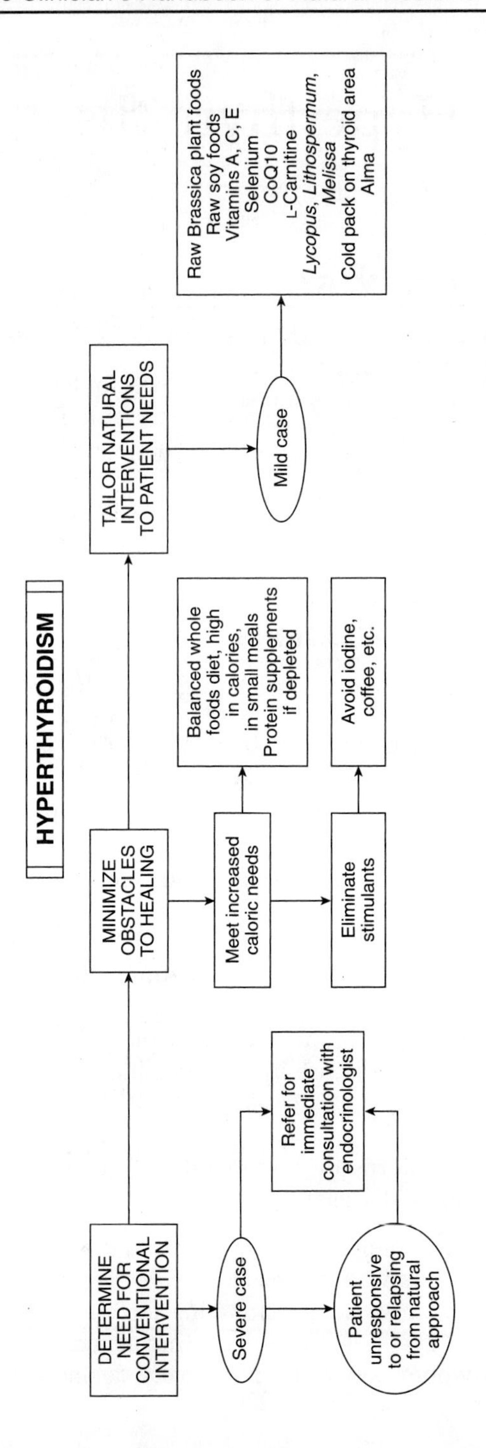
HYPERTHYROIDISM
DETERMINE NEED FOR CONVENTIONAL INTERVENTION
Severe case
Patient unresponsive to or relapsing from natural approach
Refer for immediate consultation with endocrinologist
MINIMIZE OBSTACLES TO HEALING
Meet increased caloric needs
Balanced whole foods diet, high in calories, in small meals
Protein supplements if depleted
Eliminate stimulants
Avoid iodine, coffee, etc.
TAILOR NATURAL INTERVENTIONS TO PATIENT NEEDS
Mild case
Raw Brassica plant foods
Raw soy foods
Vitamins A, C, E
Selenium
CoQ10
L-Carnitine
Lycopus, Lithospermum, Melissa
Cold pack on thyroid area
Alma

of Graves' disease often follows emotional shock—divorce, death, or difficult separation.

- **Genetics**: Graves' disease is more prevalent in some human leukocyte antigen (HLA) haplotypes ($HLA\text{-}B_8$ and $HLA\text{-}DR_3$ in whites, $HLA\text{-}Bw_{35}$ in Japanese, $HLA\text{-}Bw_{46}$ in Chinese). HLA identical twins have a 50% chance of manifesting Graves' disease if one twin is affected; fraternal twins have a 9% chance. Some haplotypes are protective against Graves' disease. Genetic haplotype does not affect clinical course of disease or response to treatment.
- **Left-handedness**: A statistical trend exists for left-handed people to manifest Graves' disease and other autoimmune diseases. Seventy percent of male Graves' patients had some degree of left-handedness compared with 24% of control subjects. Some evidence exists for a higher rate of dyslexia in Graves' patients.
- **Smoking**: a statistical correlation exists between smoking and Graves' disease, especially with ophthalmic complications. The smoking risk estimate (1.5) is less than heredity (3.6) and negative life events (6.3). The group at highest risk of increase for severe endocrine ophthalmopathy involves those with eye manifestation who continue to smoke.
- **Iodine supplementation**: dietary iodine supplementation in iodine-sufficient areas can increase incidence of thyrotoxicosis (elevated $T_4$ and suppressed TSH with both nodular and diffuse goiters) in susceptible individuals. The rate of increase for women (8.03) was much greater than for men (1.34).
- **Mercury and cadmium exposure**: exposing animals to toxic levels of cadmium (Cd) or mercury (Hg) induces immediate hyperthyroidism. Confirmatory anecdotal human clinical cases have been reported.
- **Drugs**: in older patients with hyperthyroidism, consider toxic reaction to prescription drugs. The most common causes of hyperthyroidism in the elderly are low iodine intake and higher use of amiodarone (an antihypertensive drug). Symptoms of hyperthyroidism vary in the elderly; apathy, tachycardia, and weight loss are more common.

## DIAGNOSIS

### Clinical Presentation

- **Graves' disease in young adult women**: nervousness, irritability, sweating, palpitations, insomnia, tremor, frequent stools, weight loss despite good appetite.

- **Physical examination**: smooth, diffuse, nontender goiter; tachycardia, especially after exercise; loud heart sounds (often systolic murmur); mild proptosis, lid retraction, lid lag, and tremor.
- **Other signs and symptoms**: muscle weakness and fatigue, anxiety, heat intolerance, pretibial myxedema.
- **Atypical cases (elderly)**: in apathetic thyrotoxicosis, the above symptoms are absent. In the elderly, only symptom may be depression.
- Screening lab test for suppressed TSH.
- Increased thyroid hormone can present as worsening of already present cardiac symptoms (angina pectoris, congestive heart failure, and atrial fibrillation).
- **Characteristic skin changes**: moist, warm, and finely textured; perspiration increases in response to increased body temperature; pigment changes (vitiligo) and increased pigmentation of areas (skin creases, knuckles).
- Hair may thin or fall out in patches or altogether (alopecia).
- Nails may separate prematurely from nail bed (onycholysis).
- Localized, nonpitting edema along shins (myxedema) or elsewhere, such as extensor surfaces. It is often pruritic and red.
- **Other symptoms of Graves' disease**: glucose intolerance, osteoporosis, dyspnea, polyurea and polydipsia, myopathy, paralysis, Parkinsonian or choreoathetoid affect.

## Differential Diagnosis of Hyperthyroidism

- Graves' disease is the most common diagnosis of hyperthyroidism.
- Several types of thyroiditis cause hyperthyroidism: Hashimoto's thyroiditis (early stage), subacute thyroiditis, painless thyroiditis, and radiation thyroiditis.
- Hyperthyroidism from exogenous causes: iatrogenic hyperthyroidism, factitious hyperthyroidism (dieters taking thyroxine for weight loss), and iodine-induced hyperthyroidism (Jod-Basedow disease).
- Toxic nodular goiters: toxic adenoma and multinodular goiter.
- Rare causes: thyroid carcinoma, ectopic hyperthyroidism, trophoblastic tumors (hydatidiform mole, choriocarcinoma, embryonic carcinoma of testis), excess TSH (pituitary adenoma, nonneoplastic pituitary secretion of TSH), and struma ovarii.

### Laboratory Diagnosis

Definitive diagnosis includes the following:

- Serum $T_3$, $T_4$, thyroid resin uptake, and free thyroxine usually are elevated.
- TSH assay shows low levels except in rare cases.
- TSH receptor antibodies are present in 80% of cases.
- If nodular goiter is present, use thyroid scan to rule out cancer and guide treatment.
- Serum antibodies can help rule out cancer in patients with lobular firm goiters. High antibody levels suggest chronic thyroiditis.

## THERAPEUTIC CONSIDERATIONS

The chief objective of natural treatment of Graves' disease and hyperthyroidism is to reduce symptoms while trying to reestablish normal thyroid status, but little research on natural approach has been done.

- Reduce risk factors such as stress, smoking, excess iodine intake. Stress control is the single most important action. Avoid anything that will excite the patient and increase agitation. Counseling can prevent return to stress-generating life strategies. Increase rest—daily nap after lunch plus full night's sleep.

### Diet

- **Balanced, whole-foods diet**: diet high in calories in the form of small, frequent meals to compensate for increased metabolism. Supplement protein if patient is nutritionally depleted. Avoid iodine supplements, caffeine, and other stimulants.
- **Dietary goitrogens**: substances that prevent utilization of iodine are isothiocyanates, which are similar in action and structure to propylthiouracil. Sources include turnips, cabbage, rutabagas, mustard, rapeseeds, cassava root, soybeans, peanuts, pine nuts, and millet. Goitrogens are transmitted from cow's milk to human beings. These foods are unreliable in treating hyperthyroidism.
  —Goitrogen content is quite low compared with dosages of propylthiouracil (PTU) used in hyperthyroidism (100-200 mg t.i.d. to q.i.d.).
  —Cooking inactivates goitrogens.
  —No solid evidence exists that natural goitrogens significantly interfere with thyroid function if dietary iodine is adequate.

Naturally occurring goitrogens may be used in mild cases instead of PTU and related drugs. Large amounts of these foods must be consumed raw, and iodine intake must be restricted. The highest levels of isothiocyanates are in raw soy milk (0.46-2.5 mg/dL). The Brassica family (e.g., rutabagas, cabbage, and turnips) has the highest levels, but quantity varies according to climate and soil factors. A half head of raw cabbage daily is a typical prescription. Avoid iodine sources such as kelp, other seaweeds, vegetables grown near the ocean, seafood, iodized salt, and iodine-containing nutritional supplements.

### Nutritional Supplements

- **Antioxidants**: tissues exposed to excess thyroid hormone are susceptible to free radical–mediated injury—thyrotoxic myopathy and cardiomyopathy, which are major complications of hyperthyroidism. Hyperthyroid patients have low antioxidant status. Degree of cell damage in Grave's disease directly correlates with level of oxidative stress. When given conventional therapy and antioxidants simultaneously, these patients return to euthyroid state faster. Antioxidant combination used in clinical trials: 10,000 IU beta-carotene; 200 mg vitamin C; 55 IU vitamin E; 60 μg selenium q.d. These doses are lower than typically prescribed for these antioxidants but the combination may create a synergistic effect.
  - —**Vitamin A**: large amounts inhibit thyroid function and ameliorate symptoms of Graves' disease. The exact mechanism is unknown, but iodine metabolism is altered. Animal studies suggest alteration in cellular uptake of thyroxin, capacity of nuclear $T_3$ receptors, and thyroid hormone metabolism.
  - —**Vitamin C**: experimental administration of thyroid, thyroxin, or thyrotrophic hormone reduces ascorbate in serum, blood, liver, adrenals, thymus, and kidney. Antithyroid drugs (thiourea, thiouracil) have the same effect. Hyperthyroid human beings have decreased excretion of ascorbate. Supplemental vitamin C has no direct effect on the course of disease, but supplementation is warranted to ameliorate symptoms and metabolic effects.
  - —**Vitamin E**: may protect patient from oxidative damage of hyperthyroidism. In a rat model vitamin E prevented lipid peroxidation linked to hyperthyroidism. Benefits to hyperthyroid patients are unknown, but hyperthyroid patients have low vitamin E levels.

—**Selenium (Se)**: low Se levels are common in hyperthyroidism. Subclinical hyperthyroidism may result from low Se intake, increasing serum $T_3$ and triacylglycerols with losses of body fat in healthy men fed low-Se foods. Include Se in supplement regimen.

- **Calcium (Ca)**: Ca metabolism is altered in hyperthyroidism. Graves' patients are more susceptible to osteoporosis.
- **Iodine**: dietary excess is common in developed nations. Sources include food additives (salt and iodine used to sterilize pipes in dairies) and medical products (betadine washes, iodine-containing drugs such as amiodarone, radiographic dyes). Effects of iodine in patients with hyperthyroidism include the following:
  —Temporary symptom reduction by stopping hormone synthesis (Wolff-Chaikoff effect).
  —Thyroid can remain suppressed or resume hormone synthesis at reduced, former, or increased rate (escape from Wolff-Chaikoff).
  —Excess iodine can trigger hyperthyroidism (Jod-Basedow disease) in euthyroid person or trigger overactive thyroid to return to normal.

The action of iodine is unpredictable.

- **Zinc**: red blood cell (RBC) zinc is decreased in hyperthyroid patients. Antithyroid drugs normalize RBC zinc but not until 2 months after $T_4$ and $T_3$ levels normalize. Zinc RBC in hyperthyroid patients reflects mean thyroid hormone level over preceding several months (as hemoglobin A1c indicates mean glucose levels in diabetics). Oral zinc tolerance test (get baseline zinc level after 10-hour fast followed by oral dose of 165 mg zinc sulfate heptahydrate [37.5 mg zinc] dissolved in 20 mL deionized water with blood samples drawn at 30-minute intervals over next 3 hours) indicates hyperthyroid patients have basal serum zinc similar to euthyroid persons but with greater urinary zinc excretion. This suggests zinc depletion from tissues to bloodstream caused by catabolism from hyperthyroid state. Hyperthyroidism causes lower zinc assimilation by tissues after ingestion.
- **L-Carnitine (beta-hydroxy/gamma-butyrobetaine)**: quaternary amine that transports long-chain fatty acids into mitochondrial matrix. Forms: L-carnitine is a ubiquitous nutrient in tissues. L-Carnitine is an antagonist of thyroid hormone effect in peripheral tissues by inhibiting its entry into cell nucleus. Carnitine's effect can even prevail over administered $T_4$. Because of its low toxicity,

consider carnitine for Graves' disease–induced thyrotoxicosis during pregnancy, lactation, or other conditions in which antithyroid drugs are unwanted, such as liver disease and blood disorders. Be sure to use the form L-carnitine alone or bound to either acetic or propionic acid. Never use the D form of carnitine.

- **Coenzyme $Q_{10}$ ($CoQ_{10}$) (ubiquinone)**: cofactor in electron transport chain that synthesizes adenosine triphosphate (ATP). Plasma $CoQ_{10}$ is low in adults and children with hyperthyroidism. Conventional treatments return $CoQ_{10}$ to baseline. Supplementing $CoQ_{10}$ in longstanding uncorrected hyperthyroidism and/or concomitant cardiac disease and hyperthyroidism is useful and warranted.

## Botanical Medicines

**Medicinal Plants Traditionally Used in the Treatment of Hyperthyroidism**

| Medicinal Plant | Traditional Indications |
|---|---|
| *Valeriana officinalis* (valerian) | Nervine effect |
| *Scutellaria lateriflora* (skullcap, madweed) | Nervine effect |
| *Cactus grandiflora* (night blooming cereus) | Heart tonic; use with elevated pulse |
| *Iris versicolor* (blueflag) | Traditional use for hyperthyroidism |
| *Fucus* spp. (kelp) | Use with caution; high iodine content can first improve symptoms then later cause aggravation |
| *Lycopus* spp. (e.g., bugleweed) | Blocks the TSH receptors and peripheral conversion of $T_4$ to $T_3$ |
| *Lithospermum officinale* | Blocks the TSH receptors |
| *Melissa officinalis* (lemon balm) | Blocks the TSH receptors |

Unfortunately, these plants have not been adequately evaluated in clinical studies.

- Aqueous, freeze-dried extracts of *Lycopus* spp., *Lithospermum officinale*, and *Melissa officinalis* have been studied in vivo and in vitro. Preliminary results support their use in Graves' disease; clinical research is needed.
- Inhibit effects of exogenous TSH on rat thyroid glands; block effects of TSH on TSH receptor sites on thyroid membranes;

inhibit peripheral deiodination of $T_4$ to $T_3$; and block effects of antithyroid immunoglobulins on TSH receptors.
- Oxidation products of derivatives of 3,4-dihydroxycinnamic acid are responsible for most of the effects. Blocking effects of isolated compounds of TSH receptors are reversible. None of the compounds combined irreversibly or damaged or altered TSH receptors in situ.
- Alcohol extract of *Lycopus europeus* given orally to rats caused long-lasting decrease in $T_3$ from reduced peripheral $T_4$ deiodination. TSH was reduced 24 hours later with a drop in luteinizing hormone (LH) and testosterone. Water extracts are less potent; active constituents are unoxidized alcohol-soluble phenolic compounds.
- Dosage recommendations from the British Herbal Pharmacopoeia for *Lycopus* spp. and *M. officinalis* (no mention is made of *L. officinale*) are given on the following page.
- *Emblica officinalis* (amla): Ayurvedic plant used for diabetes, cataracts, and as an anticarcinogenic agent. Fruit extract (250 mg/kg/day for 30 days) reduced $T_3$ and $T_4$ concentrations by 64% and 70% respectively, compared with PTU, which decreased hormones by 59% and 40%, respectively. *Emblica* also decreased hepatic lipid peroxidation and increased activity of superoxide dismutase and catalase, exhibiting antioxidant and hepatoprotective function. No human studies have been done.

### Other Therapies

- **Hydrotherapy**: calming hydrotherapy (neutral baths before bed) is indicated. Cold compress to throat 15 minutes every day may improve symptoms. Ice bag over heart reduces heart rate but should not be overused.
- **Acupuncture**: reported as effective treatment for hyperthyroidism. Traditional Chinese medicine views constellation of hyperthyroid symptoms as an uprising of liver fire, sometimes with accompanying qi and yin deficiency. Chinese medicine attempts to soothe the liver and clear the fire.

## THERAPEUTIC APPROACH

Acute Graves' disease is not easily treated by naturopathic methods. In severe cases no guarantee exists that natural treatments will adequately alleviate symptoms. "Thyroid storm" is a potentially fatal complication that must be treated aggressively with antithyroid drugs and/or iodine. In mild cases natural therapeutics can manage symptoms well, but monitor carefully to avoid sudden exacerbation. Relapse is quite possible. Treat mild cases symptomatically. Allow patient to return to euthyroid status if possible. If iodine is used, ablative treatment is needed; risk of escape (potential for more intense symptoms) increases with time.

- **Allopathic treatment**: three equal treatments are possible. Decision making may be difficult for the patient while in thyrotoxic state; symptomatic relief is mandatory before a decision is made. Antithyroid drugs can manage symptoms indefinitely while waiting for return to euthyroid status. If drugs are not well tolerated, consider ablative therapies. Surgery has a higher rate of euthyroid results than does radioactive iodine, but carries greater risk of serious complications. Render supportive natural treatment no matter what the choice.
- **Diet**: whole-foods diet with increased calories, micronutrients, and protein to meet increased metabolic needs. In mild cases, use large amounts of raw Brassica family foods and raw soy products and restrict iodine.
- **Supplements**:
  —Vitamin A: 50,000 IU q.d. and/or beta-carotene: 6 mg q.d.
  —Vitamin C: 2000 mg b.i.d.
  —Vitamin E: 800 IU q.d. (mixed tocopherols)
  —Se: 60 μg q.d.
  —L-Carnitine: 2-4 g q.d.
  —$CoQ_{10}$: 50-100 mg q.d.
- **Botanical medicines**:
  —*Lycopus* spp., *L. officinale,* and/or *M. officinalis*: dried herb, 1-3 g or by infusion t.i.d; tincture (1:5), 2-6 mL t.i.d.; fluid extract (1:1), 1-3 mL t.i.d.
- **Hydrotherapy**: cold packs placed over thyroid t.i.d.

# Hyperventilation Syndrome/ Breathing Pattern Disorders

## DIAGNOSTIC SUMMARY

- Pattern of overbreathing in which the depth and rate exceed the metabolic needs of the body at that time.
- Breathlessness usually occurs at rest or with only mild exercise.
- Physical, environmental, or psychologic stimuli override the automatic activity of the respiratory centers, which are tuned to maintain arterial carbon dioxide ($PaCO_2$) levels within a narrow range.

## GENERAL CONSIDERATIONS

The body's carbon dioxide ($CO_2$) production is set at a certain level by physiologic processes and feedback systems. However, the exaggerated breathing depth and rate associated with hyperventilation syndrome/breathing pattern disorders (HVS/BPD) eliminates $CO_2$ at a faster pace, resulting in a fall in $PaCO_2$ and arterial hypocapnia. The arterial hydrogen ion (pH) (acid/alkaline balance) rises to the alkaline region, thus inducing respiratory alkalosis. As a direct result of HVS/BPD, many patients have multiple symptoms, some of which mimic serious disease. However, blood tests, electrocardiograms, and thorough physical examinations may reveal nothing out of the ordinary. Up to 10% of patients in general internal medicine practice reportedly have HVS/BPD as their primary diagnosis.

More women than men have HVS/BPD, ranging from a ratio of 2:1 to 7:1. The peak age of incidence is 15 to 55 years, although other ages can be affected.

Hyperventilation can be an appropriate physiologic response to the body's metabolic needs; for example, tachypnea (rapid breathing) or hyperpnea (increase in respiratory rate proportional to increase in metabolism) may result as the respiratory centers respond automatically and appropriately to rising $CO_2$ production as a result of exercise or organic disease that may be creating acidosis.

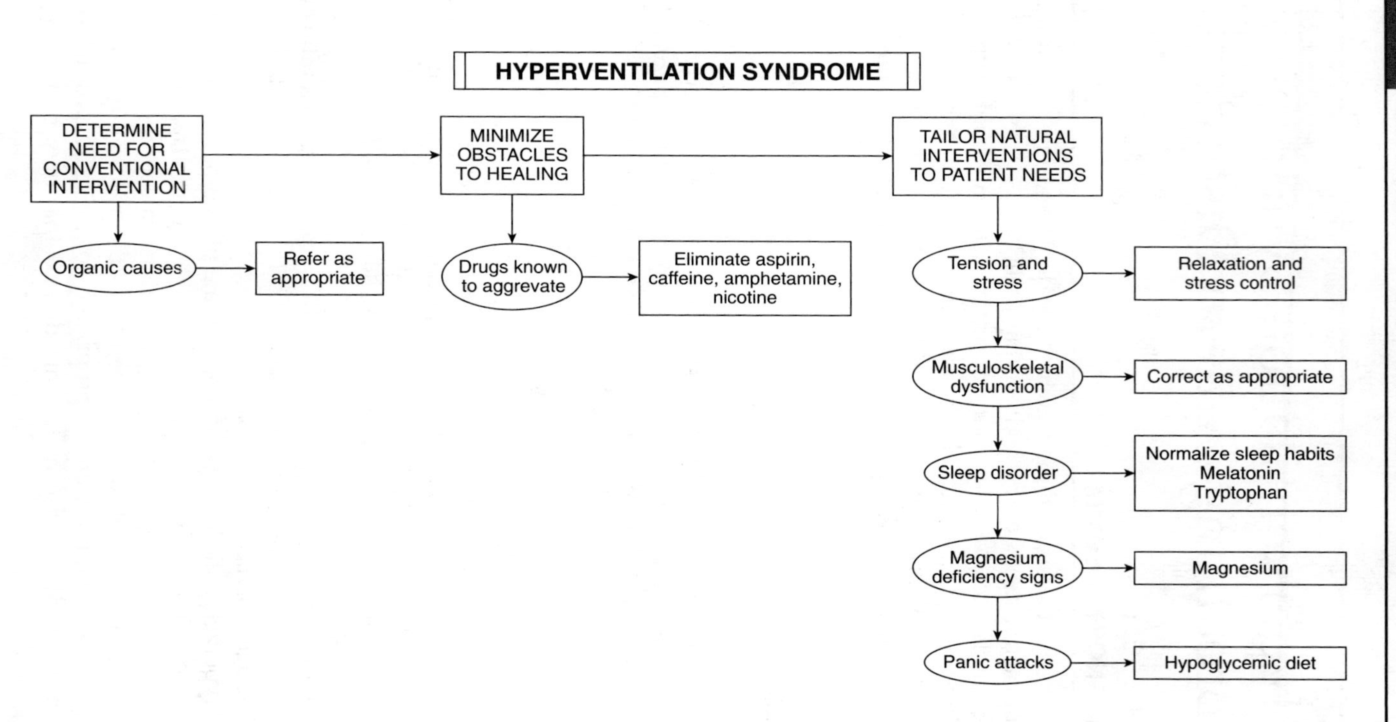
HYPERVENTILATION SYNDROME
DETERMINE NEED FOR CONVENTIONAL INTERVENTION
Organic causes
Refer as appropriate
MINIMIZE OBSTACLES TO HEALING
Drugs known to aggrevate
Eliminate aspirin, caffeine, amphetamine, nicotine
TAILOR NATURAL INTERVENTIONS TO PATIENT NEEDS
Tension and stress
Relaxation and stress control
Musculoskeletal dysfunction
Correct as appropriate
Sleep disorder
Normalize sleep habits
Melatonin
Tryptophan
Magnesium deficiency signs
Magnesium
Panic attacks
Hypoglycemic diet

## DIAGNOSTIC CONSIDERATIONS

Presenting symptoms and observation during case history should offer the alert clinician an opportunity to consider BPD as a factor or feature of the client's condition. Unless it is considered, it is unlikely to be diagnosed. Various tools are available to assist in such a diagnosis, ranging from laboratory tests to simple but effective questionnaires and palpation procedures. To recognize HVS/BPD, characteristics of a normal breathing pattern must be known.

### Normal Breathing Pattern

- The breathing rate should be 10 to 14 breaths/min, moving 3 to 5 L of air/min through the airways of the chest.
- During the active inhalation phase, air flows in through the nose, where it is warmed, filtered, and humidified before being drawn into the lungs by the downward movement of the diaphragm and outward movement of the abdominal wall and lower thoracic structures.
- The upper chest and accessory breathing muscles should remain relaxed.
- The expiratory phase is ideally effortless as the abdominal wall and lower intercostals relax downward and the diaphragm ascends back to its original domed position, aided by the elastic recoil of the lung.
- A relaxed pause at the end of exhalation briefly releases the diaphragm from the negative and positive pressures exerted across it during breathing.
- Under normal circumstances individuals are quite unaware of their breathing.
- Breathing rates and volumes increase or fluctuate in response to physical or emotional demands, but in normal subjects they return to relaxed, low chest patterns after the stimuli ceases.

### Typical Symptoms of HVS/BPD

Patients, especially those whose symptom presentation includes chronic fatigue, anxiety, or both, and who display or report a number of the following signs or symptoms, may be considered suitable candidates for respiratory treatment.

The following symptoms are indications for possible breathing pattern dysfunction:

- A feeling of constriction in the chest
- Shortness of breath

- Accelerated or deepened breathing
- Inability to breathe deeply
- Feeling tense (the Nijmegen questionnaire avoids the use of the word *anxiety*)
- Tightness around the mouth
- Stiffness in the fingers or arms
- Cold hands or feet
- Tingling fingers
- Bloated abdominal sensation
- Dizzy spells
- Blurred vision
- Feeling of confusion or losing touch with environment

Two tests of nerve hyperexcitability produced by hypocapnia-induced hypocalcaemia are Trousseau's sign and Chvostek's sign.

**Trousseau's sign** consists of occluding the brachial artery into the arm by pumping the blood pressure cuff above the systolic pressure for 2½ minutes. A positive sign occurs when paresthesia is felt severely within the period and the wrist and fingers arch in carpopedal spasm, termed *main d'accoucheur* or *obstetrician's hand.*

**Chvostek's sign** occurs if, when tapping the facial nerve as it emerges through the parotid salivary gland, a contraction of the facial muscle twitches the side of the mouth. This is also a test for magnesium deficiency.

## Organic Causes of HVS/BPD

Because hyperventilation may be an appropriate response to a metabolic disorder, organic causes that diminish arterial oxygen saturation ($PaO_2$) or elevate $PaCO_2$ levels must be excluded. Organic causes of HVS/BPD that should be excluded or identified before breathing rehabilitation is initiated include the following:

- **Respiratory**: asthma, chronic obstructive respiratory disease, pneumonia, pulmonary embolus, pneumothorax, and pleural effusion
- **Cardiovascular**: acute and chronic left heart failure, right heart failure, tachyarrhythmias
- **Hemopoietic**: anemia
- **Renal**: nephrotic syndrome, acute and chronic kidney failure
- **Endocrine**: Diabetes with ketoacidosis, pregnancy, progesterone therapy
- **Metabolic**: liver failure
- **Pharmaceutical**: aspirin, caffeine, amphetamine, nicotine

## THERAPEUTIC CONSIDERATIONS

Several models of managing HVS/BPDs are available. Assume that all organic causes of breathing pattern changes have been excluded and that coexisting problems such as asthma, chronic obstructive airway disease, chronic pain, and hormonal imbalances receive appropriate attention. Manual therapy approaches are also assumed to be incorporated as an essential element of rehabilitation. A physical therapy model of rehabilitation for HVS/BPDs includes the following:

- Breathing retraining
- Tension release through talk and relaxation
- Stress perception and management
- Enjoyable graduated exercise prescriptions
- Rest and sleep guides
- Structural normalization

Special attention is required to help the patient understand and control the causes of hyperarousal.

- **Diet**: Fluctuating blood glucose levels may trigger HVS/BPD symptoms. Patients with high simple carbohydrate diets, which produce rapid rises followed by sharp falls to fasting levels or below are at increased risk. Patients are recommended to eat breakfast that includes protein and to avoid going without food for more than 3 hours. This includes a midmorning and afternoon protein snack, as well as the usual three meals a day. This is particularly relevant to patients who experience panic attacks or have seizures, which have been shown more likely to strike when blood glucose levels are low.

## THERAPEUTIC APPROACH

- Regular assessment of breathing function based on functional evidence and palpation.
- Educate patient that the practitioner or therapist can do no more than create an environment, a possibility, for restoration of more normal function; the breathing work itself is up to the patient.
- Treatment of muscles and joints (*not* by itself able to restore normal breathing patterns without cooperative effort).
  —Manual attention to the upper fixators, accessory breathing muscles (upper trapezii, levator scapulae, scalenes,

sternocleidomastoid, pectorals, and latissimus dorsi), and diaphragm.
  —Active trigger points in these muscles may need deactivating manually or by acupuncture.
  —The thoracic spine and ribs may require mobilization (naturopathic manipulation/osteopathic or chiropractic adjustments).
- Breathing retraining (requires freeing of restricted structures).
  —Various breathing exercises should be introduced, individualized to the specific needs of the patient commonly on the basis of pursed-lip breathing and pranayama yoga methods
- Psychotherapy and counseling.
- Lymphatic pump methods may be required with evidence of stasis.
- Relaxation methods, including autogenic training, progressive muscular relaxation, both, may be introduced.
- Sleep pattern disturbances may require attention.
- Exercise of aerobic nature should be carefully introduced.
- Dietary counseling to normalize blood sugar levels and moderate fluctuations.

# Hypoglycemia

## DIAGNOSTIC SUMMARY

- Blood glucose level <40-50 mg/dL
- Normal response curve during first 2-3 hours of glucose tolerance test followed by decrease of 20 mg or more below fasting glucose level during final hours of test, with symptoms developing during decrease

## INTRODUCTION

Hypoglycemia is divided into two main categories:

- **Reactive hypoglycemia**: most common form. Symptoms of hypoglycemia occur 3-5 hours after a meal and may herald onset of early type 2 diabetes mellitus (DM). Gastric surgery may induce this condition, and anorexia nervosa may be a cause. It may also result from oral hypoglycemic drugs; these sulfa drugs (sulfonylureas) stimulate secretion of additional insulin by the pancreas and enhance tissue sensitivity to insulin. (See list of other hypoglycemic drugs below.) Some call this category "idiopathic postprandial syndrome" because symptoms exist and are related to rapid glucose drops, but absolute glucose levels are not reliable indicators of syndrome. Many asymptomatic control subjects have glucose levels <50 mg/dL and many symptomatic patients have normal postprandial glucose.
- **Fasting hypoglycemia**: rare; appears in severe disease states (pancreatic tumors, extensive liver damage, prolonged starvation, autoantibodies against insulin or its receptor, various cancers, excessive exogenous insulin in diabetics). Pregnant diabetic women taking insulin or oral glycemic drugs also can have asymptomatic hypoglycemia.

Hypoglycemia promotes untoward physiologic changes in the body. Insulin-induced hypoglycemia increases C-reactive protein, a cardiac risk factor. Glucose is the primary fuel for the brain; low levels affect brain first. Symptoms of hypoglycemia include

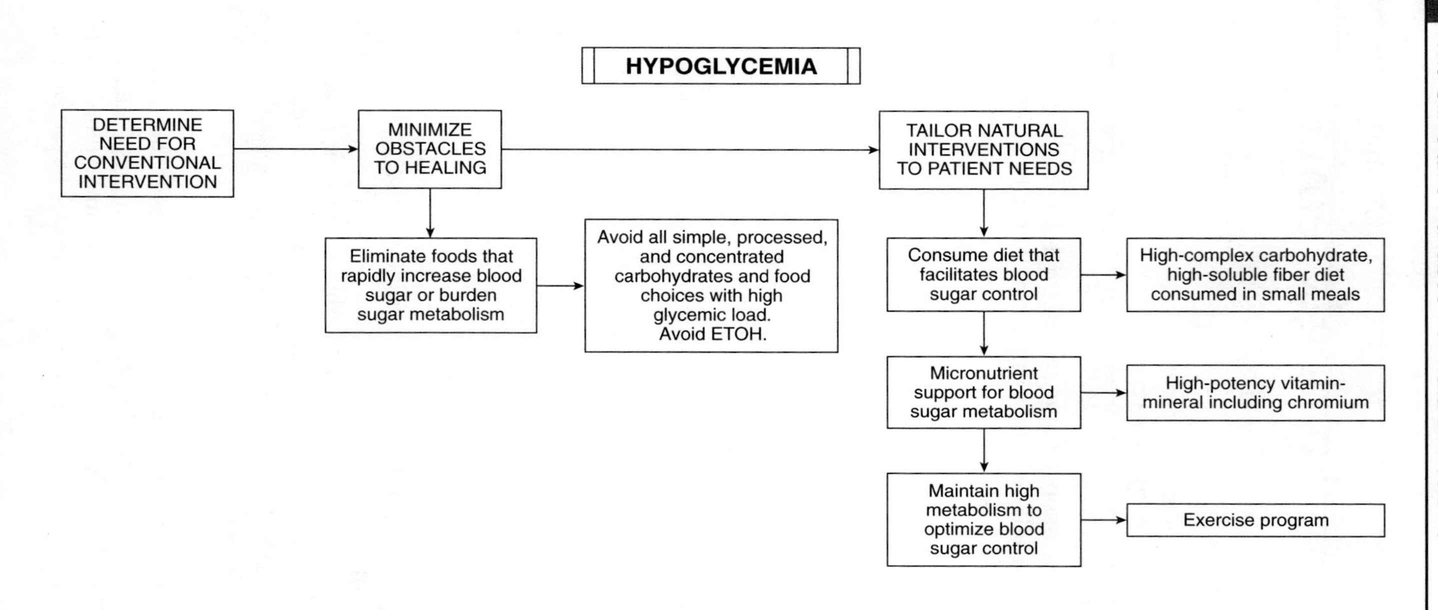
HYPOGLYCEMIA
DETERMINE NEED FOR CONVENTIONAL INTERVENTION
MINIMIZE OBSTACLES TO HEALING
Eliminate foods that rapidly increase blood sugar or burden sugar metabolism
Avoid all simple, processed, and concentrated carbohydrates and food choices with high glycemic load. Avoid ETOH.
TAILOR NATURAL INTERVENTIONS TO PATIENT NEEDS
Consume diet that facilitates blood sugar control
High-complex carbohydrate, high-soluble fiber diet consumed in small meals
Micronutrient support for blood sugar metabolism
High-potency vitamin-mineral including chromium
Maintain high metabolism to optimize blood sugar control
Exercise program

headache, depression, anxiety, irritability, blurred vision, excessive sweating, mental confusion, incoherent speech, bizarre behavior, convulsions.

## DIAGNOSTIC CONSIDERATIONS

Clinical hypoglycemia is identified by modified Whipple's criteria: (1) central nervous system symptoms of confusion, aberrant behavior, or coma; (2) simultaneous blood glucose level ≤40 mg/dL; and (3) relief of symptoms by administering glucose. Standard methods of diagnosing hypoglycemia include measuring blood glucose; normal fasting level = 65-109 mg/dL. Fasting plasma blood glucose >126 mg/dL on two separate occasions is diagnostic of DM. Blood glucose <50 mg/dL should arouse suspicion.

- **Glucose tolerance test (GTT)**: used to diagnose reactive hypoglycemia and DM, but rarely required for DM. After fasting 12+ hours, measure baseline blood glucose. Give subject glucose drink; the amount consumed is based on body weight (1.75 g/kg body weight). Measure blood sugar at 30 minutes, 1 hour, and then hourly for up to 6 hours. Levels >200 mg/dL indicate DM. Levels <50 mg/dL indicate reactive hypoglycemia (see table on p. 374).
- **Glucose-insulin tolerance test (G-ITT)**: blood sugar levels alone are often not enough to diagnose hypoglycemia; signs and symptoms of hypoglycemia occur in persons with glucose >50 mg/dL. Wide overlap exists between symptomatic patients and asymptomatic control subjects. Symptoms linked to hypoglycemia arise from increases in insulin or epinephrine (adrenaline). Measure insulin or epinephrine during GTT because symptoms often correlate better with hormones than glucose. G-ITT has greater sensitivity in diagnosing hypoglycemia and DM than does GTT. Use standard 6-hour GTT coupled with measurements of insulin. Two-thirds of subjects with suspected DM or hypoglycemia with normal GTT demonstrate abnormal G-ITT. However, G-ITT is costly.
- **Hypoglycemic index**: helps diagnose borderline hypoglycemia. The value is determined by calculating the fall in blood glucose during a 90-minute period before the lowest point divided by the value of the lowest point. Hypoglycemic index >0.8 indicates reactive hypoglycemia.
- **Hypoglycemia questionnaire**: most useful and cost-effective method of diagnosing hypoglycemia is to assess symptoms.

When symptoms appear 3-4 hours after eating and disappear with ingestion of food, consider hypoglycemia (see questionnaire on p. 375).

## GENERAL CONSIDERATIONS

Complex hormonal fluxes are largely the result of ingesting too many refined carbohydrates. Syndrome X is a cluster of abnormalities caused by a high intake of refined carbohydrates, leading to hypoglycemia, hyperinsulinemia, and glucose intolerance followed by diminished insulin sensitivity, further leading to hypertension, hypercholesterolemia, obesity, and type 2 DM. The U.S. government recommends that no more than 10% of total calories be derived from refined sugars. The average American consumes 100+ pounds of sucrose and 40 pounds of corn syrup each year.

### Health Impact of Hypoglycemia

- **Brain**: dependent on glucose as energy source. Hypoglycemia causes brain dysfunction. Hypoglycemia is involved in various psychological disorders. Depressed individuals show high percentage of abnormal GTT and G-ITT, but rarely is hypoglycemia considered and dietary therapy prescribed.
- **Aggressive and criminal behavior**: Reactive hypoglycemia is common in psychiatric patients and habitually violent and impulsive criminals. Abnormal and emotionally explosive behavior often is seen during GTT. A sugar-restricted diet reduced antisocial behavior among male juvenile inmates. Behavior improved most in those charged with assault, robbery, rape, aggravated assault, auto theft, vandalism, child molestation, arson, and possession of a deadly weapon. Dietary changes did not seem to affect female prisoners. Men may react to hypoglycemia in a different manner from women; hypoglycemia is an innate internal signal for men to hunt for food. In noncriminal men, aggressiveness often coincides with hypoglycemia.
- **Premenstrual syndrome (PMS)**: PMS-C is linked with increased appetite, craving for sweets, headache, fatigue, fainting spells, and heart palpitations. GTT on PMS-C patients 5-10 days before menses displays flattening of early part of curve and reactive hypoglycemia. GTT is normal during other parts of menstrual cycle. Flat, early part of GTT curve implies excessive insulin secretion in response to sugar consumption. Excessive secretion is hormonally regulated, but other factors are involved. Sodium

chloride ingestion enhances insulin response to sugar, and decreased magnesium in pancreas increases insulin secretion (see the chapter on premenstrual syndrome).

- **Migraine headaches**: caused by excessive dilation of blood vessels in the head. Migraines are surprisingly common (15%-20% of men and 25%-30% of women). More than half have a family history of migraine. Hypoglycemia is a common precipitating factor. Eliminating refined sugar from diets of migraine sufferers with confirmed hypoglycemia greatly improves the condition (see the chapter on migraine headaches).
- **Atherosclerosis, intermittent claudication, and angina**: reactive hypoglycemia or impaired glucose tolerance is a significant factor in atherosclerosis. High sugar intake elevates triglycerides and cholesterol. Abnormal GTT and hyperinsulinism are common in patients with heart disease. High sugar intake and reactive hypoglycemia can cause angina and intermittent claudication.
- **Syndrome X**: a set of cardiovascular risk factors (glucose or insulin disturbances, hyperlipidemia, hypertension, and android obesity). Other terms include metabolic cardiovascular risk syndrome, Reaven's syndrome, insulin resistance syndrome, and atherothrombogenic syndrome. The underlying metabolic denominator is hyperinsulinemia from elevated intake of refined carbohydrates. Development of type 2 DM is preceded by hyperinsulinemia and insulin insensitivity. In most cases these defects present themselves decades before the development of DM. Hypoglycemia, hyperinsulinemia, syndrome X, and type 2 DM are progressive stages of the same illness—maladaptation to the refined Western diet.

## THERAPEUTIC CONSIDERATIONS

### Dietary Factors

In whole, unprocessed foods, sugars are slowly absorbed because they are contained within cells and associated with fiber. A high–complex carbohydrate, high-fiber, low-sugar diet is recommended. Natural, simple sugars in fruits and vegetables have an advantage over sucrose and other refined sugars attributable to balance by a wide range of nutrients aiding the utilization of sugars. Sugars in whole, unprocessed foods are more slowly absorbed because of the integration within cells and fiber. Refining removes vitamins, trace minerals, and fiber. More than half of carbohydrates consumed in the United States are sugars added to processed foods.

- **A closer look at simple carbohydrates**: most diabetic and hypoglycemic persons can tolerate moderate amounts of fruits and fructose without a loss of blood sugar control. These foods produce less-sharp elevations in blood sugar compared with starch. Fructose decreases the amount of calories and fat consumed. Regular fruit consumption may help control sugar cravings and reduce obesity.
- **Glycemic index and glycemic load**: glycemic index expresses a rise of blood glucose after eating a particular food and serves as a guideline for dietary recommendations for people with diabetes or hypoglycemia. Glycemic index must not be the sole dietary guideline. High-fat foods (e.g., ice cream, sausage) have low glycemic indexes because fat impairs glucose tolerance and are poor food choices for hypoglycemic or diabetic patients. The standard value of 100 is based on the rise seen with ingestion of pure glucose. Glycemic index ranges from 20 for fructose and whole barley to 98 for a baked potato. Insulin response to carbohydrate-containing foods is similar to the rise in blood sugar. Avoid foods with high values and choose foods with lower values.
- **Glycemic load**: value of a food's glycemic index divided by 100, then multiplied by its available carbohydrate content. A glycemic load of 20 or more is high; 11 to 19 is intermediate; 10 or less is low. This provides more comprehensive assessment of impact of carbohydrate intake. Even though glycemic index for a food is fairly high, its glycemic load can be low, indicating that with reasonable serving sizes it does not adversely stress glycemic control. Foods containing natural soluble and insoluble fibers and minimally processed whole foods are better choices for glycemic influence and insulin response. Diets with high glycemic load are directly linked to diabetes; coronary heart disease; and colon, ovarian, and pancreatic cancer risk.
- **Fiber**: blood sugar disorders are related to inadequate dietary fiber. Increase intake of complex carbohydrate sources rich in fiber. Dietary fiber is composed of the plant cell walls plus indigestible residues from plant foods. Water-soluble forms are most beneficial to blood sugar control: hemicelluloses, mucilages, gums, and pectin. The majority of fiber in most plant cell walls is water soluble. Good sources of water-soluble fiber are legumes, oat bran, nuts, seeds, psyllium seed husks, pears, apples, and most vegetables. Daily intake of 50 g is recommended. Beneficial effects include the following:

—Slow digestion and absorption of carbohydrates, preventing rapid rises in blood sugar.
—Increase human tissue cell sensitivity to insulin, preventing hyperinsulinism.
—Improve uptake of glucose by liver and other tissues, preventing sustained hyperglycemia (*Textbook,* "Role of Dietary Fiber in Health and Disease").

- **Chromium (Cr)**: key constituent of glucose tolerance factor. Cr deficiency may be a contributing factor to hypoglycemia, DM, and obesity. Marginal Cr deficiency is common in the United States and may be a cause of many cases of reactive hypoglycemia. Cr alleviates hypoglycemic symptoms, improves insulin binding, and increases number of insulin receptors.

### Lifestyle Factors

- **Alcohol**: severely stresses blood sugar control and is a contributing factor to hypoglycemia. It induces reactive hypoglycemia by interfering with normal glucose utilization and increases secretion of insulin. Resultant drop in blood sugar produces craving for foods that quickly elevate blood sugar plus cravings for more alcohol. Increased sugar consumption aggravates reactive hypoglycemia. Hypoglycemia is a complication of short- and long-term alcohol abuse. Hypoglycemia aggravates mental and emotional problems of the withdrawing alcoholic: sweating, tremor, tachycardia, anxiety, hunger, dizziness, headache, visual disturbance, decreased mental function, confusion, and depression. Acute alcohol ingestion induces hypoglycemia. Long-term abuse leads to hyperglycemia and diabetes. The body becomes insensitive to chronic augmented insulin release caused by alcohol. Alcohol causes insulin resistance even in healthy persons. Alcohol intake is strongly correlated with DM; the higher the alcohol intake, the more likely a person will have DM.
- **Exercise**: an important part of hypoglycemia treatment and prevention. Regular exercise prevents type 2 DM and improves insulin sensitivity and glucose tolerance in existing diabetics. Exercise increases tissue chromium concentrations.

## THERAPEUTIC APPROACH

Use dietary therapy to stabilize blood sugar. Reactive hypoglycemia is not a disease, but a complex set of symptoms caused by faulty carbohydrate metabolism induced by inappropriate diet.

### GTT Response Criteria

| Diagnosis | Response |
|---|---|
| Normal | No elevation greater than 160 mg |
| | Less than 150 mg at the end of first hour |
| | Less than 120 mg at the end of second hour |
| | Never lower than 20 mg below fasting |
| Flat | No variation more than ±20 mg from fasting value |
| Prediabetic | More than 120 mg at the end of second hour |
| Diabetic | More than 180 mg during the first hour |
| | 200 mg or higher at the end of first hour |
| | 150 mg or higher at the end of second hour |
| Reactive hypoglycemia | A normal 2- or 3-hour response curve followed by a decrease of 20 mg or more from the fasting level during the final hours |
| Probable reactive hypoglycemia | A normal 2- or 3-hour response curve followed by a decrease of 10-20 mg from the fasting level during the final hours |
| Flat hypoglycemia | An elevation of 20 mg or less followed by a decrease of 20 mg or more below the fasting level |
| Prediabetic hypoglycemia | A 2-hour response identical to the prediabetic response but showing a hypoglycemic response during the final 3 hours |
| Hyperinsulinism | A marked hypoglycemic response with a value of less than 50 mg during the third, fourth, or fifth hour |

- **Diet**: avoid all simple, processed, and concentrated carbohydrates and food choices with high glycemic load. Emphasize complex-carbohydrate, high-soluble fiber foods: legumes and low-glycemic vegetables. Small meals may stabilize blood sugar more easily. Avoid alcohol (see the chapter on diabetes).
- **Supplements**: high-potency vitamin/mineral that includes Cr: 200-400 μg q.d.
- **Exercise**: graded exercise program appropriate to patient's fitness level and interest that elevates heart rate at least 60% of maximum for 30 minutes three times a week.

## G-ITT Criteria

| Pattern | Response |
|---|---|
| Pattern 1 | Normal fasting insulin 0-30 units. Peak insulin at 0.5-1 hour. The combined insulin values for the second and third hours are less than 60 units. This pattern is considered normal. |
| Pattern 2 | Normal fasting insulin. Peak at 0.5-1 hour with a delayed return to normal. Second and third hour levels between 60 and 100 units usually are associated with hypoglycemia and considered borderline for diabetes; values greater than 100 units considered definite diabetes. |
| Pattern 3 | Normal fasting insulin. Peak at second or third hour instead of 0.5-1 hour. Definite diabetes. |
| Pattern 4 | High fasting insulin. Definite diabetes. |
| Pattern 5 | Low insulin response. All tested values for insulin less than 30. If this response is associated with elevated blood sugar levels, it probably indicates insulin-dependent DM (juvenile pattern). |

## Hypoglycemia Questionnaire

| | No | Mild | Moderate | Severe |
|---|---|---|---|---|
| Crave sweets | 0 | 1 | 2 | 3 |
| Irritable if a meal is missed | 0 | 1 | 2 | 3 |
| Feel tired or weak if a meal is missed | 0 | 1 | 2 | 3 |
| Dizziness when standing suddenly | 0 | 1 | 2 | 3 |
| Frequent headaches | 0 | 1 | 2 | 3 |
| Poor memory (forgetful) or concentration | 0 | 1 | 2 | |
| Feel tired an hour or so after eating | 0 | 1 | 2 | 3 |
| Heart palpitations | 0 | 1 | 2 | 3 |
| Feel shaky at times | 0 | 1 | 2 | 3 |
| Afternoon fatigue | 0 | 1 | 2 | 3 |
| Vision blurs on occasion | 0 | 1 | 2 | 3 |
| Depression or mood swings | 0 | 1 | 2 | 3 |
| Overweight | 0 | 1 | 2 | 3 |
| Frequently anxious or nervous | 0 | 1 | 2 | 3 |
| Total | | | | |

*Scoring:* <5, hypoglycemia is not likely a factor; 6-15, hypoglycemia is a likely factor; >15, hypoglycemia is extremely likely.

## Oral Hypoglycemic Drugs

- Chlorpropamide (Diabinese)
- Glipizide (Glucotrol)
- Glibenclamide, Glyburide (DiaBeta, Micronase)
- Tolazamide (Tolinase)
- Tolbutamide (Orinase)
- Metformin (Glucophage)
- Thiazolidinediones: pioglitazone (Actos) or rosiglitazone (Avandia)
- Acarbose (Precose, Glucobay)
- Glimepiride (Amaryl)
- Gliclazide (Gen-Gliclazide)
- Nateglinide (Starlix)
- Repaglinide (Prandin)

# Hypothyroidism

## DIAGNOSTIC SUMMARY

- Depression
- Difficulty losing weight
- Dry skin
- Headaches
- Lethargy or fatigue
- Memory problems
- Menstrual problems
- Hyperlipidemia
- Recurrent infections
- Sensitivity to cold

## GENERAL CONSIDERATIONS

Hypothyroidism affects virtually all cells and body functions. Severity of symptoms in adults ranges from mild (not detectable with standard blood tests [subclinical hypothyroidism]) to severe, which can be life threatening (myxedema).

- Low thyroid hormone and elevated thyroid-stimulating hormone (TSH) levels indicate defective thyroid hormone synthesis—called "primary hypothyroidism."
- Low TSH and low thyroid hormone: pituitary gland is responsible for low thyroid function—called "secondary hypothyroidism."
- Normal blood thyroid hormone and TSH plus low functional thyroid activity (low basal metabolic rate) suggest "cellular hypothyroidism," involving impaired cellular conversion of thyroxine ($T_4$) to triiodothyronine ($T_3$).

From 1%-4% of the adult population have moderate to severe hypothyroidism. Another 10%-12% have mild hypothyroidism. The rate of hypothyroidism increases steadily with advancing age. The rate of hypothyroidism is 25% of adults and much higher in the elderly.

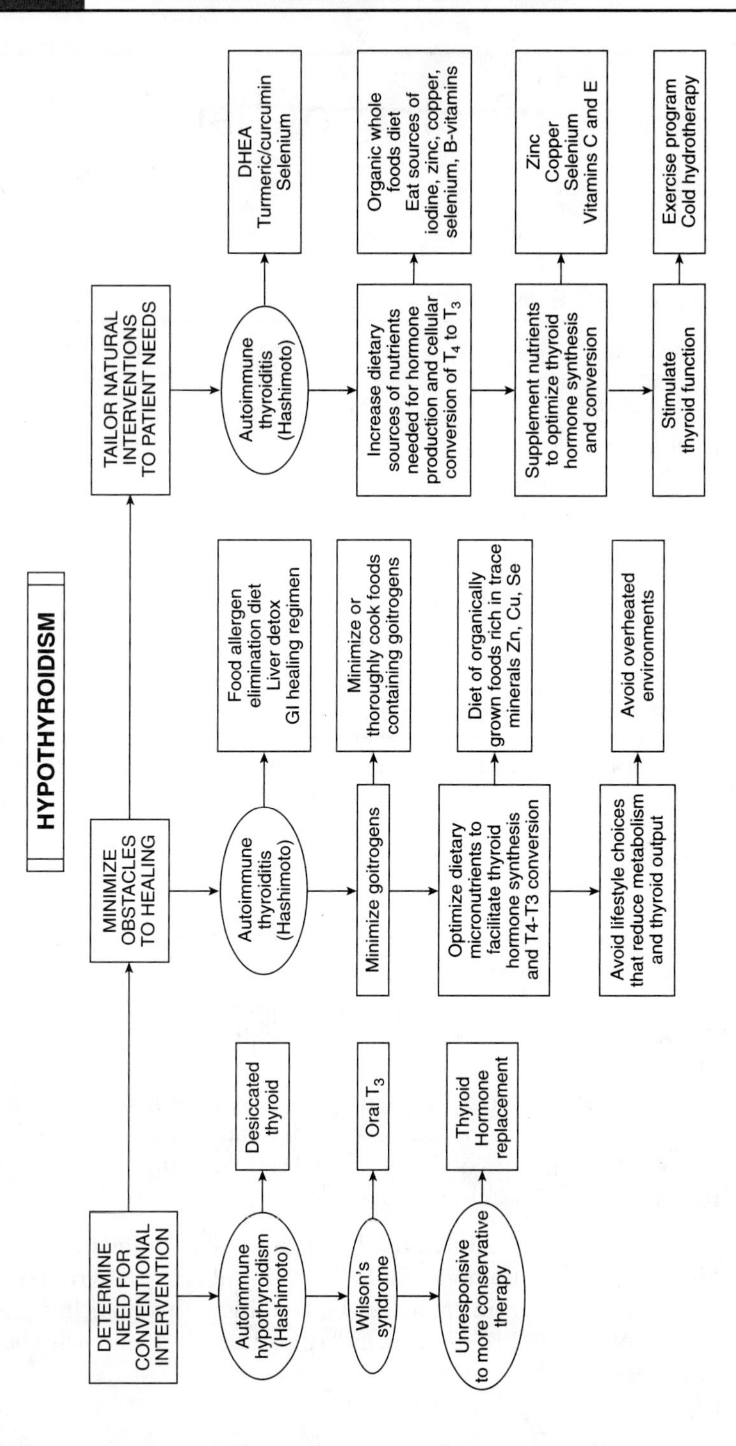
HYPOTHYROIDISM
DETERMINE NEED FOR CONVENTIONAL INTERVENTION
Autoimmune hypothyroidism (Hashimoto)
Desiccated thyroid
Wilson's syndrome
Oral $T_3$
Unresponsive to more conservative therapy
Thyroid Hormone replacement
MINIMIZE OBSTACLES TO HEALING
Autoimmune thyroiditis (Hashimoto)
Food allergen elimination diet
Liver detox
GI healing regimen
Minimize goitrogens
Minimize or thoroughly cook foods containing goitrogens
Optimize dietary micronutrients to facilitate thyroid hormone synthesis and T4-T3 conversion
Diet of organically grown foods rich in trace minerals Zn, Cu, Se
Avoid lifestyle choices that reduce metabolism and thyroid output
Avoid overheated environments
TAILOR NATURAL INTERVENTIONS TO PATIENT NEEDS
Autoimmune thyroiditis (Hashimoto)
DHEA
Turmeric/curcumin
Selenium
Increase dietary sources of nutrients needed for hormone production and cellular conversion of $T_4$ to $T_3$
Organic whole foods diet
Eat sources of iodine, zinc, copper, selenium, B-vitamins
Supplement nutrients to optimize thyroid hormone synthesis and conversion
Zinc
Copper
Selenium
Vitamins C and E
Stimulate thyroid function
Exercise program
Cold hydrotherapy

## Causes of Hypothyroidism

- **Overt hypothyroidism**: 95% of all cases of overt hypothyroidism are primary. The most common cause in the past was iodine deficiency. The thyroid gland cells add iodine to amino acid tyrosine to create thyroid hormones. Iodine deficiency leads to hypothyroidism and/or enlarged thyroid gland (goiter).
  —Goiters affect 200 million people worldwide. All but 4% are caused by iodine deficiency. Iodine deficiency is rare in industrialized countries because of iodized table salt. Goiters in the United States today are caused by excessive ingestion of goitrogens—foods that block iodine utilization: Brassica plants (turnips, cabbage, mustard, broccoli, Brussels sprouts, kale, cauliflower), cassava root, soybean, peanuts, pine nuts, millet. Cooking usually inactivates goitrogens.
  —The most frequent cause of overt hypothyroidism in the United States is the autoimmune disorder Hashimoto's disease. Antibodies are formed that bind to thyroid peroxidase enzyme, thyroglobulin, and TSH receptors and inhibit hormone synthesis. Antibodies may also bind to adrenal glands, pancreas, and acid-producing cells (parietal cells) of the stomach.
  —Thyroid surgery and ablation.
  —Postpartum hypothyroidism, a transient form that affects 5%-10% of women in the United States.
- **Subclinical hypothyroidism**: TSH is elevated and serum thyroid hormone levels are normal. The body compensates for decreased thyroid function by increasing TSH. Causes include mild autoimmune thyroid destruction and drug or surgical interventions. Subclinical hypothyroidism affects 2%-7% of adults.
- **Functional hypothyroidism**: thyroid activity is measured by functional test (Barnes test), rather than solely blood thyroid hormone levels. Incidence is 25%. Functional tests show greater incidence of low thyroid than blood tests; blood tests measure $T_4$, which accounts for 90% of hormone secreted; but $T_3$ (made by cells from $T_4$) has four times the activity of $T_4$. If cells cannot convert, the person has normal blood levels of the hormone yet is functionally thyroid deficient. Blood tests for $T_3$ miss low thyroid function in 50% of patients. Measuring thyroid effects on the body is better; measure resting metabolic rate controlled by thyroid gland. Basal body temperature is a good way of assessing basal metabolic rate. Some physicians look for high reverse $T_3/T_4$ ratio as evidence of this condition.

## DIAGNOSTIC CONSIDERATIONS

Basal body temperature (temperature of body at rest) and Achilles reflex time (reflexes are slowed in hypothyroidism) are old indicators of dysfunction. Routine blood tests may not be sensitive enough to diagnose milder, most common forms of hypothyroidism. Basal body temperature is the most sensitive functional test of thyroid function. To distinguish autoimmune Hashimoto's thyroiditis and other nonautoimmune subclinical and functional conditions, use TSH, antithyroid peroxidase, and antithyroglobulin antibody tests. Suspect Wilson's disease with low basal body temperature and high reverse $T_3/T_4$ ratio.

### Clinical Symptomatology

- **Metabolic**: hypothyroidism decreases the rate of utilization of fat, protein, and carbohydrate. Moderate weight gain and sensitivity to cold weather (cold hands or feet) are common. Cholesterol and triglycerides are increased in even mildest hypothyroidism, increasing the risk of atherosclerosis and cardiovascular disease. Hypothyroidism increases capillary permeability and slows lymphatic drainage, causing swelling of tissue (edema).
- **Endocrine**: hormonal complications are loss of libido in men and menstrual abnormalities in women. Women have prolonged and heavy menses, with a shorter menstrual cycle. Infertility is problematic; miscarriages, premature deliveries, and stillbirths are common. Rarely does a pregnancy result in normal labor and delivery in the overtly hypothyroid woman.
- **Skin, hair, and nails**: dry, rough skin covered with fine superficial scales. Hair is coarse, dry, and brittle. Hair loss can be quite severe. Nails become thin and brittle with transverse grooves.
- **Psychological**: the brain is sensitive to hypothyroidism. Depression with weakness and fatigue are first symptoms; later, difficulty concentrating and extreme forgetfulness.
- **Muscular and skeletal**: muscle weakness and joint stiffness are predominant features. Some patients have muscle and joint pain and tenderness.
- **Cardiovascular**: predisposition to atherosclerosis and myocardial infarction from induced hyperlipidemia and increased homocysteine and C-reactive protein. Hypothyroidism can also cause hypertension, reduce function of heart, and reduce heart rate.

- **Other manifestations**: shortness of breath, constipation, and impaired kidney function. Patients with dermatitis herpetiformis have significantly increased abnormalities of thyroid function tests, with significant hypothyroidism being the most common abnormality.

## Laboratory Evaluation

The American Thyroid Association recommends TSH screening every 5 years beginning at age 35. Lab diagnosis is based on results of total $T_4$, free $T_4$, $T_3$, and TSH levels. Diagnosis is straightforward in overt cases. In subclinical cases diagnosis is less clear. Elevated TSH with normal $T_4$ suggests subclinical state. Accepted normal range for TSH is quite broad: 0.35-5.50 μIU/mL (conventional approach does not treat unless TSH >10 μIU/mL). Naturopathic approach: if patient does not respond to nutritional intervention, use low-dose thyroid hormone therapy if TSH >2.5 μIU/mL—slightly higher than accepted 2.0 μIU/mL demonstrating disturbance of thyroid-pituitary axis, especially with antithyroid antibodies. Test for antithyroid antibodies in anyone with TSH >2.5 μIU/mL.

## Functional Assessment

Functional thyroid activity is estimated by measuring basal body temperature (indicator of basal metabolic rate). Barnes: normal basal body temperature is 97.6-98.2° F. Low basal metabolic rate can also indicate nutritional deficiencies and inadequate physical activity, and fever can give inaccurately high body temperature. Following are patient instructions for measuring basal body temperature:

1. Place the thermometer by the bed before going to sleep at night. If using a mercury thermometer, shake it down to below 95° F.
2. On waking, place the thermometer under armpit for a full 10 minutes. Move as little as possible. Lying and resting with the eyes closed is best. Do not get up until the 10-minute test is completed.
3. After 10 minutes, read and record the temperature and date.
4. Record the temperature for at least three mornings (preferably at the same time of day) and give the information to the physician. Menstruating women must perform the test on the second, third, and fourth days of menstruation. Men and postmenopausal women can perform the test at any time.

## THERAPEUTIC CONSIDERATIONS

### Diet and Food Allergy

A clear correlation exists among autoimmunity, intestinal permeability, and food allergy. Roughly 2% of patients with celiac disease have overt autoimmune thyroid disease. Serologic autoantibody markers become undetectable 6 months after starting a gluten-free diet. Use an elimination diet and/or detoxification regimen (see the chapter on food allergies) to decrease antigen load, strengthen gut integrity, and normalize autoantibody activity in autoimmune thyroid patients.

### Physiologic and Hormonal Considerations

Thyroid binding globulin (TBG) from the liver transports thyroid hormones, including 75% of circulating $T_4$. Factors increasing TBG include excess estrogens (as in pregnancy, oral estrogens of birth control pills and hormone replacement therapy), tamoxifen for breast cancer, and liver diseases. High TBG reduces free thyroid hormone availability, worsening hypothyroidism. Depending on clinical picture, consider moderating estrogen excess by decreasing intake of oral estrogens or using non-oral regimens to bypass the liver first pass, and/or helping liver metabolism of estrogens.

### Nutritional Considerations

Nutritionally support the thyroid gland with key nutrients required for synthesis of thyroid hormone. Avoid goitrogens.

- **Iodine, tyrosine, and goitrogens**: thyroid hormones are made from iodine and the amino acid tyrosine. The recommended daily allowance for iodine in adults is quite small: 150 μg. Average intake of iodine in the United States is >600 μg q.d. Too much iodine inhibits hormone synthesis. The only function of iodine in the body is thyroid synthesis. Dietary levels or iodine supplements should not exceed 600 μg q.d. for any length of time. Goitrogens combine with iodine, making it unavailable to thyroid. Cooking inactivates goitrogens. Goitrogenic foods should not be eaten in excess.
- **Vitamins and minerals**:
  —Zinc (Zn), vitamin E, and vitamin A function together to manufacture thyroid hormone. A deficiency of any of these reduces the amount of active hormone produced. Low zinc level is common in the elderly, as is hypothyroidism.

—Riboflavin ($B_2$), niacin ($B_3$), pyridoxine ($B_6$), and vitamin C are necessary for hormone synthesis.
—Zinc, copper (Cu), and selenium (Se) are required cofactors for iodothyronine iodinase enzyme converting $T_4$ to $T_3$. Each form requires a different trace mineral. Supplementation with zinc reestablishes normal thyroid function in zinc-deficient hypothyroid patients even though serum $T_4$ is normal.
—Areas of the world where Se is deficient have a greater incidence of thyroid disease. Se deficiency does not decrease conversion of $T_4$ to $T_3$ in thyroid or pituitary, but it does decrease conversion of $T_4$ to $T_3$ in peripheral cells. People with Se deficiency have elevated $T_4$ and TSH. Se supplements decrease $T_4$ and TSH and normalize thyroid activity. Se decreases thyroid antibodies in thyroid autoimmunity. Se is deficient in 50% of the population's diets. Se deficiency induces low cellular thyroid activity despite normal or elevated hormone.

- Antioxidants (vitamin C, vitamin E, *Curcuma longa* [turmeric] extract) increase thyroid function in animal studies, with decreased abnormal thyroid weight changes, less suppression of $T_4$ and $T_3$, and attenuated increases in cholesterol. Thyroid hormone abnormalities correlated with decreased glutathione in testicular tissues. No human studies exist to corroborate these findings; consider these safe components in an antiinflammatory antioxidant regimen.

## Exercise

Exercise stimulates thyroid secretion and increases tissue sensitivity to thyroid hormone. Many health benefits of exercise may result from improved thyroid function. Exercise is especially important in dieting overweight hypothyroid patients. A consistent effect of dieting is decreased metabolic rate as the body strives to conserve fuel. Exercise prevents decline in metabolic rate in response to dieting.

## Thyroid Hormone Replacement

If more conservative measures fail, exogenous thyroid hormones are necessary. Naturopathic physicians prefer desiccated natural thyroid complete with all thyroid hormones, not just thyroxine. Normal tissue levels of $T_4$ and $T_3$ are achieved only with infusion of $T_4$ and $T_3$, not by $T_4$ alone. Many patients treated with desiccated thyroid tend to feel better.

- **Preparations containing only $T_4$ (Synthroid, Levothyroid)**: advantages include consistent potency and prolonged duration of action. $T_3$ is rarely used alone; it is four times more potent with shorter duration of action than $T_4$.
- **Desiccated thyroid**: advantage is that it provides $T_4$ and $T_3$, plus relevant amino acids and micronutrients. Drawback: it lacks consistency of potency. By U.S. Pharmacopoeia standard, these preparations must contain at least 85% and not more than 115% of labeled amount of $T_4$ and at least 90% and not more than 110% for $T_3$; labeled amount = 38 mg $T_4$ and 9 mg $T_3$ per grain (65 mg).
- **Synthetic mixtures of $T_4$ and $T_3$ (Liotrix, Thyrolar)**: in similar ratios provide consistency that whole, natural desiccated thyroid lacks.
- **Equivalencies** (1 thyroid unit) for thyroid agents based on clinical response:
  —100 μg of $T_4$ (e.g., Synthroid)
  —20-25 μg $T_3$ (e.g., Cytomel)
  —1 Grain desiccated thyroid
  —12.5 μg $T_4$ + 50 μg $T_4$ (e.g., Thyrolar)
  (Note: 0.5 thyroid units would be equal to 50% of the values shown in the list.)
- **Food fiber**: may interfere with absorption and bioavailability of oral thyroid supplements.
- **Lifestyle and diet changes**: implement along with hormone replacement to improve lipid profile.

## THERAPEUTIC APPROACH

Natural treatment strategies are tailored to specifics of pathologic condition: autoimmunity, Wilson's syndrome, or subclinical or overt hypothyroidism.

### Treatments for Autoimmune Hypothyroidism (Hashimoto's Disease)

- **Thyroid replacement**: normalizes thyroid hormone levels and suppresses thyroid activity, decreasing autoimmune processes. Use desiccated or synthetic thyroid in high enough doses to decrease TSH at or near zero. Some literature reports TSH values ≤0.1 μIU/mL are linked to atrial fibrillation and bone density loss but not additional fracture. Desiccated thyroid stimulates blocking antibodies to antithyroid antibodies and acts as decoy for thyroid antibodies. Some patients recover from Hashimoto's after extended thyroid treatment and no longer need replacement. Some patients may not benefit from desiccated thyroid (adverse reaction to antigenic thyroid substances). Use synthetic thyroid promptly. Use frequent TSH and antibody tests to verify suppression of thyroid activity and monitor autoimmunity. Caveat: early in Hashimoto's disease hyperthyroidism often occurs. In this case, replacement is contraindicated.

- **Diet and lifestyle**: food elimination, detoxification, and gut healing options may ameliorate root factor of antigenic autoimmunity.
- **Other recommendations**:
  —Dehydroepiandrosterone (DHEA) is beneficial in autoimmunity. Clinical studies used high doses (100-200 mg q.d.), but consider much lower physiologic range of 5-10 mg q.d. or 10-20 mg q.d. in women and men, respectively. Side effects of high doses: hirsutism and acne. Start at low level; increase slowly while monitoring DHEA blood levels and clinical symptoms of excess androgens. Effects of long-term DHEA are unknown; use with caution, particularly in patients at risk for hormone-dependent cancers.
  —Turmeric (*Curcuma longa*) is an antiinflammatory antioxidant. Use 400 mg curcumin t.i.d. in capsules or liberal amounts of tumeric on food.
  —Se at 200 μg q.d. for Hashimoto's disease, especially in patients with high titers of anti–thyroid peroxidase antibodies.

## Treatment for Wilson's Syndrome

- **Thyroid replacement**: When lab reverse $T_3$ and basal body temperature suggest Wilson's syndrome (subclinical hypothyroidism), use oral $T_3$ and monitor basal body temperature until normal 98.6° F is maintained. Temperature correction will also decrease adrenal corticosteroids, mitigating fatigue, depression, and insulin resistance. Side effects of $T_3$ are antioxidant depletion, tremor, anxiety, and palpitations.
- **Other recommendations**: see thyroid support later.

## Treatments for Nonautoimmune Overt or Subclinical Hypothyroid Disorder

- **Optimize nutrients** needed for hormone production and cellular conversion of $T_4$ to $T_3$. If no response after a few months, use thyroid hormone replacement.

- **Diet:** low in goitrogens. Organic foods are richer in trace minerals needed for thyroid hormone production and activation. When eaten, these foods must be cooked to break down goitrogens. Eat sources of iodine: sea fish, sea vegetables (kelp, dulse, arame, hijiki, nori, wakame, kombu), iodized salt. Eat sources of zinc: seafood (oysters), beef, oatmeal, chicken, liver, spinach, nuts, seeds. Copper sources: liver, organ meats, eggs, yeast, beans, nuts, seeds. B vitamin sources: yeast, whole grains, liver. Se source: unshelled Brazil nuts.
- **Supplements:**
  —Zinc: 25 mg q.d.
  —Copper: 5 mg q.d.
  —Se: 200 μg q.d.
  —Vitamin C: 1-3 g q.d. in divided doses
  —Vitamin E: 400 IU q.d. (mixed tocopherols)
- **Thyroid hormones**: begin at levels ranging from 0.5 to 2 thyroid units (see above) q.d. based on patient's size and serum hormone levels. Reevaluate basal body temperature, TSH, $T_4$, $T_3$, and free $T_4$ 4-6 weeks later. Treatment goal: normalize basal body temperature and serum hormone levels. After stabilizing dosage, periodically evaluate based on individual needs or at least annually. In subclinical hypothyroidism, limit dosage to 0.5 thyroid units daily for first 3 months. Administer hormones on empty stomach to increase absorption. Avoid taking thyroid concurrently with other medicines and supplements (especially iron) that affect absorption. Once-daily dosing gives stable increases in hormone levels. Dosage during pregnancy: increased because estrogens increase serum thyroid hormone–binding globulin. Monitor carefully during pregnancy. Dosage requirements increase by 30%-50% during pregnancy and return to prepregnancy levels after delivery.
- **Exercise, physical therapy, lifestyle**: Invigorating water sports, avoidance of overheated environments, and cold hydrotherapy can stimulate thyroid function.

**Serum Thyroid Hormone Normal Values**

| | |
|---|---|
| $T_4$ | 4.8-13.2 mg/dL |
| Free $T_4$ | 0.9-2 ng/dL |
| $T_3$ | 80-220 ng/dL |
| TSH | 0.35-5.50 μIU/mL |

# Immune Support

## DIAGNOSTIC SUMMARY

- Frequent infections
- Chronic infections that do not resolve
- Cancer

## GENERAL CONSIDERATIONS

The immune system is a complex integration of synergistic segments that are continuously barraged by stimuli from both internal and external sources. Supporting the immune system is critical to good health. Conversely, good health is critical to supporting the immune system. The best approach to supporting immune function is a comprehensive plan involving lifestyle, stress management, exercise, diet, nutritional supplementation, glandular therapy, and the use of plant-based medicines.

**Psychoneuroimmunology** is the term used to describe the interactions between the emotional state, nervous system function, and the immune system. The growing body of knowledge documenting the mind's profound influence on physiology in health and disease necessitates stress management. Stress increases corticosteroid and catecholamine, which at high levels are immunosuppressive. Lymphocytes, monocytes, macrophages, and granulocytes have receptor sites for the many regulating hormones and neurotransmitters of the hypothalamic-pituitary-adrenal and the sympathetic-adrenal medullary axes. Alterations in these compounds lead to disruption of cellular trafficking, proliferation, cytokine secretion, antibody production, and cytolytic activity. For example, glucocorticoids inhibit the production of interleukin (IL)-12, interferon, tumor necrosis factor-alpha, and type 1 helper T (Th1) cells but upregulate the production of IL-4, IL-10, and IL-13 by Th2 cells. In addition to glucocorticoids, the catecholamines also play a role in stress-induced immune dysfunction.

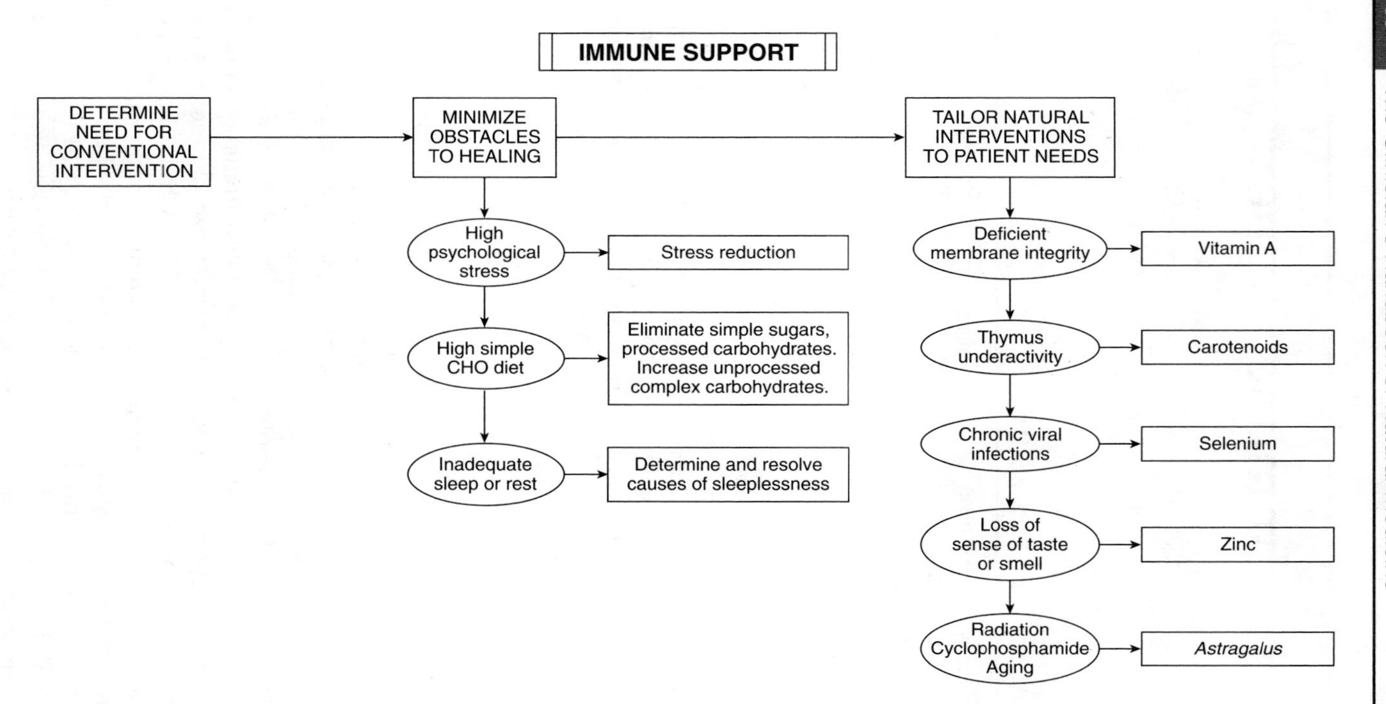
IMMUNE SUPPORT
DETERMINE NEED FOR CONVENTIONAL INTERVENTION
MINIMIZE OBSTACLES TO HEALING
TAILOR NATURAL INTERVENTIONS TO PATIENT NEEDS
High psychological stress
Stress reduction
High simple CHO diet
Eliminate simple sugars, processed carbohydrates. Increase unprocessed complex carbohydrates.
Inadequate sleep or rest
Determine and resolve causes of sleeplessness
Deficient membrane integrity
Vitamin A
Thymus underactivity
Carotenoids
Chronic viral infections
Selenium
Loss of sense of taste or smell
Zinc
Radiation Cyclophosphamide Aging
Astragalus

## THERAPEUTIC CONSIDERATIONS

### Lifestyle

Many lifestyle behaviors substantially affect immune function. Smoking suppresses immune function, as do irregular meals, simple carbohydrate consumption, excess weight, excessive alcohol consumption, inadequate sleep, and inactivity.

### Diet

Consistent with good health, optimal immune function requires a healthy diet rich in whole, natural foods such as fruits, vegetables, grains, beans, seeds, and nuts; low in fats and refined sugars; and contains adequate, but not excessive, amounts of protein.

The oral administration of 100-g portions of carbohydrate as glucose, fructose, sucrose, honey, or orange juice significantly reduces neutrophil phagocytosis, but starch has no effect. Increases of cholesterol, free fatty acids, triglycerides, and bile acids inhibit various immune functions.

Alcohol increases the susceptibility to experimental infections in animals, and alcoholics are known to be more susceptible to infections, especially pneumonia. Studies of immune function in alcoholism show a profound depression in most parameters of immunity.

### Nutrients

- **Vitamin A**: plays an essential role in maintaining the integrity of the epithelial and mucosal surfaces and their secretions. These systems constitute a primary nonspecific host defense mechanism. Vitamin A has been shown to stimulate and/or enhance numerous immune processes, including induction of cell-mediated cytotoxicity against tumors, natural killer cell activity, lymphocyte blastogenesis, mononuclear phagocytosis, and antibody response.
- **Carotenes**: have demonstrated a number of immune-enhancing effects. In addition to being converted into vitamin A, carotenes function as antioxidants. Because the thymus gland is so susceptible to damage by free radicals, beta-carotene may be more advantageous in enhancing the immune system than retinol.
- **Vitamin C**: ascorbic acid plays an important role in immune enhancement. Although vitamin C has been shown to be antiviral and antibacterial, its main effect is by improvement in host resistance. Many immunostimulatory effects have been demonstrated,

including enhancing lymphoproliferative response to mitogens and lymphotrophic activity and increasing interferon levels, antibody responses, immunoglobulin levels, secretion of thymic hormones, and integrity of ground substance. Vitamin C also has direct biochemical effects similar to those of interferon.

- **Vitamin E**: enhances both humoral immunity and cell-mediated immunity. A vitamin E deficiency results in lymphoid atrophy and decreases of lymphoproliferative response to mitogens, splenic plaque-forming colonies, antibody response, and monocyte function. Vitamin E supplementation (30-150 IU) has been shown to increase lymphoproliferative response to mitogens; prevent free radical–induced thymus atrophy; enhance helper T-cell activity; and increase splenic plaque-forming colonies, serum immunoglobulins, antibody response, peripheral mononuclear phagocytosis, and reticuloendothelial system activity.
- **Iron**: iron deficiency is a commonly encountered isolated nutritional deficiency that causes immune dysfunction in large numbers of patients. Marginal iron deficiency, even at levels that do not lower hemoglobin values, can influence the immune system. Lymphoid tissue atrophy, decreased lymphoproliferative response to mitogens, defective macrophage and neutrophil function, and decreased T-cell/B-cell ratios are common experimental and clinical findings.
- **Zinc**: zinc serves a vital role in many immune system reactions. It promotes the binding of complement to immune complex, acts as a protectant against iron-catalyzed damage by free radicals, acts synergistically with vitamin A, is required for lymphocyte transformation, acts independently on lymphocytes as a mitogen, and is a necessary cofactor in activating serum thymic factor. In vitro, zinc inhibits the growth of several viruses, including rhinoviruses, picornaviruses, togaviruses, herpes simplex virus, and vaccinia virus.
- **Selenium**: in its vital role in glutathione peroxidase, selenium affects all components of the immune system, including the development and expression of all white blood cells (WBCs). Selenium deficiency results in depression of immune function, whereas selenium supplementation results in augmentation and/or restoration of immune functions. Selenium deficiency has been found to inhibit resistance to infection through impairment of WBCs and thymus function, whereas selenium supplementation (100-200 μg/day) has been shown to stimulate WBC and thymus function.

## Botanical Medicines

- ***Echinacea***: the two most widely used species are *Echinacea angustifolia* and *Echinacea purpurea*. Both have been shown to exert profound immune-enhancing effects. One of the most important immune-stimulating components of *Echinacea* are large polysaccharides, such as inulin, that activate the alternative complement pathway (one of the immune system's nonspecific defense mechanisms) and increase the production of immune chemicals that activate macrophages. The result is increased activity of many key immune parameters: production of T-cells, macrophage phagocytosis, antibody binding, natural killer cell activity, and levels of circulating neutrophils.

  *Echinacea* strengthens the immune system even in healthy people. For example, in a study of healthy volunteers aged 25 to 40 years, the fresh-pressed juice of *E. purpurea* extract was found to increase the phagocytosis of *Candida albicans* by 30% to 40%; it also enhanced the migration of WBCs to the scene of battle by 30% to 40%.

  Besides immune support, *Echinacea* also exerts direct antiviral activity and helps prevent the spread of bacteria by inhibiting a bacterial enzyme *hyaluronidase*. This enzyme is secreted by bacteria to break through the body's first line of defense, the protective membranes such as the skin or mucous membranes.
- ***Panax ginseng***: ginseng has been shown to exert immunomodulating activity, as evidenced by its ability to enhance antibody plaque-forming cell response, circulatory antibody titer against sheep erythrocytes, cell-mediated immunity, natural killer cell activity, production of interferon, lymphocyte mitogenesis, and reticuloendothelial system proliferative and phagocytic functions.
- ***Astragalus***: the root of *Astragalus* is a traditional Chinese medicine used for viral infections. Clinical studies in China have shown it to be effective when used prophylactically against the common cold. It also has been shown to reduce the duration and severity of symptoms in acute treatment of the common cold as well as raise WBC counts in persons with chronic leukopenia. Research in animals has shown that *Astragalus* apparently works by enhancing phagocytic activity of monocytes and macrophages, increasing interferon production and natural killer cell activity, improving T-cell activity, and potentiating other antiviral mechanisms. *Astragalus* appears particularly useful in cases in which

the immune system has been damaged by chemicals or radiation. In immunodepressed mice, *Astragalus* has been found to reverse the T-cell abnormalities caused by cyclophosphamide, radiation, and aging. As with *Echinacea*, the polysaccharides contained in the root of *Astragalus membranaceus* contribute to the immune-enhancing effects.

## THERAPEUTIC APPROACH

A major challenge is to determine which intervention is the key to reactivating or supporting a patient's immune system. The regimen provided is meant as a general approach and must be tailored to the patient's specific needs to maximize the desired effects and limit unnecessary treatment.

### General Measures

- Rest (bed rest better).
- Drink large amount of fluids (preferably diluted vegetable juices, soups, and herb teas).
- Limit simple sugar consumption (including fruit sugars) to less than 50 g/day.

### Supplements

- **High-potency multivitamin and mineral formula**
- **Vitamin C**: 500 mg q2h
- **Bioflavonoids**: 1000 mg/day
- **Vitamin A**: 5000 IU/day or beta-carotene 25,000 IU/day
- **Zinc**: 30 mg/day

### Botanicals

All dosages of botanicals should be given three times per day.

- ***Echinacea* spp.**
  —Dried root (or as tea): 0.5 to 1 g
  —Freeze-dried plant: 325 to 650 mg
  —Juice of aerial portion of *E. purpurea* stabilized in 22% ethanol: 2 to 3 mL
  —Tincture (1:5): 2 to 4 mL
  —Fluid extract (1:1): 2 to 4 mL
  —Solid (dry powdered) extract (6.5:1 or 3.5% echinacoside): 150 to 300 mg
- ***Panax ginseng***: the appropriate dose of ginseng depends on the ginsenoside content; if an extract or ginseng preparation contains

high concentrations of ginsenosides (and presumably other active components), a lower dose will suffice. The standard dose for high-quality ginseng root is in the range of 4 to 6 g daily. For ginseng root extract containing 5% ginsenosides, the dose is typically 100 mg one to three times daily.

- ***Astragalus membranaceus***
  —Dried root (or as decoction): 1 to 2 g
  —Tincture (1:5): 2 to 4 mL
  —Fluid extract (1:1): 2 to 4 mL
  —Solid (dry powdered) extract (0.5% 4-hydroxy-3-methoxy isoflavone): 100 to 150 mg

# Infectious Diarrhea

## DIAGNOSTIC SUMMARY

- Increased bowel movement frequency (usually more than three bowel movements per day)
- Increased stool liquidity
- Abdominal pain
- Sense of fecal urgency
- Fecal incontinence
- Perianal discomfort
- Possible blood and/or mucus in stool

## GENERAL CONSIDERATIONS

Clinical syndromes of diarrheal disease are acute watery diarrhea, bloody diarrhea, and persistent diarrhea. Features include daily stool production of >250 g containing 70% to 95% water. More than 14 L of fluid may be lost daily in severe cases. Dysentery is defined by low volume, pain, and bloody stool. Diarrheal illness commonly causes morbidity and mortality. Intestinal infection is most common cause of diarrhea worldwide, killing 3 to 4 million persons annually, most of whom (2 million) are preschool children. Ninety percent of acute cases are mild, self-limited, and responsive within 5 days to simple rehydration or antidiarrheal agents.

## INFECTIOUS AGENTS AND SYMPTOMS

Categories of etiologic pathogens are viral, bacterial, and parasitic. Diarrhea arises from inhibition of intestinal absorption, increased secretion, and inflammatory response to promote secretory and exudative response.

### Viral Agents

In healthy adults, clinical manifestation is acute, self-limited gastroenteritis. Twenty-five different bacteria and protozoa can cause an identical clinical syndrome; >75% of diarrhea-associated cases

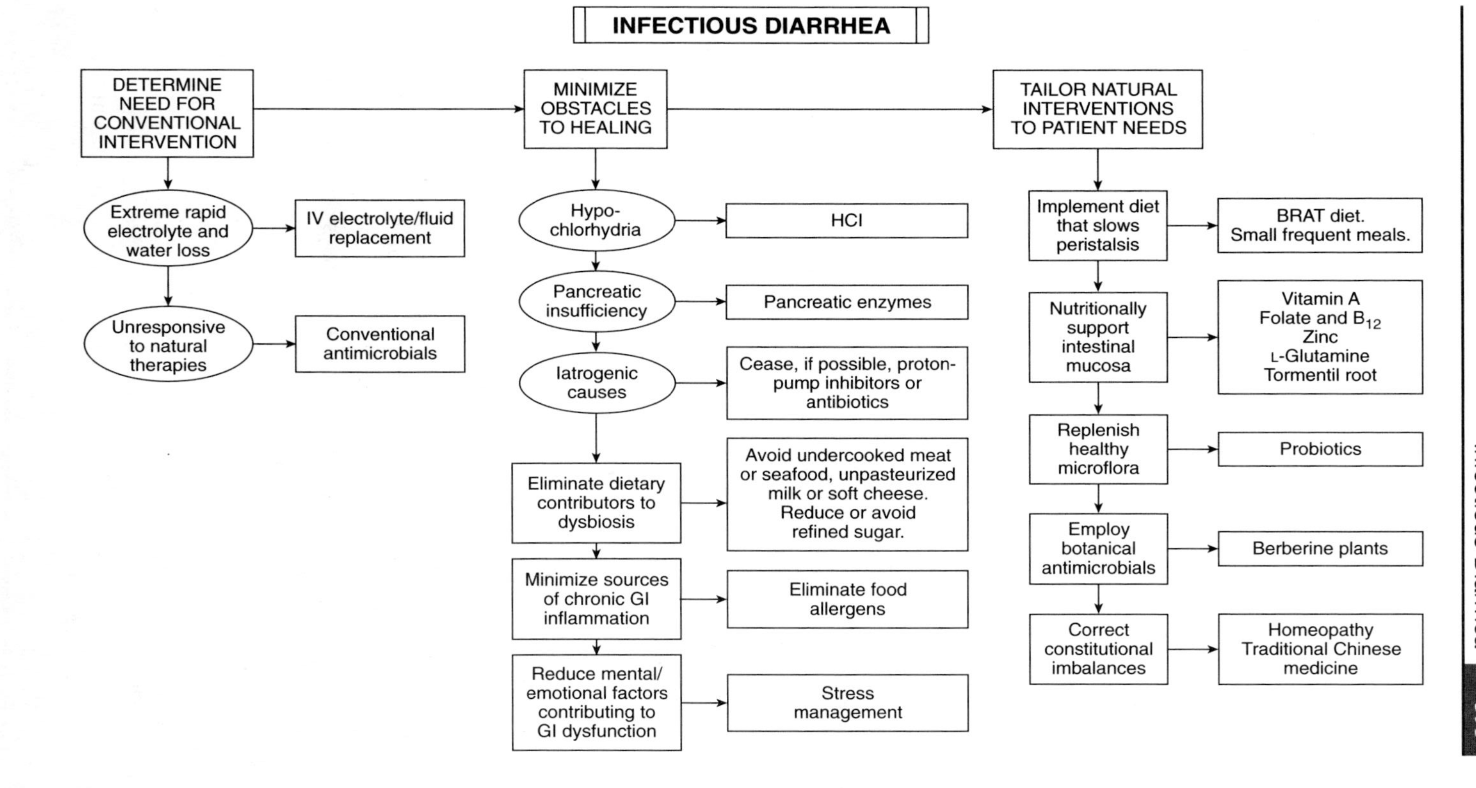
INFECTIOUS DIARRHEA
DETERMINE NEED FOR CONVENTIONAL INTERVENTION
Extreme rapid electrolyte and water loss
IV electrolyte/fluid replacement
Unresponsive to natural therapies
Conventional antimicrobials
MINIMIZE OBSTACLES TO HEALING
Hypo-chlorhydria
HCl
Pancreatic insufficiency
Pancreatic enzymes
Iatrogenic causes
Cease, if possible, proton-pump inhibitors or antibiotics
Eliminate dietary contributors to dysbiosis
Avoid undercooked meat or seafood, unpasteurized milk or soft cheese. Reduce or avoid refined sugar.
Minimize sources of chronic GI inflammation
Eliminate food allergens
Reduce mental/emotional factors contributing to GI dysfunction
Stress management
TAILOR NATURAL INTERVENTIONS TO PATIENT NEEDS
Implement diet that slows peristalsis
BRAT diet. Small frequent meals.
Nutritionally support intestinal mucosa
Vitamin A
Folate and $B_{12}$
Zinc
L-Glutamine
Tormentil root
Replenish healthy microflora
Probiotics
Employ botanical antimicrobials
Berberine plants
Correct constitutional imbalances
Homeopathy
Traditional Chinese medicine

of gastroenteritis are caused by viruses. Suspect viruses when vomiting is prominent, incubation period is >14 hours, entire illness is over in <72 hours, no warning signs of bacterial infection are present (high fever, bloody diarrhea, severe abdominal pain, more than six stools per 24 hours), and no epidemiologic clues can be gleaned from the history (e.g., travel, sexual contact, antibiotic use).

- **Rotavirus**: ubiquitous agent of acute, dehydrating diarrhea in children that causes >800,000 annual deaths of young children in developing countries. Disease is seasonal (in the United States, it begins in autumn and ends in spring in the southwest and northeast). Transmission is by the fecal-oral route, including person to person. Virions infect villous enterocytes of the small intestine, causing watery diarrhea, fever, and vomiting.
- **Parvovirus (Norwalk virus)**: caliciviruses (Norwalk-like viruses or small, round-structured viruses) cause 66% of 13.8 million cases of food-related illnesses in the United States annually. Suspect these viruses when acute gastroenteritis sweeps a semi-closed community (e.g., family, school, residential home, hospital, ship, dormitory). Transmission is by contaminated food or water or person to person. Sources of outbreaks include well water, raspberries, lunchmeat, oysters. Symptoms are nausea and vomiting, diarrhea, abdominal cramping, headache, low-grade fever, malaise, myalgias.
- **Cytomegalovirus**: presents latently in most people from birth or from sexual or parenteral exposure. It emerges from latency as a result of strong allergenic or antigenic stimulation of the immune system or severe immunodeficiency. Viral activity in the bowel wall triggers gastrointestinal disease in AIDS, transplantation, and cancer chemotherapy.
- **Epstein-Barr virus (EBV)**: almost all adults are infected by age 20 years. It infects B-cells and persists for life because B-cells proliferate indefinitely. Proliferation is controlled by virus-specific cytotoxic T-lymphocytes. EBV causes diarrhea in immunocompromised patients.

## Bacterial Agents

- ***Escherichia coli***: four varieties of diarrheogenic *E. coli* are enterotoxigenic, enterohemorrhagic, enteroinvasive, enteroadherent. In North America the most prominent is the enterohemorrhagic serotype *E. coli* O157:H7. Transmission is by contaminated ground beef. Incubation period is 1 to 8 days. Symptoms are abdominal cramping and diarrhea—mild, moderate, or severe. Bowel movements begin as loose and watery, eventually with gross blood. Some patients (children) develop life-threatening hemolytic-uremic syndrome, characterized by triad of hemolytic anemia, renal failure, and thrombocytopenia.

- ***Campylobacter jejuni***: native intestinal flora of many mammals. Transmission is by contaminated, improperly cooked meat, unpasteurized dairy, and contaminated water. Incubation period is 1 to 7 days after ingestion. Symptoms include fever, headache, and malaise followed by diarrhea and abdominal cramps within 1 to 2 days. Stools are watery to bloody. *Campylobacter* enterocolitis is usually acute and self-limited over 7 to 10 days. Rarely relapses, complications, severe disease, and death may occur.
- ***Clostridium difficile***: most common cause of infectious diarrhea in hospitalized patients, especially the elderly. It can be catalyzed by antibiotics.
- ***Salmonella* (Enterobacteriaceae)**: has 2200 known serotypes (*Salmonella enteritidis* in 85% of all *Salmonella* cases in the United States; *Salmonella typhi* and *Salmonella paratyphi,* which are responsible for typhoid fever). Transmission is by contaminated food. Symptoms of nontyphoid salmonellosis include fever, gastroenteritis-related diarrhea, localized infections of the gastrointestinal tract, endothelium, pericardium, meninges, lungs, joints, bones, urinary tract, or soft tissues. Typhoidal symptoms include gradual onset of fever, headache, arthralgias, pharyngitis, constipation, anorexia, and abdominal discomfort.
- ***Shigella* (Enterobacteriaceae)**: ingesting as few as 10 organisms may cause clinical disease. Transmission is by contaminated food or water, person to person, and flies. Incubation period is 1 to 4 days. Adult symptoms are nonbloody diarrhea with or without fever, gripping abdominal pain, urgency, relief with defecation. Episodes may increase, with mucus and blood in stool. Mild cases often spontaneously resolve in 4 to 8 days; 3 to 6 weeks may be necessary in severe cases.
- ***Yersinia enterocolitica* (Enterobacteriaceae)**: one of the less-frequent causes of bacterial enterocolitis in North America. Transmission is by fecally contaminated food or water and contaminated blood products. Incubation is 4 to 7 days. Symptoms are watery to bloody diarrhea. *Yersinia* invades lymphoid tissues, causing mesenteric lymphadenitis that mimics acute appendi-

citis. Resolution is 1 to 4 weeks, but complicating septicemia may develop in patients with underlying disease.
- ***Laribacter hongkongensis***: a novel genus and species first isolated recently from blood and empyema pus of cirrhotic patient with bacteremic empyema thoracis. It was also identified in six diarrhea patients in Hong Kong and Switzerland.

### Parasitic Agents

Diarrheal diseases caused by parasites (protozoa, helminths) are the greatest single worldwide cause of illness and death. Poor sanitation in undeveloped nations, worldwide travel, and migration to the United States are the most common cause of spread.

- ***Giardia lamblia***: most frequent cause of parasitic enteritis in the United States with history of recent hiking and drinking out of streams.
- **Waterborne infection**: in developed nations from domestic water contaminated with cysts of *Giardia intestinalis* and *Cryptosporidium parvum*.
- **Other diarrhea-linked parasites**: *Entamoeba histolytica, Microsporidia, Isospora belli, Strongyloides* spp.
- **Symptoms**: abdominal pain, cramping, explosive diarrhea, but not in every case. They can be milder. Some cases of irritable bowel syndrome, indigestion, and poor digestion are caused by parasites. Parasites are an unsuspected cause of chronic illness and fatigue.

## LAB DIAGNOSIS

- Tests include bacterial cultures using selective media, detection of pathogen-specific genes using polymerase chain reaction, electron microscopy and antigen detection for viruses, and direct examination with or without special stains for protozoa.
- Microbial cause is identified in only 50% of patients. In descending order, the most commonly identified pathogens are *Campylobacter jejuni, Salmonella, Shigella, E. coli* O157:H7.
- Important independent variables predictive of positive stool culture in adult patients with clinical picture of infectious diarrhea: month of presentation, fever, duration of abdominal pain at presentation, and requirement of intravenous fluid therapy. Neither a history of bloody diarrhea nor persistent diarrhea is associated with positive stool culture.

- Consider testing if patient is febrile or has bloody stool. With visible blood present in stool, one third of cases were caused by Shiga toxin-producing *E. coli* O157:H7.
- Ova and parasite testing has very low yield in most cases; run only in cases where diarrheal illness persists for more than 7 days.

## THERAPEUTIC CONSIDERATIONS

### Conventional Medicines

- Antibiotics and opiates are appropriate in certain cases but adversely affect gastrointestinal motility. Resistance to antimicrobials, with risk of worsened illness (hemolytic uremic syndrome with Shiga toxin-producing *E. coli* O157:H7), complicates antimicrobial and antimotility drug use, especially in children.
- Selective antibiotics treat traveler's diarrhea, shigellosis, and *Campylobacter*.
- Bismuth salts (e.g., Pepto-Bismol), for travel abroad; they coat the intestinal lining and help prevent infection.
- Antibiotic therapy in salmonellosis and *E. coli* O157:H7 remains unclear.
- Avoid antimotility agents in bloody diarrhea, especially for *E. coli* O157:H7, which could increase risk of subsequent hemolytic-uremic syndrome. In selected at-risk populations, vaccines, including oral typhoid vaccine and cholera (available only outside the United States), are recommended.
- 5-$HT_2$ and 5-$HT_3$ receptor antagonists, calcium-calmodulin antagonists, and alpha-receptor agonists may avoid adverse affects on gastrointestinal motility.

### Underlying and Predisposing Factors

Host factors that predispose illness:

- Poor digestive function, including low stomach acid and/or achlorhydria and inadequate pancreatic enzymes. Hydrochloric acid and pancreatic enzymes may be advisable.
- Immunoglobulin A (IgA) antibodies discourage epithelial adherence of pathogens. Depressed secretory IgA weakens gastrointestinal immunity. Decreased intestinal motility, caused by chronic stress and high sugar intake, allows microbes to fester. Food allergy or sensitivity encourages recurrent infectious diarrhea.

- Some pharmaceuticals increase susceptibility to infectious diarrhea: proton pump inhibitors, anti-folate drugs, and antibiotics. Hospitalized patients taking proton pump inhibitors have increased risk of *Clostridium difficile* diarrhea. Drug inhibition of stomach acid allows pathogens and undigested food to reach intestines without proper processing. Broad-spectrum antibiotics are associated with diarrhea. Antibiotics disrupt local bowel flora, allowing pathogens to flourish. (see the following section on probiotics).

## Hydration/Electrolyte Balance

- Keep diarrhea patient well hydrated; ensure electrolyte replenishment, especially in children.
- Signs of dehydration: decreased or absent urination, decreased skin turgor, dry tongue.
- Rehydrate with solutions of glucose, sodium, and potassium.
- Intravenous rehydration: severe dehydration with weight loss of >10% or unconsciousness.

## Diet

- Prevention: avoid undercooked meat or seafood, unpasteurized milk, and soft cheese.
- BRAT diet (binding foods that slow peristalsis) helps decrease gastrointestinal motility: bananas, white rice, apples, plain white toast, or bread and tea.
- Larger, less-frequent meals are more taxing to gastrointestinal digestive and absorptive capacities, prolong diarrhea, advance colonization by hemolytic enteropathogenic *E. coli*, and prolong shedding of rotavirus. Dividing same nutrient intake into small, equal portions eaten at regular intervals produces less-severe response.
- Traditional preparations for diarrhea (carrot soup, rice) are absorbent and reduce stool output and duration of diarrhea but may not diminish loss of water and electrolytes.
- For vomiting patients, small amounts of glucose can help.

## Supplements

- **Vitamin A**: 60 mg can reduce incidence of persistent diarrhea in children without changing duration or average stool frequency. Children who are not breastfed have shorter duration of diarrhea. Mean number of stools passed, proportion of episodes lasting >14 days, and percentage of children passing watery stools were lower in those treated with vitamin A.

- **Folic acid and $B_{12}$**: low levels of folic acid and vitamin $B_{12}$ correlate with increased susceptibility to diarrhea. Folate deficiency promotes malabsorption because of altered structure of intestinal mucosal cells—inflammation, atrophy, erosion, flattening of villi, lymphatic ectasia, and focal fibrosis. Anti-folate chemotherapeutic drugs (methotrexate) induce folate and $B_{12}$ deficiency, triggering diarrhea. Supplements reduce toxicity and abolish treatment-related deaths without affecting drug efficacy. Gastrointestinal disturbances (diarrhea) reduce availability of folate and $B_{12}$ to pregnant mother and fetus, increasing risk of birth defects. One or more episodes of periconceptional diarrhea increase risk of neural tube defect, independent of fever, obesity, maternal age, maternal birthplace, income, prior unproductive pregnancy, and dietary plus multivitamin folate intake. Regardless of cause of diarrhea, ensure proper folic acid and $B_{12}$ nutrition in women likely to conceive and pregnant women. Be aware that large amounts of folic acid can mask nerve damage associated with vitamin $B_{12}$ deficiency.
- **Zinc (Zn)**: diarrhea is a clinical manifestation of zinc deficiency. Zinc has antimicrobial effect on enteric pathogens (*Salmonella typhi, Salmonella, E. coli, Enterobacter, Shigella, Staphylococcus albus, Streptococcus pyogenes, Vibrio cholerae*) and may be a tool to treat diarrhea. Zinc absorption occurs throughout the small intestine, not only in the duodenum, jejunum, and ileum. Many illnesses noted for chronic diarrhea (celiac disease, cystic fibrosis) entail malabsorption of zinc. Dietary sources of Zn include meat, fish, and human milk. Acrodermatitis enteropathica (skin lesions, chronic diarrhea, recurring infections) is related to intestinal malabsorption of zinc and treated with pharmacologic doses of oral zinc. Factors influencing zinc absorption are dietary fiber and phytates (in soy, wheat bran, peas, carob, brown rice), which inhibit absorption; picolinic and citric acid facilitate it. Citric acid is the ligand linked to high bioavailability of zinc in human milk. CAUTION: Some dietary treatments for persistent postenteritis diarrhea (elimination of cow's milk, increasing fiber, carob powder, soy formula in infants) can contribute to zinc deficiency and promote persistency of diarrhea itself. Supplement zinc during diarrhea.
- **L-Glutamine**: most abundant amino acid in blood and major fuel of intestinal mucosal cells; readily available in diet and synthe-

sized in body. Supplementation improves metabolism of mucosa, stimulating regeneration. Glutamine prevents mucosal damage and decreases bacterial leakage across mucosal membranes, after damage, by stimulating repair. Applicability: enhancing repair of mucosal injury by infections, toxic agents, malnutrition, or chemotherapy- or radiation-induced enteritis. Glutamine enhances sodium and water absorption in animal models of infectious diarrhea. At dose of 0.3 g/kg/day, glutamine shortens duration of diarrhea in children. Even at high doses, it is without side effects and is well tolerated. Typical dosage is 1000 mg t.i.d. (*Textbook,* "Glutamine").

## Probiotics: *Lactobacillus* and *Saccharomyces*

- Species: *Lactobacillus acidophilus* and *Bifidobacterium bifidum* (plus *Lactobacillus casei, Lactobacillus fermentum, Lactobacillus salivarius, Lactobacillus brevis*). (See *Textbook,* "Probiotics.")
- Probiotics protect against acute diarrheal disease and treat or prevent infectious diarrhea: rotavirus, *Clostridium difficile,* traveler's diarrhea. They may prevent future nosocomial rotaviral gastorenteritis with immune-modulating effect of increasing number of cells secreting IgA.
- *Lactobacillus* species inhibit *E. coli* O157 : H7 but not *Salmonella* in refrigerated storage.
- Children are especially susceptible to infectious diarrhea and its sequelae. Supplementing formula with *B. bifidum* and *Streptococcus thermophilus* dramatically reduces risk of developing diarrhea and rotavirus shedding. Probiotics may provide protective effects similar to breast milk to prevent infection. *Lactobacillus* GG may reduce risk of nosocomial diarrhea and rotavirus gastroenteritis in children.
- *Saccromyces boulardii (Saccromyces cerevisiae)* is a nonpathogenic probiotic yeast helpful in diarrhea *of Clostridium difficile* affecting the elderly. Vancomycin is conventional treatment in severe cases. But *Saccharomyces boulardii,* alone or in combination with vancomycin, is effective for recurrent infection. Fungemia and sepsis are rare complications of *S. boulardii* in immunocompromised patients and may be contraindicated. Daily adult dose is 1 g in divided doses (500 mg b.i.d.) for 4+ weeks.
- Probiotics reduce the risk of antibiotic-induced diarrhea and reduce hospital stay from diarrhea. *L. acidophilus* corrects increase of gram-negative bacteria after broad-spectrum antibiotics, which occurs with any acute or chronic diarrhea. Mixture of

*B. bifidum and L. acidophilus* inhibits lowering of fecal flora induced by ampicillin and maintains equilibrium of intestinal ecosystem.

- Use of *L. acidophilus* during antibiotic therapy may prevent reductions of friendly bacteria and/or superinfection with antibiotic-resistant flora. Dosage is 15 to 20 billion organisms. Take probiotics as far away from antibiotics as possible.
- Antibiotics should be used only in cases in which benefits outweigh risks; adjunctive therapy may decrease untoward effects of antibiotics on gastrointestinal system.
- Choose only high-quality, lab-tested probiotics.

## Botanical Medicines

### Berberine-Containing Plants

- Goldenseal (*Hydrastis canadensis*), barberry (*Berberis vulgaris*), Oregon grape (*Berberis aquifolium*), and goldthread (*Coptis chinensis*) contain broad-spectrum antibiotic alkaloid berberine, effective against bacteria, protozoa, and fungi, including *Candida albicans.*
- Berberine's action against some pathogens is stronger than common antibiotics. Berberine prevents overgrowth of yeast. Berberine has remarkable antidiarrheal activity in even severe cases of cholera, amebiasis, giardiasis, *E. coli, Shigella, Salmonella, Klebsiella,* and chronic candidiasis.
- Dosing is based on berberine content. Standardized extracts are preferred. Dosage (t.i.d.):
  —Dried root or as infusion (tea): 2-4 g
  —Tincture (1:5): 6-12 mL (1.5-3 tsp)
  —Fluid extract (1:1): 2-4 mL (0.5-1 tsp)
  —Solid (powdered dry) extract (4:1 or 8%-12% alkaloid content): 250–500 mg
  —Note: Dosage recommendations for berberine are 25-50 mg t.i.d. or daily up to 150 mg for adults. For children, dose is based on body weight. Daily dosage: 5-10 mg berberine/kg (2.2 pounds) body weight.
- Berberine and berberine-containing plants are nontoxic at recommended dosages, but avoid during pregnancy. Higher dosages may interfere with B vitamin metabolism.

### *Potentilla tormentilla* (Tormentil Root)

- Contains >15% tannic acid, an astringent to treat infectious diarrhea, shorten rotavirus diarrhea, and decrease requirement for rehydration solutions.

- Dosing in children: 3 drops tormentil root extract per year of life t.i.d. until diarrhea ends or a maximum of 5 days.
- Dosing for adults: 60 drops of tincture b.i.d.
- Powdered herb may be more effective. Dosage: ¼ teaspoon b.i.d. for adults.

### Other Antiparasitic Botanicals

Future studies should evaluate potential benefits and toxicities of these antiparasitic herbs: *Artemisia absinthium* (wormwood), *Chenopodium abrosioides* (wormseed), *Curcuma longa* (tumeric), *Phytolacca decandra* (pokeweed, pokeroot), *Juglans* spp. (black and white walnut), and *Tanacetum vulgare* (tansy).

## THERAPEUTIC APPROACH

Natural treatments can manage most cases of non-life-threatening diarrhea. Diarrhea itself is an eliminative function that clears toxins and should not be completely suppressed. Chronic diarrhea and diarrhea causing extreme or rapid electrolyte and water loss may require conventional interventions. Maintain hydration and electrolyte balance, especially in children younger than 5 years.

Address the following underlying factors:

- Low stomach and pancreatic output; depressed IgA.
- Eliminate iatrogenic causes (proton pump inhibitors and antibiotics) if possible.
- Reduce refined sugar.
- Eliminate food allergens.
- Reduce and manage stress.

Monitor closely by standard lab methods (e.g., repeat multiple stool samples 2 weeks after initiation of therapy).

Diet: BRAT diet to discourage large volume loss in infectious diarrhea. Very small frequent meals, hourly if possible.

### Nutritional Supplements

The following dosages are for adults unless otherwise indicated:

- **Vitamin A**: 60 mg q.d. in children; up to 50,000 IU q.d. for 1 to 2 days for adults with infections. Beware doses >10,000 IU q.d. in pregnant women.
- **Folic acid**: 1 mg q.d.

- **$B_{12}$ (cyanocobalamin)**: 600-1000 μg q.d.
- **Zinc picolinate**: 30 mg q.d.
- **L-Glutamine**: 1000 mg t.i.d.
- ***Lactobacillus***: 6 billion CFU of *Lactobacillus* GG b.i.d. To prevent antibiotic-induced diarrhea: at least 15-20 billion organisms. Take as far away from antibiotic as possible. In children younger than 6 years with antibiotic-induced diarrhea, give probiotic every day of antibiotic dosing and continue for 1 week after discontinuing antibiotic.
- ***Saccharomyces bucardia***: for *Clostridium difficile* specifically. Daily adult dose: 1 g q.d. in divided doses (500 mg b.i.d.) for at least 4 weeks. Can be used adjunctively with vancomycin.

## Botanicals

- **Berberine**: 25-50 mg t.i.d. or daily dosage up to 150 mg. For children, dose is based on body weight: 5-10 mg berberine/kg (2.2 pounds) body weight.
- **Tormentil**: 60 drops tincture b.i.d. or powdered herb: ¼ teaspoon b.i.d. Children: 3 drops tormentil root extract per year of life t.i.d. until discontinuation of diarrhea, or maximum of 5 days.

# Inflammatory Bowel Disease

## DIAGNOSTIC SUMMARY

- Intermittent bouts of diarrhea, low-grade fever, and right lower quadrant pain
- Anorexia, weight loss, flatulence, and malaise
- Abdominal tenderness, especially right lower quadrant, with signs of peritoneal irritation and an abdominal or pelvic mass
- Radiographs show abnormality of terminal ileum
- Ulcerative colitis
- Bloody diarrhea with cramps in lower abdomen
- Mild abdominal tenderness, weight loss, and fever
- Rectal examination may show perianal irritation, fissures, hemorrhoids, fistulas, and abscesses
- Diagnosis confirmed by radiograph and sigmoidoscopy

## GENERAL CONSIDERATIONS

### Definition

Inflammatory bowel disease (IBD) is a general term for a group of chronic inflammatory disorders of the bowel. The two major categories are Crohn's disease and ulcerative colitis. IBD is characterized by recurrent inflammatory involvement of specific intestinal segments, resulting in diverse clinical manifestations.

- **Crohn's disease (CD)**: lesions are a granulomatous inflammatory reaction throughout entire thickness of bowel wall. In 40% of cases, granulomas are either poorly developed or totally absent. May involve buccal mucosa, esophagus, stomach, duodenum, jejunum, ileum, and colon. Crohn's disease of small intestine is called "regional enteritis"; colon involvement is called "Crohn's disease of the colon" or "granulomatous colitis" (only a portion of patients develop granulomatous lesions).
- **Ulcerative colitis (UC)**: Lesions are a nonspecific inflammatory response limited to colonic mucosa and submucosa. Well-developed granuloma formation does not occur.

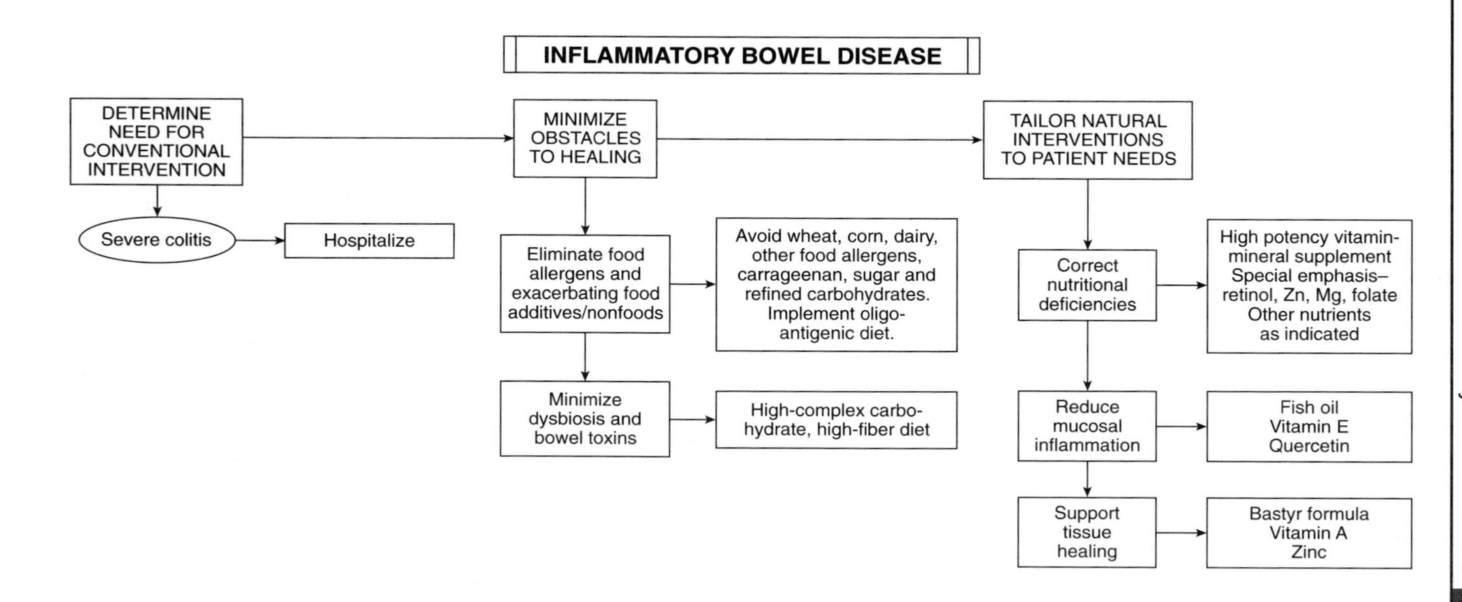
INFLAMMATORY BOWEL DISEASE
DETERMINE NEED FOR CONVENTIONAL INTERVENTION
Severe colitis
Hospitalize
MINIMIZE OBSTACLES TO HEALING
Eliminate food allergens and exacerbating food additives/nonfoods
Avoid wheat, corn, dairy, other food allergens, carrageenan, sugar and refined carbohydrates. Implement oligo-antigenic diet.
Minimize dysbiosis and bowel toxins
High-complex carbo-hydrate, high-fiber diet
TAILOR NATURAL INTERVENTIONS TO PATIENT NEEDS
Correct nutritional deficiencies
High potency vitamin-mineral supplement Special emphasis– retinol, Zn, Mg, folate Other nutrients as indicated
Reduce mucosal inflammation
Fish oil Vitamin E Quercetin
Support tissue healing
Bastyr formula Vitamin A Zinc

Common features shared by Crohn's disease and ulcerative colitis:

- Colon is frequently involved in Crohn's and invariably involved in UC.
- Although rare, patients with UC and total colon involvement may develop "backwash ileitis"; both conditions may cause changes in small intestine.
- Patients with CD often have close relatives with UC and vice versa.
- When no granuloma in CD of the colon, the two lesions may resemble each other clinically and pathologically.
- Many epidemiologic similarities exist between CD and UC: age, race, sex, and geographic distribution.
- Both conditions are associated with similar extraintestinal manifestations.
- The two conditions have etiologic parallels.
- Both conditions are associated with increased frequency of colonic carcinoma.

## Etiology

UC is more common. The incidence of UC in western Europe and the United States is six to eight cases per 100,000 and prevalence is 7-150 cases per 100,000. The incidence of CD is two cases per 100,000 and prevalence is 20-40 per 100,000. The incidence of CD is increasing in Western cultures. IBD may occur at any age but most often from ages 15 to 35 years. Women are affected slightly more frequently than men. Whites are two to five times more affected than African Americans or Asians. Jews have threefold to sixfold higher incidence compared with non-Jews. Theories about etiology of IBD include the following:

- **Genetic predisposition**: supported by ethnic distribution of incidence and multiple members of a family having CD or UC in 15%-40% of cases.
- **Infectious etiology**: The idea that a transmissible agent is responsible for IBD is a hotly debated subject. Viruses (rotavirus, Epstein–Barr virus, cytomegalovirus, and an uncharacterized RNA intestinal cytopathic virus) and mycobacteria continue to be favored candidates. Gastrointestinal (GI) infections with *Aeromonas* bacteria (*A. sobria* and *A. hydrophila*) and *Candida albi-*

*cans* can initiate and perpetuate colitis. Test all IBD patients for these infections at start of and during course of illness. Other candidates include pseudomonas-like organisms, enteric anaerobes, *Chlamydia*, and *Yersinia enterocolitica*.

- **Antibiotic exposure**: before the 1950s, CD was found in selected groups with strong genetic component. Since then, a rapid increase has occurred in developed countries and countries that previously had virtually no reported cases. CD has spread like epidemic. Wherever antibiotics are used early and in large quantities, the incidence of CD is now quite high. An infectious agent may be a normal intestinal flora suddenly producing immunostimulatory toxins or becoming invasive by sublethal doses of antibiotics that induce flora to become stronger in virility and numbers and more capable of producing toxins. Immunologic derangements are found in IBD, but whether causal of IBD or secondary to it remains unclear. Current evidence indicates that derangements are secondary to disease process.
- **Dietary factors**:
  —CD is increasing in cultures consuming a Western diet. It is virtually nonexistent in cultures consuming a primitive diet. People who have CD habitually eat more refined sugar and less raw fruit and vegetables and dietary fiber than do healthy people (122 g sugar daily vs. 65 g daily). Corn flakes have been linked to CD; they are high in refined carbohydrates and derived from common allergen (corn).
  —UC is not linked to refined carbohydrates. Food allergy is overlooked by conventional medicine.
  —Reduced intake of omega-3 oils and increased intake of omega-6 oils are linked to growing rise of CD in Japan. Genetics of the Japanese are relatively homogenous; therefore the increased incidence is from incorporation of Western foods. CD is strongly correlated with increased dietary total fat, animal fat, omega-6 fatty acids, animal protein, milk protein, and ratio of omega-6 to omega-3 fatty acids. CD is less correlated with total protein and not correlated with fish protein. CD is inversely correlated with vegetable protein. Increased animal protein is the strongest independent factor followed by increased ratio of omega-6 to omega-3 fatty acids.
- **Miscellaneous factors**: Mental and emotional stress can promote exacerbation of IBD. Thus stress management techniques may prove useful for some patients.

## THERAPEUTIC CONSIDERATIONS

### Control of Causative Factors

- **Natural history of Crohn's disease**: Many patients undergo spontaneous remission, 20% at 1 year and 12% at 2 years. "Success" of placebo therapy rises dramatically. In patients having no history of steroid therapy, 41% remitted after 17 weeks; 23% of this group continued in remission after 2 years compared with 4% of group with history of steroid use. Once remission is achieved, 75% of patients continue in remission at the end of 1 year and up to 63% by 2 years, regardless of maintenance therapy used. The key is achieving remission, which, once attained, can be maintained by conservative nondrug therapy.
- **Eicosanoid metabolism**: Prostaglandins are greatly increased in colonic mucosa, serum, and stools of IBD patients. Increased synthesis of lipoxygenase products, leukotrienes, and mono hydroxy-eicosatetraenoic acid by neutrophils amplifies inflammation and causes smooth muscle contraction. Release of lipoxygenase products is promoted by activation of alternative complement pathway. Sulfasalazine inhibits cyclooxygenase and neutrophil lipoxygenase and inhibits degranulation of mast cells. Corticosteroids inhibit phospholipase $A_2$, blocking release of arachidonic acid from membrane phospholipids. Natural flavonoid quercetin interacts with these enzymes. Formation of inflammatory compounds is decreased by reducing dietary meat and dairy while increasing omega-3 fatty acids (small wild cold-water ocean fish), containing eicosapentaenoic acid (EPA) and docosahexaenoic acid (DHA). Fish oil supplements (2.7-5.1 g total omega-3 oils daily) prevent or delay relapses in CD and UC. Flaxseed oil, which contains alpha-linolenic acid (LNA), the essential omega-3 fatty acid that the body can convert to EPA, also is of value.
- **Mucin defects in ulcerative colitis**: Mucins are high-molecular-weight, carbohydrate-rich glycoproteins responsible for viscous/elastic characteristics of secreted mucus. Alterations in mucin composition and content in colonic mucosa is noted in UC. Factors include a dramatic decrease in mucous content of goblet cells (proportional to severity of disease) and decrease in major sulfomucin subfraction. These abnormalities are not found in CD. Mucin content of goblet cells returns to normal during remission but sulfomucin deficiency does not. Specific components of sulfomucin and the cause of its lower level are unknown. Mucin

abnormalities are a major factor in increased risk of colon cancer in these patients. Many herbs effectively used to treat UC are demulcents, agents that soothe irritated mucous membranes and promote secretion of mucus.

- **Intestinal microflora** (*Textbook,* "Bacterial Overgrowth of the Small Intestine" and "Comprehensive Digestive Stool Analysis"): include 400 distinct species. Fecal flora of patients with IBD contain higher numbers of gram-positive anaerobic coccoid rods and *Bacteroides vulgatus,* a gram-negative rod. These alterations in fecal flora are not from disease. Alterations in metabolic activity of bacteria are more important than alterations in number of bacteria. Specific bacterial cell components may promote lymphocyte cytotoxic activity against colonic epithelial cells.
- **Carrageenans**: sulfated polymers of galactose and D-anhydrogalactose extracted from red seaweeds (*Eucheuma spinosum* or *Chondrus crispus*) have been used to induce IBD in animals. They are used by the food industry as stabilizing and suspending agents (ice cream, cottage cheese, milk chocolate, etc.) because of their ability to stabilize milk proteins. No correlation has been proven between human consumption of carrageenan and development of UC. Differences in intestinal bacterial flora probably are responsible for discrepancy: germ-free animals do not display carrageenan-induced damage. A bacterium linked to facilitating carrageenan-induced damage in animals is a strain of *Bacteroides vulgatus* found in much higher concentrations (six times as high) in fecal cultures of patients with IBD. Carrageenan is metabolized into nondamaging components in most human beings, but people with overgrowth of *Bacteroides vulgatus* may be at risk. Avoid carrageenan.
- **Aspirin and intestinal permeability**: first-degree relatives of CD patients had a 110% increase in intestinal permeability after acetylsalicylic acid (ASA) compared with an increase of 57% in control subjects. Thirty-five percent were hyperresponders. Familial permeability defect is a significant predisposing factor for CD because leaky gut is linked to increased incidence of food allergy and absorption of intestinal toxins (*Textbook,* "Food Allergy").
- **Endotoxemia and alternative complement pathway**: endotoxemia is linked to CD and UC. Endotoxemia-induced activation of alternative complement pathway could explain extra-GI manifestations of IBD. Whole-gut irrigation significantly reduces endotoxin pool in the gut and has a beneficial antiendotoxinemia

effect. Colonic irrigation may offer similar benefit. Colon irrigation during acute inflammatory flare is contraindicated.

## Extra-gastrointestinal Manifestations

More than 100 disorders are systemic complications of IBD. The most common extraintestinal lesion (EIL) in adults is arthritis (25% of patients).

- **Arthritis**: the more common form is peripheral arthritis that affects knees, ankles, and wrists. Arthritis is more common in patients with colon involvement. Severity of symptoms is proportional to disease activity. Arthritis may primarily affect the spine, with low back pain and stiffness, and eventual limitation of motion. This EIL occurs mainly in men with HLA-$B_{27}$ and resembles ankylosing spondylitis. It may antedate bowel symptoms by several years. A consistent underlying factor in progression of ankylosing spondylitis and IBD is likely.
- **Skin manifestations**: seen in 15% of patients. Lesions include erythema nodosum, pyoderma gangrenosum, and aphthous ulcerations. Recurrent aphthous stomatitis occurs in 10% of patients.
- **Liver**: serious liver disease (sclerosing cholangitis, chronic active hepatitis, cirrhosis) affects 3%-7% of patients with IBD from increased endotoxin load. Liver enzyme abnormalities indicate need for hepatoprotection from *Glycyrrhiza glabra* (licorice), *Silybum marianum* (milk thistle), catechin, and curcumin.
- **Other common EILs**: thrombophlebitis; finger clubbing; ocular manifestations (episcleritis, iritis, and uveitis); nephrolithiasis; cholelithiasis; and, in children, failure to grow, thrive, and mature normally.

## Malnutrition

Nutritional complications of IBD have a great influence on morbidity (and mortality).

Weight loss is prevalent in 65%-75% of IBD patients. Malabsorption arises from extensive mucosal involvement of small intestine and resection of segments of small intestine. Fat malabsorption causes a loss of calories and fat-soluble vitamins and minerals. Ileum involvement or resection causes bile acid malabsorption, and cathartic effect of bile acids on colon causes chronic watery diarrhea. Expect electrolyte and trace mineral deficiency from chronic diarrhea, plus calcium and magnesium deficiency from chronic

## Causes of Malnutrition in IBD

Decreased oral intake
- Disease-induced (pain, diarrhea, nausea, anorexia)
- Iatrogenic (restrictive diets without supplementation)

Malabsorption
- Decreased absorptive surface from disease or resection
- Bile salt deficiency after resection
- Bacterial overgrowth
- Drugs (e.g., corticosteroids, sulfasalazine, cholestyramine)
  Increased secretion and nutrient loss
- Protein-losing enteropathy
- Electrolyte, mineral, and trace mineral loss in diarrhea

Increased utilization and increased requirements
- Inflammation, fever, infection
- Increased intestinal cell turnover

---

steatorrhea. Loss of plasma proteins across damaged and inflamed mucosa may exceed the ability of the liver to replace plasma proteins. Chronic blood loss causes iron-depletion anemia. Drugs used to treat IBD (corticosteroids and sulfasalazine) increase nutritional needs.

Corticosteroids are known to do the following:

- Stimulate protein catabolism
- Depress protein synthesis
- Decrease the absorption of calcium and phosphorus
- Increase the urinary excretion of ascorbic acid, calcium, potassium, and zinc
- Increase blood glucose, serum triglycerides, and serum cholesterol
- Increase the requirements for vitamin $B_6$, ascorbic acid, folate, and vitamin D
- Decrease bone formation
- Impair wound healing

Sulfasalazine has been shown to do the following:

- Inhibit the absorption and transport of folate
- Decrease serum folate and iron
- Increase the urinary excretion of ascorbic acid

**Nutritional consequences of chronic inflammatory and/or infectious disease**: Protein requirement may be increased. Elevated sedimentation rate signifies increased protein breakdown and synthesis. IBD requires 25% more protein than usual recommended allowance.

## Prevalence of Nutritional Deficiencies

Nutritional deficiencies are quite high in hospitalized patients with IBD. Hospitalized patients have a greater incidence of nutritional deficiencies than do outpatients (more severe condition). Ambulatory patients with CD also display nutrient deficiencies: iron, $B_{12}$, folate, magnesium, potassium, retinol, ascorbate, vitamin D, zinc, vitamin K, copper, niacin, and vitamin E. Assume that most patients have micronutrient deficiency. Deficiency often is subclinical and only detected by lab investigation. Use therapeutic-potency vitamin supplements of at least five times the recommended daily allowance. Several minerals may need supplementing at similar levels. Dietary treatment is either elemental or elimination diet.

- **Elemental diet**: effective nontoxic alternative to corticosteroids as a primary treatment of acute IBD. It contains all essential nutrients: protein as predigested or free-form amino acids. It provides nutritional improvement, alters fecal flora, and serves as allergy elimination diet. The main drawback is unpalatability and hyperosmolality (causing diarrhea). Hospitalization is often required for satisfactory administration, and relapse is common when patients resume normal eating. Elimination diet may be acceptable alternative for acute flare-up of IBD, especially in chronic cases of IBD.
- **Elimination (oligoantigenic) diet**: Elimination is the primary therapy for chronic IBD. The most common offending foods are wheat and dairy. Alternative approach is to determine actual allergens by lab methods—measure reactions mediated by immunoglobulin (Ig) G and IgE. Then avoid allergens or use rotary diversified diet (*Textbook,* "Food Reactions" and "Rotation Diet: A Diagnostic and Therapeutic Tool").
- **High-complex carbohydrate, high-fiber (HFC) diet**: has a favorable effect on course of CD in direct contrast to allopathic dietary treatment, which is simply a low-fiber diet. Some foods are too "rough" to handle, so use an unrefined carbohydrate, fiber-rich diet with allergen avoidance or rotary-diversified diet. Fiber has profound effect on intestinal environment and promotes optimal intestinal flora. Avoid supplemental wheat bran.

## Minerals

- **Zinc (Zn)**: deficiency occurs in 45% of patients with CD because of low dietary intake, poor absorption, and excess fecal losses.

Many complications of CD may result from Zn deficiency: poor healing of fissures and fistulas, skin lesions (acrodermatitis), hypogonadism, growth retardation, retinal dysfunction, depressed cell-mediated immunity, and anorexia. Many patients are unresponsive to oral or intravenous Zn because of a defect in tissue transport. Zn picolinate may improve intestinal absorption and tissue transport. Patients with pancreatic insufficiency may show no improvement. Zn citrate may also be appropriate alternative. Make every attempt to ensure adequate tissue stores because disease activity correlates with Zn deficiency. Use parenteral administration as needed.

- **Magnesium (Mg)**: deficiency is prevalent in IBD. Poor correlation exists between serum levels (frequently normal) and intracellular levels (commonly decreased). Low intracellular Mg causes weakness, anorexia, hypotension, confusion, hyperirritability, tetany, convulsions, electrocardiographic or electroencephalographic abnormalities, which are responsive to parenteral Mg supplementation. Administer daily intravenous dose of 200-400 mg elemental Mg if patient is unresponsive to oral supplements. IBD may require intravenous route because of cathartic action of Mg and poor absorption in patients with short bowel. Oral supplement: Mg chelates (citrate, aspartate, etc.) are preferred rather than inorganic magnesium salts (i.e., carbonate).
- **Iron (Fe)**: iron-deficiency anemia is frequent in IBD from chronic gut blood loss. Serum ferritin is the most useful index of Fe status. Ferritin >55 ng/mL indicates adequate Fe reserves. Ferritin <18 ng/mL indicates Fe deficiency. Improve absorption with supplemental vitamin C rather than direct Fe supplements because Fe promotes intestinal infection.
- **Calcium (Ca)**: risk of Ca deficiency is from the loss of absorptive surfaces, steatorrhea, corticosteroids, and vitamin D deficiency.
- **Potassium (K)**: diarrhea is linked to $K^+$ and other electrolyte deficiencies. Symptoms of $K^+$ deficiency are rare in IBD patients, but levels are below optimum. Correcting $K^+$ deficiency reduces rates of surgical complications.

## Vitamins

- **Vitamin A**: low serum retinol occurs in 20% of patients with CD, correlated with activity of disease. Vitamin A affects metabolism and differentiation of intestinal epithelial mucosa; increases the number of goblet cells, production of mucins, and secretion of mucus; and restores normal barrier function. Vitamin A may be useful in CD, but long-term trials (at 50,000 IU b.i.d.) found no benefit in the majority of CD cases. Certain patients may respond to vitamin A. Zn supplements often normalize vitamin A metabolism because Zn is a component of retinol-binding protein.

- **Vitamin D**: deficiency is common in IBD, particularly in patients with other signs of nutritional deficiency from decreased absorption of 25-hydroxy-vitamin D. This deficit increases risk of metabolic bone diseases (osteoporosis and osteomalacia).
- **Vitamin E**: deficiency can occur in IBD with presenting symptoms: bilateral visual field scotomata, generalized motor weakness, broad-based gait with marked ataxia, brisk reflexes, bilateral Babinski response. Vitamin E inhibits leukotriene formation and reduces free radical damage.
- **Vitamin K**: deficiency results in formation of abnormal prothrombin (deficient in gamma-carboxyglutamic acid), common in patients with IBD.
- **Folic acid**: low serum levels occur in 25%-64% of cases. Sulfasalazine interferes with folate-dependent enzymes and intestinal folate transport system. Deficiency promotes malabsorption from altered structure of intestinal mucosa; cells have rapid turnover (1-4 days) versus red blood cells (3-4 months). Deficiency affects these cells earlier than red blood cells.
- **Vitamin $B_{12}$**: $B_{12}$ absorption and terminal ileal disease and/or resection are significantly correlated. Abnormal Schilling tests are seen in 48% of patients with CD. When ileal resection exceeds 90 cm, Schilling test is abnormal in all patients and never improves. If the length of resection is <60 cm, or if extent of inflammatory lesion is <60 cm, adequate absorption may occur.
- **Ascorbic acid**: low vitamin C intake is common in patients with IBD, particularly those on low-fiber diet. Serum and leukocyte ascorbic acid is much lower in patients with CD than in matched control subjects. Vitamin C is important to prevent fistulas. Patients with fistulas have lower ascorbic acid levels than those without.

A high-potency multiple vitamin/mineral formula (absolutely essential in IBD) and additional antioxidants are recommended to manage increased oxidative stress and decreased antioxidant defenses in mucosa. Two primary antioxidants in the human body are vitamins C (aqueous phase) and E (lipid phase).

- **Vitamin E (mixed tocopherols with 40% gamma-tocopherol)**: 400-800 IU
- **Vitamin C (ascorbic acid)**: 1000-3000 mg

## Botanical Medicines

- **Quercetin**: plant flavonoids are natural biologic response modifiers. Quercetin is the most pharmacologically active flavonoid. Many enzymes affected by quercetin are involved in release of histamine and other inflammatory mediators from mast cells, basophils, neutrophils, and macrophages; in the migration and infiltration of leukocytes; and in smooth muscle contraction. Quercetin antagonizes calmodulin. When Ca is bound to calmodulin, it activates enzymes involved in cyclic nucleotide metabolism, protein phosphorylation, secretory function, muscle contraction, microtubule assembly, glycogen metabolism, and Ca flux. Quercetin interacts directly with calmodulin and Ca channels. Quercetin and other flavonoids potently inhibit mast cell and basophil degranulation. It inhibits receptor-mediated Ca influx, inhibiting primary signal for degranulation. It is also active when Ca channel mechanism is not operative; therefore other mechanisms are also involved. It inhibits inflammatory processes of activated neutrophils by membrane stabilization, antioxidant effect (prevents production of free radicals and inflammatory leukotrienes), and inhibition of hyaluronidase (preventing breakdown of collagen). Its membrane-stabilizing effect prevents mast cell and basophil degranulation and decreases neutrophil lysosomal enzyme secretion. Quercetin inhibits eicosanoid metabolism by inhibiting phospholipase $A_2$ and lipoxygenase. The net result is the reduction in formation of leukotrienes. Excess leukotrienes are linked to asthma, psoriasis, atopic dermatitis, gout, possibly cancer, and IBD. Leukotrienes $C_4$, $D_4$, and $E_4$ (comprising slow-reacting substances of anaphylaxis) are 1000 times as potent as histamine in promoting inflammation. Leukotrienes cause vasoconstriction (increasing vascular permeability) and other smooth muscle contractions and promote white blood cell chemotaxis and aggregation. Reducing leukotrienes has strong antiinflammatory effects in IBD.

- **Bastyr's formula** (modified Robert's formula):
  —*Althea officinalis* (marshmallow root): demulcent, soothing to mucous membranes
  —*Baptisia tinctoria* (wild indigo): used for GI infections
  —*Echinacea angustifolia* (purple coneflower): antibacterial that normalizes immune system (*Textbook*, "*Echinacea* Species [Narrow-Leafed Purple Coneflower]")
  —*Geranium maculatum*: a GI hemostatic
  —*Hydrastis canadensis* (goldenseal): inhibits growth of many enteropathic bacteria (*Textbook*, "*Hydrastis canadensis* [Goldenseal] and Other Berberine-Containing Botanicals")
  —*Phytolacca americana* (poke root): used for healing ulcerations of intestinal mucosa
  —*Symphytum offinale* (comfrey): antiinflammatory; promotes tissue growth and wound healing
  —*Ulmus fulva* (slippery elm): demulcent
- **Other ingredients**: Cabbage powder heals GI ulcers (*Textbook*, "Peptic Ulcer—Duodenal and Gastric"). Pancreatin assists digestive process (*Textbook*, "Pancreatic Enzymes"). Niacinamide has antiinflammatory effects. Duodenal substance heals GI ulcers.

**Composition of Bastyr's Formula**

- Eight parts *Althea officinalis*
- Four parts *Baptisia tinctora*
- Eight parts *Echinacea angustifolia*
- Eight parts *Geranium maculatum*
- Eight parts *Hydrastis canadensis*
- Eight parts *Phytolacca americana*
- Eight parts *Ulmus fulva*
- Eight parts cabbage powder
- Two parts pancreatin
- One part niacinamide
- Two parts duodenal substance

## Butyrate Enemas in Ulcerative Colitis

**Short-chain fatty acids (SCFAs) and colon function**: SCFAs (acetate, propionate, and butyrate) are colon end products of bacterial carbohydrate fermentation. They function as primary energy sources for luminal colon cells, especially distal segments. Decreased levels or utilization of SCFAs impairs cellular energetics, suggesting a major role in ulcerative colitis. Enemas providing

SCFAs (butyrate only at 80-100 mmol/L or SCFA combinations with acetate 60 mmol/L, propionate 25 mmol/L, and butyrate 40 mmol/L) display excellent preliminary results in well-designed double-blind study. Butyrate and SCFA enemas may prove useful adjuncts for UC.

### Probiotics in Crohn's Disease

Probiotics are beneficial yeast and bacteria ingested for therapeutic benefit. The yeast *Saccharomyces boulardii* is safe and effective for CD, reducing diarrhea, intestinal inflammation, and risk of relapse. Dosage: 250 mg t.i.d. to q.i.d. *Lactobacillus* GG also is beneficial in CD at a dose of 10 billion CFU in enteric-coated tablets b.i.d.

## THERAPEUTIC MONITORING AND EVALUATION

- **Fecal calprotectin**: protein secreted into intestinal lumen in direct proportion to inflammation. Calprotectin in stool samples is a sensitive and specific noninvasive assessment tool for inflammatory status in IBD and for distinguishing IBD from other noninflammatory gastrointestinal conditions (irritable bowel syndrome).
- **CD activity index (CDAI)**: a monitoring tool providing uniform clinical parameters to be assessed with consistent numeric index for recording results. CDAI is calculated by adding eight variables (see p. 421). Subjective and objective information is included. A form (see p. 421) is given to patients for completion at home. Calculation of disease activity is determined. CDAI scores <150 indicate better prognosis than higher scores. CDAI is a very useful way to monitor progress.
- **Monitoring of the pediatric patient**: achieving normal growth and development is quite difficult. Growth failure occurs in 75% of pediatric patients with CD and 25% in those with UC. Evaluate at least twice yearly: pertinent history, clinical anthropometry, Tanner staging, and appropriate lab testing (see table below). Use aggressive nutritional program including supplements (enteral or parenteral methods) with doses adjusted as appropriate. CDAI is not as accurate in monitoring disease in children as in adults. Lloyd-Still and Green clinical scoring system for IBD in children: divided into five major divisions (maximal score is in parentheses): general activity (10), physical examination and clinical complications (30), nutrition (20), radiographs (15), lab (25). Elevated

score (scores in the 80s) represents good status whereas scores in the 30s and 40s represent severe disease.

## THERAPEUTIC APPROACH

- IBD is life-threatening, requiring emergency treatment in some patients. A small percentage of patients with severe colitis may have severe exacerbations requiring hospitalization (more common in patients with UC): fever of 101° F or higher; profuse, constant, loose, bloody stools; anorexia, apathy, and prostration. Abdominal signs may be normal but physical examination reveals distended abdomen, tympany, absent bowel sounds, and even rebound tenderness. IBD is typically a chronic disease requiring long-term therapy and follow-up.
- Identify and remove all factors initiating or aggravating inflammation (e.g., food allergens, carrageenan)
  —Follow diet maximizing macronutrients and micronutrients and minimizing aggravating foods and nonfood substances.
  —Use nutritional supplements to correct deficiencies in a broad-based individualized nutritional supplement plan; critical components are Zn, Mg, folate, and vitamin A.
  —Reduce inflammatory process and promote healing of damaged mucosa.
  —Use botanical medicines to promote healing and normalize intestinal flora.
- **Diet**: Eliminate all allergens, wheat, corn, dairy, and carrageenan-containing foods. Select foods high in complex carbohydrates and fiber, low in sugar and refined carbohydrates.
- **Supplements**:
  —Multivitamin and mineral supplement
  —Mg: 200 mg q.d.
  —Zn picolinate: 50 mg q.d.
  —Vitamin A: 50,000 IU q.d.
  —Vitamin E: 400-800 IU q.d. mixed tocopherols with ~40% concentration of gamma-tocopherol
  —Fish oil: 3 g q.d. of combined eicosapentaenoic acid/docosahexaenoic acid

### Botanical Medicines

- **Quercetin**: 400 mg 20 minutes before meals
- **Bastyr's formula**: two to three "00" capsules with each meal

## CDAI

Patient name: ______________________ Chart #: __________
Date: __________

| Variable | Day 1 | 2 | 3 | 4 | 5 | 6 | 7 | Sum | × Factor | = Subtotal |
|---|---|---|---|---|---|---|---|---|---|---|
| $X_1$ | | | | | | | | | 2 | |
| $X_2$ | | | | | | | | | 5 | |
| $X_3$ | | | | | | | | | 7 | |
| $X_4$ | | | | | | | | | 20 | |
| $X_5$ | | | | | | | | | 30 | |
| $X_6$ | | | | | | | | | 10 | |
| $X_7$ | | | | | | | | | 6 | |
| $X_8$ | | | | | | | | | 100 | |
| Sum of $X_1$ through $X_8$ | | | | | | | | | | |

## Independent Variables and Formula Used to Calculate CDAI

$X_1$: Number of liquid or very soft stools in 1 week

$X_2$: Sum of seven daily abdominal pain ratings: 0 = none, 1 = mild, 2 = moderate, 3 = severe

$X_3$: Sum of seven daily ratings of general well-being: 0 = well, 1 = slightly below par, 2 = poor, 3 = very poor, 4 = terrible

$X_4$: Symptoms or findings presumed related to Crohn's disease (add 1 for each category corresponding to patient's symptoms):

- Arthritis or arthralgia
- Iritis or uveitis
- Erythema nodosum, pyoderma gangrenosum, aphthous stomatitis
- Anal fissure, fistula, or perirectal abscess
- Other bowel-related fistula
- Febrile episode >100° F during past week

$X_5$: Taking Lomotil or opiates for diarrhea: 0 = no, 1 = yes

$X_6$: Abdominal mass: 0 = none, 0.4 = questionable, 1 = present

$X_7$: Men: 47 minus hematocrit; women: 42 minus hematocrit

$X_8$: 100 × (Standard weight − Body weight)/Standard weight

$CDAI = (2 \times X_1) + (5 \times X_2) + (7 \times X_3) + (20 \times X_4) + (30 \times X_5) + (10 \times X_6) + (6 \times X_7) + X_8$

## Monitoring of the Pediatric Patient With IBD

### History

- Appetite, extracurricular activities
- Type and duration of IBC, frequency of relapses
- Severity and extent of ongoing symptoms
- Medication history
- 3-day diet diary
- Physical examination
- Height, weight, arm circumference, triceps skinfold measurements
- Loss of subcutaneous fat, muscle wasting, edema, pallor, skin rash, hepatomegaly

### Laboratory Tests

- Complete blood count and differential, reticulocyte and platelet count, sedimentation rate, urinalysis
- Serum total proteins, albumin, globulin, and retinol-binding protein
- Serum electrolytes, calcium, phosphate, ferritin, folate, carotenes, tocopherol, and $B_{12}$
- Leukocyte ascorbate, magnesium, and zinc
- Creatinine height index, blood urea nitrogen/creatinine ratio

**Clinical Score in Chronic IBD**

| Measure | Score | Clinical Assessment |
|---|---|---|
| **General Activity** | 10 | Normal school attendance<br><3 bowel movements per day |
| | 5 | Lacks endurance<br>3-5 bowel movements per day<br>Misses <4 weeks school/year |
| **Physical Examination and Complications** | | |
| Abdomen | 10 | Normal |
| | 5 | Mass |
| | 1 | Distension, tenderness |
| Proctoscope | 10 | Normal, no fissures |
| | 5 | Friability, one fissure |
| | 1 | Ulcers, bleeding, fistulas, multiple fissures |

## Clinical Score in Chronic IBD—cont'd

| Measure | Score | Clinical Assessment |
|---|---|---|
| Arthritis | 5 | Nil |
| | 3 | One joint/arthralgia |
| | 1 | Multiple joints |
| Skin, stomatitis, eyes | 5 | Normal |
| | 3 | Mild stomatitis |
| | 4 | Erythema nodosum, pyoderma, severe stomatitis, uveitis |
| **Nutrition** | | |
| Height | 10 | >2 inches in/year |
| | 5 | Less than optimal % |
| | 1 | No growth |
| Radiographs | 15 | Normal |
| | 10 | Ileitis |
| | 5 | Total colon or ileocecal involvement |
| | 1 | Toxic megacolon or obstruction |
| **Laboratory** | | |
| Hematocrit | 5 | >40 |
| | 3 | 25-35 |
| | 1 | <25 |
| Erythrocyte sedimentation rate | 5 | Normal |
| | 3 | 20-40 |
| | 1 | >40 |
| White blood cell count | 5 | Normal |
| | 3 | <20,000 |
| | 1 | >20,000 |
| Albumin | 10 | Normal |
| | 5 | 3.0 g/dL |
| | 1 | <2.5 g/dL |

# Insomnia

## DIAGNOSTIC SUMMARY

- Difficulty falling asleep (sleep-onset insomnia)
- Frequent or early awakening (maintenance insomnia)

## GENERAL CONSIDERATIONS

Insomnia is an extremely common complaint with many causes.

**Causes of Insomnia***

| Sleep-Onset Insomnia | Sleep-Maintenance Insomnia |
|---|---|
| Anxiety or tension | Depression |
| Environmental change | Environmental change |
| Emotional arousal | Sleep apnea |
| Fear of insomnia | Nocturnal myoclonus |
| Phobia of sleep | Hypoglycemia |
| Disruptive environment | Parasomnias |
| Pain or discomfort | Pain or discomfort |
| Caffeine | Drugs |
| Alcohol | Alcohol |

*The boundary between the categories is not entirely distinct.

- Up to 30% of the population suffers. A total of 12.5% of the adult population uses prescribed anxiolytics or sedative hypnotics. Half of these drugs, especially benzodiazepines, are prescribed by primary care physicians.
- Psychological factors account for 50% of insomnia cases evaluated in sleep labs and are closely associated with affective disorders (see the chapter on affective disorders). Cognitive therapy is often indicated and can improve sleep quality.

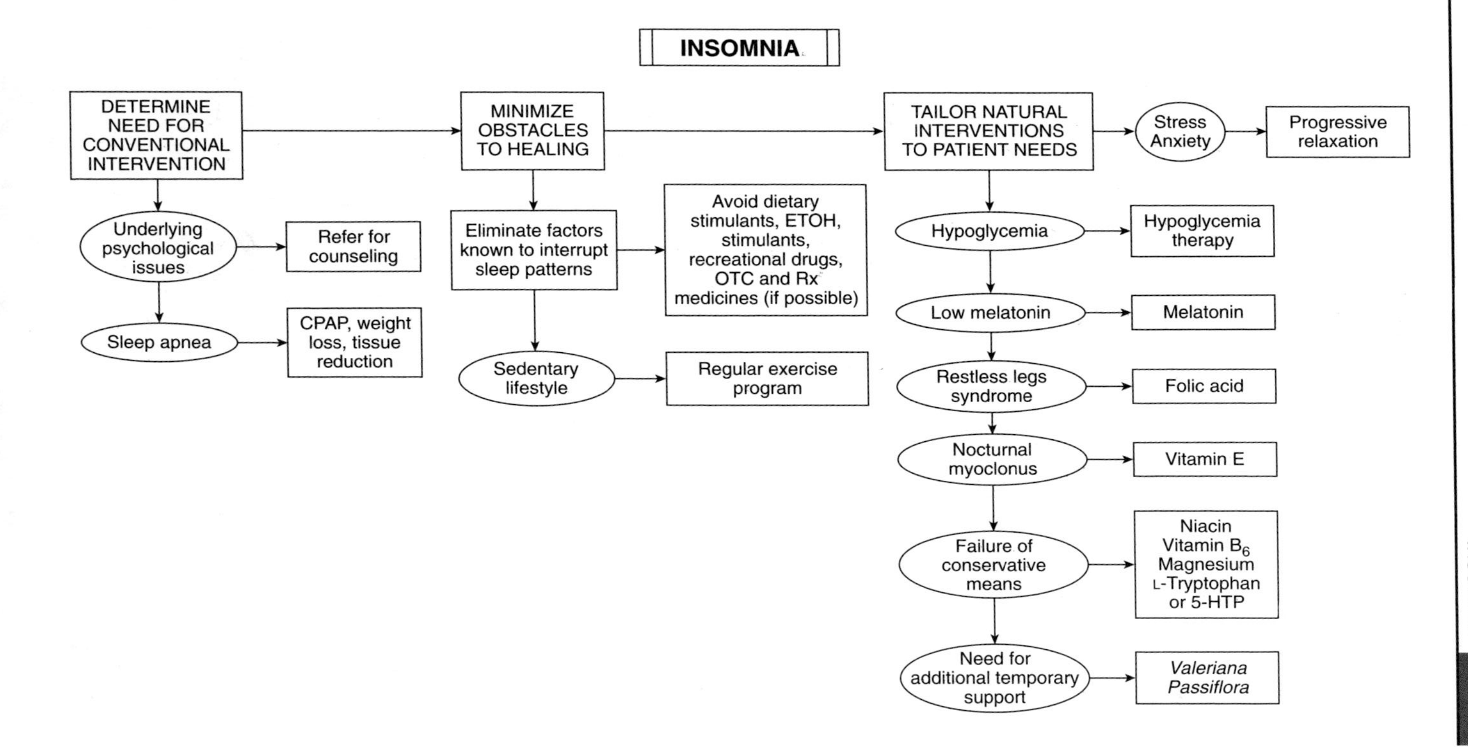
INSOMNIA
DETERMINE NEED FOR CONVENTIONAL INTERVENTION
Underlying psychological issues
Refer for counseling
Sleep apnea
CPAP, weight loss, tissue reduction
MINIMIZE OBSTACLES TO HEALING
Eliminate factors known to interrupt sleep patterns
Avoid dietary stimulants, ETOH, stimulants, recreational drugs, OTC and Rx medicines (if possible)
Sedentary lifestyle
Regular exercise program
TAILOR NATURAL INTERVENTIONS TO PATIENT NEEDS
Stress Anxiety
Progressive relaxation
Hypoglycemia
Hypoglycemia therapy
Low melatonin
Melatonin
Restless legs syndrome
Folic acid
Nocturnal myoclonus
Vitamin E
Failure of conservative means
Niacin Vitamin B6 Magnesium L-Tryptophan or 5-HTP
Need for additional temporary support
Valeriana Passiflora

- Insomnia may be a presenting symptom for a more serious condition. Conduct thorough history taking and examination, including details on recreational, prescription, and nonprescription drug use plus dietary and beverage history to identify stimulants or other agents known to interfere with sleep: thyroid preparations, oral contraceptives, beta-blockers, marijuana, alcohol, coffee, tea, chocolate.
- Consider and rule out narcolepsy and sleep apnea syndromes.

## Sleep Apnea

- Sleep apnea is the most common type of sleep disordered breathing. It is characterized by brief interruptions of breathing during sleep, with snoring between apnea episodes (not everyone who snores has this condition) or choking sensations. Frequent sleep interruptions prevent deep, restorative sleep, causing excessive daytime sleepiness and early morning headache.
- An estimated 18 million Americans suffer from sleep apnea.
- Associated issues: daytime fatigue, irregular heartbeat, hypertension, myocardial infarction, stroke, loss of memory function, other intellectual deficits.
- Patient usually is unaware and incredulous when told. Sleep partner notes heavy snoring or interrupted breathing.
- Definitive diagnosis: sleep disorder specialist in a sleep lab.
- Cause is excess fatty tissue accumulated in airway, causing it to be narrowed, leading to heavy snoring, periods of no breathing, and frequent arousals (causing abrupt changes from deep sleep to light sleep). Ingestion of alcohol and sleeping pills increases the frequency and duration of breathing pauses in people with sleep apnea. In some cases sleep apnea occurs even if no airway obstruction or snoring is present. This form of sleep apnea is called "central sleep apnea" and is caused by a loss of perfect control over breathing by the brain. In both obstructive and central sleep apnea, obesity is the major risk factor and weight loss is the most important aspect of long-term management. People with sleep apnea have periods of anoxia (oxygen deprivation of the brain) with each apneic episode, which ends in arousal and a reinitiation of breathing. Seldom does the sufferer awaken enough to be aware of the problem. However, the combination of frequent periods of oxygen deprivation (20 to several hundreds of times per night) and the greatly disturbed sleep can greatly diminish the quality of life and lead to serious problems.

The most common treatment of sleep apnea is the use of nasal continuous positive airway pressure (CPAP). In this treatment the patient wears a mask over the nose during sleep, and pressure from an air blower forces air through the nasal passages. The air pressure is adjusted so that it is just enough to prevent the throat from collapsing during sleep. The pressure is constant and continuous. Nasal CPAP prevents airway closure while in use, but apnea episodes return when CPAP is stopped or used improperly. Surgery for reducing soft tissue in the throat or soft palate should only be used as a last resort because often it does not work or can make the condition worse. Laser-assisted uvulopalatoplasty is a highly promoted surgical option. In this procedure lasers are used to surgically remove excessive soft tissue from the back of the throat and from the palate. This procedure initially works well in approximately 90% of those with sleep apnea, but within 1 year many people are the same or even worse than before because of scar tissue that invariably occurs.

## Normal Sleep Patterns

- Normal sleep patterns repeat themselves on a 24-hour cycle, of which sleep constitutes one third. Sleep tends to decrease with age, but whether this is normal is unknown. A 1-year-old baby requires 14 hours of sleep, a 5-year-old 12 hours, and adults 7-9 hours. Women require more sleep than men; the elderly sleep less at night but doze more during day than younger adults.
- Two distinct types of sleep (based on eye movement and electroencephalographic (EEG) recordings): rapid eye movement (REM) and non-REM sleep.
  —**REM sleep**: eyes move rapidly and dreaming takes place; when people are awakened during non-REM sleep, they report they were thinking about everyday matters but rarely report dreams.
  —**Non-REM sleep**: four stages graded 1-4 on the level of EEG activity and ease of arousal. As sleep progresses, it deepens and brain wave activity is slower until REM sleep, when the brain suddenly becomes much more active. In adults, the first REM cycle is triggered 90 minutes after going to sleep and lasts 5-10 minutes; EEG patterns return to non-REM for another 90-minute sleep cycle.
- Each night most adults have five or more sleep cycles; REM periods grow progressively longer as sleep continues. The last sleep cycle may produce a REM period lasting an hour. Non-

REM sleep lasts 50% of a 90-minute sleep cycle in infants and 80% in adults. With aging, in addition to less REM sleep, people tend to awaken at transition from non-REM to REM sleep.

### Importance of Adequate Sleep

- Growth hormone (GH), the anabolic anti-aging hormone, is secreted during sleep. It stimulates tissue regeneration, liver regeneration, muscle building, breakdown of fat stores, and normalization of blood sugar regulation as well as helps convert fat to muscle. Small amounts are secreted during the day, but most secretion occurs during sleep.
- Sleep is the antioxidant for the brain; free radicals are removed during this time. It is required to minimize neuronal damage from free radical accumulation during waking. Chronic sleep deprivation accelerates aging of the brain. Animal research has shown that prolonged sleep deprivation causes neuronal damage.

## THERAPEUTIC CONSIDERATIONS

Uncover causative psychological and physiologic factors; counseling and/or stress reduction techniques (biofeedback, hypnosis) are indicated in many cases.

- **Exercise**: regular physical exercise improves sleep quality; perform in the morning or early evening, not before bedtime, and at moderate intensity; 20 minutes of aerobic exercise at a heart rate between 60% and 75% of maximum (220 minus age in years).
- **Progressive relaxation**: based on simple procedure of comparing tension with relaxation; patient is taught what it feels like to relax by comparing relaxation with muscle tension. Muscle is first asked to contract forcefully for 1-2 seconds and then give way to feeling of relaxation; procedure goes progressively through all muscles of the body and eventually deep state of relaxation results. Start with contracting facial and neck muscles, then upper arms and chest, then lower arms and hands, abdomen, buttocks, thighs, calves, and feet; repeat two or three times or until asleep.
- **Nocturnal glucose levels**: low nocturnal blood glucose is the cause of maintenance insomnia; a drop in blood glucose promotes awakening by release of glucose regulatory hormones

(epinephrine, glucagon, cortisol, and GH); rule out hypoglycemia in maintenance insomnia (see *Textbook,* "Hypoglycemia").

## Serotonin Precursor and Cofactor Therapy

Serotonin is the initiator of sleep; synthesis of central nervous system serotonin depends on tryptophan.

- **L-Tryptophan**: has modest effect on insomnia with dramatic relief in some patients; it is more effective in sleep onset and less effective in sleep maintenance. An advantage of L-tryptophan over over-the-counter drugs and prescription drugs is no significant distortions of normal sleep processes, whether given one time for a prolonged period or on withdrawal. Dosages <2000 mg are ineffective. L-Tryptophan enhances melatonin synthesis and reduces sleep latency, but in normal subjects the effects are at odds with serotonin, reducing REM and increasing non-REM sleep. Some of L-Tryptophan's sleep effects do not involve serotonin or melatonin. Effects of L-tryptophan can be negated by kynurenine pathway—partially inhibited by niacin (30 mg), enhancing effects of L-tryptophan. Sleep actions of L-tryptophan are cumulative; a few nights are often necessary to start working. It should be used for 1+ week to gauge effectiveness in chronic insomnia. L-Tryptophan does exert good sleep-promoting effects with single administration (insomnia sleeping in a "strange place"); high-dose L-tryptophan (4 g) during the day can promote sleep. High tryptophan-containing foods during the day may contribute to daytime sleepiness; an evening meal high in tryptophan relative to competing amino acids may promote sleep.
- **5-Hydroxytryptophan (5-HTP)**: is one step closer to serotonin than L-tryptophan. It is not dependent on transport system for entry into the brain; it produces dramatically better results than L-tryptophan in promoting and maintaining sleep. It increases REM sleep (by 25%) and increases deep sleep stages 3 and 4 without increasing total sleep time. Sleep stages reduced to compensate for increases are non-REM stages 1 and 2, the least important stages. 5-HTP dosage for sleep promotion = 100-300 mg 30-45 minutes before retiring; start with lower dose for at least 3 days before moving up.
- **Cofactors for serotonin synthesis**: vitamin $B_6$, niacin, and magnesium are given with tryptophan to ensure conversion to serotonin; other amino acids compete for transport into the central nervous system across the blood-brain barrier, and insulin

increases tryptophan uptake by the central nervous system. Avoid protein consumption near administration, and take with a carbohydrate source (fruit or fruit juice). Niacin has sedative effect, probably from a peripheral dilating action and shunting tryptophan toward serotonin synthesis.

- **Melatonin**: modestly effective in inducing and maintaining sleep in children and adults, in those with normal sleep patterns, and those with insomnia. Sleep effects of melatonin apparent only if melatonin levels are low; melatonin is not like sleeping pill or 5-HTP; it only produces a sedative effect when melatonin levels are low. Normally, just before retiring, melatonin secretion rises; melatonin supplement is only effective as a sedative when the pineal gland's own production of melatonin is low. It is most effective for insomnia in elderly in whom low melatonin is common; dosage = 3 mg at bedtime. No serious side effects at this dosage, but melatonin supplementation could disrupt normal circadian rhythm.

## Restless Leg Syndrome and Nocturnal Myoclonus

These are significant causes of insomnia.

- Restless legs syndrome (RLS) is characterized during waking by the irresistible urge to move legs; almost all affected patients have nocturnal myoclonus.
- Nocturnal myoclonus (NM) is a neuromuscular disorder with repeated contractions of one or more muscle groups, typically of the leg, during sleep. Each jerk lasts <10 seconds. The patient is unaware of myoclonus and only reports frequent nocturnal awakenings or excessive daytime sleepiness; questioning sleep partner reveals myoclonus.
- If family history of RLS (one third of patients), high-dose folic acid (35-60 mg q.d.) is helpful but requires a prescription. The Food and Drug Administration limits the amount per capsule to 800 μg. RLS is common in patients with malabsorption syndromes.
- If no family history, measure serum ferritin, which is the best measure of iron stores; low iron (Fe) is linked to RLS. Serum ferritin is reduced in RLS patients compared with control subjects; serum Fe, $B_{12}$, folate, and hemoglobin do not differ; treatment with Fe (ferrous sulfate) at a dosage of 200 mg t.i.d. for 2 months reduced symptoms. Fe deficiency, with or without anemia, is a contributor to RLS in the elderly and Fe supplements can produce significant improvement.

- Low serum ferritin has been found in psychiatric patients experiencing "akathisia" (from the Greek word meaning "can't sit down"). Akathisia is a drug-induced agitation caused by antidepressants (e.g., Prozac, Zoloft, Paxil); the level of Fe depletion correlates with severity of akathisia. If serum ferritin <35 mg/L, try 30 mg Fe bound to succinate or fumarate b.i.d. between meals; if this therapy causes abdominal discomfort, try 30 mg with meals t.i.d.
- For NM and muscle cramps at night, magnesium (250 mg at bedtime) and/or vitamin E (400-800 IU q.d.) may help; if patient >50 years, ginkgo biloba extract (80 mg t.i.d.) may also be used.

## Botanicals With Sedative Properties

- ***Passiflora incarnata* (passion flower)**: widely used by Aztecs as diaphoretic, sedative, and analgesic; constituents are harmol, harman, harmine, harmalol, harmaline, and passicol. Harmine (called "telepathine" because of ability to induce contemplation and mild euphoria) was used by the Germans during World War II as "truth serum." Harma alkaloids are monoamine oxidase inhibitors; their use with tryptophan or 5-HTP has additive effect.
- ***Valeriana officinalis* (valerian)**: widely used in folk medicine as a sedative and antihypertensive; aqueous extract of valerian root significantly improves sleep quality. Criteria = sleep latency, night awakenings, subjective sleep quality, and sleepiness the next morning. It has the most significant effect among poor or irregular sleepers (particularly women), smokers, and those with long sleep latencies. It exerts a mild sedative effect, significantly reduces sleep latency, improves sleep quality, and reduces nighttime awakenings in insomniacs. It is as effective in reducing sleep latency as small doses of barbiturates or benzodiazepines, but these drugs increase morning sleepiness, whereas valerian reduces morning sleepiness. Compared with placebo, valerian shows significant effect, with 44% of subjects reporting perfect sleep and 89% reporting improved sleep. A combination of valerian root extract (160 mg) and *Melissa officinalis* (lemon balm) extract (80 mg) compared with benzodiazepine (triazolam 0.125 mg), and placebo: among insomniacs, the valerian preparation's effect was comparable to benzodiazepine while increasing deep sleep stages 3 and 4; the valerian preparation did not cause daytime sedation, diminished concentration, or impairment of physical performance.

## THERAPEUTIC APPROACH

Treatment should be as conservative as possible; treat psychological factors; eliminate factors known to disrupt normal sleep patterns: stimulants (coffee, tea, chocolate, coffee-flavored ice cream, etc.), alcohol, hypoglycemia, stimulant-containing herbs (e.g., ephedra, guarana), marijuana and other recreational drugs, numerous over-the-counter medications, prescription drugs. If this approach fails, use more aggressive measures; once normal sleep pattern is established, supplements and botanicals should be slowly decreased. If the patient suffers from RLS, add 5-10 mg q.d. folic acid; for NM use 400 IU q.d. natural vitamin E.

- **Lifestyle**: regular exercise program that elevates heart rate 50%-75% for 20 min q.d.
- **Supplements**: taken 45 minutes before bedtime:
  —Niacin: 100 mg (decrease dose if uncomfortable flushing interferes with sleep induction)
  —Vitamin $B_6$: 50 mg
  —Mg: 250 mg
  —Tryptophan: 3-5 g, or 5-HTP 100-300 mg
  —Melatonin: 3 mg
- **Botanical medicines**: taken 45 minutes before bedtime:
  —*Valeriana officinalis*: dried root (or as tea), 2-3 g; tincture (1:5), 4-6 mL (1-1.5 tsp); fluid extract (1:1), 1-2 mL (0.5-1 tsp); dry powdered extract (0.8% valerenic acid), 150-300 mg.
  —*Passiflora incarnata*: dried herb (or as tea), 4-8 g; tincture (1:5), 6-8mL (1.5-2 tsp); fluid extract (1:1), 2-4 mL (0.5-1 tsp); dry powdered extract (2.6% flavonoids), 300-450 mg.

# Intestinal Protozoan Infestation

## DIAGNOSTIC SUMMARY

- Systemic symptoms: depression, muscle weakness, headache, sore throat, lymphadenopathy, arthralgia, flulike symptoms, and poor exercise tolerance.
- Diagnosis confirmed by stool analysis.

## GENERAL CONSIDERATIONS

The gastrointestinal tract is the largest organ of immune surveillance in the body, home to two thirds of the total lymphocyte population. Stimulation of intestinal immune response networks by lumen-dwelling microbes may produce a variety of systemic responses independent of gastrointestinal symptoms. Immunologic hypersensitivity to *Giardia lamblia*, for example, has been shown, even in the absence of digestive symptoms, to provoke asthma, urticaria, arthritis, and uveitis.

Intestinal protozoans found in human beings include:

- ***Giardia* spp.**: chronic infection associated with deficiency of secretory immunoglobulin A (IgA), malabsorption, systemic illness, multiple nutrient deficiencies.
- ***Entamoeba histolytica***: associated with autoimmune phenomena, ulcerative colitis, and symmetrical polyarthritis very similar to rheumatoid arthritis.

## DIAGNOSTIC CONSIDERATIONS

Protozoan infection usually is diagnosed by stool examination; however, comparison of results of stool microscopy and duodenal aspiration has consistently shown that stool may fail to contain identifiable parasites even at the height of acute giardiasis. Collecting multiple specimens over several days increases the sensitivity to 85% to 90%.

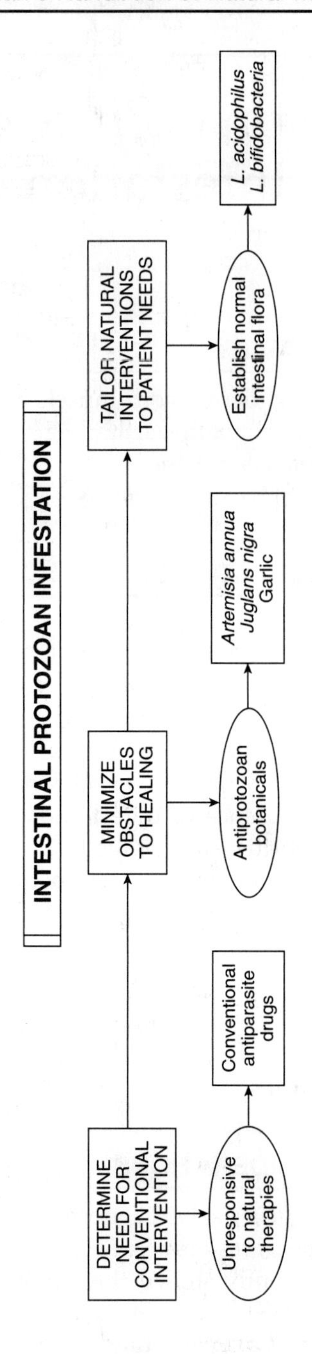
INTESTINAL PROTOZOAN INFESTATION
DETERMINE NEED FOR CONVENTIONAL INTERVENTION
Unresponsive to natural therapies
Conventional antiparasite drugs
MINIMIZE OBSTACLES TO HEALING
Antiprotozoan botanicals
*Artemisia annua*
*Juglans nigra*
Garlic
TAILOR NATURAL INTERVENTIONS TO PATIENT NEEDS
Establish normal intestinal flora
*L. acidophilus*
*L. bifidobacteria*

## THERAPEUTIC CONSIDERATIONS

**Intestinal bacterial milieu:** the intestinal bacterial milieu may be important in the treatment of protozoan infestation, especially for colonic organisms such as *Entamoeba histolytica*. Optimal treatment of protozoan infection requires administration of antimicrobial substances and strategies aimed at enhancing the function of intestinal resistance factors such as secretory IgA and phagocyte function and creating a bacterial milieu that is not parasite friendly.

### Botanical Medicines

- ***Artemisia annua*** (sweet Annie, sweet wormwood, qinghao): contains several sesquiterpene trioxane lactones, most notably artemisinin (also known as qinghaosu) but also deoxyartemisinin, artemisinic acid, and arteannuin-B. Artemisinin is thought to kill parasites through oxidation.
- **Berberine:** an alkaloid extracted from the roots of *Berberis aquifolium* (Oregon grape), *Hydrastis canadensis* (goldenseal) root, and *Coptis chinensis* (goldthread).
- ***Allium sativum* and *Juglans nigra***: have a long history of use as antimicrobials. Allicin inhibits growth of *E. histolytica* in culture and may be responsible for the antimicrobial activity of garlic. Human studies on the efficacy of garlic and black walnut in treatment of protozoan infections are lacking.

## THERAPEUTIC APPROACH

### Antiprotozoan Botanicals

- ***Artemisia annua***: sweet wormwood tea in 5 g/1 L of water, drunk in three to four divided doses
- ***Juglans nigra***: 1000 mg three times daily
- **Garlic**: 4 g or equivalent extract three times daily
- ***Lactobacillus acidophilus, Lactobacillus bifidobacteria***: to establish normal intestinal flora

# Irritable Bowel Syndrome

## DIAGNOSTIC SUMMARY

- Functional disorder of the large intestine with no evidence of accompanying structural defect.
- Characterized by some combination of:
  —Abdominal pain
  —Altered bowel function, constipation, or diarrhea
  —Hypersecretion of colonic mucus
  —Dyspeptic symptoms (flatulence, nausea, anorexia)
  —Varying degrees of anxiety or depression
- Synonyms include nervous indigestion, spastic colitis, mucous colitis, intestinal neurosis
- Splenic flexure syndrome is a variant of irritable bowel syndrome (IBS) in which gas in bowel leads to pain in lower chest or left shoulder.
- Many patients with IBS also have extraintestinal symptoms: sexual dysfunction, fibromyalgia, dyspareunia, urinary frequency and urgency, poor sleep, menstrual difficulties, lower back pain, headache, chronic fatigue, and insomnia—which increase in number with severity of IBS.

## GENERAL CONSIDERATIONS

IBS is the most common gastrointestinal (GI) disorder in general practice, accounting for 30%-50% of all referrals to gastroenterologists. Many sufferers never seek medical attention. Fifteen percent of the population have IBS symptoms; women predominate 2:1 (men do not report symptoms as often). Etiology is attributed to physiologic, psychological, and dietary factors. IBS often is a diagnosis of exclusion, but clinical judgment is needed to determine extent of diagnostic process. Detailed history and physical examination can eliminate vagueness in diagnosing IBS. Distension, relief of pain with bowel movements, and onset of loose or more frequent bowel movements with pain correlate best with diagnosis

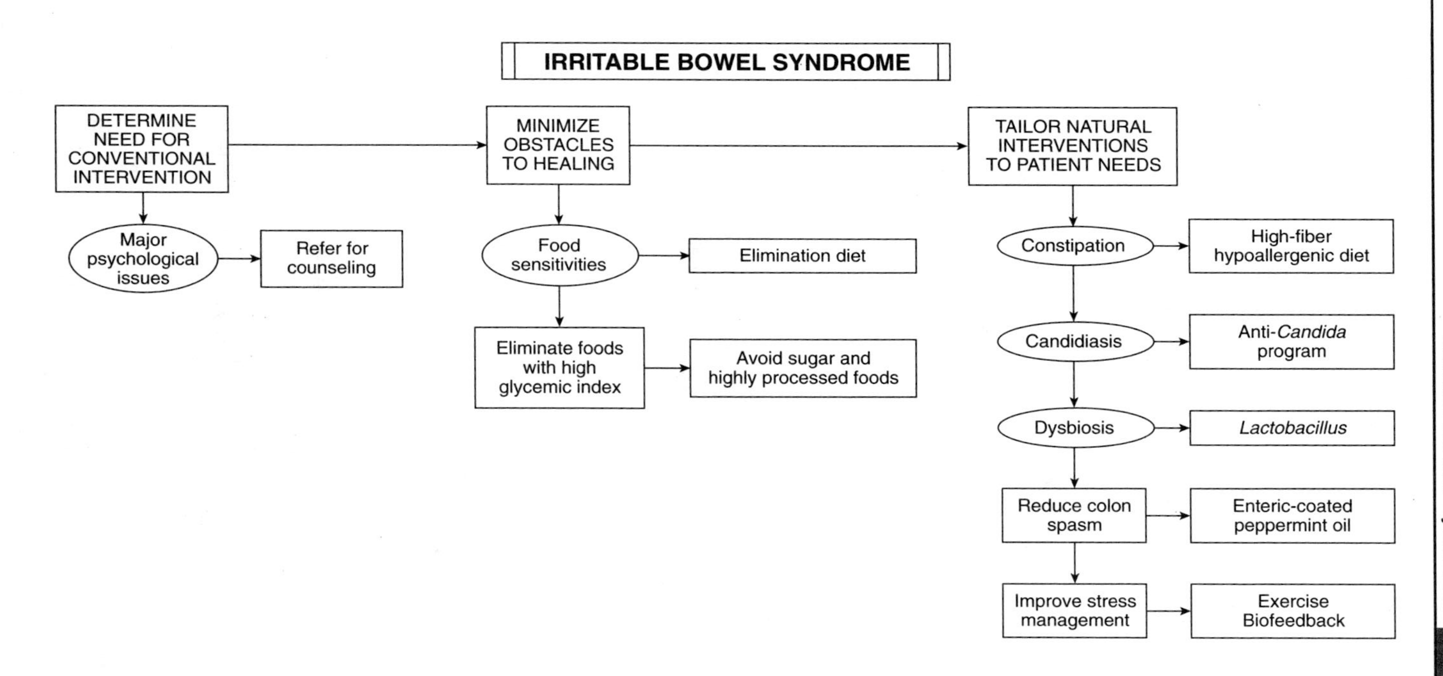
IRRITABLE BOWEL SYNDROME
DETERMINE NEED FOR CONVENTIONAL INTERVENTION
Major psychological issues
Refer for counseling
MINIMIZE OBSTACLES TO HEALING
Food sensitivities
Elimination diet
Eliminate foods with high glycemic index
Avoid sugar and highly processed foods
TAILOR NATURAL INTERVENTIONS TO PATIENT NEEDS
Constipation
High-fiber hypoallergenic diet
Candidiasis
Anti-*Candida* program
Dysbiosis
*Lactobacillus*
Reduce colon spasm
Enteric-coated peppermint oil
Improve stress management
Exercise Biofeedback

of IBS. Comprehensive stool and digestive analysis (*Textbook,* "Comprehensive Digestive Stool Analysis 2.0"), complete blood count, erythrocyte sedimentation rate, thyroid stimulating hormone, and serum protein concentration are necessary to determine diagnosis. If diarrhea is the predominant symptom, consider antiendomysial antibody test to rule out celiac disease (see the chapter on celiac disease). If no discernible cause is identified, screening for fecal occult blood and flexible sigmoidoscopy are indicated in patients <50 years and colonoscopy in patients >50 years old.

### Conditions That Can Mimic IBS

- Gastrogenic dietary factors: excessive tea, coffee, carbonated beverages, simple sugars
- Infectious enteritis: amebiasis, giardiasis
- Inflammatory bowel disease
- Lactose intolerance
- Laxative abuse (An easy test exists to rule out this possibility: add a few drops of NaOH solution to stool specimen. Most laxatives contain phenolphthalein, causing the stool to turn red.)
- Intestinal candidiasis
- Disturbed bacterial microflora as a result of antibiotic or antacid usage
- Malabsorption diseases: pancreatic insufficiency, celiac disease
- Metabolic disorders: adrenal insufficiency, diabetes mellitus, hyperthyroidism
- Mechanical causes (e.g., fecal impaction)
- Diverticular disease
- Neoplasm

## THERAPEUTIC CONSIDERATIONS

Three major treatments to consider: (1) increasing dietary fiber, (2) eliminating allergic or intolerant foods, and (3) controlling psychological components (*Textbook,* "Food Reactions," "Irritable Bowel Syndrome," and "Role of Dietary Fiber in Health and Disease").

- **Dietary fiber**: patients with constipation are more likely to respond to dietary fiber than are those with diarrhea. Food allergy has been ignored in studies of fiber. Wheat bran is usually contraindicated because food allergy is a significant factor in IBS. Fiber from fruit and vegetables, rather than cereals, is more beneficial in some patients. In certain cases, especially diarrhea cases, fiber may aggravate diarrhea. Cooked vegetables in small quantities at first may be most helpful (*Textbook,* "Role of Dietary Fiber in Health and Disease"). Partially hydrolyzed guar gum

(PHGG), from the ancient guar plant *Cyamopsis tetragonolobus* of India and Pakistan, is a natural, water-soluble fiber that decreases frequency of IBS symptoms—flatulence, abdominal spasms, and tension. At a dosage of 5 g q.d. PHGG works well for altered intestinal motility and is easy to use because of its nongelling properties, unlike unhydrolyzed gum.

- **Food allergy**: the type of food sensitivity most significant in IBS is nonimmunologic—food intolerance rather than food allergy (*Textbook,* "Food Allergy"). Two thirds of patients with IBS have food intolerances. Foods rich in carbohydrates and fats, coffee, alcohol, and hot spices are problematic. The most common allergens are dairy (40%-44%) and grains (40%-60%). The reaction arises from prostaglandin synthesis or immunoglobulin (Ig) G rather than IgE mediation; thus skin tests and IgE radioallergosorbent test are poor indicators of intolerances. Enzyme-linked immunosorbent assay ACT or ELISA IgE/$IgG_4$ may be better indicators. Many sensitivities are undetectable by current lab procedures. Elimination diets can give marked clinical improvement. Many patients with IBX have associated symptoms of vasomotor instability (palpitation, hyperventilation, fatigue, excessive sweating, headache) consistent with food allergy or intolerance reactions.
- **Sugar**: meals high in refined sugar contribute to IBS and small intestinal bacterial overgrowth by decreasing intestinal motility. A rapid rise in blood sugar slows GI tract peristalsis. Glucose is primarily absorbed in the duodenum and jejunum; hence the message affects this portion of GI tract the strongest; the duodenum and jejunum become atonic.

## Nutritional Supplements

- ***Lactobacillus***: dysbiosis in IBS has not been well investigated. Some benefits attributed to fiber may be mediated by alterations in colon bacteria. *Lactobacillus* improves IBS symptoms, with normalization of stool frequency in constipated patients (see *Textbook*, "Probiotics").
- **L-Tryptophan**: This amino acid and its derivative 5-hydroxytryptophan (5-HTP) are considered for IBS because of their relation to serotonin, the neurotransmitter produced in the digestive tract and brain. Because comorbidity of psychiatric conditions (depression or anxiety) correlates highly with IBS, modulation of serotonin pathway with tryptophan seems indicated and needs further investigation.

## Botanical Medicines

- **Enteric-coated volatile oils**: peppermint oil and similar volatile oils inhibit GI smooth muscle action in lab animals and human beings. Peppermint oil reduces colonic spasm during endoscopy; enteric-coated peppermint oil is used to treat IBS.
- Enteric coating is necessary because menthol and other monoterpenes in peppermint oil are rapidly absorbed, limiting effects to upper intestine and causing relaxation of cardiac esophageal sphincter with esophageal reflux and heartburn.
- Symptoms reduced: abdominal pain and distension, stool frequency, borborygmi, flatulence.
- Transient hot burning sensation in rectum on defecation (unabsorbed menthol) is noted in some patients.
- Dosage: 0.2 mL b.i.d. between meals.
- Improves rhythmic contractions of intestinal tract and relieves intestinal spasm.
- Effective against *Candida albicans*. Overgrowth of *C. albicans* may be an underlying factor in cases unresponsive to dietary advice and in patients consuming large amounts of sugar. Nystatin (600,000 IU q.d. for 10 days) given to patients unresponsive to elimination diet produced dramatic improvement.
- Safe and effective in children with moderate pain from IBS.
- Herbal formulas

  **Robert's formula**: has a long history of use in this condition (see the chapter on peptic ulcers).

  **Tibetan herbal formula Padma Lax**: effective for constipation-predominant IBS. It may cause loose stools in some patients, which is easily remedied by lowering the dosage.

  **Asian medicines**: individualized therapies with Chinese herbal medicines, acupuncture, and Ayurvedic herbal preparations improve bowel and global symptoms and recurrence rate.

## Miscellaneous Considerations

- **Psychological factors**: mental and/or emotional problems (anxiety, fatigue, hostile feelings, depression, sleep disturbances) are reported by almost all patients with IBS. Symptom severity and frequency correlate with psychological factors. Anxiety predicts a high degree of food-related symptoms in IBS. Poor sleep quality increases symptom severity.
- **Theories linking psychological factors to IBS**: (1) Learning model: when exposed to stressful situations, some children learn to develop GI symptoms to cope with stress. (2) IBS is a mani-

festation of depression, chronic anxiety, or both. IBS sufferers have higher anxiety and more feelings of depression. (3) IBS is either secondary to bowel disturbances (malabsorption) or the result of common etiologic factors (stress, food allergy, or candidiasis).

- **Increased colonic motility during stress**: occurs in normal subjects and patients with IBS. This accounts for increased abdominal pain and irregular bowel functions seen in IBS and normal subjects during emotional stress. Those with IBS may have difficulty adapting to life events. Psychotherapy (relaxation therapy, biofeedback, hypnosis, counseling, or stress management training) reduces symptom frequency and severity and enhances results of conventional treatment of IBS. Hypnosis, practiced at home with audio compact disc recording equipment, reduces fasting colonic motility and rectal sensitivity. Anxiolytic drugs (tranquilizers, antispasmodics, antidepressants) have not yielded effective results.
- **Physical medicine**: increasing physical exercise is helpful; daily leisurely walks markedly reduce symptoms.

## THERAPEUTIC APPROACH

IBS is a multifactorial disease requiring consideration and integration of many factors: dietary fiber, determination and elimination of food allergies and intolerances, stress reduction, and exercise. Peppermint oil and Robert's formula temporarily ameliorate symptoms. Because diagnosis is made by exclusion, careful diagnostic workup is always indicated.

- **Diet**: increase fiber-rich foods (*Textbook*, "Role of Dietary Fiber in Health and Disease"). Eliminate allergenic foods, refined sugar, and highly processed foods.
- **Supplements**:
  —*Lactobacillus acidophilus*: 1-2 billion live organisms q.d.
- **Botanical medicine**:
  —Enteric-coated volatile oil preparations (peppermint oil): 0.2-0.4 mL b.i.d. between meals.
- **Exercise**: take daily, leisurely 20-minute walks.
- **Counseling**: helps patient develop effective stress reduction program. Biofeedback is particularly useful for these patients.

# Kidney Stones

## DIAGNOSTIC SUMMARY

- Usually asymptomatic.
- Diagnosed adventitiously or by acute symptoms of urinary tract obstruction.
- Excruciating intermittent radiating pain originating in flank or kidney.
- Nausea, vomiting, abdominal distension.
- Chills, fever, and urinary frequency if infection is present.

## GENERAL CONSIDERATIONS

- In the past, stone formation was almost exclusively in the bladder; today most stones form in upper urinary tract. Ten percent of all men have kidney stone during their lifetime. Annual incidence is 0.1%-6.0% of the general population. Incidence is steadily increasing, paralleling rise in other diseases linked to a Western diet (e.g., ischemic heart disease, cholelithiasis, hypertension, diabetes).
- In the western hemisphere, kidney stones usually are composed of calcium salts (75%-85%), uric acid (5%-8%), or struvite (10%-15%).
- Mutations in genes can lead to hypercalciuria, excess urinary excretion of oxalate, cystine, and uric acid.
- Incidence varies geographically, reflecting environmental factors, diet, and components of drinking water.
- Men are affected more than women. Most patients are older than 30 years.
- Human urine is supersaturated with calcium oxalate, uric acid, and phosphates. They remain in solution because of pH control and secretion of inhibitors of crystal growth.
- Primary and secondary metabolic diseases can cause kidney stones; they must be ruled out early in the clinical process (e.g., hyperparathyroidism, cystinuria, vitamin D excess, milk-alkali syndrome, destructive bone disease, primary oxaluria, Cushing's syndrome, sarcoidosis.

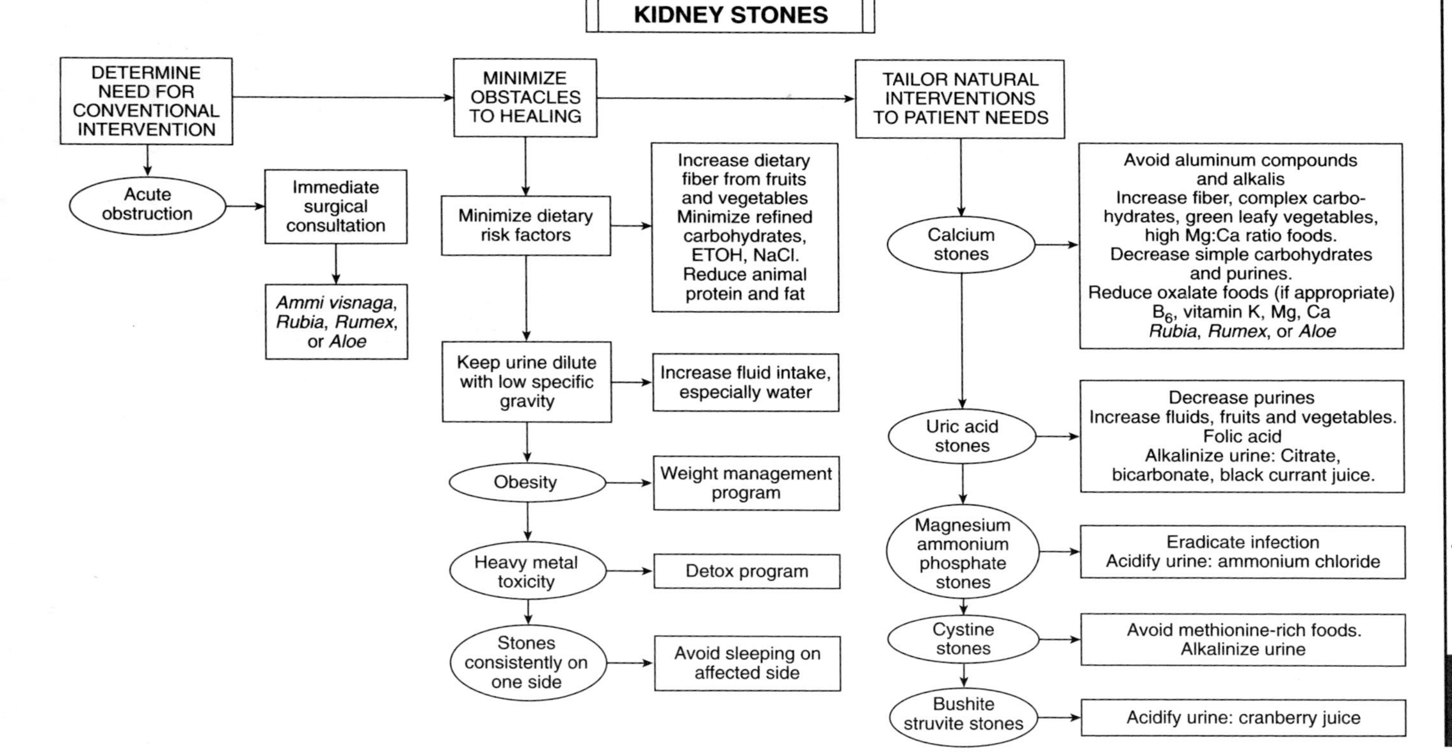
KIDNEY STONES
DETERMINE NEED FOR CONVENTIONAL INTERVENTION
Acute obstruction
Immediate surgical consultation
Ammi visnaga, Rubia, Rumex, or Aloe
MINIMIZE OBSTACLES TO HEALING
Minimize dietary risk factors
Increase dietary fiber from fruits and vegetables Minimize refined carbohydrates, ETOH, NaCl. Reduce animal protein and fat
Keep urine dilute with low specific gravity
Increase fluid intake, especially water
Obesity
Weight management program
Heavy metal toxicity
Detox program
Stones consistently on one side
Avoid sleeping on affected side
TAILOR NATURAL INTERVENTIONS TO PATIENT NEEDS
Calcium stones
Avoid aluminum compounds and alkalis Increase fiber, complex carbohydrates, green leafy vegetables, high Mg:Ca ratio foods. Decrease simple carbohydrates and purines. Reduce oxalate foods (if appropriate) $B_6$, vitamin K, Mg, Ca Rubia, Rumex, or Aloe
Uric acid stones
Decrease purines Increase fluids, fruits and vegetables. Folic acid Alkalinize urine: Citrate, bicarbonate, black currant juice.
Magnesium ammonium phosphate stones
Eradicate infection Acidify urine: ammonium chloride
Cystine stones
Avoid methionine-rich foods. Alkalinize urine
Bushite struvite stones
Acidify urine: cranberry juice

## DIAGNOSTIC CONSIDERATIONS

Conditions favoring stone formation include the following:

- **Factors increasing concentration of stone crystalloids**: reduced urine volume (dehydration) and increased excretion of stone constituents.
- **Factors favoring stone formation at normal urinary concentrations**: urinary stasis, pH changes, foreign bodies, reduction of normal substances that solubilize stone constituents.

### Causes of Excessive Excretion of Relatively Insoluble Urinary Constituents

| Constituent | Cause of Excess Secretion | Laboratory Findings |
|---|---|---|
| Calcium | (>250 mg/day excreted) | |
| | Absorptive hypercalciuria | Low serum $PO_4$<br>30%-40% of all stone formers |
| | Renal hypercalciuria (renal tubular acidosis) | High serum PTH<br>High urinary cAMP |
| | Primary hyperparathyroidism | High serum calcium<br>High $1,25(OH)_2D_3$ |
| | Hyperthyroidism | |
| | High vitamin D intake | High serum calcium |
| | Excess intake of milk and alkali | |
| | Aluminum salt intake | Low serum phosphate<br>High $1,25(OH)_2D_3$ |
| | Destructive bone disease | |
| | Sarcoidosis | |
| | Prolonged immobility | |
| Oxalate | Familial oxaluria | Rare |
| | Ileal disease, resection, or bypass | |
| | Steatorrhea | |
| | High oxalate intake | |
| | Ethylene glycol poisoning | |
| | Vitamin C excess (extremely unlikely) | Vitamin $B_6$ deficiency or abnormal oxalate metabolism |
| | Methoxyflurane anesthesia | |
| Uric acid | (>750 mg/day excreted) | |
| | Gout | |
| | Idiopathic hyperuricosuria | |
| | Excess purine intake | |
| | Anticancer drugs | Rapid cell destruction |
| | Myeloproliferative disease | |
| Cysteine | Hereditary cystinuria | |

*PTH*, Parathyroid hormone; *cAMP*, cyclic adenosine monophosphate.

**Physical Changes in the Urine and Kidney**

| Condition | Possible Cause |
|---|---|
| Increased concentration | Dehydration<br>Stasis<br>Obstruction<br>Foreign body concretions |
| Urinary pH | Low—uric acid, cystine<br>High—calcium oxalate and $PO_4$ |
| Infection | Proteus—struvite |
| Uricosuria | Crystals of uric acid initiate precipitation of calcium oxalate from solution |
| Nuclei for stone formation | Cells bacteria, blood, etc. initiate precipitation |
| Sponge kidney | Horseshoe kidney |
| Deformities of kidney | Caliceal obstruction or defect |

## THERAPEUTIC CONSIDERATIONS

- **Stone composition**: diagnosing the type of stone is critical to therapy. Evaluate the following criteria to determine stone composition if one is not available for analysis: diet; underlying metabolic or disease factors; serum and urinary calcium, uric acid, creatinine, and electrolyte levels; urinalysis; urine culture.
- **Dietary factors**: calcium (Ca)-containing stones are calcium oxalate, calcium oxalate mixed with calcium phosphate, or (very rarely) calcium phosphate alone. High incidence of Ca stones in affluent societies is linked to a diet low in fiber and high in refined carbohydrates, alcohol, animal protein, fat, high-Ca food, and vitamin D-enriched food.
  - —Dietary factors induce hyperuricemia, hypercalciuria, and stone formation, building a cumulative effect.
  - —Vegetarians have a decreased risk of developing stones. Among meat eaters, those eating more fresh fruits and vegetables have a lower incidence of stones. Bran supplements and changing to whole wheat bread lower urinary calcium.
  - —Dietary factors in acidifying or alkalinizing urine: depending on stone type, the ability to alter urine pH may help treat

and prevent stones. Cranberry juice decreases urine pH and increases oxalic acid excretion and relative supersaturation for uric acid. Blackcurrant juice increases urine pH, excretion of citric acid, and oxalic acid loss. Blackcurrant juice may treat or prevent uric acid stones by alkalizing urine. Cranberry juice acidifies urine and may treat brushite and struvite stones and urinary tract infections.

- **Weight and carbohydrate metabolism**: Excess weight and insulin insensitivity induce hypercalciuria and higher risk. After glucose ingestion, urinary calcium rises along with decreased phosphate reabsorption. Low plasma phosphate stimulates 1,25-dihydroxy-cholecalciferol (active vitamin D) production, increased intestinal absorption of Ca, and hypercalciuria. Sucrose and other simple sugars cause exaggerated increase in urinary calcium oxalate in 70% of recurrent kidney stone formers.
- **Gut flora**: oxalate homeostasis depends in part on the colon anaerobe bacterium *Oxalobacter formigenes*. Its absence (from prolonged antibiotic use) predisposes idiopathic calcium oxalate kidney stones from increased hyperoxaluria and calcium-oxalate stone formation. *O. formigenes* therapy repopulates gut and reduces urinary oxalate after oxalate load, thereby reducing calcium oxalate stone formation. Supplementing deficient persons may protect against future kidney stones.

## Nutrients

- **Magnesium (Mg) and vitamin $B_6$**: Mg-deficient diet accelerates renal tubular Ca deposition in rats. Mg increases solubility of calcium oxalate and inhibits precipitation of calcium phosphate and calcium oxalate. Low urinary Mg/Ca ratio is an independent risk factor in stone formation. Supplemental Mg alone prevents recurrences. Mg plus vitamin $B_6$ have even greater effect. Induced $B_6$ deficiency in rats produces oxaluria and calcium oxalate lithiasis (prevented by Mg supplementation).
- **Pyridoxine (vitamin $B_6$)**: reduces endogenous production and urinary excretion of oxalates. Patients with recurrent oxalate stones show abnormal EGPT, EGOT, UGPT, and UGOT activation levels, indicating clinical insufficiency of $B_6$ and impaired glutamic acid synthesis. Levels normalize after 3 months of treatment.
- **Glutamic acid**: decreased glutamic acid (from $B_6$ deficiency or other reasons) is linked to kidney stones; increased glutamic acid in urine reduces calcium oxalate precipitation. Glutamic acid supplementation in rats reduces incidence of calculi but may be superfluous with adequate vitamin $B_6$.

- **Calcium**: Ca restriction enhances oxalate absorption and stone formation absorption. Ca supplements reduce oxalate excretion. Kidney stone risk is higher in persons with lowest daily Ca intakes compared with those with highest. Ca supplementation (300-1000 mg q.d.) may be preventive.
- **Citrate**: low urinary citrate excretion is a risk for nephrolithiasis. Urinary Ca rises in patients taking Ca-citrate, but citrate reduces urinary saturation of calcium oxalate and calcium phosphate. It retards nucleation and crystal growth of Ca salts. Potassium and sodium citrate for recurrent calcium oxalate are quite effective; they cease stone formation in 90% of subjects. Mg citrate may offer the greatest benefit.
- **Vitamin K**: urinary glycoprotein inhibitor of calcium oxalate monohydrate growth requires posttranscription carboxylation of glutamic acid to form gamma-carboxyglutamic acid. Vitamin K is an essential for this carboxylation. Impairment of glutamic acid formation or vitamin K deficiency reduces this glycoprotein. Vitamin K in green leafy vegetables may be one reason vegetarians have a lower incidence of kidney stones.
- **Uric acid metabolism**: dietary purine intake is linearly related to rate of urinary uric acid excretion. Hyperuricosuria is a causative factor in recurrent Ca oxalate stones. High supplemental folic acid promotes purine scavenging and xanthine oxidase inhibition, decreasing excretion of uric acid (see the chapter on gout).

## Botanicals

- Anthraquinones isolated from *Rubia* (madder root), *Cassia* (senna), and *Aloe* species bind Ca and reduce growth of urinary crystals when used in oral doses lower than laxative dose. *Rubia tinctura, Rumex* (yellow dock), *Rheum* (rhubarb), *Polygonum aviculare, Aloe, Senna, Rhamnus alnus,* and *Mitchella repens* (squaw vine) are sources of anthraquinones, which are used to prevent formation and, during acute atacks, reduce the size of stones.
- Furanocoumarin-containing herb *Ammi visnaga* (khella), is unusually effective at relaxing the ureter and allowing stone to pass. Ca channel–blocking capabilities act primarily on the ureters. Atropine and papaverine have similar, but less active, smooth muscle–relaxing effects. *Peucedanum, Leptotania, Ruta graveolens* (rue, bitterword), and *Hydrangea* contain similar furanocoumarins promoting smooth muscle relaxation, justifying historic uses in kidney stones.

### Lifestyle

- **Sleep position**: patients with recurrent renal calculi often have calculi on the same side. Sleep posture may affect renal hemodynamics. The side of the stone is identical to dependent sleep side in 76% of cases with positive predictive values of right and left side down posture for ipsilateral stone at 82% and 70%, respectively.
- **Stress**: events of intense emotional impact with apprehension and distress, for at least 1 week in duration, increase risk of kidney stone formation. These events may encourage loss of litholytic urinary constituents (Mg, citrate). Sympathetic fight-or-flight response may increase vasopressin, causing more hypertonic urine.

### Miscellaneous

- **Hair mineral analysis**: heavy metals (mercury, gold, uranium, and cadmium) are nephrotoxic. Cadmium (elevated serum cadmium) increases incidence of kidney stones.
- **Vitamin C**: in persons not on hemodialysis or suffering from recurrent kidney stones, severe kidney disease, or gout, high-dose vitamin C will not cause kidney stones. Vitamin C up to 10 g q.d. has no effect on urinary oxalate levels.
- **Inositol hexaphosphate ($IP_6$)**: a naturally occurring compound in whole grains, cereals, legumes, seeds, and nuts that is known for antineoplastic activity. Inadequate intake may increase calcium oxalate in urine, predisposing urolithiasis.
- **Salt**: decrease sodium chloride intake. Urinary Ca excretion increases 1 mmol (40 mg) for each 100 mmol (2300 mg) increase in dietary sodium in normal adults. Renal Ca stone formers with hypercalcemia have greater increase in urinary Ca per 100 mmol increase in salt intake.

## THERAPEUTIC APPROACH

Accurately differentiate stone types. Recognize and control underlying metabolic diseases or structural abnormalities of the urinary tract. The goal is to prevent recurrence. Dietary management is effective, inexpensive, and free of side effects. Specific treatment is determined by type of stone. Possible interventions include the following:

- Reducing urinary calcium
- Reducing purine intake

- Avoiding high oxalate–containing foods
- Increasing foods with a high Mg/Ca ratio
- Increasing vitamin K–rich foods.

For all types of stones, increase urine flow with increased intake of pure water to dilute urine. Maintain specific gravity <1.015 and daily urinary volume of 2000+ mL. If stones occur on one side only, avoid sleeping on that side. Consider stress reduction techniques and counseling for patients with stones and a history of significant stress.

### Acute Obstruction

Surgical removal or lithotripsy may be necessary.

- *Ammi visnaga* (khella) extract (12% khellin content): 250 mg t.i.d.
- *Rubia tinctura, Rumex crispus* (yellow dock), or *Aloe vera* at below-laxative doses.

### Calcium Stones

- **Diet**: increase fiber, complex carbohydrates, and green leafy vegetables. Decrease simple carbohydrates and purines (meat, fish, poultry, yeast). Increase high Mg/Ca ratio foods (barley, bran, corn, buckwheat, rye, soy, oats, brown rice, avocado, banana, cashew, coconut, peanut, sesame seed, lima beans, potato). If stones are oxalate, reduce oxalate foods (black tea, cocoa, spinach, beet leaves, rhubarb, parsley, cranberry, nuts). Limit dairy products.
- **Supplements**:
  —Vitamin $B_6$: 25 mg q.d.
  —Vitamin K: 2 mg q.d.
  —Magnesium: 600 mg q.d. in divided doses.
  —Calcium: 300-1000 mg q.d.
- **Botanicals**: use any of the following in a dose below the laxative effect:
  —*Rubia tinctura*
  —*Rumex crispus*
  —*Aloe vera*
- **Miscellaneous**: avoid aluminum compounds and alkalis.

### Uric Acid Stones

- **Diet**: decrease purines (listed previously); ensure adequate fluid (pure water) intake and a high alkali load with plenty of fruits and vegetables.
- **Supplements**: folic acid at 5 mg q.d.

- **Miscellaneous**: alkalinize urine with citrate, bicarbonate, black-currant juice.

### Magnesium Ammonium Phosphate Stones

- Eradicate infection (*Textbook,* "Immune Support")
- Acidify urine: ammonium chloride (100-200 mg t.i.d.).

### Cystine Stones

- **Diet**: avoid methionine-rich foods (eggs, soy, wheat, dairy products [except whole milk], fish, meat, lima beans, garbanzo beans, mushrooms, and all nuts except coconut, hazelnut, and sunflower seeds).
- **Miscellaneous**: alkalinize urine; optimal pH is 7.5-8.0.

### Bushite and Struvite Stones

- Acidify urine: cranberry juice

**Chemical and Physical Characteristics of Urinary Stones**

| Composition | Crystal Name | Frequency | X-ray Appearance | Urine Characteristics | Crystal Characteristics |
|---|---|---|---|---|---|
| Calcium oxalate | Whewellite | 30%-35% | Opaque | Nonspecific | Small, hempseed or mulberry shaped, brown or black color |
| Calcium oxalate + calcium phosphate | | 30-35 | Opaque | pH >5.5 | Small, hempseed or mulberry shaped, brown or black color |
| Calcium phosphate | Apatite | 6-8 | Opaque | pH >5.5 | Staghorn configuration, light color |
| Magnesium ammonium phosphate | Struvite | 15-20 | Opaque | pH >6.2 | Staghorn configuration, light color |
| | Triple phosphate | | | Infection | |
| Uric acid | | 6-10 | Translucent | pH <6.0 | Ellipsoid, tan or red-brown |
| Cystine | | 2-3 | Opaque | pH <7.2 | Multiple, faceted, maple sugar color |

# Leukoplakia

## DIAGNOSTIC SUMMARY

- Adherent white patch or plaque appearing anywhere on oral mucosa.
- Asymptomatic until ulceration, fissuring, or malignant transformation.
- Diagnosis confirmed by biopsy.

## GENERAL CONSIDERATIONS

Leukoplakia is the clinical term for a white plaquelike lesion anywhere on the oral mucosa. It is a reaction to irritation (cigarette smoking, tobacco, betel nut chewing) and early sign in HIV infection. It most frequently occurs in men aged 50-70 years. In 90% of cases, it represents epithelial hyperkeratosis and hyperplasia. In 10% of cases epithelial dysplasia also is present; these lesions are considered precancerous.

Oral cancer is a common malignant neoplasm; 50,000 new cases and 12,000 deaths occur in the United States alone each year. Survival rates with chemotherapy, radiation, and surgery are unchanged in the past few decades. Prevent death by preventing occurrence with abstinence from tobacco and increased intake of antioxidants.

## THERAPEUTIC CONSIDERATIONS

Remove all irritants. Electrodesiccation, cryosurgery, and proteolytic enzymes have not given predictably favorable results.

- **Vitamin A and beta-carotene**: clinically effective for leukoplakia. The micronucleus test is a useful indicator of cancerous tendency of epithelial cells, giving immediate information on genotoxic damage. Micronuclei are formed during chromatid or chromosomal breakage; the rate of formation is linked to oral carcinogenesis. It is a good predictor of cancer, which takes years to

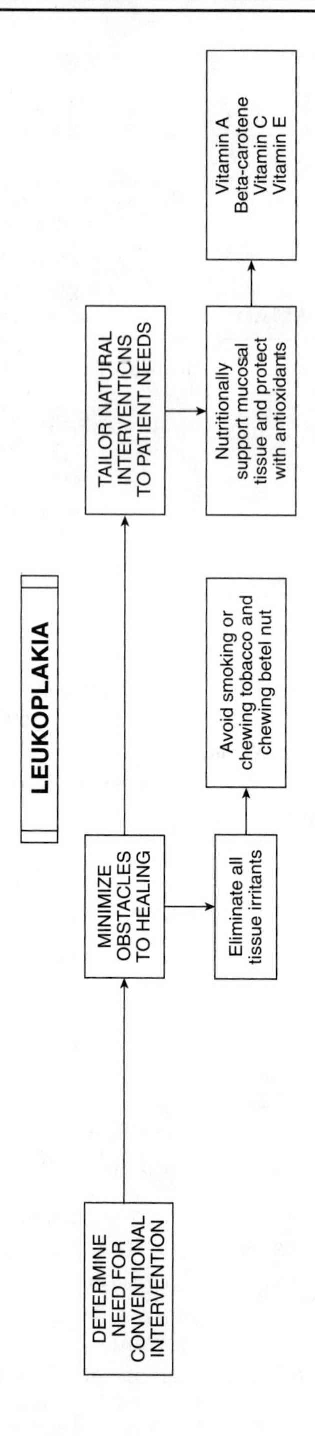
LEUKOPLAKIA
DETERMINE NEED FOR CONVENTIONAL INTERVENTION
MINIMIZE OBSTACLES TO HEALING
Eliminate all tissue irritants
Avoid smoking or chewing tobacco and chewing betel nut
TAILOR NATURAL INTERVENTICNS TO PATIENT NEEDS
Nutritionally support mucosal tissue and protect with antioxidants
Vitamin A
Beta-carotene
Vitamin C
Vitamin E

develop recognizable signs. Beta-carotene is quite effective in decreasing the mean proportion of cells with micronuclei on buccal mucosa in Asian betel nut and tobacco chewers. (Subjects continued to chew betel nut and tobacco during the study.) Evidence documenting the protective effect of carotenoids and retinoids against epithelial cancers is overwhelming (*Textbook,* "Beta-carotene and Other Carotenoids"). An inverse relation exists between serum retinol and carotene levels and cancer incidence holds true for oral carcinomas. Studies on leukoplakia used very high but effective retinol dosages (150,000-900,000 IU q.d.). Beta-carotene is as effective as retinol in decreasing micronuclei with much higher therapeutic index. (Note: vulvar leukoplakia is responsive to retinol and perhaps beta-carotene.) Head-to-head comparative study found an advantage with retinol. Homogeneous leukoplakia and smaller lesions respond better than did nonhomogeneous and larger lesions. No major toxicities were observed even with prolonged vitamin A supplementation.

- **Other antioxidants**: vitamin E (400 mg q.d.) produces a 65% response rate. Use a combination of antioxidants to accommodate their interactions and limitations. A combination of vitamin C (1000 mg q.d.), beta-carotene (30 mg q.d.), and vitamin E (400 mg q.d.) gives encouraging results.

## THERAPEUTIC APPROACH

Leukoplakia is caused by a combination of excessive carcinogenic irritation and marginal or low levels of vitamin A. Eliminate all sources of irritation. Establish optimal vitamin A, beta-carotene, and antioxidant levels. The main irritants are tobacco smoking and chewing, betel nut chewing, and ultraviolet exposure.

### Supplements

- **Vitamin A**: 5000 IU q.d.
- **Beta-carotene**: 30-90 mg q.d.
- **Vitamin C**: 1,000-3000 mg q.d.
- **Vitamin E**: 400 IU q.d. (mixed tocopherols)

# Lichen Planus

## DIAGNOSTIC SUMMARY

- **History**: pruritus (can be severe); rash or skin eruption.
- **Physical examination**: skin lesions are flat topped, violaceous to purple, polygonal or oval papules from 1-10 mm wide with edges that are sharply defined and shiny. Lesions may be grouped, linear (Koebner phenomenon), annular, or disseminated when generalized. White lines (Wickham's striae) are possible. Use handheld lens; apply clear oil over lesion to intensify visibility of Wickham's striae. In dark-skinned patients appears as postinflammatory hyperpigmentation. Lesion location: flexor surfaces of wrists, lumbar region, eyelids, shin, scalp, glans penis, mouth, but may occur anywhere. An uncommon presentation is plaque-size lesions. Location is on nails and hair follicles, with dystrophic changes and scarring.
- **Oral lesions**: inflammation and leukohyperkeratoses generating reticulated, white puncta or papules and lines in a lacelike pattern. Plaques may occur. Inflammation may cause erosions with blisters. Location is on buccal mucosa; bilateral in nearly all patients on tongue, lips, and gingiva. Skin lesions occur in 10%-60% of oral cases.
- **Other locations**: genitalia; papular, annular, or erosive lesions on penis, scrotum, labia majora, labia minor, and vagina. On the scalp, atrophic skin and scarring alopecia; on the nails, destruction of nail fold and nail bed with longitudinal splintering.
- **Biopsy**: if doubt exists or if blisters, plaques, or erosions occur in the oral form.

## GENERAL CONSIDERATIONS

Lichen planus (LP) is an inflammatory, pruritic disease of the skin and mucous membranes and can be generalized or localized. Characteristic features include distinctive purplish, flat-topped papules (discrete or coalescent into plaques) on the trunk and flexor surfaces.

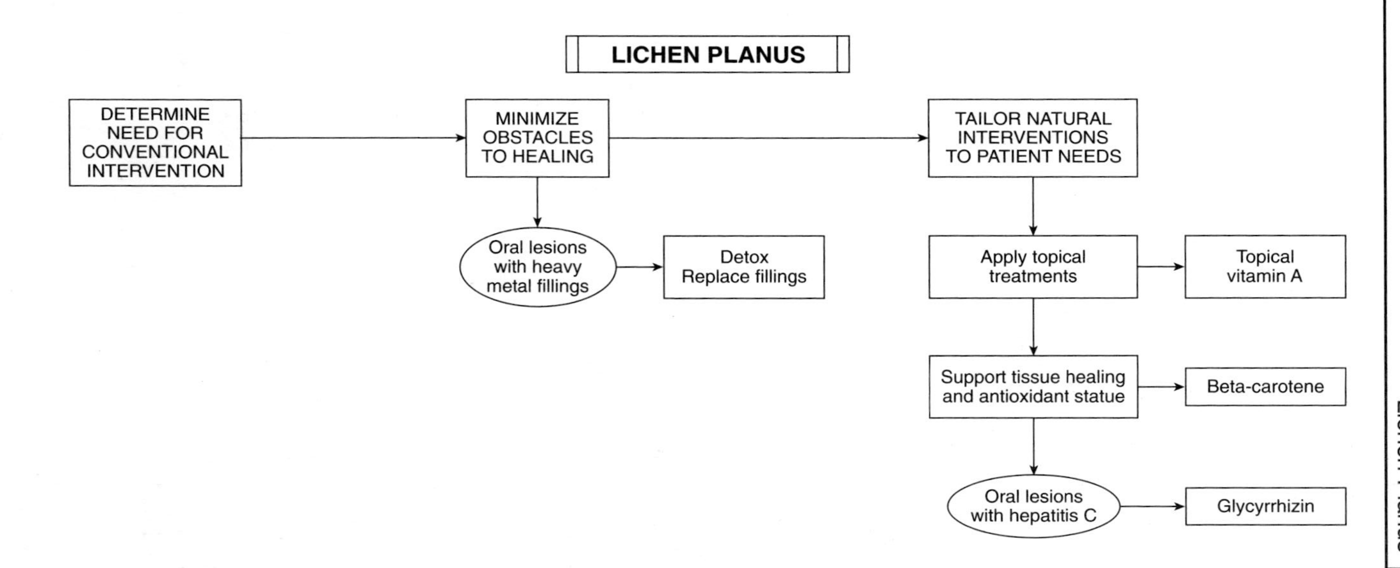
LICHEN PLANUS
DETERMINE NEED FOR CONVENTIONAL INTERVENTION
MINIMIZE OBSTACLES TO HEALING
Oral lesions with heavy metal fillings
Detox
Replace fillings
TAILOR NATURAL INTERVENTIONS TO PATIENT NEEDS
Apply topical treatments
Topical vitamin A
Support tissue healing and antioxidant statue
Beta-carotene
Oral lesions with hepatitis C
Glycyrrhizin

- **Etiology**: unknown. Metals (gold, mercury), or infection (hepatitis C virus) altering cell-mediated immunity may play a role. Human leukocyte antigen genetic susceptibility may exist.
- **Epidemiology**: higher prevalence of hepatitis C virus infection in patients with LP, but a pathogenic relation has not been established. LP affects women more than men. Age of onset is 30-60 years. Hypertrophic LP is more common in African Americans.
- **Variants**
  - —**Hypertrophic**: large, thick plaques on foot and shins; more common in African-American men. Hypertrophic lesions may become hyperkeratotic rather than smooth.
  - —**Follicular**: individual keratotic-follicular papules and plaques leading to cicatricial alopecia. Graham Little syndrome is a complex of spinous follicular lesions, any lichen planus, and cicatricial alopecia.
  - —**Vesicular**: vesicular or bullous lesions within or independent of lesions. Direct immunofluorescence reveals bullous pemphigoid; patients have bullous pemphigoid immunoglobulin G (IgG) autoantibodies.
  - —**Actinicus**: papular lesions in sun exposed areas (e.g., dorsum of hands and arms).
  - —**Ulcerative**: therapy-resistant ulcers (soles) requiring skin grafting.
  - —**Oral/mucous membranes**: reticular, hyperkeratotic, erosive, plaque type, atrophic, bullous types
- **Incidence**: six per 1000 dermatology patients, or 4.4 per 1000 people in the United States per year. Oral LP is the most common cause of oral white lesions, occurring in 0.5%-1% of dental patients. Oral LP occurs alone or with skin lesions.
- **Onset**: acute or insidious. Lesions remain for months to years. Lesions are asymptomatic or mildly to severely pruritic; they are more painful on mucous membranes and worse with ulceration.
- **Course of oral LP**: chronic from months to years; two thirds of cases undergo spontaneous resolution within 1 year. Recurrence is uncommon (<20% of patents). Mucous membrane cases have much more prolonged course, but 50% remit in 2 years. Incidence of oral squamous cell carcinoma in patients with oral LP is increased by 5%.

LP-like eruptions can occur from graft-versus-host disease, dermatomyositis, and as cutaneous manifestations of malignant lymphoma and certain drugs.

## THERAPEUTIC CONSIDERATIONS

The underlying mechanism of LP is unknown. The immune system's role is evidenced by the presence of immunoglobulin (Ig) M (possibly IgA, IgG) and complement at the dermal/epidermal junction in 95% of LP lesions; certain drug eruptions and graft-versus-host reactions in bone marrow transplant recipients mimic LP. Primary immune factor is cell-mediated processes. Activated $T_H$ cells in early lesions target basal cells, which may have antigenic alterations. $T_s$ cells predominate in older lesions.

- **Dental amalgams**: oral LP is more resistant to therapy than are skin lesions. Dental amalgams are linked to oral LP. Replacing mercury amalgam fillings with alternative substances dramatically improves chronic lichenoid reactions. The greatest effect is noted with gold crowns versus palladium-based crowns. If gold crowns are present, have the patient patch tested for gold allergy; consider removal if positive. (Note: many patch test–negative patients still respond to amalgam removal.)
- **Antifungal griseofulvin therapy**: in a double-blind, controlled study, 70.6% of patients treated with griseofulvin showed regression of symptoms compared with 35.3% on placebo. Biopsy of griseofulvin responders and placebo responders revealed uniform histologic changes.
- **Photodynamic therapy**: a case report showed LP of the penis resistant to steroids (and initially diagnosed as intraepidermal carcinoma). Photodynamic therapy was preceded by topical 5-aminolevulinic acid (20%) ointment (4 hours before treatment). Irradiate with a Paterson-Whitehurst lamp (Paterson Institute, Christie Hospital, Manchester, U.K.) at center wavelength of 630 and rectangular pass band of 27 nm. Dose gradually increased to 50 $J/cm^2$ at fluence rate of 55 $mW/cm^2$ to prevent edema and phimosis. Treatment was repeated after 6 weeks. Lesions completely resolved after another 4 weeks, with no recurrence at 6 months. Biopsy: mild changes identifying condition as LP.

### Supplements and Botanical Medicines

Vitamin A and beta-carotene:

- Topical retinoic acid (0.1% in petroleum jelly base) applied three times a day over a 3-week period to hypertrophic LP of the palms or soles caused irritation because of the frequency of application. When applied every other day two to three times per day, it

induced regression after 2 to 3 weeks. A slight recurrence arose after 3-4 months.
- Topical retinoic acid 0.05% was not as effective as fluocinolone acetonide 0.1% applied q.i.d. to various stages of oral LP.
- Patients with mucosal dysplasia (leukoplakia, LP, erythroplasia, leukokeratosis) are low-normal for serum vitamin A, beta-carotene, and cis-retinoic acid. Of 18 patients receiving beta-carotene (30 mg q.i.d.), one deteriorated, nine remained stable, and eight improved (six completely). The addition of isotretinoin (Accutane) 10 mg t.i.d. caused three stable patients to improve. Response to treatment was much higher in smokers (30 pack-years or more) than nonsmokers.
- Vitamin A can be applied with folic acid in an adhesive base (Orabase).

### Glycyrrhizin

Of nine patients with oral LP and hepatitis C receiving intravenous glycyrrhizin (40 mL 0.2% solution of glycyrrhizin q.d. for 4 consecutive weeks), six improved clinically. They had only mildly raised alanine aminotransferase and aspartate aminotransferase levels. (Note: Scientific Botanicals *Glycyrrhiza* SE is standardized to 17% glycyrrhizin. A comparable oral dose is 500 mg solid extract.)

## THERAPEUTIC APPROACH

Because the cause of LP is undetermined, curative approaches are unclear. For oral lesions and significant metal-based fillings, consider heavy metal detoxification and replacement of metal fillings.

### Supplements

- **Vitamin A (0.1% solution)**: topical application q.i.d.
- **Beta-carotene**: 30 mg q.i.d.
- **Glycyrrhizin**: topical application

# Macular Degeneration

## DIAGNOSTIC SUMMARY

- Progressive visual loss caused by degeneration of the macula.
- Ophthalmologic examination may reveal spots of pigment near macula and blurring of macular borders.

## GENERAL CONSIDERATIONS

The macula is the area of the retina where most images focus and the portion of the retina responsible for fine vision. Macular degeneration (MD) is the leading cause of severe visual loss in the United States and Europe in persons aged 55 years and older; it is second to cataracts as the leading cause of decreased vision in persons older than 65 years. More than 150,000 Americans are legally blind from age-related MD (ARMD); 20,000 new cases arise each year. The number of ARMD cases will double in the next 25 years.

- **Major risk factors**: smoking, aging, atherosclerosis, and hypertension. Degeneration results from free radical damage. Decreased blood and oxygen supply to the retina are a harbinger of MD.
- **Other factors**: region of chromosome 10 may be linked to ARMD but the diversity in phenotype and late onset of disease complicate feasibility of linkage. Higher birth weight and lower head circumference/birth weight ratio are associated with increased risk.

### Types of Age-Related Macular Degeneration

In either form, patients experience blurred vision. Straight objects appear distorted or bent. A dark spot appears near or around the center of the visual field. While reading, parts of words are missing. The two types of ARMD are:

- **Atrophic "dry" ARMD**: 80%-95% of people with ARMD have the dry form. Primary lesions are atrophic changes in retinal pigmented epithelium (RPE) (innermost layer of retina). Cells of RPE gradually accumulate, throughout life, sacs of cellular debris

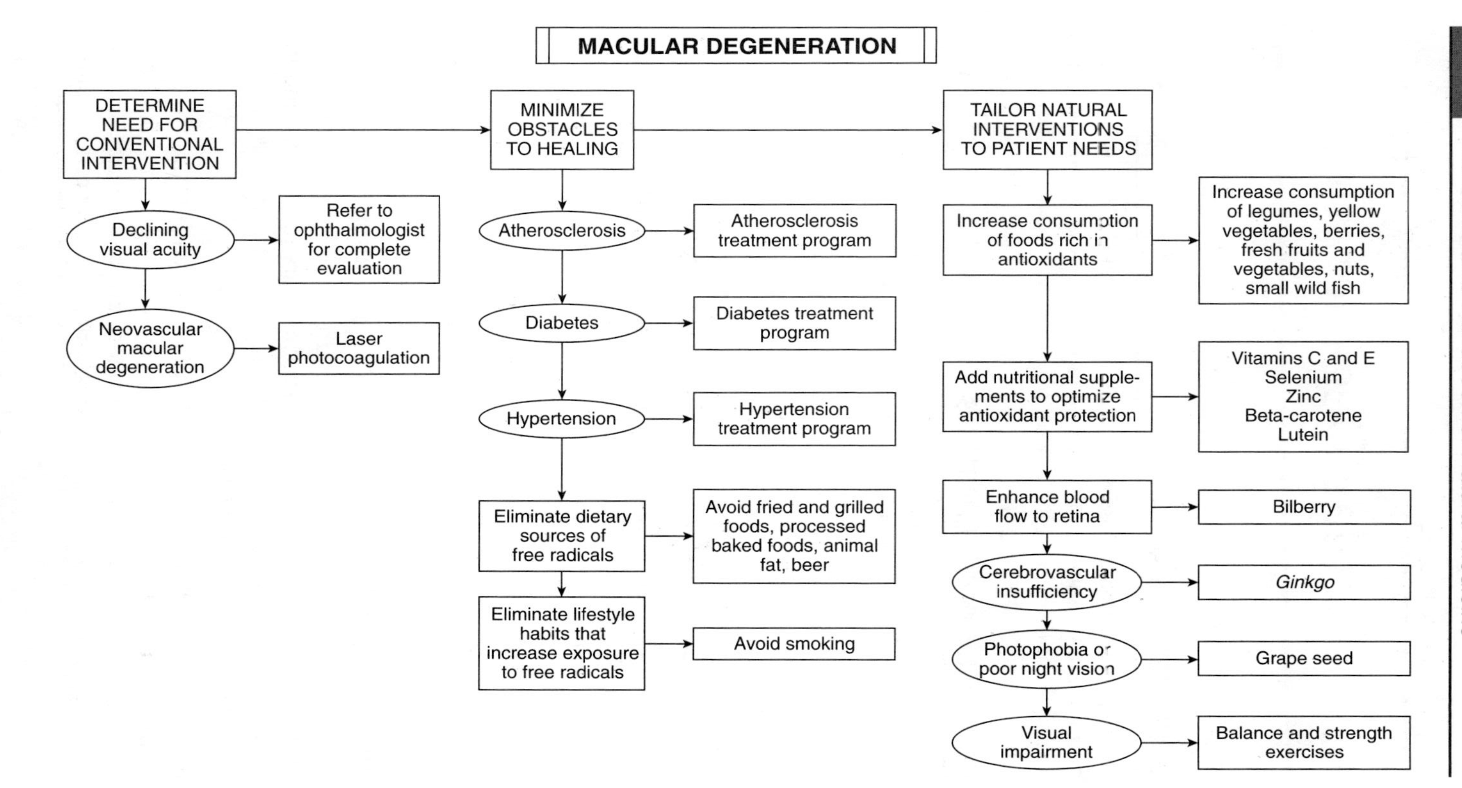
MACULAR DEGENERATION
DETERMINE NEED FOR CONVENTIONAL INTERVENTION
Declining visual acuity
Refer to ophthalmologist for complete evaluation
Neovascular macular degeneration
Laser photocoagulation
MINIMIZE OBSTACLES TO HEALING
Atherosclerosis
Atherosclerosis treatment program
Diabetes
Diabetes treatment program
Hypertension
Hypertension treatment program
Eliminate dietary sources of free radicals
Avoid fried and grilled foods, processed baked foods, animal fat, beer
Eliminate lifestyle habits that increase exposure to free radicals
Avoid smoking
TAILOR NATURAL INTERVENTIONS TO PATIENT NEEDS
Increase consumption of foods rich in antioxidants
Increase consumption of legumes, yellow vegetables, berries, fresh fruits and vegetables, nuts, small wild fish
Add nutritional supplements to optimize antioxidant protection
Vitamins C and E
Selenium
Zinc
Beta-carotene
Lutein
Enhance blood flow to retina
Bilberry
Cerebrovascular insufficiency
Ginkgo
Photophobia or poor night vision
Grape seed
Visual impairment
Balance and strength exercises

(lipofuscin)—remnants of degraded molecules from damaged RPE or phagocytized rod and cone membranes. Progressive lipofuscin engorgement of RPE cells extrudes tissue components (hyaline, sialomuccin, cerebroside). Hallmark excrescences beneath RPE seen on ophthalmoscopic examination are called drusen. The disease progresses slowly and only central vision is lost; peripheral vision remains intact. Total blindness from dry ARMD is rare. No standard medical treatment exists.

- **Neovascular "wet" ARMD**: neovascular form affects 5%-20% of those with ARMD. It involves growth of abnormal blood vessels and can be treated effectively in the early stages with laser photocoagulation. The disease rapidly progresses to a point at which surgery is ineffective; perform surgery as soon as possible.

## THERAPEUTIC CONSIDERATIONS

Treatment for wet form is laser photocoagulation. New treatments include photodynamic therapy with photosensitive drugs (verteporfin) and low-powered laser and low-dose radiation.

Treating the dry form and preventing the wet form involve antioxidants and natural substances that correct underlying pathophysiology—free radical damage and poor oxygenation of macula. Reduce risk factors for atherosclerosis; increase dietary fresh fruits and vegetables and use nutritional and botanical antioxidants.

- **Reducing and preventing atherosclerosis**: atherosclerosis is a risk factor for MD. In subjects younger than 85 years, plaques in carotid bifurcation indicate 4.7-fold increased prevalence of MD; lower extremity atherosclerosis indicates a 2.5 times greater risk (see the chapter on atherosclerosis).
- **Dietary fruits and vegetables**: a diet rich in fruits and vegetables offers a lower risk for ARMD by increasing intake of antioxidants. Non–provitamin A carotenes lutein, zeaxanthin, and lycopene and flavonoids are more protective against ARMD than traditional nutritional antioxidants. The macula (and central portion, the fovea) owes its yellow color to a high concentration of lutein and zeaxanthin that prevent oxidative damage to the retina and protect against MD. Individuals with lycopene in the lowest quintile are twice as likely to have ARMD. Persons with lowest plasma concentrations of zeaxanthin have a 2.0 odds ratio for risk of ARMD. Risk is increased in people with lowest plasma

lutein plus zeaxanthin and with lowest lutein, but neither of these relations was statistically significant.

- **Animal fat**: animal fat and processed baked goods intake carried a twofold increased risk of progression of ARMD. Higher fish intake lowers risk of progression among subjects with lower linoleic acid intake. Nuts are protective. Egg yolks are an excellent source of bioavailable lutein and zeaxanthin, but increase low-density lipoprotein by 8% to 11%. Other studies found no change in cholesterol in healthy volunteers with moderate egg consumption and that only those with concomitant high plasma cholesterol and triglycerides are subject to hyperlipidemic increases when eating foods with dietary cholesterol, such as eggs.
- **Alcohol**: moderate wine consumption decreases MD risk. Red-purple foods contain protective anthocyanin antioxidants. Avoid beer because it increases drusen accumulation and risk of exudative MD.
- **Nutritional supplements**: antioxidants (vitamin C, selenium, beta-carotene, vitamin E) are important for treatment and prevention. Combinations are better than any single nutrient alone because none alone accounts for impaired antioxidant status in ARMD. Decreased antioxidant status reflects decreases in combinations of nutrients.
- **Antioxidant preparations**: progression of dry ARMD was halted (but not reversed) with a commercial antioxidant combination. Another antioxidant containing beta-carotene, vitamins C and E, zinc, copper, manganese, selenium, and riboflavin was able to maintain or improve visual acuity in these patients.
- **Lutein**: the Lutein Antioxidant Supplementation Trial studying atrophic ARMD found that patients receiving lutein (10 mg) alone or in combination with other vitamins and minerals in a broad-spectrum formula improved mean eye macular pigment optical density, Snellen equivalent visual acuity, and contrast sensitivity.
- **Zinc (Zn)**: essential in metabolism of retina; the elderly have a high risk for Zn deficiency. Supplementing 200 mg q.d. Zn sulfate (80 mg elemental Zn) reduces visual loss. Age-Related Eye Disease Study used 500 mg vitamin C, 400 IU vitamin E, 15 mg beta-carotene, 80 mg Zn (Zn oxide), and 2 mg copper (cupric oxide) to reduce risk of developing advanced ARMD. Researchers recommended combination of Zn and antioxidants for patients older than 55 years at risk for ARMD. These results were not confirmed in a study of wet ARMD.

- **Flavonoid-rich extracts**: *Vaccinium myrtillus* (bilberry), *Ginkgo biloba*, and *Vitis vinifera* (grapeseed) are beneficial in preventing and treating ARMD. These excellent antioxidants improve retinal blood flow and function. They can halt progressive visual loss of dry ARMD and may even improve visual function. Bilberry extracts standardized to 25% anthocyanidins are most useful. *Vaccinium* anthocyanosides have very strong affinity for RPE, the functional portion of retina affected by ARMD, reinforcing collagen structures of the retina and preventing free radical damage. *Ginkgo biloba* extract (24% *Ginkgo* flavonglycoside and 6% terpenoids) is a better choice if patient also has signs of cerebrovascular insufficiency. Grapeseed extract is most useful with photophobia or poor night vision.
- **Lifestyle**: because oxidant exposure is the major factor in MD, smoking increases risk in men and women. Currently smoking 25+ cigarettes daily carries a relative risk of 2.4 for ARMD compared with nonsmokers. Past smokers of 25+ cigarettes daily have a twofold increased risk relative to never-smokers. Risk did not return to control until after not smoking for 15 years.
- **Exercise**: may not play a role in reversing or preventing ARMD, but strength and balance training can minimize risk of falling in visually impaired patients.

## THERAPEUTIC APPROACH

Prevention or treatment at an early stage is most effective. The treatment for wet form of ARMD is laser photocoagulation as soon as possible. For the dry form, use antioxidants and promote retinal blood flow. Refer any patient 55 years or older with visual loss to an ophthalmologist for complete evaluation, especially if visual loss is progressing rapidly. Investigate and treat underlying diabetes and/or hypertension (see the chapters on diabetes mellitus and hypertension).

- **Diet**: avoid fried and grilled foods and other sources of free radicals; animal fat; processed baked goods; beer. Increase legumes (high in sulfur-containing amino acids), yellow vegetables (carotenes), flavonoid-rich berries (blueberries, blackberries, cherries), vitamin E– and vitamin C–rich foods (fresh fruits and vegetables), nuts, and small wild fish. Moderate red wine intake is advised for those without contraindications to alcohol.

- **Supplements**:
  - —Vitamin C: 1 g t.i.d.
  - —Vitamin E: 600-800 IU q.d. (mixed tocopherols)
  - —Selenium: 400 μg q.d.
  - —Zinc: 30 mg q.d.
  - —Beta-carotene (mixed carotenoids): 50,000 IU q.d.
  - —Lutein: 15 mg q.d.
- **Botanical medicines (choose one)**:
  - —*Ginkgo biloba* extract (24% ginkgo heterosides): 40-80 mg t.i.d.
  - —*Vaccinium myrtillus* (bilberry) extract (25% anthocyanidin content): 40-80 mg t.i.d.
  - —Grapeseed extract (95% procyanidolic oligomer content): 150-300 mg q.d.
- **Exercise**: balance training and strength exercises, especially for those who are visually impaired.

# Male Infertility

## DIAGNOSTIC SUMMARY

- Inability to conceive child after 6 months of unprotected sex in the absence of female causes.
- Total sperm count <5 million/mL
- Presence of >50% abnormal sperm
- Inability of sperm to impregnate egg as determined by postcoital or hamster egg penetration tests

## GENERAL CONSIDERATIONS

- In the United States, 18% of couples have difficulty conceiving a child. In one third of cases the man is responsible; in another third both are responsible; in another third the woman is responsible. Six percent of men aged 15-50 years are infertile.
- Most male infertility reflects abnormal sperm count (oligospermia) or quality. Natural barriers in the female reproductive tract allow only 40 of 20 million ejaculated sperm to reach the vicinity of the egg. The number of sperm in ejaculate correlates strongly with fertility. In 90% of oligospermia cases, the reason is deficient sperm production; in 90% of these cases the cause for decreased sperm formation is unidentified and known as "idiopathic oligospermia" or "azoospermia." Azoospermia is the complete absence of living sperm in semen.

## DIAGNOSTIC CONSIDERATIONS

Semen analysis is the most widely used test of male fertility potential. Semen is analyzed for concentration of sperm and sperm quality. Sperm count and quality in the male population has deteriorated over the last few decades. Men now supply 40% of the number of sperm per ejaculate compared with 1940 levels.

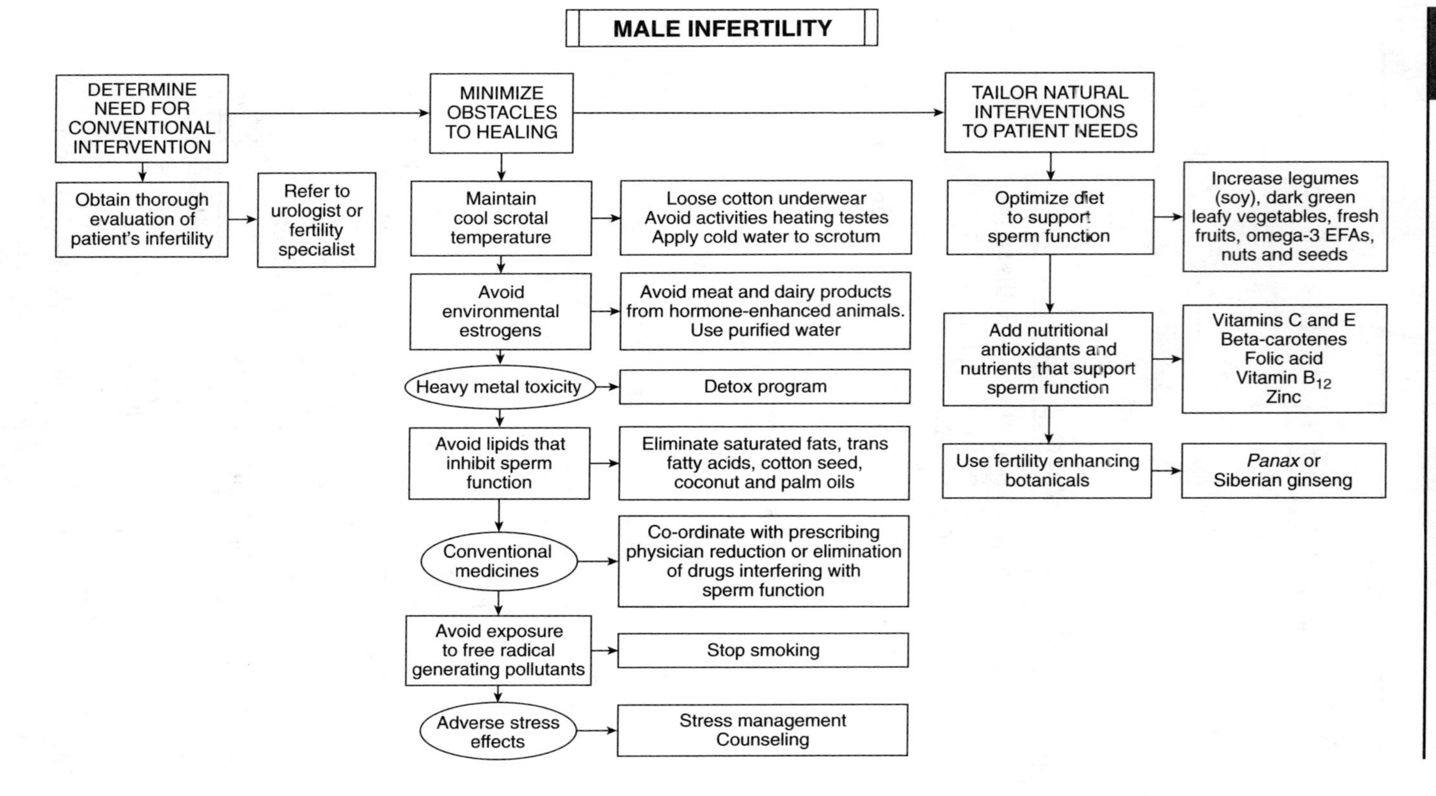
MALE INFERTILITY
DETERMINE NEED FOR CONVENTIONAL INTERVENTION
Obtain thorough evaluation of patient's infertility
Refer to urologist or fertility specialist
MINIMIZE OBSTACLES TO HEALING
Maintain cool scrotal temperature
Loose cotton underwear
Avoid activities heating testes
Apply cold water to scrotum
Avoid environmental estrogens
Avoid meat and dairy products from hormone-enhanced animals.
Use purified water
Heavy metal toxicity
Detox program
Avoid lipids that inhibit sperm function
Eliminate saturated fats, trans fatty acids, cotton seed, coconut and palm oils
Conventional medicines
Co-ordinate with prescribing physician reduction or elimination of drugs interfering with sperm function
Avoid exposure to free radical generating pollutants
Stop smoking
Adverse stress effects
Stress management
Counseling
TAILOR NATURAL INTERVENTIONS TO PATIENT NEEDS
Optimize diet to support sperm function
Increase legumes (soy), dark green leafy vegetables, fresh fruits, omega-3 EFAs, nuts and seeds
Add nutritional antioxidants and nutrients that support sperm function
Vitamins C and E
Beta-carotenes
Folic acid
Vitamin $B_{12}$
Zinc
Use fertility enhancing botanicals
*Panax* or Siberian ginseng

## Causes of Male Infertility

Deficient sperm production
Ductal obstruction
- Congenital defects
- Postinfectious obstruction
- Cystic fibrosis
- Vasectomy

Ejaculatory dysfunction
- Premature ejaculation
- Retrograde ejaculation

Disorders of accessory glands
- Infection
- Inflammation
- Antisperm antibodies
- Coital disorders
- Defects in technique
- Premature withdrawal
- Erectile dysfunction

## Possible Causes of Falling Sperm Counts

Increased scrotal temperature
- Tight-fitting clothing and briefs
- Varicoceles are more common

Environmental
- Increased pollution
- Heavy metals (e.g., lead, mercury, arsenic)
- Organic solvents
- Pesticides

Dietary
- Increased saturated fats
- Reduced intake of fruits, vegetables, and whole grains
- Reduced intake of dietary fiber
- Increased exposure to synthetic estrogens

Environmental, dietary, and lifestyle changes in recent decades interfere with a man's ability to manufacture sperm. As sperm counts have declined, the line differentiating infertile and fertile men has been reduced progressively from 40 million/mL to 5 million/mL. Quality is more important than quantity; a high sperm count is meaningless if the percentage of healthy sperm is not also high.

### "Normal" Spermatogenesis

| Criteria | Value |
|---|---|
| Volume | 1.5-5.0 mL |
| Density | >20 million sperm/mL |
| Motility | >30% motile |
| Normal forms | >60% |

If most sperm are abnormally shaped or nonmotile, the man is infertile despite normal sperm concentration. Low sperm count does not always mean a man is infertile.

### Causes of Temporary Low Sperm Count

- Increased scrotal temperature
- Infections, the common cold, the flu
- Increased stress
- Lack of sleep
- Overuse of alcohol, tobacco, or marijuana
- Many prescription drugs
- Exposure to radiation
- Exposure to solvents, pesticides, and other toxins

**Conventional semen analysis**: must be interpreted with caution. Functional tests are indicated especially when screening couples for in vitro fertilization.

### Male Fertility Tests

| Test | Fertility Prediction Accuracy |
|---|---|
| Semen analysis | 30% |
| Hamster egg penetration test | 66% |

- **Postcoital test**: measures ability of sperm to penetrate cervical mucus after intercourse.
- **Hamster egg penetration test**: human sperm can, under appropriate conditions, penetrate hamster eggs. Fertile males have a range of penetration of 10%-100%; penetration <10% indicates infertility. This test predicts fertility in 66% of cases compared with 30% for conventional semen analysis.

- **Antisperm antibodies**: those produced by men attack the tail of sperm, impeding motility and penetration of cervical mucus. Antibodies produced by women attack the head. Antibodies in semen are a sign of past or current infection in the male reproductive tract.

## THERAPEUTIC CONSIDERATIONS

- Standard medical treatment of oligospermia is effective when the cause is known (increased scrotal temperature, chronic infection of male sex glands, pharmaceuticals, endocrine disturbances such as hypogonadism and hypothyroidism), but 90% of cases are idiopathic. Azoospermia caused by ductal obstruction is surgically correctable.
- Rational approach is to enhance factors promoting spermatogenesis. Sperm formation is linked to scrotal temperature and nutritional status. Eat a healthful diet and use nutritional factors: antioxidants, essential fats and oils, zinc, vitamin $B_{12}$, carnitine, arginine. Avoid dietary sources of estrogens. Use botanicals that increase sperm counts and glandular therapy.

### Controlling Sperm-Damaging Factors

#### Scrotal Temperature

Normal temperature is between 94° and 96° F. Above 96° F, sperm production is inhibited or halted. Mean scrotal temperature is higher in infertile men than in fertile men. Reducing scrotal temperature may be enough to make them fertile. Best methods are to avoid tight-fitting underwear, tight jeans, and hot tubs. Avoid exercises that raise scrotal temperature while wearing synthetic fabrics, tight shorts, or tight bikini underwear, such as rowing machines, simulated cross-country ski machines, treadmills, and jogging.

- Allow testicles to hang free to recover from heat buildup. Wear boxer-type underwear.
- Apply cold shower or ice to scrotum. Use "testicular hypothermia device" or "testicle cooler," which must be worn daily during waking hours. It is fairly comfortable and easy to conceal.
- Rule out varicocele that can increase temperatures high enough to inhibit sperm production and motility. Surgical repair may be necessary, but try scrotal cooling first.

## Genitourinary Infections

Genitourinary infections play a major role in many cases. Many infections are asymptomatic. Antisperm antibodies are good indicators of chronic infection. A wide range of microbes can infect the male genitourinary system.

- *Chlamydia* is the most common and serious and a major cause of acute nonbacterial prostatitis and urethritis. Symptoms are pain or burning on urination or ejaculation. More serious is *Chlamydia* infection of the epididymis and vas deferens; scarring and blockage can occur. Antibiotics are essential—tetracyclines and erythromycin. Because *Chlamydia* live within host cells, total eradication is difficult. Chronic infections can be asymptomatic. 28%-71% of infertile men have evidence of chlamydial infection. Antibiotics typically provide only limited improvements in sperm count and quality, but isolated cases of tremendous improvement after antibiotics have occurred. Both partners should take the antibiotic but only if evidence of chronic infection is present. Antisperm antibodies may indicate chronic *Chlamydia* infection. In the absence of a positive culture, rectal ultrasonography and anti-*Chlamydia* antibodies confirm diagnosis.

## Avoiding Estrogens

- The "virtual sea of estrogens" in the environment increases exposure to estrogens during fetal development and reproductive years. This is is a major cause of increased disorders of development and function of the male sexual system.
- Avoiding hormone-fed animal and milk products is important for male sexual vitality, especially in oligospermia and hypotestosteronemia.
- Estrogens have been detected in drinking water and are harmful to male sexual vitality. These are presumably recycled synthetic estrogens (birth control pills), which are more potent because they do not bind to sex-hormone-binding globulin. Use purified or bottled water.
- Weakly estrogenic xenobiotics (polychlorinated biphenyls, dioxin, dichlorodiphenyltrichloroethane) resist biodegradation and are recycled in the environment and interfere with spermatogenesis.
- Greatest impact is during fetal development. Estrogens inhibit multiplication of Sertoli cells, the number of which is directly proportional to the number of sperm produced. Sertoli cell mul-

tiplication occurs during fetal life and before puberty under control of follicle-stimulating hormone. Estrogens inhibit follicle-stimulating hormone (FSH) secretion, causing a reduced number of Sertoli cells and reduced sperm counts.

- Fiber: a low-fiber, high-fat diet is linked to higher levels of estrogens because estrogens excreted in bile are reabsorbed because they are not being bound by fiber.
- Phytoestrogens: if testosterone is low or marginal, or if estrogens are elevated, legumes (beans), especially soy foods, may be of benefit. Soy is a good source of isoflavonoid phytoestrogens. Soy isoflavonoids have 0.2% of estrogen activity of estradiol. Isoflavones bind to estrogen receptors. Their weak estrogenic action is antiestrogenic, preventing binding of endogenous estrogen to receptors. Phytoestrogens may reduce effects of estrogens by stimulating production of sex hormone binding globulin that binds estrogens.
- Phytosterols: soy, other legumes, nuts, and seeds are good sources of phytosterols that aid steroid hormone synthesis, including testosterone.
- Heavy metals: sperm are susceptible to damage by heavy metals (lead, cadmium, arsenic, mercury). Hair mineral analysis is indicated on all men with oligospermia.

## Nutritional Considerations

- Antioxidants: free radical/oxidative damage to sperm is the major cause of idiopathic oligospermia in many cases. Free radicals are abundant in semen of 40% of infertile men.
- Three factors combine to render sperm susceptible to free radical damage: (1) high membrane concentration of polyunsaturated fatty acids, (2) active generation of free radicals, and (3) lack of defensive enzymes.
- Health of sperm depends on antioxidants. Men exposed to increased levels of free radicals are more likely to have abnormal sperm and sperm counts. Sperm are sensitive to free radicals, which depend on integrity and fluidity of the cell membrane for proper function. Improper membrane fluidity activates enzymes that impair motility, structure, and viability of sperm. The major determinant of membrane fluidity is concentration of omega-3 polyunsaturated fatty acids (alpha-linolenic acid [LNA], eicosapentaenoic acid [EPA], docosahexaenoic acid [DHA]), which are susceptible to free radical damage.

- Sperm have low superoxide dismutase and catalase to neutralize free radicals and generate free radicals abundantly to break through barriers to fertilization.
- Sources of oxidants: smoking and pollutants, linked to decreased sperm counts and motility plus increased abnormal sperm.
- **Antioxidants** (vitamin C, beta-carotene, selenium, vitamin E) protect sperm. Vitamin C protects sperm DNA. Ascorbate is much higher in seminal fluid compared with other body fluids, including blood. Low dietary vitamin C is likely to lead to infertility. Smoking reduces vitamin C throughout the body. Sperm quality in smokers improves with ascorbate supplementation. Nonsmokers benefit from vitamin C as much as smokers.
- Sperm become agglutinated when antibodies bind to them. Antibodies to sperm are linked to chronic genitourinary tract or prostatic infection. When >25% of sperm are agglutinated, fertility is unlikely. Vitamin C reduces percentage of agglutinated sperm. Vitamin C is very effective in treating male infertility because of antibodies against sperm.
- **Vitamin E** is the main antioxidant in sperm membranes. It inhibits free radical damage to polyunsaturated fatty acids, enhances ability of sperm to fertilize egg in vitro, and decreases malondialdehyde in sperm pellet suspensions. Supplementation is indicated on the basis of its physiologic effects alone. It exerts more beneficial effects on sperm counts or motility at higher dosages (600-800 IU q.d.) and in combination with selenium (100-200 μg q.d.).
- **Lycopene** is in high concentrations in testes and seminal plasma; levels are decreased in infertile men. In idiopathic nonobstructive oligozoospermia, asthenozoospermia, and teratozoospermia, 2 mg lycopene b.i.d. for 3 months improved sperm concentration by 22 million/mL, motility by 25%, and morphology by 10%.
- **Proanthocyanidins** (200 mg q.d. for 90 days) improved capacitated sperm morphology and functionally normal sperm.
- Antioxidant supplements produce clinical results only when increased oxidative stress is a primary factor.
- **Fats and oils**: saturated fats; hydrogenated oils; trans fatty acids; and cotton, coconut, and palm oil should be avoided. Coconut and palm oils are saturated. Cottonseed contains toxic pesticide residues. It also contains gossypol, a substance that inhibits sperm function and may be used as male antifertility agent ("male birth control pill"), leading to low sperm counts followed

by total testicular failure. Saturated fats decrease membrane fluidity and interfere with sperm motility. Increase omega-3 polyunsaturated fatty acids. Instruct patients to read food labels carefully and avoid all sources of cottonseed oil, saturated fats, and hydrogenated fats.

- **Zinc (Zn)**: most critical trace mineral for male sexual function—works in hormone metabolism, sperm formation, and sperm motility. Zn deficiency decreases testosterone and sperm counts. Zn levels are much lower in infertile men with oligospermia. Zn supplementation (60 mg elemental Zn q.d. for 45-50 days) is indicated for oligospermia with low testosterone levels. Results of one study showed Zn supplements increased testosterone and sperm counts in men with infertility >5 years and resulted in impregnation of wives. Recommended daily allowance is 15 mg. Sources include whole grains, legumes, nuts, and seeds. Supplement dosage: 45-60 mg q.d.
- **Vitamin $B_{12}$**: involved in cellular replication. $B_{12}$ deficiency reduces sperm counts and motility. Supplementation without deficiency improves sperm counts in men with <20 million/mL or motility rate <50%. Experimental dosage: 1000 to 6000 μg q.d.
- **L-Carnitine**: antioxidant with greatest amount of clinical research for treating male infertility. It is essential for transporting fatty acids into mitochondria; deficiency decreases fatty acid levels in mitochondria and reduces energy production. Carnitine levels are high in epididymis and sperm. Epididymis gets most of its energy from fatty acids, as do sperm during transport through epididymis. After ejaculation, sperm motility correlates with carnitine content; the higher the carnitine content, the more motile are the sperm. Carnitine deficit impairs sperm development, function, and motility. With 3000 mg L-carnitine q.d. for 4 months, among patients with poorest sperm motility motile sperm increased from 19.3% to 40.9% and sperm with rapid linear progression increased from 3.1% to 20.3%. Because L-carnitine is expensive, try other nutritional measures first. Optimal dosage: 1000 mg t.i.d.
- **L-Arginine**: required for replication of cells and essential in sperm formation. It may be an effective treatment of male infertility. The critical determinant is the level of oligospermia, if counts <20 million/mL, arginine is less beneficial. Dosage: 4+ g q.d. for 3 months. Reserve it for use after other nutritional measures have been tried.

## Botanical Medicines

- **Ginseng**: *Panax ginseng* (Chinese or Korean ginseng) and *Eleutherococcus senticosus* (Siberian ginseng) are effective in male infertility. They have long histories of traditional use as male tonics. *Panax* promotes growth of testes, increases sperm formation and testosterone levels, and increases sexual activity and mating behavior in studies with animals. Siberian ginseng increases reproductive capacity and sperm counts in bulls. *Panax* has more potent effects (stimulant) than *Eleutherococcus*. Siberian contains no ginsenosides; therefore it is not a true ginseng. But it has many of the same, but milder, effects as *Panax*.
- ***Pygeum africanum***: improves fertility if diminished prostatic secretion plays significant role. It increases prostatic secretions and improves composition of seminal fluid by increasing total seminal fluid, alkaline phosphatase, and protein. It is most effective if alkaline phosphatase activity is reduced (<400 IU/$cm^3$) with no evidence of inflammation or infection (no white blood cells or immunoglobulin A [IgA]). Lack of IgA in semen is a good indicator of potential clinical success. It improves capacity to achieve erection in patients with benign prostatic hypertrophy or prostatitis as determined by nocturnal penile tumescence. (Benign prostatic hypertrophy and prostatitis often are linked to erectile dysfunction and other sexual disturbances.)

## THERAPEUTIC APPROACH

Refer to a urologist or fertility specialist for complete evaluation. Achieve scrotal cooling by wearing loose cotton underwear, avoiding activities that elevate testicular temperature (e.g., hot tubs), and applying cold water to testes. Optimize nutrition (antioxidants and zinc). Identify and eliminate environmental pollutants. Use fertility-enhancing botanicals.

- **General measures**
  —Maintain scrotal temperatures between 94° and 96° F
  —Avoid exposure to free radicals
  —Identify and eliminate environmental pollutants
  —Stop or reduce, in coordination with prescribing physicians, all drugs (antihypertensives, antineoplastics [cyclophosphamide] and antiinflammatories [sulfasalazine])
- **Stress-reduction techniques** and psychological counseling, if needed.

- **Diet**
  - —Avoid dietary free radicals, saturated fats, hydrogenated oils, trans fatty acids, and cottonseed oil
  - —Increase legumes (soy for phytoestrogens and phytosterols), dietary antioxidant vitamins, carotenes, and flavonoids (dark-colored vegetables and fruits), essential fatty acids, and zinc (nuts and seeds)
  - —Eat 8-10 servings of vegetables, 2-4 servings of fresh fruits, and half a cup of raw nuts or seeds daily
- **Nutritional supplements**
  - —Multiple vitamin/mineral
  - —Vitamin C: 1000-3000 q.d. in divided doses
  - —Vitamin E: 600-800 IU q.d. (mixed tocopherols)
  - —Beta-carotene: 100,000-200,000 IU q.d. (mixed carotenoids)
  - —Folic acid: 400 μg q.d.
  - —Vitamin $B_{12}$: 1000 μg q.d.
  - —Zinc: 30-60 mg q.d.
- **Botanical medicines**
  - —*Panax ginseng* (t.i.d.): high-quality crude ginseng root, 1.5-2 g q.d.; standardized extract (5% ginsenosides), 500 mg
- *Eleutherococcus senticosus* (t.i.d.): dried root: 2-4 g; tincture (1:5), 10-20 mL; fluid extract (1:1), 2.0-4.0 mL; solid (dry powdered) extract (20:1), 100-200 mg

Dosage of ginseng is based on ginsenoside content. The typical dose (taken three times daily) should contain saponin content of at least 25 mg ginsenosides with ratio of Rb1 to Rg1 of 2:1 (for high-quality ginseng root extract containing 5% ginsenosides, dose is 500 mg). The response to ginseng is individually unique; observe for possible ginseng toxicity (*Textbook, "Panax ginseng* [Korean Ginseng]"). Begin at lower doses and increase gradually. Russian approach for long-term *Panax* or Siberian ginseng is cyclic use: 15-20 days on followed by 2 weeks off.

# Menopause

## DIAGNOSTIC SUMMARY

- Last spontaneous menstrual period 12 months prior.
- Average age of onset is 51 years.
- Symptoms can, but do not necessarily, include hot flashes, night sweats, palpitations, headache, insomnia, mood swings, anxiety, vaginal dryness, urinary incontinence, rheumatism, fatigue, hair thinning, skin dryness, acne, facial hair, low libido, bladder infections, vaginal infections, nausea, and mild cognitive changes (irregular bleeding with perimenopause).
- Physical examination: vaginal thinning, hair thinning and facial hair, height, weight, abdominal fat, general physical.
- Lab analysis: increase in follicle-stimulating hormone (FSH).
- Lab analysis and imaging may assess risks for osteoporosis and cardiovascular disease.

## GENERAL CONSIDERATIONS

Cessation of menstruation usually occurs at approximately 51 years. Perimenopause is the period before menopause. Postmenopause is the period after menopause. During the perimenopausal period, many women ovulate irregularly, indicating changes in menstrual cycle, with or without other symptoms.

- **Causes of menopause**: thought to occur when no eggs are left in the ovaries. At birth a female has approximately 1 million eggs (ova) which drop to 300,000-400,000 at puberty. Only 400 actually mature during the reproductive years. The absence of active follicles reduces estrogen and progesterone, causing the pituitary to increase follicle-stimulating hormone (FSH) in large and continuous quantities. Luteinizing hormone (LH) and FSH cause ovaries and adrenals to secrete androgens, which can be converted to estrogens by fat cells of the hips and thighs. Converted androgens are the source of most circulating estrogen in postmenopausal women. Total estrogen is still far below reproductive levels.

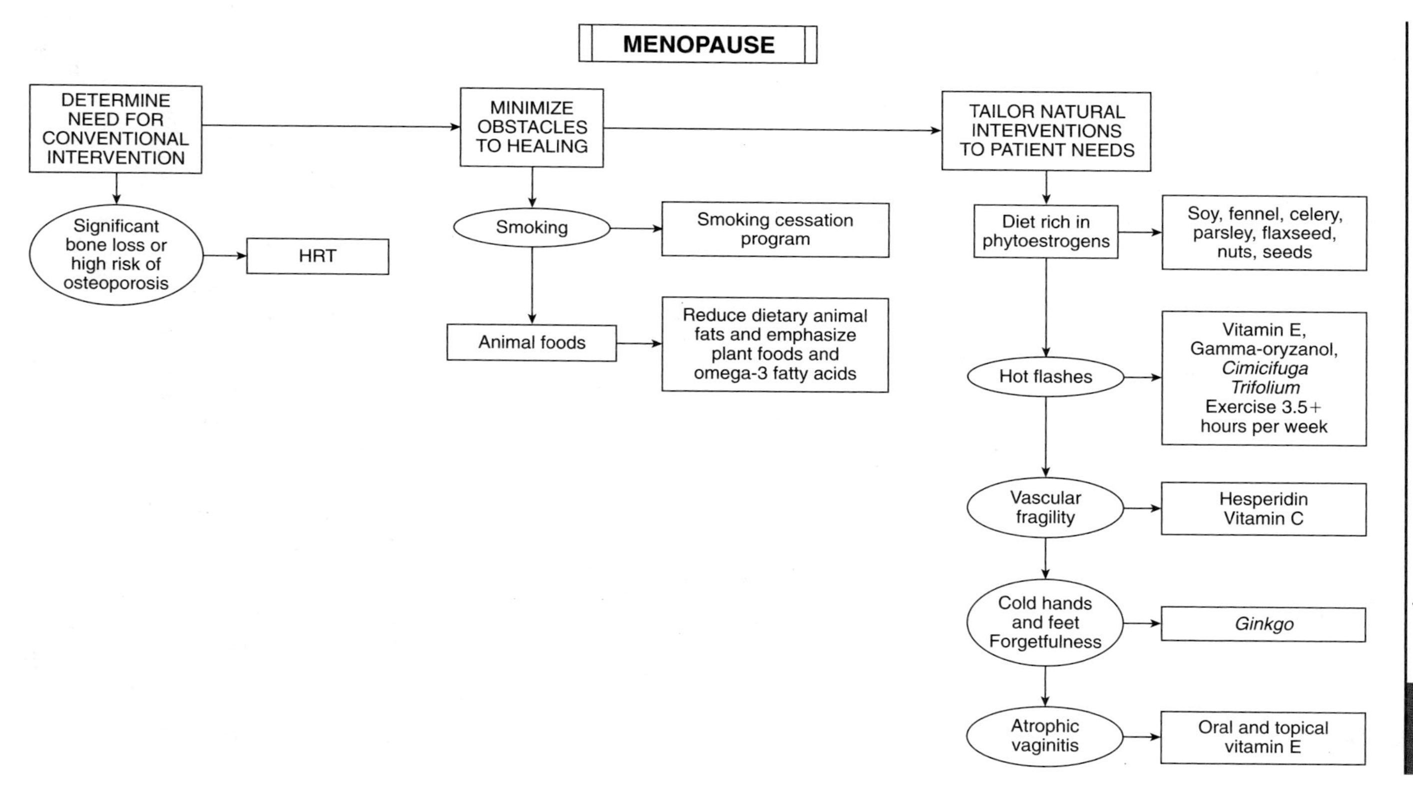
MENOPAUSE
DETERMINE NEED FOR CONVENTIONAL INTERVENTION
Significant bone loss or high risk of osteoporosis
HRT
MINIMIZE OBSTACLES TO HEALING
Smoking
Smoking cessation program
Animal foods
Reduce dietary animal fats and emphasize plant foods and omega-3 fatty acids
TAILOR NATURAL INTERVENTIONS TO PATIENT NEEDS
Diet rich in phytoestrogens
Soy, fennel, celery, parsley, flaxseed, nuts, seeds
Hot flashes
Vitamin E, Gamma-oryzanol, *Cimicifuga* *Trifolium* Exercise 3.5+ hours per week
Vascular fragility
Hesperidin Vitamin C
Cold hands and feet Forgetfulness
*Ginkgo*
Atrophic vaginitis
Oral and topical vitamin E

- **Menopause as social construct**: social and cultural factors contribute greatly to how women react to menopause. Modern society values allure of everlasting youth, culturally devaluing of older women. The cultural view of menopause is directly related to symptoms of menopause. If the cultural view is negative, symptoms are common; if menopause is viewed in a positive light, symptoms are less frequent. In a study of rural Mayan Indians, no women had hot flashes or any other symptoms, and no women showed evidence of osteoporosis despite hormonal patterns identical to postmenopausal women in the United States. Mayan women saw menopause as a positive event, providing acceptance as a respected elder as well as relief from childbearing.
- **Options for managing menopause**: diet, exercise, stress management, nutrition, botanicals, natural hormones, conventional hormones, additional pharmaceuticals.

## Estrogen Replacement Therapy

The key question: "Is hormone replacement therapy necessary?" Estrogen replacement therapy (ERT) without appropriate progestogen increases the risk of endometrial cancer. Hormone replacement therapy (HRT) combines estrogen with a progestogen (either progestin or oral micronized progesterone) to reduce the risk of endometrial cancer such that it is lower than a natural perimenopause transition without HRT. Current conventional medical treatment involves short-term HRT (1-5 years) for menopause symptoms.

## Benefits and Risks of Conventional HRT (cHRT) and Natural HRT (nHRT)

- **Reasons to discontinue cHRT**: uterine bleeding, mood changes, breast tenderness, bloating and weight gain, fear of breast cancer, misunderstanding or disbelief in need for long-term use, lack of patient education.
- **Benefits of continuing cHRT**: symptomatic relief from hot flashes, night sweats, vaginal dryness, insomnia, mood swings, depression, incontinence, infections. ERT controls vasomotor symptoms and genitourinary symptoms. Vaginal estrogen is as efficacious as oral or transdermal estrogen for genitourinary symptoms and advantageous because of local delivery and effect. Sex steroids affect sleep, libido, cognitive function, motor coordination, and pain sensitivity. In perimenopause or early

menopause, depression and mood disorders are more common than in reproductive years. HRT benefits many women.

- **Osteoporosis**: inhibits age-related bone loss, reduces risk of vertebral and hip fracture, decreases bone resorption, prevents osteoporosis, and reduces fractures. But ERT is no longer approved by the Food and Drug Administration for treating osteoporosis in deference to drugs such as bisphosphonates (risedronate and alendronate). Continuous-combined estrogen-progestogen therapy reduced relative risk for hip, vertebral, other osteoporotic, and total fractures. Estrogen agents approved for prevention of osteoporosis are:
  —Oral micronized estradiol: 1.0 mg
  —Conjugated equine estrogens: 0.625 mg
  —Ethinyl estradiol: 5 μg
  —Transdermal estradiol: 50 μg
  —Esterified estrogen: 0.3 mg
  Dual-energy x-ray absorptiometry scans provide the most reliable objective information on the status of bone mineral density and efficacy of dosing.

## Risks

- **Colorectal cancer**: ERT reduces risk of colorectal cancer and risk of dying from colon cancer.
- **Endometrial cancer**: unopposed ERT is linked to increased risk of endometrial cancer by a factor of 8 to 10 over 10+ years. Risk decreases after discontinuing ERT but remains elevated after 10+ years. Proven dose/delivery progestogen (progestins or progesterone), opposing estrogen, minimizes risk and helps prevent endometrial hyperplasia and cancer. Oral micronized progesterone (OMP) and cyclic OMP (200 mg q.d. for 12 days per month) protect endometrium. OMP is equally appropriate to use as medroxyprogesterone acetate (MPA) to protect endometrium. Compounded OMP and Prometrium are indicated products.
- **Venous thromboembolism**: deep vein thromboembolism is complication expected of HRT. For women at risk for thromboembolism or those who are older, absolute risks of HRT are higher.

## Coronary Heart Disease

ERT reduces plasma low-density lipoprotein (LDL) and increases plasma high-density lipoprotein (HDL) cholesterol. ERT reduces lipoprotein A, inhibits oxidation of LDL, improves endothelial vascular function, reduces fibrinogen, and reduces thickening in arterial walls. But ERT may increase triglycerides, clotting, and C-reactive protein, thereby overriding the beneficial effects. HRT does not reduce overall rate of coronary heart disease (CHD), but actually increases it.

Consider cardioprotective effects of nutrition, exercise, stress management, and selected nutrients (vitamin $B_3$, red yeast rice, magnesium, fish oils, pantethine, vitamin C, vitamin E, folic acid, vitamin $B_{12}$, vitamin $B_6$, garlic, soy, hawthorne, gugulipid, and policosanols).

Problem with HRT and CAD: HRT (conjugated equine estrogens [Premarin] and MPA [Provera]) for women with established CHD is linked to a similar myocardial infarction (MI) death rate and nonfatal MIs as placebo, with 50% increase in risk of CHD events (thromboembolism) and early risk of blood clots in legs and lungs, MIs and stroke.

A subgroup of women could be predisposed to hyperinsulinemia, hypertension, hyperhomocysteinemia, increased C-reactive protein and lipoprotein A, obesity, and elevated LDL. Rate of CHD and thromboembolic events after 1 year is much lower in HRT plus statin users than in those who did not use statins.

Neither estrogen alone nor estrogen plus progestin affect progression of coronary atherosclerosis. In women with CAD, MPA does not cancel out beneficial effects of ERT. HRT does not affect the progression of atherosclerosis in women with established heart disease. HRT (transdermal natural estradiol alone or with progestin norethindrone) may slightly increase rates of cardiovascular events during the first 2 years.

Unopposed natural (human) estradiol halts or mildly regresses thickening of arteries. Concurrent lipid-lowering drugs made no difference in rate of progression with either estrogen or placebo.

HRT does not appear to reduce risk of cardiovascular events in postmenopausal women who already have CAD.

Most common HRT in the United States (0.625 mg Premarin + 2.5 mg Provera = PremPro) increases the risk of CHD combined with increased risk of breast cancer. Estrogen plus progestin does not confer a benefit for preventing CHD among women with a uterus.

## Stroke

No excess risk of stroke occurred with an estrogen plus progestin group in the first year but does arise in the second year and persists. The mechanism is not related to increased blood pressure. Estrogen plus progestin increases risk of strokes in women determined to be healthy.

### Gallstones

The risk of gallstones or cholecystecomy is increased in postmenopausal women taking ERT.

### Areas of Uncertainty

- **Breast cancer**: no data clearly and consistently demonstrate an increased risk of breast cancer associated with HRT. An analysis of 90% of postmenopausal women who had ever used HRT had a small but statistically significant increase in risk compared with those who never used HRT. Among current users or recent users, relative risk increased by factor of 1.02 to 1.04 for each year of use. After not using HRT for 5 years, no significant excess risk remains. Breast cancers diagnosed in HRT users tend to be less advanced and more localized. No studies found an increased risk of breast cancer with short-term use of HRT. If long-term use increases risk, it is a small increase.
- **Cognitive function**: HRT may prevent or delay Alzheimer's disease (AD). In women symptomatic from menopause, ERT improves verbal memory, vigilance, reasoning, and motor speed, but no consistent effects were seen on visual recall, working memory, complex attention, mental tracking, mental status, or verbal functions. ERT does not enhance asymptomatic women's performance. HRT may decrease the risk of dementia. Efficacy of preparations or doses, progestin use, and duration of treatment have not been assessed because of insufficient data. Prior use of HRT reduces risk of AD, but duration of use specifically affects benefit. No apparent benefit is found with currently using HRT unless use exceeds 10 years.
- **Ovarian cancer**: a weak possible positive association exists between HRT and ovarian cancer risk. Women currently using HRT may have higher death rates from ovarian cancer than those who had never used HRT. Given the low incidence of ovarian cancer, even if relative risk increases significantly, it may not affect absolute risk. Ovarian cancer mortality rate in postmenopausal women is extremely low, and 7+ years of oral contraceptive use during the reproductive age lowers the incidence of ovarian cancer. A twofold increased risk exists among long-term users of HRT and ERT. Users of ERT for >10 years have a much

increased risk of ovarian cancer, with a relative risk of 1.8. Users of ERT for 20+ years have a relative risk of 3.2 . Users of short-term combination HRT are not at increased risk.

## Natural Hormones

The natural compounded estrogens are estriol, estrone, or estradiol. Estriol is unique; it has one quarter the potency of estradiol and estrone. Natural compounded estrogens are used in lower doses because of the combined effect of weaker estriol plus estradiol and/or estrone. Natural estrogens may be metabolized differently by the body, have a shorter half-life, are customizable for dosing and potency, and are adjustable stronger or weaker in small units to taper someone off or onto hormones. Bioidentical and nonbioidentical hormones may have different metabolic consequences: cytotoxicity to estrogen-sensitive tissues, alteration of binding of other hormones to receptors, or the alteration of liver metabolism of carcinogens.

Natural progesterone has fewer adverse effects on the cardiovascular system than synthetic progestins (e.g., MPA). It lowers HDL less than MPA, is less atherogenic, and does not cause coronary artery spasm as MPA does.

Natural estradiol is used in a half-strength dose (0.5 mg total q.d.) because it is combined with weaker estriol. Estriol acts as an antiestrogen in the breast with little impact on the cardiovascular system.

Holistic approach includes hormones plus other strategies to reduce risk of breast cancer and heart disease: soy, flaxseed, cabbage family foods, and supplements to promote metabolism of estrogens to anticarcinogenic metabolites. Use breast cancer and heart disease prevention diets with nutrients and botanicals: vitamins E and C, carotenes, soy, coenzyme $Q_{10}$, green tea, garlic.

Women using CEE and MPA should consider natural regimens or nonhormonal approaches. Women using natural estrogens and progesterone should reevaluate their regimen to find the lowest dose to achieve benefits and minimize risks. Reconsider yearly continuation of use on an individual basis. Women without a uterus only need estrogen.

Black cohosh, red clover, soy, bioflavonoids, kava, and the proprietary formula Women's Phase II have proven scientific efficacy for menopausal symptoms. Many women need only nonhormonal supplements for symptom relief and never need HRT. Others may be able to lower the dose of cHRT or natural hormones while using them in combination with herbal and nutritional supplements.

### Task Force Recommendations

Following are basic recommendations from the Scientific Advisory Panel of the North American Menopause Society:

1. Treatment of menopause symptoms is the primary indication for HRT and ERT.
2. The only menopause-related indication for chronic progestogen use appears to be endometrial protection from unopposed estrogen therapy. For all women with an intact uterus using estrogen therapy, prescribe adequate progestogen; women without a uterus should not be prescribed a progestogen.
3. No HRT should be used for primary or secondary prevention of CHD. Use proven alternate cardioprotective regimens. The effect of ERT on CHD is not yet clear. Until confirming data are available, ERT should not be used for primary or secondary prevention of CHD.
4. The Women's Health Initiative and the Heart and Estrogen/Progestin Replacement Study data cannot be directly extrapolated to symptomatic perimenopausal women or to women experiencing early menopause (40-50 years of age) or premature menopause (<40 years).
5. Many HRT and ERT products are approved by the Food and Drug Administration for the prevention of postmenopausal osteoporosis; however, because of risks, alternatives should also be considered, weighing risks and benefits.
6. Use of HRT or ERT should be limited to the shortest duration consistent with treatment goals, benefits, and risks for the individual woman.
7. Lower-than-standard doses of HRT and ERT should be considered. The Women's Health, Osteoporosis, Progestin, Estrogen (HOPE) trial demonstrated equivalent symptom relief and preservation of bone density without an increase in endometrial hyperplasia with lower doses of HRT.
8. Alternate routes of administration of HRT may offer advantages, but the long-term risk/benefit ratio has not been demonstrated.
9. An individual risk profile is essential for every woman contemplating any regimen of HRT or ERT. Women should be informed of known risks.

Recent recommendations from the U.S. Preventive Task Force (www.ahrq.gov/clinic/prevenix.htm): Estrogen and progestin should not be routinely used to prevent chronic conditions in postmenopausal women; evidence is insufficient to recommend for or against unopposed estrogen for prevention in postmenopausal women who have had a hysterectomy. Estrogen plus progestin therapy (EPT) has harmful effects that exceed chronic disease prevention benefits in most women. Although risks outweigh benefits, the absolute increase in risk associated with EPT is modest. Benefits include increased bone mineral density, reduced risk for fracture, and reduced risk for colorectal cancer. Harms include increased risk for breast cancer, venous thromboembolism, coronary heart disease, stroke, and cholecystitis.

The two most valid indications are menopausal symptoms and prevention or treatment of osteoporosis. Educate the patient on nutritional, botanical, and hormone options; review benefits and risks of HRT; discuss side effects; acknowledge lack of certainty in some areas; discuss differences (known and hypothetical) among synthetic hormones, horse urine estrogens, plant-derived nonbioidentical hormones, and plant-derived bioidentical "natural" hormones.

Low-dose, compounded, plant-derived natural hormones can manage menopause symptoms and lower the risk of fractures. The combination of low-dose natural hormones, for individually determined amount of time, plus breast cancer and heart disease prevention strategies is the safest, most gentle, and least invasive form of HRT. Each woman should be reevaluated at least on a yearly basis for benefits versus risks.

## Types of HRT

General consensus: use the lowest dose possible for the shortest duration possible. Current recommendations from the North American Menopause Society: 2-3 years for symptom management, then decrease and/or discontinue. Assess benefits and risks for long-term therapy.

For women with an intact uterus, estrogen is given in combination with progestin or oral progesterone, either in cyclical fashion or continuously.

- **Cyclical approach**: estrogen for 25 to 30 days and progestin or OMP for last 10-12 days of cycle. A 3- to 6-day hormone-free interval follows for planned bleeding. Menstruation continues in 90% of women.

- **Combined cHRT**: prevents monthly bleeding. Estrogen and progestin/progesterone are given daily without hormone-free interval. Give lowest dose of estrogen possible plus 2.5 mg MPA or 100 mg OMP.

### Advantages of Combined Continuous Hormone Replacement Therapy

- Avoidance of cyclical bleeding
- Continuous protection of the endometrium against the cancer-causing effects of estrogen
- Lower daily and cumulative amounts of progestins required
- Avoidance of symptoms of premenstrual syndrome that often accompany estrogen
- Prolongation of the synergistic effects of estrogen and progesterone on bone integrity
- Prevention of rare conceptions by promoting endometrial atrophy
- Greater convenience and patient compliance

### Forms of Estrogens

- Bioidentical natural hormones, manufactured from compounds of either soybeans or Mexican wild yam root, that are biochemically identical to endogenous estradiol, estrone, or estriol. Two main sources:
  1. Compounded estradiol, estrone, or estriol from a compounding pharmacy
  2. Pharmaceutical company version with bioidentical estradiol or estrone but with patentable binder, filler, preservative, adhesive, or dye. Examples: Estrace, Gynediol, Estraderm, Vivelle, Climara, Alora, Esclim, Orthoest, Ogen cream, Vagifem cream, Estrace cream, Estring.
- Hormones derived from natural substances but not biochemically identical to endogenous estrogens. Examples: conjugated equine estrogens (Premarin, Premarin cream) and esterified plant estrogens (Estratab, Menest).
- Hormones of synthetic origin and not bioidentical. Example: Cenestin.
- Combination estrogen/progestin and, in some cases, testosterone products.

### Major Symptoms of Perimenopause and Menopause

- Irregular bleeding (perimenopause)
- Hot flashes

- Atrophic vaginitis
- Mood changes
- Cognitive changes
- Body aches
- Sleep disturbances
- Others: fatigue, sexual dysfunction, hair thinning, facial hair, headache, dry skin, joint pains, bladder infections, urinary incontinence.
- **Atrophic vaginitis**: avoid substances that dry mucous membranes, such as antihistamines, alcohol, caffeine, diuretics. Keep well hydrated. Clothes made from natural fibers, such as cotton, allow skin to breathe, decreasing the incidence of vaginal infections. Regular intercourse helps increase blood flow to vaginal tissues, improving tone and lubrication. Use lubricant oil or K-Y Jelly. Atrophic vaginitis is a strong indication of the need for HRT or vaginal estrogens: estriol cream or suppositories (compounding pharmacy), estradiol cream (Estrace cream), conjugated equine estrogens cream (Premarin cream), vaginal estradiol tablet (Vagifem), or estradiol ring (Estring).
- **Bladder infections**: enhance normal host protection against urinary tract infections. Increase urine flow with optimal hydration; promote pH that inhibits growth of microbes by using vaginal estrogens that help maintain vaginal pH and tone and anatomy of urethra; prevent bacterial adherence to bladder endothelial cells. Use botanical medicines recommended in the *Textbook* ("Cystitis").
- **Cognition**: estrogen, progesterone, and testosterone modulate brain function by the neurotransmitters acetylcholine, serotonin, noradrenalin, dopamine. Estrogen affects memory and learning with acetylcholine. Concentration and memory also may be impaired by sleep disturbances, hot flashes, and stressors.

## THERAPEUTIC CONSIDERATIONS

Seven levels of intervention:

1. Diet, exercise, stress management
2. Nutritional supplementation
3. Botanicals
4. Natural hormones (nHRT)
5. Friendlier conventional hormones (fcHRT): bioidentical but with filler, binder, preservative, dye, or adhesive patented by pharmaceutical manufacturer

6. Less-friendly conventional hormones (cHRT)
7. Condition-specific nonestrogen pharmaceuticals (for symptom relief or disease prevention and/or treatment)

- Three fundamental goals in treatment: symptom relief and disease prevention and/or treatment.
- Subjectively and objectively assess for scope and severity of symptoms: risks of osteoporosis, heart disease, breast cancer, AD, colorectal cancer, and other chronic health problems.
- Baseline evaluation of menopausal women: (some of these tests are routine either initially or annually. Other tests are chosen on health history, disease risks, current health problems, and family history.)
- Detailed personal medical history, including chief complaint, review of other systems, medical history, past and present medications, family history, dietary habits and history, exercise habits and history, social history, occupation.
- General physical examination
- Breast examination
- Pelvic examination
- Laboratory tests to consider: complete blood count, blood chemistry panel, lipid panel, thyroid function panel, FSH, homocysteine, C-reactive protein, lipoproteins
- Screening mammography
- Bone density testing
- Pap smear
- Electrocardiography
- Colonoscopy

## Diet

Increase plant foods high in phytoestrogens and fruit and vegetables. Reduce animal foods.

- **Phytoestrogen-containing foods**: Phytoestrogens are ubiquitous nonsteroidal plant compounds derived by metabolism of precursors. They have only a fraction of the strength of endogenous or typically exogenous doses of estrogen, allowing them to act as both estrogen agonists and estrogen antagonists depending on target organ, dose, nature of estrogen receptor (alpha or beta), total body estrogen load, and kind of phytoestrogen. They are nature's alternatives to the selective estrogen receptor modulators tamoxifen and raloxifene. Food sources include soybeans, flaxseed, apples, carrots, fennel, celery, parsley, other legumes. Phytoestrogens also decrease incidence of breast, colon, and prostate cancer.

- **Soy phytoestrogens**: isoflavones genistein, daidzein, and glycitein bind to estradiol receptors in uterus, breast, brain, bone, and arteries. They can weakly mimic estrogens in some tissues; in others they block the effect of estrogens. Look for isoflavone content on product labels. Each gram of unprocessed soy protein containts 1.2 mg genistein, 0.5 mg daidzein, and small quantities of glycitein. Genestein has a sixfold greater affinity for beta estrogen receptor than for alpha receptor. It may act as proestrogen in bones but antiestrogen in the breast. Fermented products are preferred to minimize digestive difficulties. Avoid thyroid synthesis inhibition by keeping isoflavones intake to <200 mg per day, including supplements. Asian diet includes 30-80 mg isoflavones daily or 1 to 3 servings daily. Benefits include reduction in hot flashes and/or night sweats; stabilization of bone density; decreased total cholesterol, LDL, triglycerides, homocysteine, blood pressure.
- **Flaxseed**: richest plant source of lignans. Benefits are antitumor, antioxidant, weak estrogenic, antiestrogenic. Flaxseed has minimal impact on menopause symptoms and limited reduction in vaginal dryness and hot flashes or night sweats.
- **Disease prevention diet**: high in fruits, vegetables, whole grains, vegetarian proteins, nuts, seeds, legumes; low in saturated fats, trans fats, simple carbohydrates, fast foods.

## Nutritional Supplements

- **Vitamin E**: relieves hot flashes and menopausal vaginal symptoms; improves blood supply to vaginal wall when taken for 4+ weeks. Dose: 400 IU q.d. for atrophic vaginitis. Vitamin E oil, creams, ointments, or suppositories are used topically for atrophic vaginitis.
- **Hesperidin and vitamin C**: hesperidin improves vascular integrity and relieves capillary permeability. Combined with vitamin C, hesperidin and other citrus flavonoids may relieve hot flashes. Dosage: 900 mg hesperidin, 300 mg hesperidin methyl chalcone (citrus flavonoid), and 1200 mg vitamin C q.d. Side effect: slightly offensive body odor and perspiration-discoloring clothing.
- **Gamma-oryzanol (ferulic acid)**: growth-promoting substance in grains and isolated from rice bran oil. It enhances pituitary function and endorphin release by the hypothalamus. It is effective even in surgically induced menopause. It also lowers cholesterol and triglycerides. It is an extremely safe natural substance with no significant side effects. Dosage: 300 mg q.d.

## Botanical Medicines

Plants that tone the female glandular system are termed "uterine tonics." Phytoestrogens improve blood flow to female organs and nourish and tone female glands and organ system. Plants for specific symptoms: valerian (sedative) for insomnia and chaste tree (increases luteinizing hormone with indirect progesterone-like effect) for dysfunctional uterine bleeding. Herbal phytoestrogens have no side effects and inhibit mammary tumors.

### Sources of Phytoestrogens

| Phytoestrogen | Plant Source |
|---|---|
| Lignans | Vegetables, fruits, nuts, cereals, spices, seeds (especially flaxseeds) |
| Isoflavones | Spinach, fruits, clovers, peas, beans (especially soy) |
| Flavones | Beans, green vegetables, fruits, nuts |
| Chalcones | Licorice root |
| Diterpenoids | Coffee |
| Triterpenoids | Licorice root, hops |
| Coumarins | Cabbage, peas, spinach, licorice, clover |
| Acyclics | Hops |

Phytoestrogens in medicinal herbs, compared with estrogen, are at most only 2% as strong. Modulating effect: if estrogens are low, they increase estrogen effect; if estrogens are high, binding of phytoestrogens to receptors decreases estrogens' effects.

- ***Trifolium pretense* (red clover)**: constituents include flavonoid glycosides, coumestans, volatile oils, L-dopa caffeic acid conjugates, polysaccharides, resins, fatty acids, hydrocarbons, alcohols, chlorophylls, minerals, and vitamins. A 40-mg standardized extract reduces hot flashes. Other effects: no endometrial thickening; increased HDL; no abnormalities in liver function tests, complete blood count, or estradiol; reduced coronary vascular disease by increasing arterial elasticity.
- ***Cimicifuga racemosa* (black cohosh)**: single most important herb for menopausal symptoms. It relieves hot flashes, night sweats, headache, insomnia, mood swings. It improves fatigue, irritability, vaginal dryness. It may not work in the presence of an antiestrogen, such as tamoxifen. Other characteristics: no

phytoestrogens have been identified, no significant changes in levels of female hormones, no estrogenic effect on vaginal cytology, and no estrogenic effect but nevertheless decreases Kupperman index for menopause symptoms.

- ***Panax ginseng* (Korean or Chinese ginseng)**: contains 13 triterpenoid saponins (ginsenosides); reduces mental and physical fatigue, enhances ability to cope with physical and mental stressors by supporting adrenal glands, treats atrophic vaginal changes from estrogen loss.
- **Combination products**: contain dong quai, motherwort, licorice root, burdock root, and wild yam root. Dosage: 2 caps t.i.d. Effects: after 3 months, it reduced symptoms and total number of symptoms; greatest benefit for hot flashes, mood changes, insomnia; mild decrease in estrogens and progesterone; no effects on HDL, triglycerides, or total cholesterol.
- ***Ginkgo biloba* extract**: improves blood flow for cold hands and feet; forgetfulness that accompanies menopause; peripheral vascular disease of extremities, such as Raynaud's syndrome; cerebral vascular insufficiency. It increases blood flow to the brain, enhances energy production in the brain, increases uptake of glucose by brain cells, and improves transmission of nerve signals. It may take 12+ weeks to see clinical efficacy. Although most report benefits within a 2- to 3-week period, some individuals may take longer to respond. The longer the treatment is continued, the more obvious and lasting the result.

## Natural Topical Preparations

- **Natural progesterone cream**: can be quite effective in perimenopause by regulating menstrual cycle, hot flashes, night sweats, mood swings, sleep disruption, premenstrual syndrome symptoms. Transdermal progesterone cream (¼ tsp containing 20 mg progesterone applied daily to skin) plus multivitamin and 1200 mg calcium for 1 year improved or resolved hot flashes in 83% of women. Some researchers conclude that transdermal progesterone is not sufficiently absorbed into the bloodstream to achieve biologic effects.

## Lifestyle Factors

- **Exercise**: hypothesis is that impaired endorphin activity in hypothalamus may provoke hot flashes. Regular physical exercise decreases frequency and severity of hot flashes. Exercise may obviate need for HRT. Women with no hot flashes spent 3.5

hours/week exercising. Exercise also elevates mood. Benefits are derived for women both on and off HRT.

- **Cigarette smoking**: increases risk of early menopause and doubles the risk of menopause between ages of 44 and 55 years. Former smokers have lower risk, indicating a partial reversal of effect.

## THERAPEUTIC APPROACH

Natural measures can help alleviate most common symptoms. In most cases, HRT either is not necessary or is only needed for 1-4 years. HRT may be indicated in women at high risk for osteoporosis who already had significant bone loss and menopause symptoms or who do not tolerate osteoporosis medicines. For women with intolerable menopause symptoms, try nHRT, fcHRT, or cHRT with periodic attempts at reducing or discontinuing hormones.

### Diet

- Increase soy foods, legumes, flaxseeds, fennel, celery, parsley.

### Supplements

- **Vitamin E (mixed tocopherols)**: 800 IU q.d. until symptoms have improved, then 400 IU q.d.
- **Hesperidin**: 900 mg q.d.
- **Vitamin C**: 1200 mg q.d.
- **Gamma-oryzanol**: 300 mg q.d.

### Botanical Medicines

- ***Cimicifuga racemosa* (black cohosh)**: standardized extract based on content of 27-deoxyacteine: 20 mg of 27-deoxyacteine b.i.d.
  —Powdered rhizome: 1-2 g
  —Tincture (1:5): 4-6 mL
  —Fluid extract (1:1): 3-4 mL (1 tsp)
  —Solid (dry powdered) extract (4:1): 250-500 mg
- ***Ginkgo biloba* extract**
  —24% *Ginkgo* flavonglycoside content: 40 mg
- ***Trifolium pretense* (red clover)**: 40 mg isoflavones extract b.i.d.

### Lifestyle

- **Regular exercise program**: at least 30 minutes four times a week.

# Menorrhagia

## DIAGNOSTIC SUMMARY

- Excessive menstrual bleeding (blood loss >80 mL) occurring at regular cyclical intervals (cycles are usually, but not necessarily, of normal length).
- May be caused by dysfunctional uterine bleeding (no organic cause) or local lesions (e.g., uterine myomas [fibroids], endometrial polyps, endometrial hyperplasia, endometrial cancer, adenomyosis, and endometritis). Other causes include bleeding disorders and hypothyroidism.
- Key to diagnosis begins with history and physical examination. Pelvic ultrasound, hysterosonography, hysteroscopy, Pap smear, thyroid function studies, pregnancy test, complete blood count, ferritin, liver function or coagulation studies, follicle-stimulating hormone/luteinizing hormone (LH), serum progesterone, testosterone, dehydroepiandrosterone sulfate, sexually transmitted disease testing, endometrial biopsies or dilation and curettage—used for diagnosis and management as needed.

## GENERAL CONSIDERATIONS

Other patterns of abnormal bleeding are oligomenorrhea (interval >35 days), polymenorrhea (interval <21 days), metrorrhagia (irregular or frequent intervals with excessive flow and duration), menometrorrhagia (prolonged heavy bleeding at irregular intervals), and intermenstrual bleeding (variable amounts occurring between regular menses).

Normal menstrual cycle: length of 28 days (± 7 days), duration of 4 days (± 4 days), blood loss of 40 mL (± 20 mL).

Menorrhagia is largely subjective; an objective measure of blood loss is rarely done. Measured blood loss correlates poorly with patient assessment of bleeding. Patients with menorrhagia have increased menstrual blood flow during first 3 days (up to 92% of total menses lost at this time), indicating that mechanisms

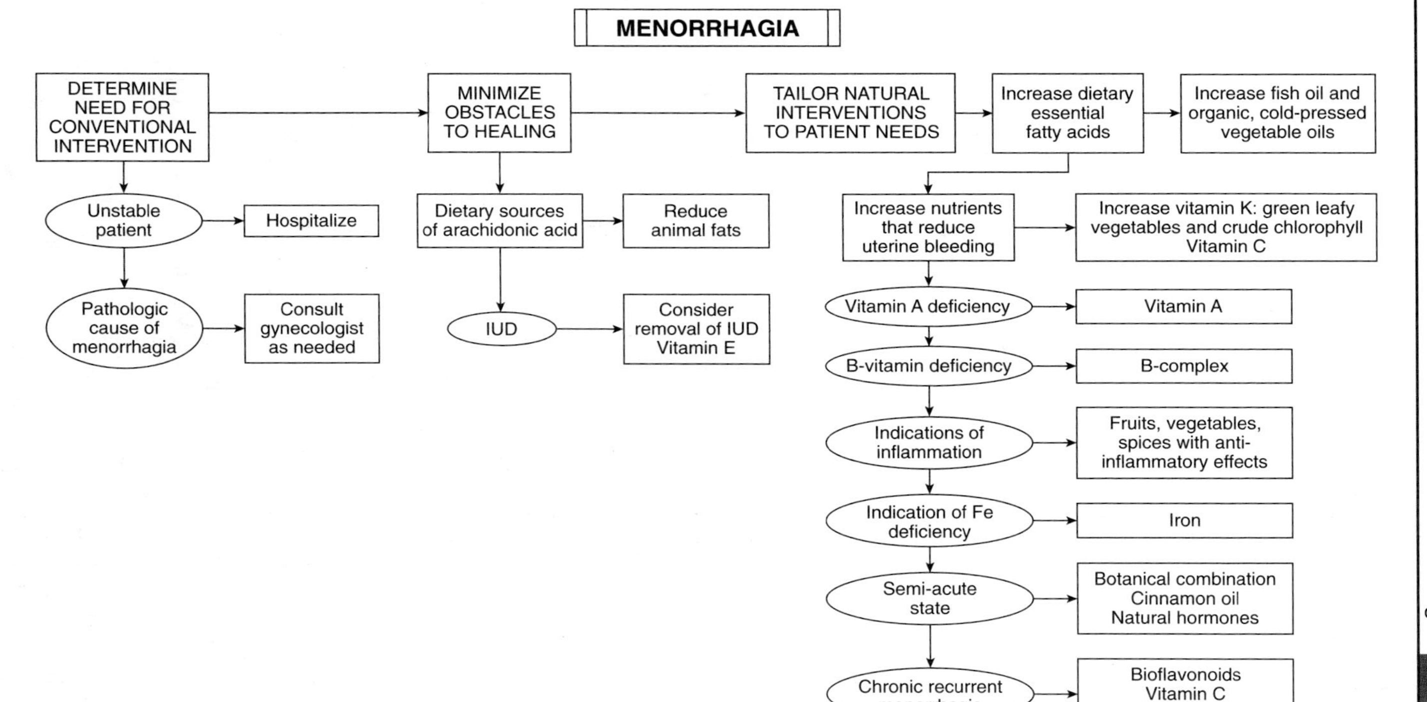
MENORRHAGIA
DETERMINE NEED FOR CONVENTIONAL INTERVENTION
MINIMIZE OBSTACLES TO HEALING
TAILOR NATURAL INTERVENTIONS TO PATIENT NEEDS
Increase dietary essential fatty acids
Increase fish oil and organic, cold-pressed vegetable oils
Unstable patient
Hospitalize
Dietary sources of arachidonic acid
Reduce animal fats
Increase nutrients that reduce uterine bleeding
Increase vitamin K: green leafy vegetables and crude chlorophyll
Vitamin C
Pathologic cause of menorrhagia
Consult gynecologist as needed
IUD
Consider removal of IUD
Vitamin E
Vitamin A deficiency
Vitamin A
B-vitamin deficiency
B-complex
Indications of inflammation
Fruits, vegetables, spices with anti-inflammatory effects
Indication of Fe deficiency
Iron
Semi-acute state
Botanical combination
Cinnamon oil
Natural hormones
Chronic recurrent menorrhagia
Bioflavonoids
Vitamin C
Chaste tree

responsible for ceasing menses are as effective in women with menorrhagia as in normal women, despite high blood loss.

## Etiology

Consult gynecology textbook to rule out pathologic causes. Realize scope of causes and do not assume dysfunctional uterine bleeding (DUB).

- **DUB definition**: abnormal uterine bleeding without demonstrable organic cause. DUB includes menorrhagia, oligomenorrhea, polymenorrhea, metrorrhagia, menometrorrhagia, and intermenstrual bleeding.
- **Abnormal bleeding categories**: hormonal, mechanical, and clotting abnormalities. Not all cause menorrhagia, but rather other abnormal bleeding patterns.
- **Hormonal causes**: anovulation and luteal phase defects and stress (DUB), exogenous hormones, hypothyroidism, ovarian cysts.
- **Mechanical causes**: uterine polyps, uterine fibroids, uterine cancer, intrauterine devices, ectopic pregnancy, pregnancy, endometriosis, endometritis.
- **Clotting abnormalities**: vitamin K deficiency, drug-induced hemorrhage (heparin, warfarin, aspirin), dysproteinemias, disseminated intravascular coagulation, severe hepatic disease, primary fibrinolysis, circulating inhibitors of coagulation.
- **Abnormalities in prostaglandin metabolism**: menorrhagic endometrium excessively incorporates arachidonic acid into neutral lipids and inadequately incorporates it into phospholipids. Increased arachidonic acid release during menses increases production of series 2 prostaglandins—a major factor in excess menstrual bleeding and dysmenorrhea. Excessive bleeding during first 3 days is caused by vasodilation by prostaglandin (PG) $E_2$ and $PGI_2$ and antiaggregating activity of $PGI_2$; pain of dysmenorrhea is caused by excess $PGF_{2alpha}$.
- **Thyroid abnormalities**: overt hypothyroidism and hyperthyroidism are linked to menstrual disturbances. Minimal, subclinical insufficiency (thyroid stimulation test) may cause menorrhagia and other menstrual disturbances. Minimal hypothyroid patients with menorrhagia may respond dramatically to thyroxine. Consider thyroid-stimulating hormone testing for patients with longstanding menstrual dysfunction (with no obvious uterine pathosis). This is preferred to empirical use of thyroid hormone.

## Estimating Menstrual Blood Loss

- Assessing blood loss by asking for an estimate of number of pads or tampons used during each period and duration of period is inaccurate. Forty percent of women losing >80 mL considered their periods only moderately heavy or scanty; 14% with loss of <20 mL judged their periods to be heavy.
- Serum ferritin is best indicator of blood loss but may be impractical for immediate information. Attempt to understand blood loss. Be concerned about excess bleeding >7 straight days, more frequently than every 21 days, new pad or tampon every hour for more than half a day. Changing pad or tampon every half hour or less requires urgent attention; it may be an emergency. Any bleeding in postmenopausal women is abnormal.

**Pathologic Causes of Menorrhagia**

| Cause | Possible Etiology |
|---|---|
| Anovulation | Excessive estrogen<br>Failure of mid-cycle surge of LH<br>Hypothyroidism<br>Hyperprolactinemia<br>Polycystic ovarian disease |
| Intrauterine structural defects | Fibroids<br>Polyps<br>Cancer<br>Ectopic pregnancy<br>Intrauterine devices |
| Bleeding disorders | See table on hemorrhagic disorders |

- **Abnormalities of prostaglandin metabolism**: menorrhagic endometrium incorporates arachidonic acid (AA) into neutral lipids to much greater extent than normal while incorporation into phospholipids is decreased; increased AA release during menses increases production of series 2 prostaglandins, a major factor in excess bleeding and dysmenorrhea; excess bleeding during first 3 days from the vasodilatory properties of $PGE_2$ and $PGI_2$ and antiaggregating activity of $PGI_2$; pain of dysmenorrhea is due to overproducing $PGF_{2a}$.
- **Other contributing factors**: iron deficiency, hypothyroidism, vitamin A deficiency, intrauterine devices, local factors (uterine myomas, endometrial polyps, adenomyosis, endometrial hyperplasia, salpingitis, endometritis).

## THERAPEUTIC CONSIDERATIONS

Needless hysterectomies have been performed because of inadequate management of heavy menses. Factors to consider for hysterectomy: inability to manage menorrhagia, patient safety and health, lack of clear diagnosis, stress and fatigue wearing on patient. Hysterectomy is needed in selected circumstances, but most cases of menorrhagia can be treated without surgery with botanicals, nutriceuticals, hormones, and pharmaceuticals. Less-permanent surgical procedures may spare the uterus—dilation and curettage, hysteroscopic resections and ablations, and uterine artery embolization.

- **Psychological stress**: directly affects bleeding patterns by influencing the hypothalamic/pituitary/ovarian axis. This causes anovulation and subsequent lack of progesterone. Endometrium is in estrogen-dominant state with plump thickening without opposing, stabilizing progesterone, causing heavy bleeding at next menses. Adolescents account for many of these cases; remainder are perimenopausal women.
- **Iron (Fe) deficiency**: blood loss >60 mL per period causes negative Fe balance. Chronic Fe deficiency can cause menorrhagia:
  - —Many patients without organic pathosis respond well to Fe supplements alone.
  - —High rate of organic pathosis (fibroids, polyps, adenomyosis) in patients unresponsive to Fe supplements.
  - —Serum Fe levels rise in many patients given Fe supplements.
  - —Fe therapy is less effective when initial serum Fe is high.
  - —Menorrhagia correlates with depleted tissue Fe stores (bone marrow) irrespective of serum Fe level.
  - —Seventy-five percent of patients on Fe supplements improve compared with 32.5% on placebo.

  Hematologic screening and serum ferritin (first indicator of decreased Fe stores, whereas hemoglobin concentration, mean corpuscular volume, and mean corpuscular hemoglobin may be normal) are essential. Iron supplementation dose: 100 mg elemental Fe q.d. as prophylactic therapy to prevent menorrhagia and depletion of Fe-containing enzymes before hematologic changes are observed. Decreased serum ferritin is a good indicator of need for Fe supplementation.
- **Vitamin A**: serum retinol is significantly lower in women with menorrhagia than healthy control subjects. A dosage of 60,000 IU

vitamin A for 35 days can reduce or normalize blood loss in such patients.

- **Vitamin C and bioflavonoids**: capillary fragility is believed to play a role in many cases of menorrhagia. Ascorbate and bioflavonoids strengthen capillary walls. Bioflavonoids may also reduce heavy bleeding because of their antiinflammatory effect, as with antiinflammatory drugs. Vitamin C (200 mg t.i.d.) and bioflavonoids can reduce menorrhagia. Vitamin C increases Fe absorption; the therapeutic effect also may be from enhanced Fe absorption.
- **Vitamin E**: free radicals may play a causative role in endometrial bleeding, particularly with an intrauterine device. Vitamin E (100 IU every 2 days) has improved patients within 10 weeks. Vitamin E may work by antioxidant activity or prostaglandin metabolism.
- **Vitamin K and chlorophyll**: although bleeding time and prothrombin levels usually are normal in menorrhagia, vitamin K (crude preparations of chlorophyll) has clinical and limited research support. Also, some women may have inherited or acquired bleeding disorder.

**Acquired Generalized Hemorrhagic Disorders**

| Factor | Possible Cause |
|---|---|
| Deficiency of vitamin K | Low intake, impaired absorption, antimicrobial inhibition of gut flora that synthesize vitamin K |
| Drug-induced hemorrhage | Heparin, warfarin administration |
| Dysproteinemias | Myeloma, macroglobulinemia |
| Disseminated intravascular coagulation | |
| Severe hepatic disease | |
| Circulating inhibitors of coagulation | |
| Primary fibrinolysis | |

- **Essential fatty acids**: the majority of tissue AA is derived from the diet. Reducing dietary animal products and increasing linoleic, linolenic, and dihomo-gamma-linolenic acid may curtail blood loss by decreasing AA. Increasing fish, nuts, and seeds in the diet may alter production of AA. Fish oils, flax oil, and other seed oils used as supplements may produce faster results.

- **Vitamin B complex**: menorrhagia may correlate with B-vitamin deficiency. The liver loses its ability to inactivate estrogen in B-complex deficiency. Some cases of menorrhagia are caused by an excessive estrogen effect on endometrium. Supplementing B vitamins may normalize estrogen metabolism. B complex can give prompt improvement in menorrhagia and metrorrhagia. Preparations used: thiamin 3-9 mg, riboflavin 4.5-9 mg, and up to 60 mg niacin.

## Botanicals

- ***Zingiber officinale* (ginger)**: inhibits prostaglandin synthesis, linked to altered $PG_2$ ratio associated with excessive menstrual loss. Inhibition of PG and leukotriene formation explains traditional use of ginger as an antiinflammatory.
- ***Vitex agnus castus* (chaste tree)**: best-known herb in Europe for hormonal imbalances and abnormal bleeding in women; most important herb to normalize menstrual flow, but not a fast-acting herb. Results may not be achieved for 3 to 4 months. Seeds are the part used. It acts on the hypothalamus/pituitary axis to increase LH and mildly inhibit release of FSH. Result: shift in ratio of estrogen and progesterone, causing progesterone-like action. It improves amenorrhea, polymenorrhea, oligomenorrhea, and menorrhagia. In polymenorrhea, time between periods lengthened from 20.1 days to 26.3 days; the number of heavy bleeding days was shortened. Dose: 15 drops chaste tree liquid extract.
- **Astringent herbs**: reduce blood loss from reproductive tract, gastrointestinal tract, respiratory tract, and skin. Astringents for uterine blood loss are high in tannins (not the only helpful constituents). Major astringent and hemostatic herbs used in chronic and acute menorrhagia (used in combination formulations for weeks and months to bring about results):
  —Yarrow (*Achillea millefolium*)
  —Ladies' mantle (*Alchemilla vulgaris*)
  —Cranesbill (*Geranium maculatum*)
  —Beth root (*Trillium erectum*)
  —Greater periwinkle (*Vinca major*)
  —Horsetail (*Equisetum arvense*)
  —Goldenseal (*Hydrastis canadensis*)
  —Shepherd's purse (*Capsella bursa pastoris*): was traditionally used to manage obstetric and gynecologic hemorrhage. Intravenous and intramuscular injections have been effective in menorrhagia because of functional abnormalities and

fibroids. Its hemostatic action may arise from high levels of oxalic and dicarboxylic acids.

- **Traditional uterine tonics**: used to ease menstrual flow. Traditionally and empirically, if the uterus is hypotonic, heavy bleeding may be occurring. Improving uterine tone may normalize or regulate menstrual bleeding. Uterine tonics and/or amphoterics that regulate tone and potentially reduce bleeding include:
  —Blue cohosh (*Caulophyllum thalictroides*)
  —Helonia (*Chamaelirium luteum*)
  —Squaw vine (*Mitchella repens*)
  —Raspberry leaves (*Rubus idaeus*)
  —Life root (*Senecio aureus*)
- **Astringent and uterine tonic herbs**: can be used in formulations for weeks to several months as tea, liquid extract, or powdered capsule.
- **Traditional herbs for semiacute or acute blood loss in a stable patient**: some of these herbs have dose-specific toxicities; use only after consulting botanical reference text to ensure proper dosing. Cinnamon essential oil dose: 1-5 drops every 3-4 hours. Other herbs: do not exceed 20 drops every 2 hours or 1 capsule every 4 hours.
  —Cinnamon essential oil (*Cinnamomum verum*)
  —Life root (*Senecio aureus*)
  —Canadian fleabane (*Erigeron canadensis*)
  —Greater periwinkle (*Vinca major*)
  —Shepherd's purse (*Capsella bursa pastoris*)
  —Yarrow (*Achillea millefolium*)
  —Savin (*Sabina officinalis*)
  —Beth root (*Trillium erectum*)

**Use these botanicals only in women who are stable. In unstable patients, use them as adjuncts to intravenous estrogens, other pharmaceuticals, or surgical interventions.** They can be used for patients with chronic menorrhagia who are stable and for semiacute blood loss or acute blood loss if patient shows no signs of instability and improves within 12-24 hours.

## Natural Hormones

Natural estradiol and progesterone can effectively manage menorrhagia, just as conjugated equine estrogens (CEE) or synthetic estrogens/progestins are used in conventional medicine. To control an acute bleeding episode, natural estradiol should be just as effective as CEE. These hormones are prescription items administered by qualified practitioners. Cyclic natural progesterone can correct recurring menorrhagia; a short course of natural progesterone can be used in acute menorrhagia. Natural progesterone creams are not as effective as higher dose pills or oral micronized natural progesterone.

## THERAPEUTIC APPROACH

- Unstable patients (hypotensive, dizzy, loss of consciousness, chills or fever, or passage of large amounts of tissue) require transfer to hospital for intravenous estrogens, dilation and curettage, hysterectomy, or uterine ablation.
- First step in treating menorrhagia is to control the cause: correct prothrombin time, hematologic status, or thyroid function.. Mechanical causes, such as endometrial polyp or uterine fibroid, may be managed without removing cause; but if no improvement occurs, consider conventional treatment, including surgery. Endometrial hyperplasia requires definitive, proven progesterone and progestin with biopsy-proven improvement. Endometrial cancer requires hysterectomy. Uterine infections need appropritate treatment. Ectopic pregnancy with or without bleeding requires immediate conventional intervention. In chronic menorrhagia or effectively managed episodic acute blood loss, complete blood count and serum ferritin can monitor anemia status.
- Diet: low in sources of AA (animal fats) and high in fish oils, linolenic and linoleic acids (vegetable oils), green leafy vegetables, and other sources of vitamin K. Fruits, vegetables, and spices with antiinflammatory effects: garlic, onions, cumin, pineapple, citrus.
- Supplements:
  —Vitamin C: 1000-3000 mg q.d.
  —Bioflavonoids: 250-2000 mg q.d.
  —Vitamin A: 25,000-30,000 IU b.i.d. for limit of 3 months. CAUTION: Ensure the woman is not pregnant or likely to get pregnant. High levels of vitamin A are a known teratogen.
  —Vitamin E (mixed tocopherols): 200-800 IU q.d.
  —Chlorophyll: 25 mg q.d. (use a crude form)
  —Iron succinate or fumarate: 30 mg b.i.d. or iron sulfate 325 mg q.d. to b.i.d.

## Botanical Medicine

Chronic recurring menorrhagia:

- **Bioflavnoids**: 1000 mg b.i.d.
- **Vitamin C**: 1-3 g q.d.
- **Chaste tree**: tincture 1/2-1 tsp q.d. or standardized extract 175 mg q.d.

Semiacute:

- **Botanical combination tincture** of equal parts of each herb: (20-30 drops every 2-3 hours)
  —Yarrow
  —Greater periwinkle
  —Shepherd's purse
  —Life root
- **Cinnamon oil**: 1-5 drops every 3-4 hours

## Natural Hormones

- **Oral micronized progesterone**: 100 mg b.i.d. 7-12 days per month for recurring menorrhagia. A dosage of 200-400 mg q.d. for 7-12 days may be used for semiacute blood loss.
- **Progesterone cream**: ¼ to ½ tsp b.i.d. for 12 days per month for mild recurring menorrhagia. Use a product containing at least 400 mg progesterone per ounce.
- **Natural estradiol**: one high-dose regimen for acute bleeding—2 mg estradiol every 4 hours for 24 hours, single daily dose for 7-10 days, followed by oral micronized progesterone 200 mg before bed for 7-12 days.

# Migraine Headache

## DIAGNOSTIC SUMMARY

- Recurrent, paroxysmal attacks of headache.
- Headache typically is pounding and unilateral but may become generalized.
- Attacks often preceded by psychological or visual disturbances (auras) accompanied by anorexia, nausea, and gastrointestinal upset and followed by drowsiness.
- Physical examination reveals no focal neurologic deficit.

## GENERAL CONSIDERATIONS

Lifetime prevalence of migraine headache is 18%. Women are more frequently affected than men. More than half of patients have a family history of migraine.

- Auras: migraines can come without warning but often have symptoms (auras) a few minutes before onset of pain: blurring or bright spots of vision, anxiety, fatigue, disturbed thinking, unilateral peripheral numbness or tingling.
- Migraine headaches are caused by excessive dilation of blood vessels in the head; they affect 15%-20% of men and 25%-30% of women.
- Vascular headache pain (e.g., migraine): throbbing or pounding sharp pain; nonvascular headache (tension headache) pain: steady, constant, dull pain starting at base of skull or in forehead and spreading over entire head, giving sensation of pressure or vise grip applied to skull. Pain of headache comes from outside the brain because brain tissue is insensate. Pain arises from meninges and scalp, large cranial vessels, proximal intracranial vessels, and scalp vasculature and muscles when stretched or tensed.
- Most common nonvascular headache is the tension headache, caused by tightened muscles of the face, neck, or scalp, resulting from stress or poor posture. Tightened muscles pinch nerves or

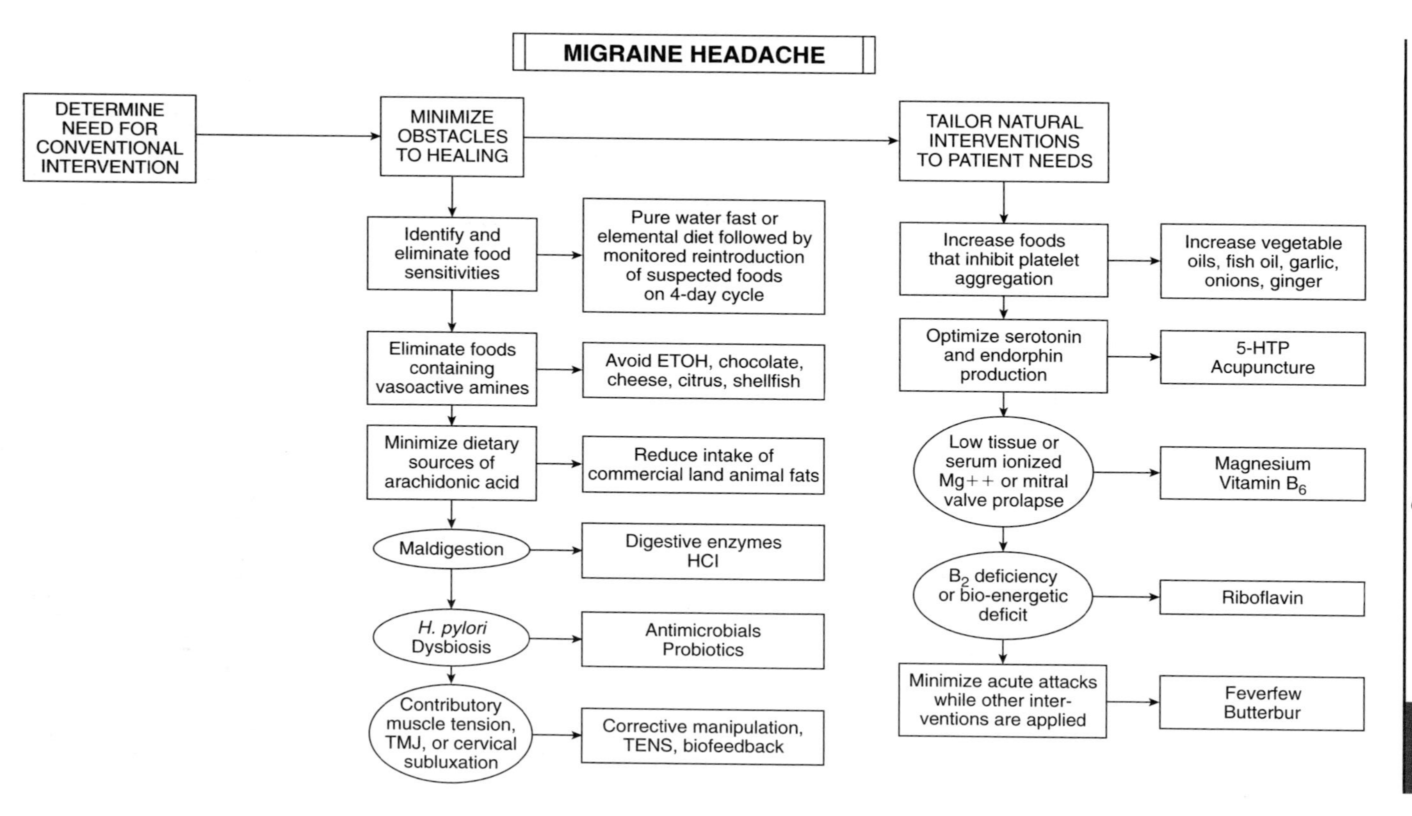
MIGRAINE HEADACHE
DETERMINE NEED FOR CONVENTIONAL INTERVENTION
MINIMIZE OBSTACLES TO HEALING
Identify and eliminate food sensitivities
Pure water fast or elemental diet followed by monitored reintroduction of suspected foods on 4-day cycle
Eliminate foods containing vasoactive amines
Avoid ETOH, chocolate, cheese, citrus, shellfish
Minimize dietary sources of arachidonic acid
Reduce intake of commercial land animal fats
Maldigestion
Digestive enzymes HCl
H. pylori Dysbiosis
Antimicrobials Probiotics
Contributory muscle tension, TMJ, or cervical subluxation
Corrective manipulation, TENS, biofeedback
TAILOR NATURAL INTERVENTIONS TO PATIENT NEEDS
Increase foods that inhibit platelet aggregation
Increase vegetable oils, fish oil, garlic, onions, ginger
Optimize serotonin and endorphin production
5-HTP Acupuncture
Low tissue or serum ionized Mg++ or mitral valve prolapse
Magnesium Vitamin B6
B2 deficiency or bio-energetic deficit
Riboflavin
Minimize acute attacks while other interventions are applied
Feverfew Butterbur

their blood supply, causing pain and pressure. Relaxation of muscle usually brings immediate relief.

## Classification and Diagnosis

### Migraine Classification

| | Common | Classic | Complicated |
|---|---|---|---|
| Incidence | 80% | 10% | 10% |
| Pain | Frontal, unilateral or bilateral | Unilateral | Unpredictable, may be absent |
| Aura | Unusual | Half-hour before striking | Neurologic aura, vertigo, syncope, diplopia, hemiparesis |
| Duration of headache | 1-3 days | 2-6 hours | Unpredictable |
| Physical examination | Unhappiness | Pallor, vomiting | Mild neurologic signs, speech disorder, hemiparesis, unsteadiness, cranial nerve III palsy |

- **Cluster headache** was once considered migraine-type because vasodilation is a key component. It is now separately classified. It is also called histamine cephalgia, Horton's headache, or atypical facial neuralgia. It is much less common than migraine.
- **Chronic daily headache** (CDH) (also called chronic tension headache, migraine with interparoxysmal headache, transformed migraine, evolutive migraine, mixed headache syndrome, tension-vascular HA): affects 40% of patients in headache clinics.

### Types of Chronic Daily Headache

Transformed migraine
- Drug-induced
- Non-drug-induced

Chronic tension-type headache
New daily persistent headache
Posttraumatic headache

## Pathophysiology

Migraine is linked to vasomotor instability but the mechanisms are unknown. It is not simply a primary vascular event.

- **Vasomotor instability theory**: superficial temporal vessels are visibly dilated. Local compression of these vessels or carotid artery temporarily relieves pain. Other types of extracranial vasodilation (heat or exercise induced) are not problematic. Patients are pale during headache despite extracranial vasodilation, and lower skin temperature of the affected side suggests constriction of small vessels. Focal or diffuse cerebral or brainstem dysfunction is attributed to intracranial vasoconstriction. Blood flow is greatly reduced during the prodromal stage, followed by a stage of increased blood flow persisting for >48 hours. Aura may be caused by cortical spreading depression, a process producing transient depression of spontaneous and evoked neuronal activity. During this time, the brain fails to maintain normal ionic homeostasis and efflux of excitatory amino acids from neurons. Cortical spreading depression may be linked to decreased cerebral blood flow during aura. This stage may be followed by phase of increased blood flow that can persist for >48 hours. Migraine patients may have functional abnormality of vasomotor control, suggested by orthostatic symptoms and abnormal sensitivity to vasodilatory effects of physical and chemical agents. Migraineurs experience heightened central nervous system activity, which appears to be mediated by the trigeminovascular system.
- **Platelet disorder theory**: migraine platelets show increased spontaneous aggregation, aberrant manner of serotonin release, and aberrant platelet composition. Hanington theory: most common precipitant of migraine is emotional stressor causing increased plasma catecholamine, triggering serotonin release, platelet aggregation, and vasoconstriction. Migraineurs' platelets aggregate more readily than normal, both spontaneously and when exposed to serotonin, adenosine diphosphate (ADP), and catecholamines, similar to transient cerebral ischemic attacks (TIA). TIA symptoms resemble prodromal phase of migraine headache. Attack onset is accompanied by elevated plasma serotonin, followed by increased urinary 5-hydroxyindoleacetic acid (5-HIAA), a breakdown product of serotonin metabolism. Blood serotonin is normally stored in platelets and released by aggregation and in response to stimuli (catecholamines). Total serotonin

content in normal and migraine platelets is identical. Quantity of serotonin released by migraine platelets, in response to serotonin stimulation, is normal (or subnormal) after attack but progressively higher as next attack approaches. Plasma serotonin elevation may not be causative; it may be self-defense mechanism or epiphenomenon produced by neurogenic inflammation. Yet platelet deactivating agents (aspirin, feverfew, essential fatty acids) help prevent migraines. Platelet hypothesis evidence: classic migraine patients have twofold increase in incidence of mitral valve prolapse. Prolapsing mitral valve damages platelets and increases aggregation and possibly release of serotonin and other vasoactive substances.

- **Neuronal disorder theory**: trigeminovascular neurons, which innervate pial arteries, release peptide substance P either in direct response to initiators or secondarily to changes in the central nervous system. Substance P is a mediator of pain released into arteries, linked to vasodilation, mast cell degranulation, and increased vascular permeability. Arterial endothelial cells may respond to substance P by releasing vasoactive substances; functional changes within the noradrenergic system may be the threshold for migraine activation. Potentiators may exert effects by modulating sympathetic activity. Chronic stress is a potentiator in this model.
- **Migraine as a "serotonin deficiency" syndrome**: 5-HIAA increases in urine during migraine arising from increased breakdown of serotonin from increased activity of monoamine oxidase. Migraine sufferers have low tissue serotonin (low serotonin syndrome). Low serotonin may cause decreased pain threshold. Positive clinical results are seen with serotonin precursor 5-hydroxytryptophan (5-HTP) (*Textbook*, "5-Hydroxytryptophan"). Link between low serotonin and headache is the basis of many migraine prescription drugs. Monoamine oxidase inhibitors (which increase serotonin) prevent headaches. Increasing serotonin relieves chronic migraines. Effects of 5-HTP and drugs on the serotonin system are complex because of the multiple types of serotonin receptors. Binding to 5-$HT_{1c}$ receptors triggers migraines; inhibiting 5-$HT_{1c}$ prevents migraines. Binding receptor 5-$HT_{1d}$ may prevent and stop migraines. 5-$HT_{1c}$ receptors are desensitized, that is, they lose affinity for serotonin, by increasing serotonin exposure by using 5-HTP. Serotonin binds instead to 5-$HT_{1d}$ receptor, decreasing headaches. Evidence for theory: 5-HTP is more effective over time (after 60 days of use rather than after

30). Antimigraine triptan drugs are 5-$HT_{1b}$ and 5-$HT_{1d}$ receptor agonists that constrict blood vessels, and block neurogenic inflammation and neural peptide release. They may also inhibit neuronal activity within the trigeminovascular system. Safety issue: triptans activate serotonin receptors on cerebral vessels and coronary arteries; avoid in patients with ischemic heart disease, uncontrolled hypertension, or cerebrovascular disease. Avoid using triptans, ergotamine-based drugs, and selective serotonin reuptake inhibitors (SSRIs) concurrently, although risk of serotonin syndrome is low. Some practitioners use 5-HTP successfully with SSRIs, but caution is advised. Although SSRIs are used for migraine prophylaxis, their biochemical effect is unknown, quality of evidence is poor, and clinical impact is low.

- **Unified hypothesis**: migraine has a three-stage process: initiation, prodrome, and headache. Initiation depends on accumulation over time of several stressors that ultimately affect serotonin metabolism. At a critical point of susceptibility (or threshold), a cascade event is initiated. Susceptibility is a combination of decreased tissue serotonin, platelet changes, altered responsiveness of key cerebrovascular end organs, increased sensitivity of intrinsic noradrenergic system of the brain, and buildup of histamine, arachidonic acid metabolites, or other mediators of inflammation. Platelet changes: increased adhesiveness, enhanced tendency to release serotonin, and increased membrane arachidonic acid. When platelets are stimulated to secrete serotonin, platelet aggregation, vasospasm, and inflammatory processes cause local cerebral ischemia. This is followed by rebound vasodilation and release of peptide substance P and other mediators of pain.

## THERAPEUTIC CONSIDERATIONS

Pharmaceuticals tend to be inadequate because they fail to address underlying cause. Identify precipitating factors. Food intolerance or allergy is the most important, but many other factors are primary causes or contributors. Assess role headache medicines play, especially in chronic headaches.

### Drug Reaction

Seventy percent of patients with CDH suffer from drug-induced headaches. Two main forms of drug-induced CDH are analgesic rebound headache (ARHA) and ergotamine rebound headache

(ERHA). Withdrawal of medicine induces prompt improvement in most cases.

**ARHA**: should be suspected in any patient with chronic headaches who is taking large quantities of analgesics and experiencing daily predictable headache. Critical dosage leading to ARHA is 1000 mg acetaminophen or aspirin. Analgesic medicines typically contain additional substances (caffeine or a sedative such as butabarbital) that further contribute to the problem and may lead to withdrawal headache, nausea, abdominal cramps, diarrhea, restlessness, sleeplessness, and anxiety. Withdrawal symptoms start at 24-48 hours and subside in 5-7 days.

**ERHA**: ergotamine is a widely used drug for severe acute migraine and cluster headaches. It works by constricting blood vessels of head, preventing or relieving excessive dilation responsible for headache pain. It is administered intramuscularly, by inhalation, or by suppository; it is poorly absorbed if given orally. It is quite effective but associated with side effects. Symptoms of acute ergotamine poisoning include vomiting, diarrhea, dizziness, rise or fall of blood pressure, slow or weak pulse, dyspnea, convulsions, and loss of consciousness.

- Symptoms of chronic poisoning result from blood vessel contraction and reduced circulation (numbness and coldness of extremities, tingling, chest pain, heart valve lesions, hair loss, decreased urination, and gangrene of fingers and toes) and those resulting from nervous system disturbances (vomiting, diarrhea, headache, tremors, contractions of facial muscles, and convulsions).
- Regular ergotamine use in migraine is linked to dependency syndrome—severe chronic headache with increased intensity—on ceasing medicine. Most migraines rarely occur more than once or twice a week; presence of daily migraine-type headache in persons taking ergotamine is a good clue for ERHA. Dosage can be a clue: weekly dosages >10 mg (some patients take 10-15 mg q.d.).
- Stopping ergotamine causes predictable, protracted, debilitating headache with nausea and vomiting within 72 hours and may last another 72 hours. Improvement after cessation is common. Ginger may lessen ergotamine withdrawal symptoms.

## Diet

Food allergy or intolerance plays role in many cases. Detection and removal of allergens or intolerant foods eliminate or greatly reduce symptoms in the majority of patients (success ranges from 30% to 93%). Incidences of food allergy are similar for the three major types of migraine. Mechanism is unknown, but several theories have been proposed:

- Idiopathic response to a pharmacologically active substance, such as tyramine
- Monoamine oxidase deficiency
- Platelet phenolsulfotransferase deficiency; immunologically mediated food allergy
- Platelet abnormalities

**Egger theory**: chronic alteration of nonspecific responsiveness of cerebral vascular end organ from long-term antigenic stimulation (analogous to asthmatic response of bronchioles to exercise or cold after antigen contact). Food allergies cause platelet degranulation and serotonin release. Lab detection of food allergies is most convenient for patient. Challenge testing is most reliable but has a delayed response, requiring several days of repeated challenge. Ingestion of large amounts of several foods is needed to detect the marginally reactive.

**Dietary amines**: chocolate, cheese, beer, and wine precipitate migraines because they contain histamine and/or other vasoactive compounds, triggering migraines in sensitive individuals by causing blood vessels to expand.

- **Red wine** is more problematic than white wine because it has 20-200 times the amount of histamine, and it stimulates release of vasoactive compounds by platelets. Being much higher in flavonoids, it inhibits enzyme (phenolsulfotransferase), which breaks down serotonin and other vasoactive amines in platelets. Migraine sufferers have much lower levels of this enzyme. High vasoactive amine foods (cheese, chocolate) worsen the problem.
- Standard treatment of histamine-induced headache is a histamine-free diet plus vitamin $B_6$.
- Enzyme diamine oxidase, which breaks down histamine in small intestine mucosa before absorption into circulation, influences whether a person reacts to dietary histamine. Persons sensitive to dietary histamine have less of this enzyme than control subjects. Diamine oxidase is vitamin $B_6$ dependent. Compounds inhibiting $B_6$ (that also inhibit diamine oxidase): food coloring agents (hydrazine dyes: FD&C yellow #5), drugs (isoniazid, hydralazine, dopamine, penicillamine), birth control pills,

alcohol, and excessive protein intake. Yellow dye #5 (tartrazine) is consumed in greater quantities (15 mg q.d.) than the recommended daily allowance for vitamin $B_6$ (2.0 mg for males and 1.6 mg for females).

- **Vitamin $B_6$** (1 mg/kg body weight) improves histamine tolerance, presumably by increasing diamine oxidase activity. Women have lower diamine oxidase. This may explain the higher incidence of histamine-induced headaches among women. Women are more frequently intolerant of red wine. Level of diamine oxidase in women increases by more than 500 times during pregnancy; women with histamine-induced headaches commonly have complete remission during pregnancy.
- Diet-related triggers: hypoglycemia can trigger migraine and is correctable by dietary manipulation. Hypoglycemia may arise from refined carbohydrate intake, especially when insulin becomes elevated. Excessive sodium intake may increase antiotensin in response to sodium ingestion. For lactose intolerance, avoiding dairy may afford improvement. Aspartame, a common sweetener, may increase migraine incidence.
- Dysbiosis and detoxification: migraine is not just food intolerance; digestive and detoxification aberrations complicate matters. Metabolic waste of pathogenic organisms may produce headache. Correct intestinal dysbiosis is identified clinically or by stool culture, organic acids analysis, or intestinal permeability assessment. *Helicobacter pylori* was detected in 40% of migraine patients; eradication of the bacterium improved headache intensity, duration, and frequency in 100% of patients treated. Toxic overload or suboptimal function of detoxification enzymes may trigger headache. Susceptibility to toxicity is produced by excessive environmental exposures, genetic polymorphisms in detoxification enzyme production, and depletion of nutrient cofactors catalyzing phase I and/or phase II detoxification reactions.

## Nutritional Supplements

- **5-HTP**: increases serotonin (see earlier). It also increases endorphins and is at least as effective as pharmaceuticals used to prevent migraine but much safer and better tolerated. Dosage: 200-600 mg q.d.
- **Essential fatty acids (EFAs) and arachidonic acid**: have received little research attention for migraine. Platelet aggregation and arachidonic acid metabolites play a major role mediating events causing prodromal cerebral ischemia. Manipulating dietary EFAs

may be very useful. Reducing animal fats and increasing fish significantly change platelet and membrane EFA ratios and decrease platelet aggregation. Sixty percent of the brain is composed of lipids. Omega-3 fatty acids can reduce headache frequency and intensity. Fish oil and olive oil improve migraine frequency, duration, and severity. Proposed mechanisms of action of omega-3s: reduced platelet serotonin release, modulation of prostaglandin synthesis, and diminution of cerebral vasospasm. Elevated blood lipids and free fatty acids are associated with increased platelet aggregability, decreased 5-HT, and increased prostaglandin levels. Biologic states that produce increased free fatty acids and lipids: high fat intake, obesity, insulin resistance, vigorous exercise, hunger, intake of alcohol and caffeine, oral contraceptives, tobacco abuse, and stress.

- **Riboflavin (vitamin $B_2$)**: Another hypothesis states that migraines are caused by reduced energy production within mitochondria of cerebral blood vessels. $B_2$ is the precursor of flavin mononucleotide and flavin adenine dinucleotide, which are required for activity of flavoenzymes of electron transport chain. Riboflavin can increase mitochondrial complex I and II activity in mitochondrial energy metabolism without changing neuronal excitability—allowing excellent tolerance and lack of central nervous system adverse effects. Dosage for prophylaxis: 400 mg q.d. for 3+ months. It improved patients 68.2% as determined by migraine severity score used by researchers. Diarrhea and polyuria may be associated with administration of high-dose $B_2$. Advantages: well tolerated, inexpensive, reduces brain oxidative toxicity. Other prophylactic B vitamins: folic acid.
- **Magnesium (Mg)**: low Mg is linked to migraine and tension headache. Low brain and tissue Mg levels are found in patients with migraines. Key Mg functions are to maintain tone of the blood vessels and prevent overexcitability of nerve cells. Mg supplements may only be effective in patients with low tissue or low ionized levels of Mg. Low tissue Mg is common in migraine patients but is unnoticed because serum Mg is normal. Serum Mg, however, is an unreliable indicator because most body Mg stores are intracellular. Low serum Mg is an end-stage deficiency. Use red blood cell (erythrocyte) Mg and ionized $Mg^{2+}$ (most biologically active form) in serum. Patients with acute migraine and low serum ionized Mg (<0.54 mmol/L) are more likely to respond to intravenous $MgSO_4$ than patients with higher serum ionized Mg. Pain relief lasts at least 24 hours in patients with serum ionized

Mg <0.54 mmol/L. Average ionized Mg in patients most relieved by intravenous Mg is significantly lower than in less-responsive patients. Intravenous Mg is extremely effective in some cases of acute migraine, tension, and cluster headaches. Dosage of 1-3 g intravenous Mg (over 10-minute period) has 90% success rate in patients with low ionized Mg. $MgSO_4$ completely eliminates migraine-associated symptoms of nausea and photosensitivity. Adverse effects include a brief flushed feeling. Mg improves mitral valve prolapse that can damage platelets, causing release of histamine, platelet-activating factor, and serotonin. Eighty-five percent of patients with mitral valve prolapse have chronic Mg deficiency. Oral Mg improves mitral valve prolapse. Mg bound to citrate, malate, aspartate, or other Krebs cycle compound is better absorbed and tolerated than inorganic forms with laxative effect. Use 50 mg vitamin $B_6$ q.d. to increase intracellular Mg.

## Physical Medicine

Effective in shortening duration and decreasing intensity of an attack, especially those with significant muscular contraction component, but relatively ineffective in curing true migraine.

- **Cervical manipulation**: has no influence on frequency of recurrence, duration, or disability but can reduce pain associated with attacks.
- **Temporomandibular joint dysfunction syndrome (TMJ)**: incidence of migraine in patients with TMJ is similar to that in the general population; incidence of headache from muscle tension is much higher. Correction of TMJ dysfunction may be useful in treating migraine, but it is far more important in muscle tension headaches.
- **Transcutaneous electrical stimulation (TENS)**: TENS is effective in migraine and muscle tension headaches (55% responded to treatment vs. 18% placebo response). Inappropriately applied TENS (TENS applied below perception threshold) is ineffective.
- **Acupuncture**: relieves migraine pain. Mechanism of relief is not endorphin mediated. Acupuncture increases endorphins in control subjects, but low levels of serum endorphins in migraine patients do not increase with treatment. Mechanism may be by normalization of serotonin levels. It is effective in relieving pain when it normalizes serotonin levels, but ineffective in relieving pain and raising serotonin in patients with very low serotonin. It offers some success reducing frequency of migraine attacks;

40% of subjects experienced a 50%-100% reduction in severity and frequency in one study; five treatments (over a period of 1 month) decreased recurrence in 45% of patients over a period of 6 months.

- **Biofeedback and relaxation therapy**: most widely used nondrug therapy for migraine headaches is thermal biofeedback and relaxation response training. Thermal biofeedback uses feedback gauge to monitor hand temperature. Patient consciously raises (or lowers) temperature using the device feedback. Relaxation training produces a relaxation response—a physiologic state that opposes stress response. These approaches are as effective as drugs but without side effects.

## Botanical Medicines

- ***Tanacetum parthenium* (feverfew)**: most popular antimigraine botanical. Seventy percent of surveyed migraine sufferers eating feverfew leaves q.d. for prolonged periods claimed decreased frequency and/or intensity of attacks (many of these patients were unresponsive to orthodox medicines). It has been claimed to inhibit serotonin release, inhibit prostaglandin synthesis and platelet aggregation, inhibit polymorphonuclear leukocyte degranulation and phagocytosis of neutrophils, inhibit mast cell release of histamine, promote cytotoxic activity against human tumor cells, and possess both antimicrobial activity and antithrombotic potential. Studies indicate feverfew treats and prevents migraine by inhibiting release of serotonin from platelets. Constituents: sesquiterpene lactone (e.g., parthenolide). Avoid or use with caution in patients on anticoagulants because of platelet inhibition. Side effects: well tolerated; oral ulceration (from chewing feverfew leaves) and gastrointestinal symptoms are the most common adverse events, but these effects are mild and reversible with discontinuation. It is in same family as ragweed and chamomile; avoid in allergic persons.
- ***Zingiber officinalis* (ginger)**: ginger root has significant effects against inflammation and platelet aggregation. Much anecdotal information on migraine exists but little experimental evidence. Most active antiinflammatory components are found in fresh preparations and ginger oil.
- **Butterbur (*Petasites hybridus*)**: vascular wall antispasmodic, especially for cerebral vessels. It inhibits leukotriene synthesis and lipoxygenase activity. Active principles petasine and isopetasine also produce vasodilation. This plant can decrease

migraine frequency by 60% (while improving dysmenorrhea). Use prophylactically as daily supplement for 4-6 months; taper until migraine incidence begins to increase. It is well tolerated. Side effects: diarrhea in some patients. No drug interactions have been identified, but it is not known to be safe during pregnancy or lactation. Pyrrolizidine alkaloids are hepatotoxic and carcinogenic; use only extracts from which these have been removed. Adult dosage: 50-100 mg b.i.d. with meals.

## Hormones

- **Melatonin**: downstream metabolite of dietary tryptophan. Ninety percent of serotonin is produced in the walls of the gastrointestinal tract, stored in platelets, and distributed to the rest of the body except the central nervous system (serotonin cannot cross the blood-brain barrier). Tryptophan and 5-HTP cross the blood-brain barrier to be converted into serotonin in the pineal gland, which contains 90% of CNS serotonin and most of the melatonin. The pineal gland is the interface between the environment and CNS and is involved in triggering external and internal factors—certain foods, toxins/odors, flickering lights, sleep deprivation, travel through time zones, menses. Migraine patients have decreased plasma and urinary melatonin. Melatonin deficit excessively stimulates the trigeminovascular system. Melatonin therapy helps migraineurs with delayed sleep phase syndrome and may resynchronize circadian rhythms to lifestyle, relieving triggers and symptoms. Melatonin produces headache in susceptible persons. Regular sleep, regular meals, exercise, avoidance of excessive stimulation and relaxation, and evasion of dietary triggers help reduce activation.
- **Sex steroid hormones**: onset of migraine rises with menarche. Migraines are linked to menstruation in 60% of female migraineurs (menstrual migraine) and improve with pregnancy (sustained estrogens). Oral contraceptives can induce, improve, or exacerbate migraine. Incidence tends to decrease with advancing age but either regress or worsen during menopause. Headaches occur during and after simultaneous decline of both estrogen and progesterone. Falling estrogen levels are linked to menstrual migraine. Estrogens given premenstrually can delay migraine but not menstruation; progesterone given premenstrually delays menstruation but not migraine. Percutaneous estradiol gel perimenstrually reduces headaches. Estrogens increase number of progesterone, muscarinic, and serotonin (5 HT-2) receptors and

decrease number of 5-HT1 and beta-adrenergic receptors. Estrogens increase trigeminal mechanoreceptor receptive fields, increasing receptive input from trigeminal system. Progesterone blocks estrogen-induced increase in 5-HT2 receptors. Transdermal progesterone therapy can prevent migraine for some patients. Hysterectomy or oophorectomy has not been helpful.

## THERAPEUTIC APPROACH

Migraine is a multifaceted disorder that may be a symptom rather than a disease. Determine which factors are responsible for each patient's migraine process. Identifying and avoiding precipitating factors reduce frequency and cumulative effect of initiators.

- **Identify problematic foods**: high incidence (80%-90%) of food allergy or intolerance in migraine warrants 1 week of careful avoidance of all foods to which patient may be allergic or intolerant; follow a pure water fast or elemental diet. (Oligoantigenic diet may be used but is less desirable because allergens may be inadvertently included.) Avoid all other possible allergens (vitamin preparations, unnecessary drugs, herbs). Food-sensitive patients will exhibit strong exacerbation of symptoms early in the week, followed by almost total relief by the end of fast or modified diet. This sequence is caused by the addictive characteristic of reactive foods. When patient is symptom free, one new food is reintroduced (and eaten several times) daily with symptoms carefully recorded. Some recommend reintroduction on 4-day cycle. Suspected foods (symptom onset ranges from 20 minutes to 2 weeks) are eliminated, and apparently safe foods are rotated through the 4-day cycle (*Textbook,* "Food Allergy Testing"). When symptom-free period of at least 6 months is established, 4-day rotation diet is no longer necessary.
- **Oligoantigenic diet**: effective in some patients, but a longer trial (4-8 weeks) is necessary, depending on frequency of episodes. Eliminate dairy, gluten, eggs, corn, chocolate, peanuts, coffee, black tea, soft drinks, alcohol, and processed foods. Food allergy immunoglobulin testing gives mixed results.
- **Optimize digestive function**, as needed.
- **Correct intestinal dysbiosis**, including *Helicobacter pylori.*
- **Reduce toxic overload** and support detoxification enzymes.
- **Diet**: eliminate food allergens. Use 4-day rotation diet until patient is symptom-free for 6 months. Eliminate foods containing vasoactive amines and reintroduce carefully after symptoms are

controlled. Eliminate alcohol, cheese, chocolate, citrus fruits, and shellfish. Reduce sources of arachidonic acid (land animal fats). Increase foods inhibiting platelet aggregation (olive and flaxseed oils, fish oils, garlic, onion).

- **Supplements**:
  - —Magnesium: 250-800 mg q.d. in divided doses; titrate to symptoms and bowel tolerance
  - —Vitamin $B_6$: 50-75 mg tq.d. balanced with vitamin B complex
  - —5-HTP: 100-200 mg q.d. to b.i.d.
  - —Vitamin $B_2$ (riboflavin): 400 mg q.d., balanced with vitamin B complex

## Hormonal Therapies

- Trial of melatonin: 0.3-3 mg at bedtime.
- Trial of transdermal progesterone or estradiol, carefully individualized to clinical picture.
- Botanical medicines:
  - —*Tanacetum parthenium* (feverfew): 0.25-0.5 mg parthenolide b.i.d.
  - —*Zingiber officinalis* (ginger): fresh ginger approximately 10 g q.d. (6-mm slice); dried ginger, 500 mg q.i.d.; extract standardized to contain 20% of gingerol and shogaol, 100-200 mg t.i.d. for prevention and 200 mg every 2 hours (up to six times daily) in the treatment of an acute migraine.
  - —*Petasites hybridus* (butterbur): 50-100 mg b.i.d. with meals.
- Physical medicine:
  - —TENS to control secondary muscle spasm
  - —Acupuncture to balance meridians
- Biofeedback (The Association for Applied Psychophysiology and Biofeedback, 10200 West 44th Avenue, Suite 304, Wheat Ridge, CO 80033, (303) 422-8436)
- Guided imagery (The Academy for Guided Imagery, PO Box 2070, Mill Valley, CA 94942, (800)-726-2070)

## Patient Resources

- *Headache Help: A Complete Guide to Understanding Headaches and the Medicines that Relieve Them,* by Lawrence Robbins, MD, and Susan S. Lang, Houghton Mifflin Company, Boston/New York, 2000.
- *Headache Relief for Women,* by Alan M. Rapoport, LittleBrown, Boston, 1996.
- *Managing Your Migraine; A Migraine Sufferer's PracticalGuide,* by Susan L. Burks, Humana Press, New Jersey, 1994.
- *The Hormone Headache: New Ways to Prevent, Manage, and Treat Migraines and Other Headaches,* by Seymour Diamond, MD, with

Bill Still and Cynthia Still, Simon & Schuster Macmillan Company, New York, 1995.

- *Taking Control of Your Headaches: How to Get the Treatment You Need,* by P.N. Duckro, PhD, W. D. Richardson, MD, J.E. Marshall, RN, et al, Guilford Press, New York, 1995.
- *Headache Free,* by Roger Cady, MD, and Kathleen Farmer, PsyD, Bantam Books, New York, 1996.
- *Migraine: Everything You Need to Know About Their Cause and Care,* by Arthur H. Elkind, MD, Avon Publishing, 1997.
- *The Headache Alternative: A Neurologist's Guide to Drug-Free Relief,* by Alexander Mauskop, MD, and Marietta Abrams Brill, Dell Publishing, 1997.
- *Headache and Diet: Tyramine-Free Recipes,* by Seymour Diamond, MD, Bill Still, and Cynthia Still, International University Press, 1990.
- *Headaches in Children,* by Leonardo Garcia-Mendez, MD, Lemar Publishing, 1996.

## Primary Classifications of Headache

Vascular headache

- Migraine headache
- Classic migraine
- Common migraine
- Complicated migraine
- Variant migraine

Cluster headache

- Episodic cluster
- Chronic cluster
- Chronic paroxysmal hemicrania

Miscellaneous vascular headaches

- Carotidynia
- Hypertension
- Exertional
- Hangover
- Toxins and drugs
- Occlusive vascular disease
- Nonvascular
- Tension headache
- Common tension headache
- TMJ dysfunction
- Increased or decreased intracranial pressure
- Brain tumors
- Sinus infections
- Dental infections
- Inner or middle ear infections

## Factors That Trigger Migraine Headaches

- Low serotonin levels
- Genetics
- Shunting of tryptophan into other pathways
- Foods
- Food allergies
- Histamine-releasing foods
- Histamine-containing foods (alcohol, especially red wine)
- Chemicals
- Nitrates
- Monosodium glutamate
- Nitroglycerin
- Withdrawal from caffeine or other drugs that constrict blood vessels
- Stress
- Emotional changes, especially letdown after stress, and intense emotions such as anger
- Hormonal changes such as menstruation, ovulation, birth control pills
- Too little or too much sleep
- Exhaustion
- Poor posture
- Muscle tension
- Weather changes, such as barometric pressure changes, exposure to sun
- Glare or eyestrain

## Foods That Most Commonly Induce Migraine Headaches

| Food | Egger et al (%) | Hughes et al (%) | Monro et al (%) |
|---|---|---|---|
| Cow's milk | 67 | 57 | 65 |
| Wheat | 52 | 43 | 57 |
| Chocolate | 55 | 57 | 26 |
| Egg | 60 | 24 | 22 |
| Orange | 52 | — | 13 |
| Benzoic acid | 35 | — | — |
| Cheese | 32 | — | — |
| Tomato | 32 | 14 | — |
| Tartrazine | 30 | — | — |
| Rye | 30 | — | — |
| Rice | — | — | 30 |
| Fish | 22 | 29 (shell) | 17 |

### Foods That Most Commonly Induce Migraine Headaches—cont'd

| Food | Egger et al (%) | Hughes et al (%) | Monro et al (%) |
|---|---|---|---|
| Grapes | 12 | 33 | — |
| Onion | — | 24 | — |
| Soy | 17 | 24 | — |
| Pork | 22 | — | 17 |
| Peanuts | 12 | 29 | — |
| Alcohol | — | 29 | 9 |
| Monosodium glutamate | — | 19 | — |
| Walnuts | — | 19 | — |
| Beef | 20 | 14 | — |
| Tea | 17 | — | 17 |
| Coffee | 15 | 19 | 17 |
| Nuts | 12 | 19 (cashew) | 17 |
| Goat's milk | 15 | 14 | — |
| Corn | 20 | 9 | — |
| Oats | 15 | — | — |
| Cane sugar | 7 | 19 | — |
| Yeast | 12 | 14 | — |
| Apple | 12 | — | — |
| Peach | 12 | — | — |
| Potato | 12 | — | — |
| Chicken | 7 | 14 | — |
| Banana | 7 | — | — |
| Strawberry | 7 | — | — |
| Melon | 7 | — | — |
| Carrot | 7 | — | — |

### Factors Involved With Histamine-Induced Headaches

Histamine levels increased by:

- Histamine in alcoholic beverages (particularly red wine)
- Histamine in food
- Histamine-releasing foods
- Food allergy
- Vitamin $B_6$ deficiency

Histamine breakdown inhibited by:

- Vitamin $B_6$ antagonists
- Alcohol
- Drugs
- Food additives (e.g. yellow dye #5, monosodium glutamate)
- Vitamin C deficiency

Histamine release prevented by:

- Disodium cromoglycate
- Quercetin
- Antioxidants (e.g., vitamin C, vitamin E, selenium)

Histamine breakdown promoted by:

- Vitamin $B_6$
- Vitamin C

# Multiple Sclerosis

## DIAGNOSTIC SUMMARY

- Episodic neurologic symptoms depending on the parts of the central nervous system affected
- Typically occurs between 20 and 55 years of age
- Symptoms not consistent with a single neurologic lesion

## GENERAL CONSIDERATIONS

- Multiple sclerosis (MS) is a central nervous system (CNS) disease characterized by relapses and remissions, a variety of symptoms (depending on parts of the CNS are affected), and permanent disability. MS is the most common disabling neurologic disease of young and middle-aged adults in North America and Europe.
- MS is an inflammatory disorder of multifocal destruction of myelin sheaths (demyelination) and axons within the brain, spinal cord, and optic nerves. Areas of demyelination are termed plaques. Destruction of the myelin sheath around axons occurs with relative sparing of the axons, but axon damage also occurs. Macrophages and lymphocytes are present in active demyelination within plaques.
- Neurologic problems depend on location and severity of plaques.
- In 85% of cases, relapsing MS begins with a remitting course—relapses or attacks of a new problem, return of an old problem that had resolved, or worsening of preexisting symptoms. Relapses develop over a few days or weeks; improvement and stability then ensue, averaging one relapse every 2 years. Between relapses the patient is clinically stable but the effects of previous relapses are permanent. Relapses causing symptoms are the tip of the iceberg of disease activity. Asymptomatic new lesions appear within the brain five to 10 times more commonly than symptomatic lesions. Asymptomatic relapses cause permanent damage.

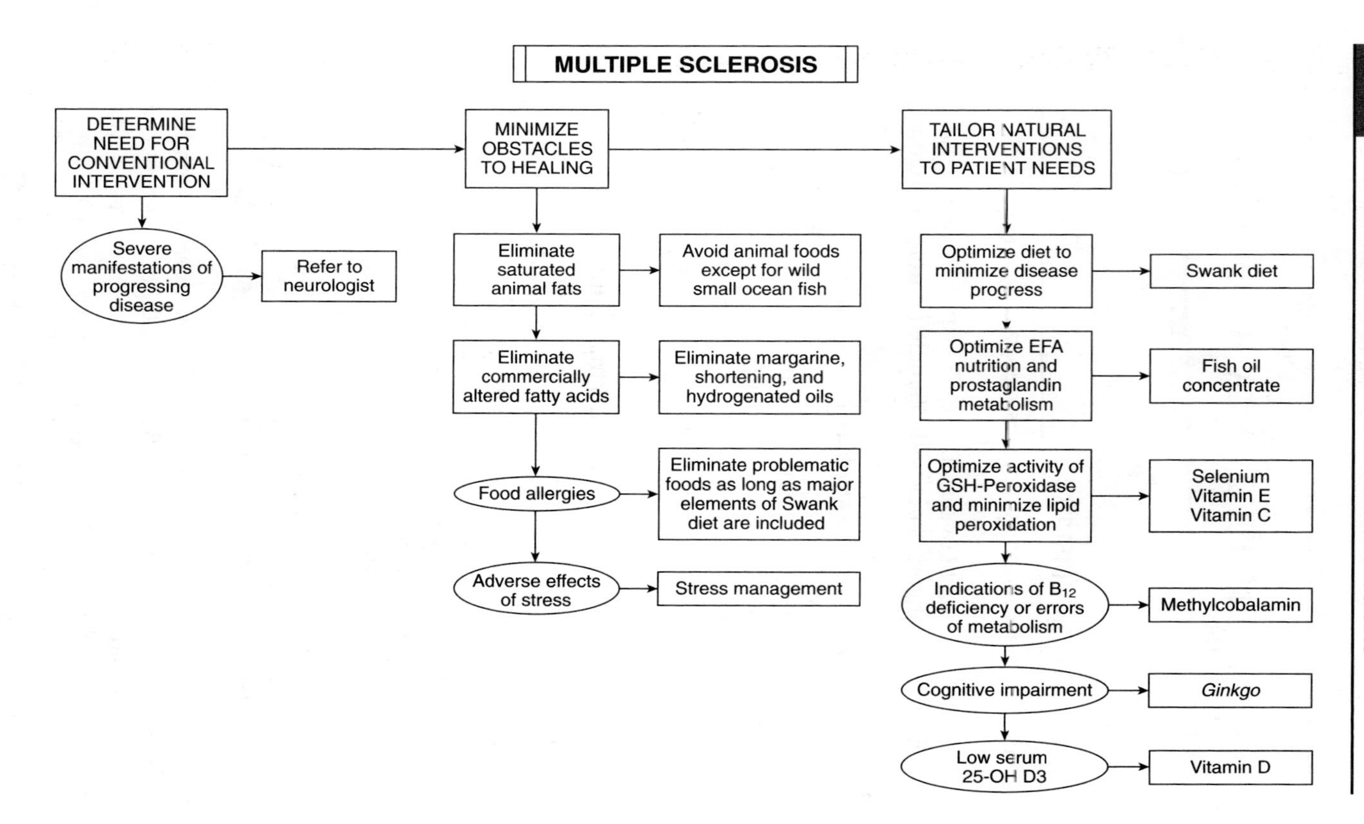
MULTIPLE SCLEROSIS
DETERMINE NEED FOR CONVENTIONAL INTERVENTION
Severe manifestations of progressing disease
Refer to neurologist
MINIMIZE OBSTACLES TO HEALING
Eliminate saturated animal fats
Avoid animal foods except for wild small ocean fish
Eliminate commercially altered fatty acids
Eliminate margarine, shortening, and hydrogenated oils
Food allergies
Eliminate problematic foods as long as major elements of Swank diet are included
Adverse effects of stress
Stress management
TAILOR NATURAL INTERVENTIONS TO PATIENT NEEDS
Optimize diet to minimize disease progress
Swank diet
Optimize EFA nutrition and prostaglandin metabolism
Fish oil concentrate
Optimize activity of GSH-Peroxidase and minimize lipid peroxidation
Selenium
Vitamin E
Vitamin C
Indications of $B_{12}$ deficiency or errors of metabolism
Methylcobalamin
Cognitive impairment
*Ginkgo*
Low serum 25-OH D3
Vitamin D

- Fifty percent of patients with relapsing/remitting MS enter a progressive phase (secondary progressive MS) 5-15 years after onset characterized by steady worsening with or without relapses. Fifteen percent of patients have progressive worsening from disease onset (primary progressive MS).
- MS is rarely fatal but is disabling; one third of patients lose the ability to walk 15-20 years after onset.
- Benign forms (up to 15% of patients) never develop permanent disability from MS but develop varying degrees of permanent disability.

## Epidemiology

- Incidence: 1 person per 1000 in the United States, Canada, and Northern Europe.
- Begins typically between ages 20 and 55 years but may occur at any age.
- Women are more commonly affected than men; 60% of cases are female.
- Racial influence: most common among whites of Northern European descent; rare among Asians and black Africans; relatively common among African Americans. Genetic predisposition is linked to risk of MS.
- Geographic distribution: highest prevalence in higher latitudes of northern and southern hemispheres where a person lives his or her first 2 decades of life. Environmental exposure in first 2 decades of life influences risk.

## Pathogenesis

- Pathologic features: demyelination of axons and, to a lesser extent, loss of axons.
- T-lymphocytes, macrophages, and plasma cells cause destruction during development of acute plaques.
- Subset of T-lymphocytes initiates acute lesions, recognizes antigens within CNS, becomes activated, and initiates inflammatory cascade that injures myelin and axons.
- Mediators of tissue damage: macrophages releasing soluble inflammatory mediators, cytokines, and free radicals or stripping myelin from axon sheath. Activated T-cells can release cytokines. Antimyelin antibodies can damage myelin by initiating complement cascade or facilitating macrophage phagocytosis of myelin.

- Disease process is "turned off" by apoptosis of initiating T-cells and by recruitment of regulatory T-cells into the CNS.

### Role of Free Radicals

- Oxygen and nitrogen free radicals are implicated in myelin and axon damage and upregulating proinflammatory tumor necrosis factor-alpha, inducible nitric oxide, and nuclear transcription factor-kappaB.
- They are also implicated in activating matrix metalloproteinase (MMP), a mediator of T-lymphocyte trafficking into CNS.
- Metabolites of oxidative and nitrosative stress are elevated in the cerebrospinal fluid (CSF) of patients with MS, who also have decreased reduced glutathione and increased oxidized glutathione in the CSF. A specific genotype for glutathione S-transferase is linked to an increased number of active lesions and impaired ability to detoxify oxidized lipids and DNA.

### Viruses and Autoantigens

- Categories of targets initiating inflammation of MS: viruses and autoantigens.
- Currently no convincing evidence links any infectious agent and MS. Lack of evidence does not exclude the possibility.
- Primary targets of pathogenic immune response are myelin antigens, indicating autoimmunity. MS patients are immunologically sensitized to a variety of myelin antigens.
- Viral infections may induce an autoimmune response in genetically susceptible persons that ultimately results in MS.

## ETIOLOGY

- Why people develop MS remains uncertain. Genes and the environment influence risk.

### Genes

- Having a first-order relative (parent or sibling) increases risk fivefold to tenfold.
- Twins in which one has MS: for nonidentical twins, chances of the second twin having MS are 1%-2% (similar to nontwin siblings). For identical twins, the chance of the second twin having MS is 25%.
- Ten to 15 different genes affect risk, including HLA-DR2 among northern Europeans.

### Environment

- One review study found risk of MS is correlated with: consumption of animal fat, animal protein, and meat from nonmarine mammals.
- Another study found that intake of omega-3 linolenic acid, but not fish oils or docosahexaenoic acid (DHA), was associated with a lower risk for MS.
- No relation between intake of fruits and vegetables and risk of MS has been found.
- A protective effect of cereals and breads, vegetable protein, dietary fiber, vitamin C, thiamin, riboflavin, calcium, and potassium for all cases and fish in cases of women only has been identified.

## DIAGNOSTIC CONSIDERATIONS

- Only neurologists have sufficient training and experience to make an accurate diagnosis.
- Diagnosis of MS rests on objective demonstration of two or more areas of demyelination in CNS occurring at more than one time point. It is not solely based on patient's symptoms.
- Evidence: neurologic exam, magnetic resonance imaging of brain and spinal cord as well as electrophysiologic tests, called evoked potentials, that assess visual, auditory, and somatosensory pathways.
- CSF exam for plasma cells producing immunoglobulins—qualitative (oligoclonal bands) and quantitative (total immunoglobulin (Ig) G, IgG index, and IgG synthesis rate) changes.
- Rule out other disorders: unusual causes of cerebrovascular disease, vitamin $B_{12}$ deficiency, spinal cord compression from tumors, herniated disks or spinal canal stenosis, vascular malformations of spinal cord, Lyme disease.
- MRI allows diagnosis at early stages and helps exclude other diseases.

## THERAPEUTIC CONSIDERATIONS

### Allopathic Treatments

- Medicines that help decrease disease activity in relapsing/remitting MS: human recombinant interferon-beta (Avonex, Betaseron, and Rebif) and glatiramer acetate (Copaxone), a random polymer of four amino acids that stimulates protective T-cells. These agents decrease relapse rate by one third, decrease new lesion formation in the brain, and decrease risk of permanent neurologic disability. Corticosteroids, such as methylprednisolone, in high doses can decrease duration of relapses but do not affect degree of eventual recovery from relapses. The immunosuppressant/chemotherapy agent mitoxantrone (Novantrone) decreases disease activity in rapidly progressive forms.

## Natural Medicine

Interventions used in combination with appropriate allopathic therapies:

- Dietary therapy
- Nutritional supplements
- Exercise
- Stress management

## Diet Therapy

### Dr. Roy Swank Diet

- Diet low in saturated fats over a long period can retard disease process, reduce number of attacks, and decrease mortality rate. A low-fat diet supplemented with cod liver oil decreased the incidence of MS in populations eating diets low in animal fats and high in cold-water fish.
  —Saturated fat intake: <15 g q.d.
  —Unsaturated fat intake: 20-50 g q.d.
  —No red meat for first year (including dark meat of turkey and chicken); only 3 oz/week red meat thereafter.
  —White meat poultry, fish, and shellfish in any amounts if low in saturated fats
  —Eliminate dairy containing 1% butterfat or more
  —1 tsp or 4 capsules nonconcentrated cod liver oil; one multiple vitamin/mineral
- Benefits: antiinflammatory and neuron membrane–stabilizing effects of omega-3 fatty acids eicosapentaenoic acid (EPA) and docosahexaenoic acid (DHA).
- Recent uncontrolled open-label study diet for newly diagnosed relapsing remitting MS: low in saturated fats; increased intake of fish plus fish oil, vitamin B complex, and vitamin C; reduced intake of sugar, coffee, tea, and alcohol; no smoking. Over a 2-

year period, plasma omega-3 increased and plasma omega-6 decreased, with a reduction in both relapse rates and disability.

## Nutritional Supplements

### Linolenic Acid (Omega-3 Fatty Acids)

- "Marine lipids" EPA and DHA: MS patients have increased proinflammatory cytokines, tumor necrosis factor-alpha (TNF-alpha), interferon-gamma (IFN-gamma), and interleukin-2 (IL-2), mediators of immunopathogenesis of MS linked to disease activity in peripheral blood, CSF, and brain lesions. MMPs are also implicated. These proteases aid in remodeling extracellular matrix, basement membrane, and other tissues by digesting collagen components. MMPs play a role in transmigration of inflammatory cells into the CNS by disrupting the blood-brain barrier. MS patients have elevated serum levels of MMP-9.
- Omega-3s decrease mRNA and protein levels of cytokines: TNF-α, IFN-γ, IL-1, IL-2, and vascular cell adhesion molecule-1. Fish oil supplements decrease proinflammatory cytokines participating in pathogenesis of MS in patients and healthy control subjects. Fish oil decreases gene expression and protein levels of proinflammatory cytokines and MMPs.
- Omega-3s help treat depression in MS. Inflammatory cytokines are correlated with depression in MS. Gene expression levels of TNF-α and IFN-γ positively correlate with scores on depression inventory (high score indicating greater depression) in MS patients during relapses. Depression is common in MS. Ethyl-EPA significantly improves primary depression in non-MS patients. Dose: 1 to 4 g q.d. Omega-3 supplementation might help in conjunction with counseling and, when indicated, antidepressant drugs.

### Linoleic Acid (Omega-6 Fatty Acids)

- Supplementing omega-6 increased transforming growth factor beta-1 (TGF beta-1) in peripheral blood mononuclear cells of healthy subjects. TGF beta-1 is an antiinflammatory cytokine that might be beneficial for MS. Animal study models of MS report that supplementing linoleic acid decreases severity of disease and reduces inflammation in the CNS.
- MS patients supplemented with linoleic acid had a smaller increase in disability and reduced severity and duration of relapses compared with patients supplemented with olive oil.

Dose: sunflower seed oil emulsion at sufficient dosage to provide daily 17.2 g linoleic acid.

- Evening primrose oil (EPO) contains omega-6 gamma-linoleic acid (GLA). GLA might be more effective than linoleic acid because of easier incorporation into brain lipids and greater effect on immune function. But EPO contains low levels of GLA and is expensive; EPO also showed no benefit in a clinical trial. EPO is not recommended for MS.

### Antioxidants

- **Selenium (Se)**: MS patients have inadequate glutathione peroxidase (GSH-Px) activity in red blood cells and white blood cells. Impaired glutathione S-transferase genotype is linked to increased numbers of active lesions. Se is a component of selenoproteins, including GSH-Px enzymes. Supplementing MS patients with 6 mg q.d. sodium selenite, 2 g q.d. vitamin C, and 480 mg q.d. vitamin E for 5 weeks increased GSH-Px fivefold. However, clinical parameters were not evaluated.
- **Vitamin C and E**: decrease lipid peroxidation. Isoprostane, a measure of lipid peroxidation, is increased in MS and Alzheimer's, Huntington's, and Creutzfeldt-Jakob diseases. Isoprostane is increased in CSF of MS patients. Both vitamin supplements decrease isoprostane levels.
- **Alpha lipoic acid (ALA)**: ALA and its reduced form, dihydrolipoic acid (DHLA), are potent antioxidants with multiple modes of action. ALA/DHLA regenerates other antioxidants (GSH-Px, vitamins C and E), scavenges reactive oxygen species, repairs oxidative damage, and chelates oxidizing metallic ions. DHLA restores reduced GSH. ALA is absorbed in the diet and synthesized de novo, converted intracellularly to DHLA, and crosses the blood-brain barrier. Both ALA and DHLA are present in extracellular and intracellular environments. At doses of 10-100 mg/kg/day, ALA suppressed an animal model of MS by inhibiting T-lymphocyte trafficking into the spinal cord.

### Vitamin $B_{12}$

Acquired vitamin $B_{12}$ deficiency and inborn errors of metabolism involving $B_{12}$ cause demyelination in the CNS. Vitamin $B_{12}$ deficiency can mimic MS. Reports that $B_{12}$ levels in serum are low in MS are conflicting. A decrease in binding capacity of unsaturated $B_{12}$ may occur. Massive oral doses of $B_{12}$ (60 mg q.d.) in severe progressive MS have improved visual and brainstem auditory evoked potentials by 30%, but motor function did not improve.

### Vitamin D

Recent research has shown dramatic benefit when large doses of vitamin D (2000-3000 IU/day) are used. Vitamin D is now known as an immune system modulator with low levels resulting in excessive immune activation. Vitamin D deficiency is surprisingly common, especially in those with dark skin and residing in more northern latitudes. Monitor with serum 1-OH cholecalciferol.

### Botanical Medicine

- ***Ginkgo biloba* (GB)**: has antioxidant and antiplatelet activities. GB blocks platelet activating factor (PAF). Overproduction of PAF is implicated in neurodegeneration. MS patients have elevated PAF in plasma and CSF; PAF elevation correlates positively with number of active lesions seen by magnetic resonance imaging. In the treatment of animals with MS-like disease PAF increased disease progression; PAF antagonists suppressed disease progression. Ginkgolide B (terpenoid of GB) is an antagonist of PAF. Whether GB extract, with both antioxidant and antiplatelet activities, is effective in treating relapses or as long-term treatment of MS is not known. GB may help manage cognitive dysfunction. Significant cognitive impairment occurs in 40%-60% of MS patients; no allopathic symptomatic therapies exist. GB modestly slows progression in Alzheimer's disease. GB (240 mg q.d.) has given modest benefit to MS patients with mild cognitive impairment.

## OTHER CONSIDERATIONS

- **Exercise**: benefits MS patients by lessening fatigue and improving quality of life and well-being. T'ai Chi/Qi Gong—the practice of mindfulness of movement—does not improve measures of balance but does improve measures of MS-related symptoms, walking speed, hamstring flexibility, and subjective sense of well-being and quality of life. No reports on yoga for MS have been published.
- **Stress**: worsens MS symptoms and triggers exacerbation. Increased conflicts and disruptions in routine are followed by increased risk of developing new brain lesions 8 weeks later. But stress at a point in time does not reliably predict clinical

exacerbations in individual patients. Distraction moderates effect of stress on new lesions. Emotional preoccupation is linked to increased relation between stress and new lesions. Coping can moderate effect of stress on MS disease activity. Stress management training decreases anxiety and somatization. Patients are less preoccupied with physical symptoms after undergoing stress management training. Approaches to stress management include exercise, yoga, T'ai Chi, prayer, meditation, massage therapy. Meditation lowers stress and improves symptoms in patients with chronic illnesses. Experienced meditators have enhanced biochemical and physiologic functioning compared to those who did not meditate.

- **Food allergy**: although no convincing evidence exists that gluten-free or allergy elimination diets are beneficial in MS, food allergens should be eliminated as long as other dietary measures are also included (e.g. low-fat diet, Swank diet).
- **Malabsorption**: Forty-two percent of MS patients studied have fat malabsorption, 42% have high levels of undigested meat fibers in feces, 27% have abnormal D-xylose absorption, and 12% had malabsorption of vitamin $B_{12}$. Multiple subclinical deficiencies may result from inability to absorb nutrients.
- **Hyperbaric oxygen (HBO)**: no significant improvement was seen during trials, except for subjective improvement in bowel and bladder functions in one study. HBO was supplied at pressures of 1.75-2 ATA during 20 sessions of 90 minutes over a period of 4 weeks. Side effects: ear and visual problems. Given expense of HBO and lack of proven efficacy in MS, HBO should not be recommended.

## THERAPEUTIC APPROACH

Diet, nutritional supplementation, exercise, and stress reduction comprise the natural medicine approach to MS. This approach also can be used in conjunction with allopathic therapies.

### Diet

Swank's dietary protocol is recommended:

- A daily unsaturated fat intake between 20 g and 50 g
- No red meat consumption for the first year (including the dark meat of turkey and chicken); after the first year only 3 oz of red meat per week

- White meat poultry, fish, and shellfish are permissible in any amounts as long as they contain low saturated fats
- Elimination of dairy products containing 1% butterfat or more
- One multiple vitamin/mineral supplement

Although the Swank diet calls for 1-4 capsules of nonconcentrated cod liver oil, substitute fish oil concentrate (see Nutritional Supplements below). Emphasize fresh whole plant foods; reduce or avoid animal foods (except small wild cold-water fish).

## Nutritional Supplements

- **Fish oil concentrate**: 1.8 g q.d. EPA and 1.0 g q.d. DHA
- **Selenium**: 200 μg q.d.
- **Vitamin E (mixed tocopherols)**: 800 IU q.d.
- ***Ginkgo biloba* extract** (24% ginkgo flavonglycosides, 6% terpenoids): 40-80 mg t.i.d. for patients with cognitive impairment
- **Vitamin $D_3$**: 2000 IU/day

### Symptoms of MS and Their Neurologic Causes

| Symptoms | Cause |
|---|---|
| Weakness, numbness, and tingling in legs and arms; stiffness in legs | Spinal cord lesions |
| Urinary urgency, retention, incontinence, and recurrent infections | Spinal cord lesions |
| Constipation | Spinal cord lesions; diet |
| Sexual dysfunction | Spinal cord lesions |
| Blurred vision and blindness | Optic nerve lesions |
| Double vision | Brainstem lesions |
| Imbalance | Spinal cord and cerebellar lesions |
| Tremor of arms | Cerebellar lesions |
| Impaired memory and concentration | Cerebral lesions |
| Fatigue | Effects of inflammatory cytokines on neuronal function; nerve fiber fatigability resulting from demyelination |
| Heat sensitivity | Sensitivity of demyelination to elevations in body temperature |
| Depression and other mood disorders | Cerebral lesions and changes in neurotransmitters |

### Exercise and Stress Management

- **Exercise**: type and amount tailored for patient. Mild to moderate exercise for 30+ minutes, three times per week. Types: walking, stretching, bicycling, low-impact aerobics, stationary bicycle, swimming or water aerobics, yoga, T'ai Chi.
- **Stress** management: tailored for patient. Stress reduction therapies recommended for MS: exercise, meditation, deep breathing or breath exercises, prayer.

# Nausea and Vomiting of Pregnancy

## DIAGNOSTIC SUMMARY

- Morning or evening nausea and vomiting occurring during the first trimester of pregnancy.

## GENERAL CONSIDERATIONS

- Nausea and vomiting of pregnancy (NVP) ("morning sickness") occurs in 75% of pregnancies. A higher incidence occurs in the first trimester, but only 50% of cases resolve by week 14; 90% resolve by week 22. Eighty percent of women have nausea lasting all day.
- Hyperemesis gravidarum (HG) is NVP with severe vomiting, weight loss, and dehydration. HG is serious, life threatening, and may require inpatient care.

### Diagnostic and Etiologic Summary

- The cause of NVP is a mystery. Possible factors include hormonal or digestive changes, blood and Qi imbalances, altered thyroid function, emotional blocks, improper nutrition, stress, and lifestyle habits.
- Address individual mother rather than condition: physiologic and metabolic change (reduced gastric motility, oxidative stress or carbohydrate/vitamin B deficiency). Consider environment, emotional status, family, relationship, job or financial stress.

## THERAPEUTIC CONSIDERATIONS

### Psychological, Emotional, and Lifestyle Aspects

- Both physiologic and psychological factors contribute.
- Discuss whether pregnancy was planned and emotions of anger, fear, ambivalence, doubt, resentment, disgust, denial, or unresolved conflict.
- Ask questions about family, relationship, job and finances, or stressors—environmental toxicity exposure.

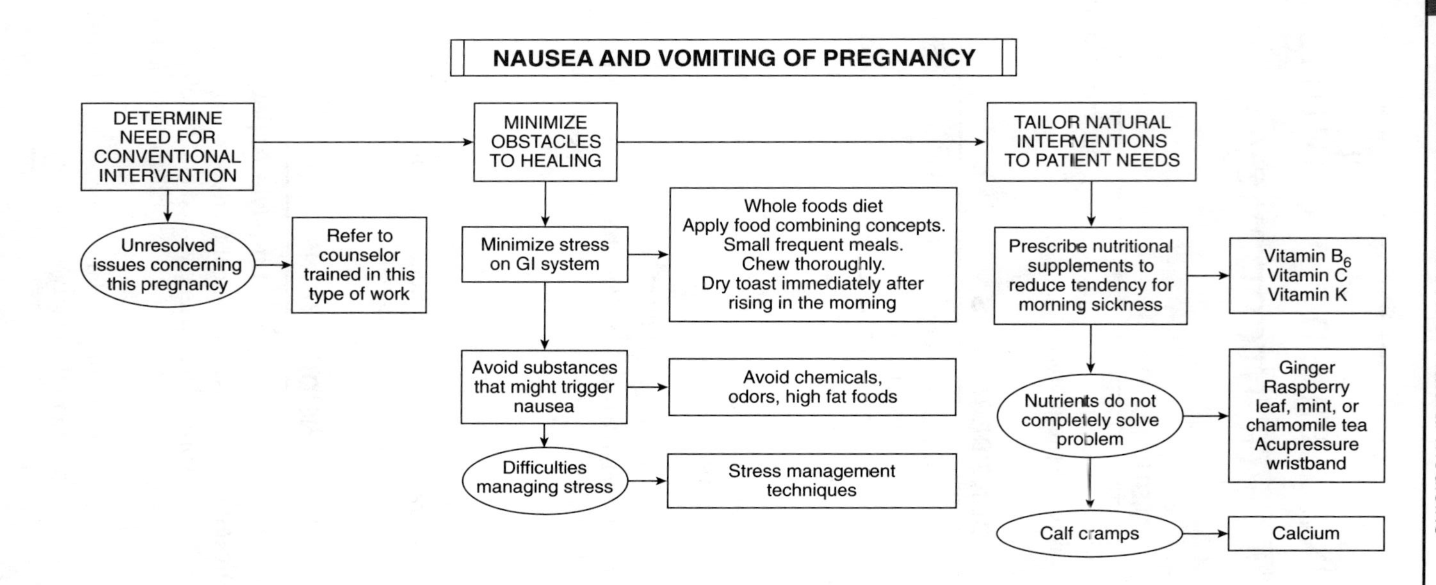
NAUSEA AND VOMITING OF PREGNANCY
DETERMINE NEED FOR CONVENTIONAL INTERVENTION
Unresolved issues concerning this pregnancy
Refer to counselor trained in this type of work
MINIMIZE OBSTACLES TO HEALING
Minimize stress on GI system
Whole foods diet
Apply food combining concepts.
Small frequent meals.
Chew thoroughly.
Dry toast immediately after rising in the morning
Avoid substances that might trigger nausea
Avoid chemicals, odors, high fat foods
Difficulties managing stress
Stress management techniques
TAILOR NATURAL INTERVENTIONS TO PATIENT NEEDS
Prescribe nutritional supplements to reduce tendency for morning sickness
Vitamin B6
Vitamin C
Vitamin K
Nutrients do not completely solve problem
Ginger
Raspberry leaf, mint, or chamomile tea
Acupressure wristband
Calf cramps
Calcium

## Nutrition and Nutrients

- Balanced whole foods diet.
- Eat small regular meals to prevent stomach from completely emptying and blood sugar from dropping; both are linked to nausea and vomiting.
- Drink plenty of fluids to prevent dehydration, another contributing factor.
- HG, postpartum depression, and lactation failure are linked to deficiencies of zinc, magnesium, vitamin $B_6$, essential fatty acids.
- **Prenatal multivitamin** is needed to supplement even a healthy diet. Multivitamins decrease nausea and vomiting.
- **Pyridoxine (vitamin $B_6$)**: $B_6$ can improve or relieve NVP. Study dosage: 30 mg q.d. to 25 mg vitamin $B_6$ every 8 hours. Combinations of $B_6$, ginger, and acupressure are being studied.
- **Vitamins K and C**: effective clinically when used together. Ninety-one percent of patients in one study had complete remission within 72 hours. Both vitamins alone show little effect.

## Botanical Medicines

- ***Zingiber officinale* (ginger)**: traditional common remedy and effective antiemetic. Decreases nausea and vomiting induced by surgery and anesthesia, chemotherapy, seasickness, and NVP. Ginger root powder at dosage of 250 mg q.i.d. has provided significant relief. Ginger is as effective as metoclopramide to control vomiting. Of all herbal remedies, the only one that has undergone successful clinical or scientific investigation with regards to NVP is ginger.
- ***Rubus idaeus* (raspberry leaf)**: used as a general support for pregnant women in China, Europe, and North America. Constituents: vitamins A, B complex, C and E; calcium, iron, phosphorus, potassium. Tannins provide astringent properties. It also is a uterine tonic. It is not implicated in childbirth complications; no evidence of long-term toxic or teratogenic effects.
- Herbs that stimulate liver function and improve gastrointestinal tone help nausea and vomiting. Carminative herbs have calming and soothing effect. *Mentha piperita* (peppermint) tea has been used. Documented research is inadequate. Concern exists over safety of botanical medicines for pregnancy. Currently no documented research proves that any of the herbs mentioned have caused detrimental side effects to pregnant women or fetuses.

### Other Therapies

- **Acupressure, acupuncture, and Chinese herbal formulas**: widely used for NVP in China for centuries. Most research has been done on one specific point, Pericardium 6 (P6) (Neiguan point) and its efficacy in relieving nausea and vomiting. Acupressure wristbands have helped relieve morning sickness, anxiety, depression, behavioral dysfunction, and nausea. Acupressure at P6 helps reduce nausea and vomiting after laparoscopic surgery. Commercially available adjustable acupressure wristbands put pressure on P6 point, relieve symptoms of motion sickness, and reduce gastric tachyarrhythmia, the abnormal electrical activity of the stomach that is a reliable physiologic marker for motion sickness. Nonadjustable wristbands have failed, perhaps because insufficient pressure was applied to specific P6 point. Some bands provide electrical stimulation to P6 and are adjustable. Eighty-seven percent of pregnant women had improvement of NVP versus 43% with placebo device.

## THERAPEUTIC APPROACH

### Psychological, Emotional, and Lifestyle Support

Guidance to provide the pregnant woman:

- Create strong support system for pregnancy—people and activities you can rely on to keep you balanced and healthy.
- Discuss unresolved conflicts about pregnancy with counselor trained in this type of work.
- Use stress management techniques: meditation, quality sleep, relaxation, play time.
- Exercise and/or stretching practice with deep breathing to enhance circulation.
- Avoid or minimize contact with chemicals and cigarette smoke.
- Stay well hydrated with cool water, electrolyte drinks without refined sugars, diluted juices, teas, and broths. Apply cool cloths to face and spend time in fresh air (outdoors or in rooms with good natural ventilation). Avoid recirculated air or stuffy, enclosed rooms.

### Diet

- Fresh vegetables, especially green leafy vegetables; balanced proteins; complex carbohydrates; fiber.

- Apply food-combining techniques; avoid combining protein with starch, starchy vegetables, or processed sugary foods/ drinks in the same meal.
- Eat small, frequent meals slowly. Chew thoroughly. Eat main meal in middle of the day. Avoid liquids with meals.
- Eat small amounts of complex carbohydrates (biscuit or dry toast) especially when waking while still lying down (helps settle stomach). Sit up slowly and drink lemon or ginger and honey in water, herbal tea, or a tablespoon of apple cider vinegar in a cup of warm water with or without a tablespoon of honey.
- Keep small, easily digested snack in the bathroom to keep blood sugar normal and stomach from getting empty in middle of the night.
- Identify and avoid odors or spices that might trigger nausea. Reduce saturated fats or high-fat foods; eat more protein or adjust diet according to blood type.

## Nutritional Supplementation

Whole foods, easy to digest, prenatal vitamin, and the following additions depending on individual needs:

- **Vitamin $B_6$**: 25 mg b.i.d. to t.i.d.
- **Vitamin C**: 250-1000 mg b.i.d. to t.i.d.
- **Vitamin K**: 5 mg q.d.
- **Extra calcium** (especially for calf cramps)
- **Essential fatty acids**: 1-2 tbsp flaxseed oil or 2-4 capsules purified fish oil q.d.

## Botanical Medicine

Avoid almost all botanical medicines in the first trimester except the following:

- **Ginger**: 1-2 g as dry powder, decoction, extract, or natural ginger ale
- **Raspberry leaf, mint, or chamomile tea**: 1-3 cups q.d.

Use ginger, raspberry leaf, mint, and other safe botanicals throughout pregnancy when indicated.

# Obesity

## DIAGNOSTIC SUMMARY

- Body mass index (BMI) >30
- Body fat >30% for women and >25% for men

## GENERAL CONSIDERATIONS

- Obesity is a major contributor to mortality risk. Definition: excessive body fat distinguished from being overweight (excess body weight relative to height). A muscular athlete may be overweight but have a low body fat percentage. Body weight alone is not an index of obesity. BMI is the standard for classifying body composition. BMI correlates well to total body fat. BMI calculation:

$$BMI = (pounds \times 703)/square\ inches\ (height)$$

$$Metric: BMI = kilograms/square\ meters\ (height)$$

### Classification of Body Mass Index

| | |
|---|---|
| Underweight | <18.5 |
| Normal | 18.5-24.9 |
| Overweight | 24.9-29.9 |
| Obesity | 30.0-39.9 |
| Extreme obesity | >40.0 |

Height and weight indexes are still used to determine obesity; tables of desirable weights for height provided by the Metropolitan Life Insurance Company are criticized for three shortcomings:

- Stated weight ranges merely reflect weights of those with lowest mortality rate of insured persons, which may not reflect U.S. population.

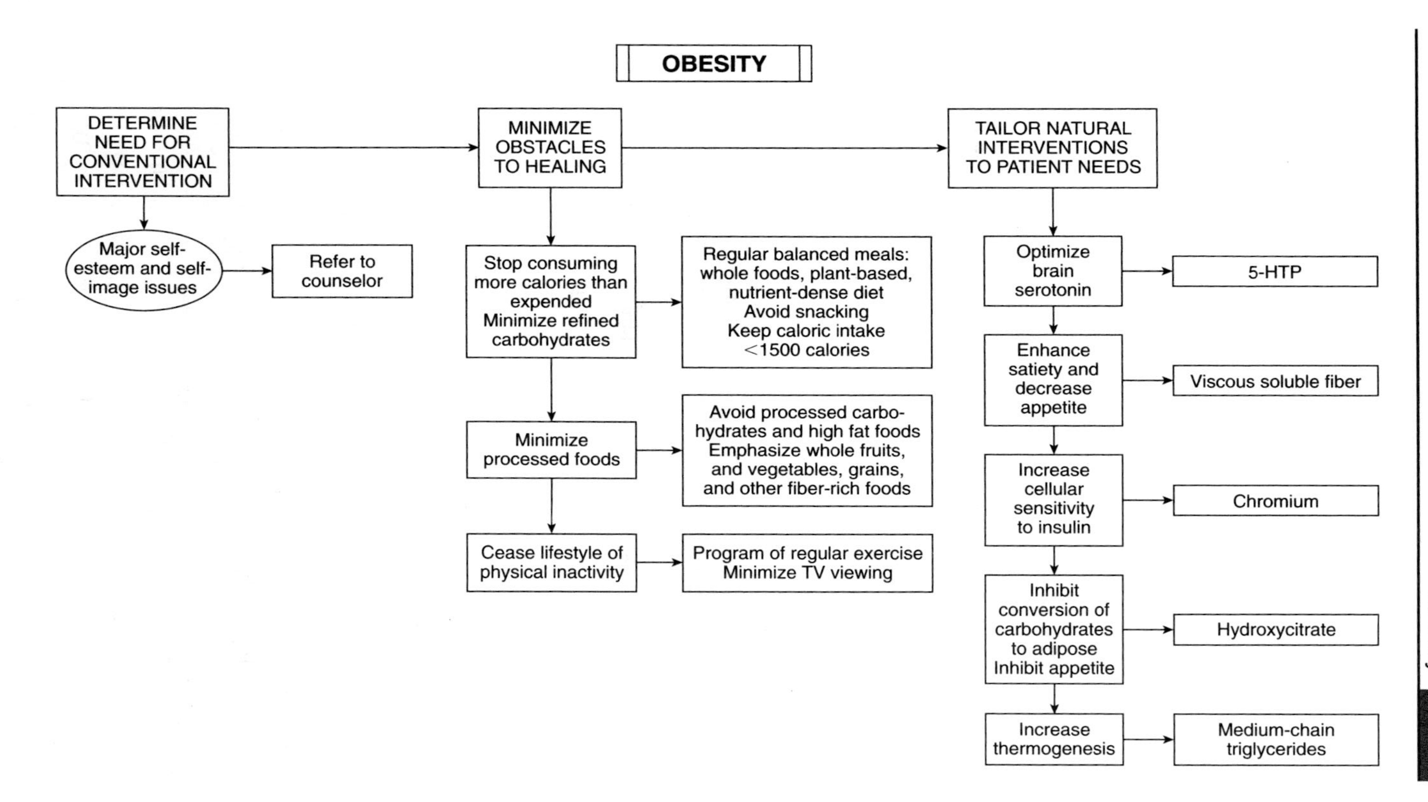
OBESITY
DETERMINE NEED FOR CONVENTIONAL INTERVENTION
Major self-esteem and self-image issues
Refer to counselor
MINIMIZE OBSTACLES TO HEALING
Stop consuming more calories than expended
Minimize refined carbohydrates
Regular balanced meals: whole foods, plant-based, nutrient-dense diet
Avoid snacking
Keep caloric intake <1500 calories
Minimize processed foods
Avoid processed carbohydrates and high fat foods
Emphasize whole fruits, and vegetables, grains, and other fiber-rich foods
Cease lifestyle of physical inactivity
Program of regular exercise
Minimize TV viewing
TAILOR NATURAL INTERVENTIONS TO PATIENT NEEDS
Optimize brain serotonin
5-HTP
Enhance satiety and decrease appetite
Viscous soluble fiber
Increase cellular sensitivity to insulin
Chromium
Inhibit conversion of carbohydrates to adipose
Inhibit appetite
Hydroxycitrate
Increase thermogenesis
Medium-chain triglycerides

- Weight ranges for lowest mortality rate do not necessarily reflect optimal healthy weight for height.
- Standard values make assessing degree of obesity difficult; a person within proper weight range may have excess fat and lower than optimal lean body mass, and a person with increased musculature may be "overweight" despite low body fat percentage.

## Prevalence

- Obese persons have 50%-100% increased risk of death from all causes. Most of the risk is from cardiovascular causes: type 2 diabetes mellitus (DM), elevated cholesterol, hypertension, and atherosclerosis.
- Determination of body composition: obesity is defined as body fat percentage >30% for women and >25% for men. Indirect methods of measurement must be used.
- Visual observation: qualitative analysis of obesity. Classifying by body types (somatotyping) is the physical anthropologic classification of physique based on body size and proportion:
  —**Endomorph**: relatively large body, short arms and legs
  —**Mesomorph**: large muscular chest that dominates abdomen, prominent bony joints
  —**Ectomorph**: relatively small frame (slender, delicate bone structure), long arms and legs
  Endomorphs are at greatest risk for obesity; mesomorphs are at moderate risk and ectomorphs are extremely unlikely to develop obesity.
- Distribution of body fat: gynecoid (female) and android (male). See the section on the types of obesity.
- Skinfold/fat fold thickness: measuring thickness of subcutaneous fat (skinfold or fat fold thickness) with skinfold calipers at several sites to improve accuracy—triceps, biceps, subscapular, suprailiac skinfolds. Limitations: inability to control intersubject and intrasubject variation in skinfold compressibility; inability to palpate fat/muscle interface; impossibility of obtaining interpretable measurements on very obese persons; interobserver variability; errors from use of different types of calipers. Skinfold measurements give easiest and least expensive method for estimating fat percentage. More precise tools: bioelectrical impedance, ultrasound, total body electrical conductivity, hydrostatic weighing.

**Body Fat Rating Chart for Use With a Body Fat Measuring Scale**

| Age (Years) | Risky | Excellent | Good | Fair | Poor |
|---|---|---|---|---|---|
| **Male** | | | | | |
| 19-24 | <6% | 10.8% | 14.9% | 19.0% | 23.3% |
| 25-29 | <6% | 12.8% | 16.5% | 20.3% | 24.4% |
| 30-34 | <6% | 14.5% | 18.0% | 21.5% | 25.2% |
| 35-39 | <6% | 16.1% | 19.4% | 22.6% | 26.1% |
| 40-44 | <6% | 17.5% | 20.5% | 23.6% | 26.9% |
| 45-49 | <6% | 18.6% | 21.5% | 24.5% | 27.6% |
| 50-54 | <6% | 19.8% | 22.7% | 25.6% | 28.7% |
| 55-59 | <6% | 20.2% | 23.2% | 26.2% | 29.3% |
| 60+ | <6% | 20.3% | 23.5% | 26.7% | 29.8% |
| **Female** | | | | | |
| 19-24 | <9% | 18.9% | 22.1% | 25.0% | 29.6% |
| 25-29 | <9% | 18.9% | 22.0% | 25.4% | 29.8% |
| 30-34 | <9% | 19.7% | 22.7% | 26.4% | 30.5% |
| 35-39 | <9% | 21.0% | 24.0% | 27.7% | 31.5% |
| 40-44 | <9% | 22.6% | 25.6% | 29.3% | 32.8% |
| 45-49 | <9% | 24.3% | 27.3% | 30.9% | 34.1% |
| 50-54 | <9% | 26.6% | 29.7% | 33.1% | 36.2% |
| 55-59 | <9% | 27.4% | 30.7% | 34.0% | 37.3% |
| 60+ | <9% | 27.6% | 31.0% | 34.4% | 38.0% |

- Measurement of body density: quantitative measure of body fat determined from specific gravity by measuring different weights of body in and out of water. Weigh patient under water and out of water, taking into account residual volume of lungs. Factual basis: fat is lighter than water; other tissues are heavier than water. This is the gold standard of body composition determination. Limitation of hydrostatic weighing: requires subject cooperation to exhale completely and then submerge completely under water up to 10 times—impossible for elderly, ill, or hospitalized patients.
- Bioelectrical impedance: measures conduction of applied electrical current through body tissues. In biologic structures, constant

low-level AC current results in impedance to flow of current that is frequency dependent, according to type of tissue. Fluids act as electrical conductors; cell membranes act as electrical condensers. At low frequencies (1 kHz), current mainly passes through extracellular fluids; at higher frequencies (500-800 kHz), it penetrates intracellular and extracellular fluids. Fat-free mass has greater conductivity than fat does, explaining the strong relation between conductance and lean body mass. This method is safe, noninvasive, and rapid. Home scales with bioelectrical impedance are available for $50-$200.

### Types of Obesity

Categories based on size and number of fat cells and how fat is distributed in the body (e.g., abdomen vs. hips):

- **Hyperplastic obesity**: increased number of fat cells throughout body; dependent on the diet of the mother while in utero and early infant nutrition. Excess calories during early stages of development increase number of fat cells for life. Hyperplastic obesity begins in childhood and is linked to fewer serious health effects.
- **Hypertrophic obesity**: increased size of fat cells; linked to DM, heart disease, hypertension. Fat distribution is around waist, considered male patterned or android. Android obesity is a waist larger than hips. In female-patterned or gynecoid obesity, the hips are larger. Waist/hip ratio: measure waist circumference one half inch above navel; measure hips circumference at the greatest protrusion of buttocks. Divide waist circumference by hip circumference. Ratio >1.0 for men and >0.8 for women is linked to metabolic syndrome (syndrome X) and increases risk of type 2 DM, hypertension, coronary heart disease, stroke, and gout.
- **Hyperplastic-hypertrophic obesity**: increase in number and size of fat cells.

## CAUSES OF OBESITY

- Tendency to be overweight is inherited. Yet even high-risk persons can avoid obesity; dietary and lifestyle factors (physical inactivity) are responsible.
- Psychological factors: insensitivity to internal signals for hunger and satiety plus extreme sensitivity to external stimuli (sight, smell, taste), increasing appetite. Watching television: linked to

onset of obesity with dose-related effect; linked to obesity in children and smoking and hypercholesterolemia in adolescence and adulthood. Time spent watching television is positively linked to risk of obesity and type 2 DM. Each 2-hour increment in television watching daily is linked to a 23% increase in obesity and 14% increase in risk of DM. Each 2-hour increment in sitting at work daily is linked to a 5% increase in obesity and 7% increase in DM. Physiologic effects of watching television: reducing physical activity and lowering resting (basal) metabolic rate to a level during trance states.

## Physiologic Factors

- **Theory**: obese persons are extremely sensitive to specific internal cues for dysfunctional appetite control because of genetic, dietary, and lifestyle factors. Central issue: insulin resistance as a conditioned reaction to a high-glycemic diet. Vicious positive feedback cycle of obesity: insulin resistance, central adiposity, alterations in adipokine secretion by adipocytes and gut-derived hormones, impaired diet-induced thermogenesis, and low brain serotonin. Obesity is an adaptive physiologic response.
- **"Set point"**: weight that a body tries to maintain by regulating food and calories consumed. Each person has programmed set point weight. Fat cells may control set point: when enlarged fat cells in obese persons become smaller, they either send messages to brain to eat or they block action of appetite-suppressing compounds (leptin). Signals are too strong to ignore indefinitely, causing rebound overeating and set point at a higher level, increasing difficulty for weight loss—known as a ratchet effect or yo-yo dieting. Key to overcoming fat cells' set point: increase sensitivity of fat cells to insulin by exercise, specially designed diet, and key nutritional supplements. Diet that does not improve insulin sensitivity will fail to provide long-term results.
- **Fat cell engorgement**: when fat cells (especially in the abdomen) become full of fat, they secrete resistin, leptin, tumor necrosis factor, and free fatty acids that dampen the effect of insulin, impair glucose utilization in skeletal muscle, and promote liver gluconeogenesis. Increased number and size of fat cells induce reduced secretion of compounds that promote insulin action—adiponectin (novel protein produced by fat cells). Adiponectin improves insulin sensitivity, is antiinflammatory, lowers triglycerides, and blocks development of atherosclerosis. Fat cells severely stress blood sugar control and promote a complication

of DM—atherosclerosis. Adipose tissue is now considered part of the endocrine system.

- **Adiponectin and gut-derived hormone alterations**: obese persons are more sensitive to internal signals to eat. Appetite, for human survival during famine, is extremely biased toward weight gain. People who survived famines were more adept at storing fat with a built-in tendency to overeat. Normal physiologic processes that curb appetite must be advanced. The hypothalamus controls appetite and eating. Adipokines (e.g., leptin, triggering appetite control) originate in the gastrointestinal (GI) tract. GI nerve signals feed back to the central nervous system; gut-derived hormones and peptides (neuropeptide Y, ghrelin, cholecystokinin [CCK]). Peptide YY 3-36 (PYY) dramatically reduces appetite in obese and normal persons. Stomach-derived hormone ghrelin increases appetite, with highest levels when the stomach is empty and during calorie restriction. Obese persons have elevated ghrelin, which rises while dieting. Gastroplasty may succeed because of reduced ghrelin production.
- **Human compensatory actions**: may negate the effect of appetite regulators. A perfect agent should increase insulin sensitivity, reduce factors that increase appetite, and increase factors that decrease appetite. Highly viscous dietary fiber blends may be useful.
- **Gut-derived appetite regulators**: main hormones inhibiting food intake are CCK, glucagon-like peptide (GLP-1), oxyntomodulin (OXM), and PYY. Hormonal stimulators of appetite are ghrelin and orexin A. Enteroendocrine cell function is regulated by the presence or absence of viscous dietary fiber; the main target for these neurotransmitters are vagal afferent neurons, and the appetite-inhibiting effects of CCK are enhanced by the mechanical effects of dietary fiber (gastric distension). Gut-derived appetite regulators include the following:
  —**CCK**: controls gastric emptying and delivery of enzymes from the pancreas. It inhibits appetite, and its effect is enhanced with moderate gastric distension triggering gastric mechanoreceptors. Viscous dietary fiber increases CCK secretion.
  —**GLP-1**: distal intestinal peptide GLP (7-36)-1 is derived from different regions of glucagon precursor. It inhibits food intake, decreases sensations of hunger, and inhibits plasma ghrelin. Secretion of GLP-1 is influenced by food intake, but specifics are unknown.

—**OXM**: released from gut postprandially in proportion to food volume and energy content. OXM is elevated during anorexia and suppresses ghrelin. Elevated OXM is linked to GI disorders and may contribute to anorexia.
—**PYY**: secreted by enteroendocrine cells of the ileum and colon; the related compound pancreatic polypeptide is secreted by the pancreas. Plasma PYY in obese subjects, basal and postprandial, is subnormal. PYY inhibits food intake, with long-term action. Viscous dietary fiber raises PYY.
—**Ghrelin**: peptide from X-cells in stomach lining. It makes the stomach "rumble" and is a powerful appetite stimulator. Plasma ghrelin is depressed in anorexia nervosa and elevated in obesity. Ghrelin levels decline on feeding, especially fiber. Effect is mediated by insulin; insulin resistance is associated with higher ghrelin levels.
—**Orexin A**: peptide in hypothalamus, enteric neurons, and gut endocrine cells (enterochromaffin cells). It stimulates appetite and inhibits CCK-stimulated excitation of vagal afferent fibers (negating appetite-suppressing effect of CCK). Plasma orexin A increases with fasting. It may contribute to overeating during or immediately after a meal by suppressing satiety signaling by CCK.

## Diet-Induced Thermogenesis

- In lean persons, a meal stimulates up to a 40% increase in diet-induced thermogenesis; overweight persons display up to a 10% increase. In the obese food energy is stored, not converted to heat.
- Insulin insensitivity contributes to decreased thermogenesis. Enhancing insulin sensitivity may restore thermogenesis and normal set point. Even after weight loss, obesity-prone persons still have decreased diet-induced thermogenesis.
- Brown fat cells: contain multiple fat storage compartments localizing triglycerides into smaller droplets surrounding numerous mitochondria. Blood vessel network and density of mitochondria give the brown color and increased capacity to metabolize fats. Brown fat does not metabolize fatty acids to adenosine triphosphate efficiently, causing increased heat production. Lean people may have a higher ratio of brown fat to white fat than overweight people have. The amount of brown fat in human beings is extremely small (0.5%-5% of body weight). It has a profound

effect on thermogenesis; just 1 oz of brown fat (0.1% of body weight) makes the difference between stable body weight or adding an extra 10 pounds per year.

- For overfed lean persons to increase and maintain excess weight, caloric intake must increase by 50% over previous intake. To maintain a reduced weight, formerly obese persons must restrict intake to 25% less than a lean person of similar weight and body size.
- Decreased diet-induced thermogenesis worsens weight gain on a high-fat diet compared with lean people; it increases intake of fat and decreases exercise tendency.

### Low Serotonin Theory

- Diets deficient in tryptophan induce increased appetite, causing binge eating of carbohydrates. Tryptophan deficit causes low brain serotonin and brain sense of starvation that stimulates appetite control centers, with a preference for carbohydrates. Carbohydrate foods increase tryptophan delivery to the brain, elevating serotonin synthesis.
- Carbohydrate craving may play a major role in obesity.
- Blood tryptophan and brain serotonin levels plummet with dieting. Brain starvation signals cannot be ignored; this is why most diets fail.
- Upper end of spectrum of carbohydrate addiction is bulimia, a serious eating disorder of binge eating and purging by forced vomiting or laxatives. Medical consequences of bulimia: rupture of stomach, erosion of dental enamel, and heart disturbances from the loss of potassium.

## THERAPEUTIC CONSIDERATIONS

- Only 5% of obese persons attain and maintain "normal" body weight for a year or more; 66% of those a few pounds overweight do.
- Basic foundations: positive mental attitude, healthy lifestyle (regular exercise), health-promoting diet, supplements.
- To lose weight, energy intake must be less than energy expenditure; decrease caloric intake and increase metabolizing of calories.
- To lose 1 lb, a person must consume 3500 fewer calories than expended. Loss of 1 lb/week requires a negative caloric balance

of 500 calories/day—achievable by decreasing calories and/or increasing exercise.

- Reducing intake by 500 calories/day or increasing metabolism by 500 calories/day by exercise (45-minute jog, playing tennis for 1 hour, or brisk walk for 1.25 hours) is a challenge. Sensible approach: both diet and exercise.
- Weight loss begins at a caloric intake <1500 calories/day with exercise for 15-20 minutes three to four times per week.
- Starvation and crash diets: rapid weight loss (muscle and water) with rebound weight gain.
- Most successful approach: gradual weight reduction (0.5-1 lb/week) by long-term dietary and lifestyle habits.
- Even modest weight reductions help: 5%-10% reduction in weight improves cholesterol, blood pressure, blood glucose.

## Behavioral Therapy

- Despite behavioral approaches, lost weight is generally regained; most patients return to pretreatment weight within 3 years.
- Main behavioral characteristics have been identified of persons who avoid weight regain:
  —High level of physical activity
  —Low-fat diet
  —Active monitoring of body weight
- Boost to self-esteem and self-confidence plus improving appearance, feeling more attractive, and being able to wear more fashionable clothing give motivation for continued weight loss until goals or effective maintenance of weight loss is achieved.
- Majority of people want to lose weight for changes in physical appearance, not health benefits. Key to success: identify primary goals of weight loss.

## Dietary Strategies

### Atkins Diet

- High-protein, high-fat, low-carbohydrate diet: unlimited amounts of all meats, poultry, fish, eggs, most cheeses.
- Four phases:
  —Induction phase (first 14 days): carbohydrates limited to <20 g/day. No fruit, bread, grains, starchy vegetables, or dairy, except cheese, cream, and butter.
  —Ongoing weight loss phase: dieters experiment with levels of carbohydrate intake to find most liberal level of

carbohydrate intake that allows continued weight loss. Dieters maintain this level until weight loss goals are met.
—Premaintenance and maintenance phases: dieters determine level of carbohydrate intake that allows stable weight. Dieters must stick to this level of intake for life.

- Diets high in sugar and refined carbohydrates cause weight gain and obesity. Atkins dieters are spared feelings of hunger and deprivation of other regimens, but this diet is not conducive to long-term health.
- In the long term, Atkins dieters gain back all the weight lost plus more. Findings from clinical trials indicate that although strictly adhering to the Atkins diet (dramatically reducing carbohydrates while allowing high-fat, high-protein foods) can lead to more weight loss in the first 6 months, a healthier diet is equally effective long term with fewer risks. High protein level in the Atkins diet stresses liver and kidneys.

**Natural Weight Loss Aids**

- **5-Hydroxytryptophan (5-HTP)**: genetically decreased activity of tryptophan hydroxylase, which converts tryptophan to 5-HTP, itself subsequently converted to serotonin, is linked to overeating and obesity in animals. Many human beings are genetically predisposed to obesity. Preformed 5-HTP can bypass this genetic defect to increase serotonin synthesis (*Textbook,* "5-Hydroxytryptophan"). 5-HTP reduces calorie intake and promotes weight loss in women despite no conscious effort to lose weight. Weight loss during 5-week period of 5-HTP support: 3 pounds. 5-HTP helps overweight people adhere to dietary recommendations. It promotes early satiety. Dosage: 300 mg t.i.d. Side effects: mild nausea during first 6 weeks of therapy; never severe enough to stop therapy.
- **Meal replacement formulas**: are a popular strategy; effectiveness confirmed in several clinical trials; improve dietary compliance and convenience. Formulations should contain high-quality nutrition low in glycemic load and high in viscous, soluble fiber.
- **Fiber supplements**: dietary fiber promotes weight loss. Best supplements for weight loss: glucomannan, gum karaya, psyllium, chitin, guar gum, pectin—rich in water-soluble fibers. Taken with water, they form a gelatinous mass, inducing satiety. Benefits: enhanced glycemic control, decreased insulin levels, reduced calories absorbed. They can reduce number of calories

absorbed by 30-180 calories/day, inducing a 3- to 18-pound weight loss in a year.

—Avoid products that contain a lot of sugar or sweeteners to camouflage taste.

—Drink adequate amounts of water with fiber supplement, especially in pill form.

- **Guar gum (water-soluble fiber from Indian cluster bean [*Cyamopsis tetragonoloba*])**: 10 g of guar gum immediately before lunch and dinner induced loss of 9.4 pounds in 2 months, with reductions in cholesterol and triglycerides. Soluble fiber reduces cholesterol and weight in a dose-dependent fashion. Dosage: as high as possible. Water-soluble fibers are fermented by colon bacteria, producing gas, flatulence, and abdominal discomfort. Start with dosage of 1 to 2 g before meals and at bedtime; gradually increase to 5 g.
- **Chromium**: essential to glycemic control and insulin sensitivity. No recommended dietary allowance exists, but optimal health requires 200 μg/day. Chromium levels are depleted by refined sugars and flour and lack of exercise. Chromium decreases fasting glucose, improves glucose tolerance, lowers insulin, decreases total cholesterol and triglycerides, increases high-density lipoprotein. It is effective in DM and hypoglycemia, improving glucose tolerance and number of insulin receptors on red blood cells. Chromium supplements lower body weight yet increase lean body mass by increasing insulin sensitivity. Results are most striking in elderly and in men. Dosage: in picolinate form 400 μg is more effective than 200 μg q.d. Greater muscle mass means greater fat-burning potential. Women in an exercise program did not show significant changes in body composition. Effects of chromium arise from increased insulin sensitivity. Forms: chromium picolinate, chromium polynicotinate, chromium chloride, and chromium-enriched yeast.
- **Medium-chain triglycerides (MCTs)**: saturated fats (from coconut oil) in six to 12 carbon chains. The body uses MCTs differently from long-chain triglycerides (LCTs) in common fats found in nature. LCTs are storage fats in human beings and plants with 18 to 24 carbons. MCTs promote weight loss rather than weight gain by increasing thermogenesis and energy expenditure. LCTs are stored in fat deposits; their energy is conserved. A diet high in LCTs decreases metabolic rate. Excess energy of MCTs is not efficiently stored as fat, but wasted as heat. MCT oil given over a 6-day period can increase diet-induced thermogenesis by 50%.

LCTs elevate blood fats by 68%; MCTs have no effect on blood fat level. To benefit from MCTs, keep diet low in LCTs. Use MCTs as oil for salad dressing, bread spread, or as supplement. Dosage: 1-2 tbsp/day. Closely monitor diabetics and persons with liver disease when using MCTs; they may develop ketoacidosis.
- **Hydroxycitrate (HCA)**: natural substance isolated from fruit of Malabar tamarind *(Garcinia cambogia)*, a yellowish fruit the size of an orange, with thin skin and deep furrows similar to acorn squash. It is native to southern India, where it is dried and used in curries. Dried fruit has 30% HCA. HCA is powerful lipogenic inhibitor in animals, reducing food intake and weight gain in rats. It also suppresses appetite. Still maintain a low-fat diet; it only inhibits conversion of carbohydrates into fat. Dosage: 1500 mg t.i.d.

## THERAPEUTIC APPROACH

Implement four cornerstones of good health:

- Proper diet: whole foods, plant-based, nutrient-dense diet
- Adequate exercise is critical (*Textbook,* "The Exercise Prescription")
- Psychological support: consider referral for counseling to heal assaults on self-esteem and self-image; maintain positive mental attitude
- Support body through natural measures

### Supplements

- **5-HTP**: begin at 50-100 mg 20 minutes before meals for 2 weeks; then double dosage (to maximum of 300 mg) if weight loss is <1 lb/week. Higher dosages of 5-HTP (e.g., 300 mg) are associated with nausea, but this symptom disappears after 6 weeks of use.
- **Viscous, soluble fiber**: 5 g before meals
- **Chromium**: 200-400 μg q.d.
- **MCTs**: incorporate 1-2 tbsp into diet

### Botanical Medicines

- **HCA *(Garcinia cambogia)***: 1500 mg t.i.d.

### Indirect Methods of Analyzing Body Fat Composition

- Visual observation (somatotypes)
- Anthropometric measurements

- Height and weight
- Circumferences and diameters
- Skinfold thickness
- Isotope or chemical dilution
- Body water
- Body potassium
- Body fat
- Body density and body volume
- Conductivity
- Total body electrical conductivity
- Bioelectric impedance
- Neutron activation
- Imaging techniques
- Ultrasound
- Computer tomography
- Nuclear magnetic resonance
- Nuclear magnetic spectroscopy

# Osteoarthritis

## DIAGNOSTIC SUMMARY

- **Symptoms**: mild early morning stiffness, stiffness after periods of rest, pain that worsens on joint use, and loss of joint function.
- **Signs**: local tenderness, soft tissue swelling, joint crepitus, bony swelling, restricted mobility, swelling of Heberden's (proximal interphalangeal joints) and/or less common Bouchard's (distal interphalangeal joints) nodes, and other signs of degenerative loss of articular cartilage.
- **Radiographic findings**: narrowed joint space, osteophytes, increased density of subchondral bone, subchondral sclerosis, bony cysts, soft tissue swelling, and periarticular swelling.

## GENERAL CONSIDERATIONS

Osteoarthritis (OA) characteristics include joint degeneration, loss of cartilage, and alterations of subchondral bone. It is the most common form of arthritis, with the highest morbidity rate of any illness. It primarily affects the elderly, but 35% of its incidence in the knee starts as early as age 30 years (often diagnosed as chondromalacia patellae). The incidence dramatically increases with age. More than 40 million Americans have OA, including 80% of persons older than 50 years. Men and women are equally affected, but symptoms occur earlier and appear to be more severe in women.

- Diseases thought to be OA of specific joints: hands (Heberden's and Bouchard's nodes), hips (malum coxae senilis), temporomandibular (Costen's syndrome), knees (chondromalacia patellae), and spine (ankylosing hyperostosis, interstitial skeletal hyperostosis).
- Weight-bearing joints and peripheral and axial articulations are principally affected. Hyaline cartilage destruction is followed by hardening and formation of large bone spurs (calcified

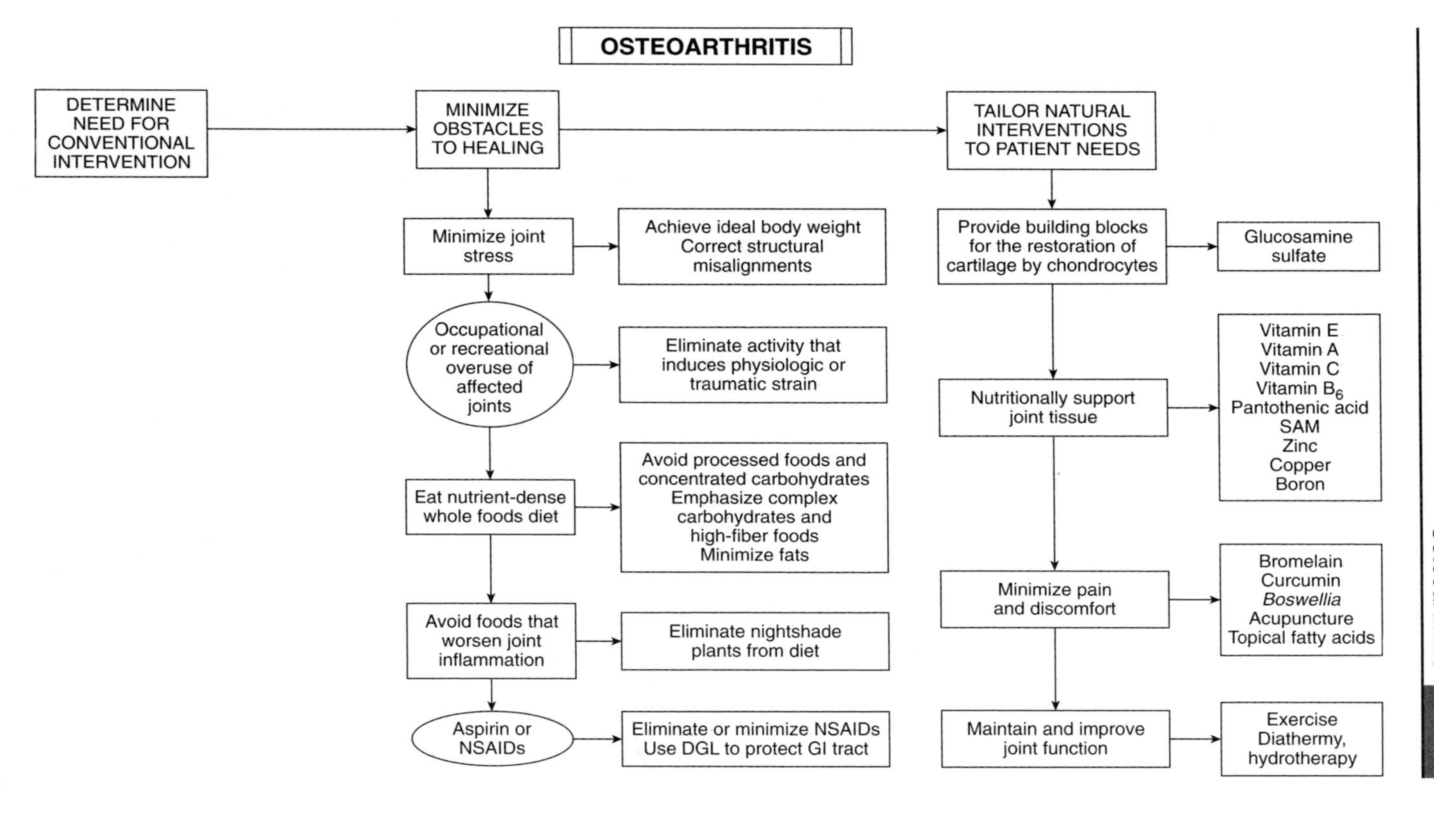
OSTEOARTHRITIS
DETERMINE NEED FOR CONVENTIONAL INTERVENTION
MINIMIZE OBSTACLES TO HEALING
TAILOR NATURAL INTERVENTIONS TO PATIENT NEEDS
Minimize joint stress
Achieve ideal body weight
Correct structural misalignments
Occupational or recreational overuse of affected joints
Eliminate activity that induces physiologic or traumatic strain
Eat nutrient-dense whole foods diet
Avoid processed foods and concentrated carbohydrates
Emphasize complex carbohydrates and high-fiber foods
Minimize fats
Avoid foods that worsen joint inflammation
Eliminate nightshade plants from diet
Aspirin or NSAIDs
Eliminate or minimize NSAIDs
Use DGL to protect GI tract
Provide building blocks for the restoration of cartilage by chondrocytes
Glucosamine sulfate
Nutritionally support joint tissue
Vitamin E
Vitamin A
Vitamin C
Vitamin $B_6$
Pantothenic acid
SAM
Zinc
Copper
Boron
Minimize pain and discomfort
Bromelain
Curcumin
*Boswellia*
Acupuncture
Topical fatty acids
Maintain and improve joint function
Exercise
Diathermy, hydrotherapy

osteophytes) in joint margins, causing pain, deformity, and limited joint motion. Inflammation usually is minimal.

- Two categories of OA: (1) primary OA arises from wear and tear after the fifth and sixth decades, with no predisposing abnormalities. The cumulative effects of decades of use stress collagen matrix. Damage releases enzymes that destroy collagen components. With aging, the ability to synthesize restorative collagen decreases. (2) Secondary OA entails predisposing factors for degeneration. Factors include congenital abnormalities in joint structure or function (e.g., hypermobility and abnormally shaped joint surfaces), trauma (obesity, fractures along joint surfaces, surgery), crystal deposition, presence of abnormal cartilage, previous inflammatory disease of joint (rheumatoid arthritis [RA], gout, septic arthritis).

## DIAGNOSIS

Onset is subtle; morning joint stiffness is the first symptom, then pain on joint motion worsened by prolonged activity and relieved by rest. No signs of inflammation are present. Clinical picture varies with joint(s) involved. Disease of the hands causes pain and limitation of use; knee involvement causes pain, swelling, and instability; hip OA has local pain and limp; spinal OA (very common) involves compression of nerves and blood vessels, causing pain and vascular insufficiency. RA is associated with much more inflammation of surrounding soft tissues. After a complete medical history, the best diagnostic tool is a radiograph of the suspected joint, which should reveal joint space narrowing, loss of cartilage, and presence of bone spurs (osteophytes).

### Causes of Misdiagnosis of Osteoarthritis

Source of pain is not OA, but:

- Arthritis of other origin
- Pathologic changes of adjacent bone (tumor, osteomyelitis, metabolic bone disease)
- Mechanical injuries
- Pathologic fractures
- Referred pain of neuritis, neuropathy, or radiculopathy
- Other neurologic disorders causing stiffness of joints

Source of pain is OA but not at joint suspected:

- OA of hip, pain localized to knee
- OA of cervical spine, causing pain in shoulder
- OA of lumbar spine, causing pain in hip, knee, or ankle
- OA of shoulder, causing pain in elbow

Source of pain is caused by secondary soft tissue alterations of OA:

- Tendonitis or ligamentitis (especially of knee)
- Enthesopathy, tendinopathy from joint contracture
- Bursitis

Misinterpretation of deformity:

- Pseudohypertrophic osteoarthropathy
- Psoriatic arthritis
- Flexion contracture of joints
- Mucopolysaccharidoses
- Neurogenic arthropathies
- Calcium pyrophosphate dihydrate crystal deposition disease
- Genu varum and valgum

Misinterpretation of x-ray films:

- Arthritis with previous OA changes
- Initial stage of OA, may have normal radiograph
- Flexion contracture can cause virtual loss of joint space width
- Neurogenic and metabolic arthropathies
- Pain: severity of OA (by radiograph) does not correlate with degree of pain. Forty percent of patients with the worst radiographic classification for OA are pain free. The cause of pain in OA is still not well defined. Depression and anxiety increase OA pain.

## THERAPEUTIC CONSIDERATIONS

Cellular and tissue response is purposeful and aimed at repair of anatomic defects. Disease process is arrestable and sometimes reversible. Therapeutic goal: enhance collagen matrix repair and regeneration by chondrocytes. Studies to determine natural course of OA show marked clinical improvement and radiologic recovery of joint space in almost 50% of cases with no therapy. Medical intervention may promote disease progression.

## Conventional Pharmacologic Treatment

Conventional treatment attempts to decrease inflammation to relieve pain. Yet in OA inflammation is mild and involves only periarticular tissues. Antiinflammatory drugs can only be marginally effective at reducing pain and are ineffective in enhancing repair.

- Aspirin (ASA) and nonsteroidal antiinflammatory drugs (NSAIDs): ASA is effective in relieving pain and inflammation and is inexpensive. Therapeutic dose is high (2-4 g q.d.) and toxicity is frequent, including tinnitus and gastric irritation. Side effects of other NSAIDs are gastrointestinal upset, headache, and dizziness. They are only recommended for short periods. Unexpected side effects may increase the rate of cartilage degeneration; they inhibit collagen matrix synthesis and accelerate cartilage destruction. NSAID use is associated with acceleration of OA. NSAIDs suppress symptoms but accelerate OA progression.

Main drug categories and individual drugs used to treat OA:

- NSAIDs: salicylates (aspirin), propionic acids (ibuprofen [Motrin], naproxen [Anaprox], oxaprozin [Daypro], flurbiprofen [Ansaid], ketoprofen [Orudis]), acetic acids (diclofenac [Voltaren], tolmetin [Tolectin], etodolac [Lodine], sulindac [Clinoril], indomethacin [Indocin]), and oxicams (piroxicam [Feldene])
- Cyclooxygenase inhibitors
- Irritants and counterirritants: capsaicin 0.025% cream
- Hyaluronic acids: hylan G-F 20 (Synvisc), sodium hyaluronate (Hyalogen)
- Glucocorticoids: prednisone

Pharmaceutical treatment is moderately effective for pain relief but offers little help for tissue repair.

## Hormonal Considerations

Endocrine forces may initiate or accelerate OA by altering the chondrocyte's microenvironment; all hormones act on connective tissue cells: fibroblasts, osteoblasts, and chondrocytes.

- **Estrogen**: higher prevalence of OA in women suggests estrogen involvement. Estradiol worsens OA. The antiestrogen drug tamoxifen improves experimental OA by decreasing erosive lesions; this suggests a therapeutic role for estrogen blockade.

Botanicals (e.g., *Glycyrrhiza glabra* and *Medicago sativa*) used for OA contain phytoestrogens that bind to estrogen receptors, acting as estrogen antagonists. Food sources of phytoestrogens include soy, fennel, celery, parsley, nuts, whole grains, and apples. Insulin, growth hormone (GH), and somatomedin (SMM): diabetics have greater incidence and more severe OA than non-diabetics. DM features causing OA: insulin insensitivity or deficiency, increased GH, and decreased SMMs (insulinlike growth factors secreted by liver in response to GH). Insulin stimulates chondrocytes to increase synthesis and assembly of proteoglycans. The most prominent early changes in articular cartilage are decreased proteoglycans and state of aggregation; thus insulin insensitivity or deficiency predisposes to OA. Excessive GH is detrimental to bone and joint structures; and increased incidence of OA is found in acromegaly. Women with primary osteoporosis have higher basal GH levels than do control subjects. GH is detrimental to chondrocytes. SMMs mediate normal chondrocyte activity. Impaired hepatic function, diabetes, and malnutrition suppress liver secretion of SMMs in response to GH, increasing risk of OA.

- **Thyroid**: hypothyroidism increases risk of OA compared with age- and sex-matched population samples.

## Dietary and Exercise Considerations

- Achieve normal body weight to minimize stress on weight-bearing joints affected with OA. Lack of exercise decreases hydration of joint cartilages and retards diffusion of nutrients into the affected area. OA pain causes reduced activity, decreasing muscle strength. Muscle weakness increases joint wear; inactivity causes weight gain, exacerbating OA and the cycle of degeneration. Diabetics and cardiovascular patients increase risks as their exercise diminishes. Weight loss, dieting, and exercise independently decrease causative factors of OA.
- Healthy diet rich in complex carbohydrates and dietary fiber (*Textbook,* "Role of Dietary Fiber in Health and Disease").
- Regimens combining diet and exercise are superior to protocols using only one, not both.
- Nightshade vegetables: Childers' theory is that genetically susceptible individuals might develop arthritis from long-term, low-level consumption of the solanum alkaloids found in *Solanaceae* (nightshade) plants: tomatoes, potatoes, eggplant, peppers, and tobacco. Alkaloids may inhibit normal collagen repair. This

theory is as yet unproven, but diet is beneficial to some patients.

## Nutritional Supplements

Americans spend more on natural remedies for osteoarthritis than for any other medical condition.

- **Antioxidant nutrients**: Framingham Osteoarthritis Cohort Study showed that high intake of antioxidant nutrients, especially vitamin C, gave a threefold reduced risk of cartilage loss and OA disease progression in the middle and highest tertiles of vitamin C intake. Advocate diet rich in plant-based antioxidants.
- **Glucosamine sulfate (GS)**: stimulates manufacture of glycosaminoglycans (GAGs) by chondrocytes and promotes incorporation of sulfur into cartilage. With age comes a reduced ability to synthesize sufficient glucosamine; cartilage loses its gel-like nature and ability to absorb shock. Inability to manufacture glucosamine may be the major factor leading to OA. GS was significantly more effective than placebo in improving pain and movement after 4 weeks (1500 mg q.d.) in a double-blind crossover study. Longer GS use gives greater therapeutic benefit. Rate and severity of GS side effects are not different from placebo. Head-to-head studies: GS gives better long-term results than NSAIDs in relieving OA pain and inflammation despite little direct antiinflammatory or analgesic effect from GS. NSAIDs offer only symptomatic relief and may promote disease process. GS treats root cause (cartilage synthesis), improving symptoms and helping the body repair damage. Higher dosages may be required for heavy or obese patients. Patients with peptic ulcers should take GS with food. Individuals taking diuretics may need an increased dosage to compensate for reduced efficacy. Improvement with GS lasts 6-12 weeks after end of treatment. GS should be taken for long periods or in repeated short-term courses. GS has high safety and excellent tolerability and is suitable for long-term use (*Textbook*, "Glucosamine"). Glucosamine hydrochloride at 2000 mg q.d. for 5 months provided significant pain relief and improved function after 8 weeks. With respect to concerns about effects on blood sugar in diabetics, 1500 mg of glucosamine (and 1200 mg of chondroitin) given daily to diabetics, most on antiglycemic medicines, had no effect on hemoglobin A1c after a 90-day trial.

- **Chondroitin sulfate (CS), shark cartilage, bovine cartilage extracts, sea cucumber**: contain a mixture of intact or partially hydrolyzed glycosaminoglycans (GAGs) of molecular weights 14,000 to 30,000. CS is composed of repeating units of derivatives of GS. Absorption rate of GS is 90%-98%; absorption of intact CS is 13%. CS is 50-300 times larger than GS. Key reason why GS is effective is its small molecular size, allowing diffusion through joint cartilage to chondrocyte. CS levels typically are elevated in synovial tissues of OA patients; CS is less effective than GS. Any benefit from CS is likely from the absorption of sulfur or smaller GAG molecules broken down by the digestive tract. No evidence exists that shows using both GS and CS together is more effective than either alone. GS gives more impressive results; it is faster acting and has greater overall benefit. Evidence of modifying joint space pathology makes CS a reasonable addition to GS regimen for OA.
- **Niacinamide**: Kaufman and Hoffer treatment of RA and OA with high-dose niacinamide (900-4000 mg q.d. in divided doses) improves joint function, range of motion, muscle strength and endurance, and sedimentation rate. Benefits are noted within 1-3 months of use; peak benefits occur after 1 to 3 years of continuous use. A dosage of 3000 mg q.d. in six divided doses resulted in a 29% improvement in global arthritis impact versus 10% worsening with placebo. Pain levels did not change, but niacinamide patients reduced NSAID use. It reduced erythrocyte sedimentation rate by 22% and increased joint mobility by 4.5 degrees over control subjects (8 vs. 3.5 degrees). No other changes in blood chemistry were noted. Side effects were mild GI complaints, managed by taking with food or fluids. High doses can result in significant side effects (e.g. glucose intolerance and liver damage); strict supervision is required.
- **S-adenosylmethionine (SAM)**: is formed in the body by converting the essential amino acid methionine to adenosyl-triphosphate. SAM deficiency in joint tissue causes loss of gel-like nature and shock-absorbing qualities of cartilage. SAM is important in the synthesis of cartilage components. Supplemental SAM increases cartilage formation (determined by magnetic resonance imaging) in osteoarthritis of the hands. It shows mild analgesic and antiinflammatory effects in animal studies. SAM induces similar reductions in pain scores and clinical symptoms to NSAIDs. SAM administered orally at dose of 1200 mg q.d. is significantly more effective than NSAIDs (physicians' and

patients' judgments). It is better tolerated than placebo. Its efficacy has been described as very good or good in 71% of cases, moderate in 21%, and poor in 9%. Tolerance was assessed as very good or good in 87%, moderate in 8%, and poor in 5% of cases. SAM offers significant advantages over NSAIDs. Side effects: occasional GI disturbances, mainly diarrhea.

- **Superoxide dismutase (SOD)**: intraarticular injections of SOD have significant therapeutic effects. Whether SOD is absorbed orally is yet to be determined; preliminary indications are unfavorable.
- **Vitamin E**: 600 IU q.d. is significantly beneficial because of its antioxidant and membrane-stabilizing actions. In vitro, it inhibits activities of lysosomal enzymes and stimulates increased deposition of proteoglycan.
- **Vitamin C**: deficient intake is common in the elderly, causing altered collagen synthesis and compromised connective tissue repair. In vitro, vitamin C has anabolic effect on cartilage. Excess of ascorbic acid is needed in human chondrocyte protein synthesis. In vivo study of experimental OA in guinea pigs found cartilage erosion is much less, and overall histologic and biochemical changes in and around OA joint are much milder, in animals on high doses of vitamin C. Vitamins C and E have synergistic effects that enhance stability of sulfated proteoglycans in cartilage.
- **Vitamin D**: the Framingham Heart Study found low intake and low serum levels of vitamin D are both linked to increased risk for progression of OA of knee. Low serum vitamin D predicts loss of cartilage, indicated by joint space and osteophyte growth. Sunlight and sufficient intake in childhood and young adulthood may decrease risk of OA. Whether increasing vitamin D intake helps decrease or reverse already established OA is not known.
- **Pantothenic acid**: acute deficiency in rats causes pronounced failure of cartilage growth and lesions similar to OA. It clinically improves OA symptoms at a dosage of 12.5 mg. Results often do not manifest until 7-14 days. A larger, double-blind study of RA patients found no significant benefit at dosage at 500 mg q.d.
- **Vitamins A and E, pyridoxine, zinc, copper, and boron**: required for synthesis of collagen and maintenance of normal cartilage. Deficiency of any one of these allows accelerated joint degeneration. Supplements at appropriate potencies may promote cartilage repair. Boron has been used to treat OA in Germany since the mid-1970s. At a dosage of 6 mg boron q.d.

(sodium tetraborate decahydrate), 71% of patients improved compared with 10% on placebo. Open trial: boron at 6-9 mg q.d. gave effective relief in 90% of arthritis patients, including OA, juvenile arthritis, and RA. Boron is of value in arthritis; many OA patients experience complete resolution.

### Physical Therapy

- Skewed musculoskeletal dynamics play a role in abnormally stressing involved joints. Patients with varus alignment have a fourfold increased risk of medial OA progression; those with valgus alignment have five times the risk of lateral OA progression. Decline is greater for those with more extensive misalignments. Consider musculoskeletal dynamics when evaluating any patient with OA. Misalignments may need manual manipulation, orthotics, and extremity adjustments plus massage to relax hypertonic muscles. Assessing and treating younger persons may reduce risk of OA later on in life.
- Exercise, heat, cold, diathermy, and ultrasound often improve joint mobility and reduce pain in OA, especially when administered regularly. Benefit of physical therapy is achieving proper hydration within the joint capsule.
- Short-wave diathermy may be of greatest benefit. Combining short-wave diathermy with periodic ice massage, rest, and appropriate exercises may be the most effective approach. Ultrasound and laser therapy also are helpful.
- Best exercises are isometrics and swimming; they increase circulation to joints and strengthen surrounding muscles without excess strain on joints. Increasing quadriceps strength improves clinical features and reduces pain in knee OA. Walking helps improve functional status and relieve pain in knee OA.

### Magnetic Therapies

- Used to treat a wide variety of chronic pain syndromes. Magnetic fields may stimulate chondrocyte proliferation and synthesis of proteoglycans. Studies support use in knee OA.
- Low-frequency and low-amplitude pulsed fields improve pain, functionality, and physician global evaluation of patients' condition.
- High-strength magnetic knee sleeve treatment for 4 hours in a monitored setting and self-treatment 6 hours daily for 6 weeks decreased pain scores.

## Relaxation

- Relaxation techniques, such as meditation, deep breathing, and guided imagery, are applied to many types of pain.
- Daily listening to music of Mozart for 20 minutes over a 14-day period caused patients to have less pain compared with those who sat quietly for 20 minutes and did not listen to music. Pain decreased incrementally over a 14-day study period.

## Botanical Medicines

When inflammation is present, botanicals and nutritional factors possessing antiinflammatory activity are indicated, such as bromelain, curcumin, and ginger.

- ***Yucca:*** double-blind trial found saponin extract of yucca has positive therapeutic effect. Results are gradual with no direct joint effects. Improvement is caused by indirect effects on GI flora. Bacterial lipopolysaccharides (endotoxins) depress the biosynthesis of proteoglycans. *Yucca* may decrease bacterial endotoxin absorption, reducing inhibition of proteoglycan synthesis. Other saponin-containing herbs and other ways of reducing endotoxin load may be useful.
- ***Harpagophytum procumbens*** **(devil's claw)**: in experimental animal models of inflammation, Devil's claw has an antiinflammatory and analgesic effect comparable to phenylbutazone. Other studies indicate little, if any, antiinflammatory effect. Equivocal research may reflect a mechanism of action inconsistent with current antiinflammatory models or failure to use quality-controlled (standardized) extracts. Main components of Devil's claw are saponins; the therapeutic effect in OA may be similar to that of yucca.
- ***Boswellia serrata***: large branching tree native to India with exudative gum resin (salai guggul) used for centuries. Newer preparations, concentrated for active components (boswellic acids), give better results. Boswellic acid extracts have antiarthritic effects in animal models. Mechanisms of action: inhibit inflammatory mediators, prevent decrease in GAG synthesis, and improve blood supply to joint tissues. Herbal formulas with Boswellia yield good clinical results in OA and RA. Dosage for boswellic acids in arthritis is 400 mg t.i.d. No side effects from boswellic acids have been reported.
- ***Zingiber officinalis*** **(ginger)**: ginger extract had moderate effect on symptoms of knee OA, reducing need for acetaminophen and reducing knee pain on standing and after walking. Side effect:

mild GI upset. Other studies indicate no benefit. More research is needed.

### Topical Applications

- **Fatty acids**: cetylated fatty acids are similar to omega 3-fatty acids. Omega-3s have been used for both internal and topical treatment of OA. Cetylated fatty cream was applied bilaterally to anterior, posterior, and lateral surfaces of knees for 30 days of two treatments daily. Compared with placebo, fatty acids significantly decreased timing for stair climbing and getting up from a chair after initial treatment and at 1 month. Range of motion also improved.

## THERAPEUTIC APPROACH

Clinical study of comprehensive, integrated program for OA has yet to be conducted. Therapeutic approach: reduce joint stress, promote collagen repair, and eliminate foods and other factors that inhibit collagen repair. Control all diseases or predisposing factors. Avoid NSAIDs as much as possible. If aspirin is used, deglycyrrhizinated *Glycyrrhiza glabra* (licorice) (DGL) may protect GI tract from damaging effects and ASA should be discontinued as soon as possible.

- **Diet**: avoid simple, processed, and concentrated carbohydrates. Emphasize complex-carbohydrate, high-fiber foods. Minimize fats. Eliminate *Solanaceae* foods (tomatoes, potatoes, eggplant, peppers, and tobacco). Liberally consume flavonoid-rich berries or extracts.
- **Supplements**:
  —Glucosamine sulfate: 1500 mg q.d.
  —Niacinamide: 500 mg six times/day (under strict supervision; monitor liver enzymes)
  —Vitamin E: 600 IU q.d. (mixed tocopherols)
  —Vitamin A: 5000 IU q.d.
  —Vitamin C: 1000-3000 mg q.d.
  —Vitamin $B_6$: 50 mg q.d.
  —Pantothenic acid: 12.5 mg q.d.
  —SAM: 400 mg t.i.d.
  —Zinc: 45 mg q.d.
  —Copper: 1 mg q.d.
  —Boron: 6 mg q.d.

- **Botanical medicines**:
  —*Medicago sativa* (alfalfa): equivalent to 5-10 g q.d.
  —*Yucca* leaves: 2-4 g t.i.d.
  —*Harpagophytum procumbens*: dried powdered root, 1-2 g t.i.d.; tincture (1:5), 4-5 mL t.i.d.; dry solid extract (3:1), 400 mg t.i.d.
  —*Boswellia serrata*: equivalent to 400 mg boswellic acids t.i.d.; topical application, cetylated fatty acid cream applied to affected area b.i.d.
- **Physical therapy and exercise**: avoid physical activity that induces physiologic or traumatic strain (occupational or recreational overuse). Normalize posture; orthopedically correct structural abnormalities to limit joint strain. Prescribe monitored daily nontraumatic exercise (isometrics and swimming). Use short-wave diathermy, hydrotherapy, and other physical therapy modalities that improve joint perfusion.

# Osteoporosis

## DIAGNOSTIC SUMMARY

- Usually asymptomatic until severe backache
- Most common in postmenopausal (PM) white women
- Spontaneous fractures of the hip and vertebra
- Decrease in height
- Defined as a T-score at or below a bone mineral density of –2.5 standard deviations below that of a young normal adult

## GENERAL CONSIDERATIONS

- Osteoporosis (OP) is the most common bone disease in human beings and is a health threat for PM women. Features include low bone mass, deterioration of microarchitecture of bone tissue, fragility of bones, and increased risk of fracture. Approximately 1.5 million OP fractures occur each year in the United States, of which 250,000 are hip fractures. Twenty percent of women with hip fractures die of complications within a year; an additional 25% require long-term nursing care. Half the women who have a hip fracture are unable to walk without assistance.
- Vertebral fractures of the thoracic and/or lumbar region cause pain, height loss, and exaggerated kyphosis or deformity of thoracic spine, with restricted range of motion, changes in posture, restricted lung function, and digestive problems.
- Depression, anxiety, low self-esteem, and tooth loss are also caused by OP.

### Pathophysiology

- Bone remodeling is process of bone resorption (breakdown) and bone formation. Osteoclasts induce enzymatic dissolution of minerals and protein for bone resorption. Osteoblasts create protein matrix of collagen for remineralization and bone formation. Bone remodeling is normally a balance of resorption and formation. Imbalance between removal and replacement causes bone loss and risk of fracture.

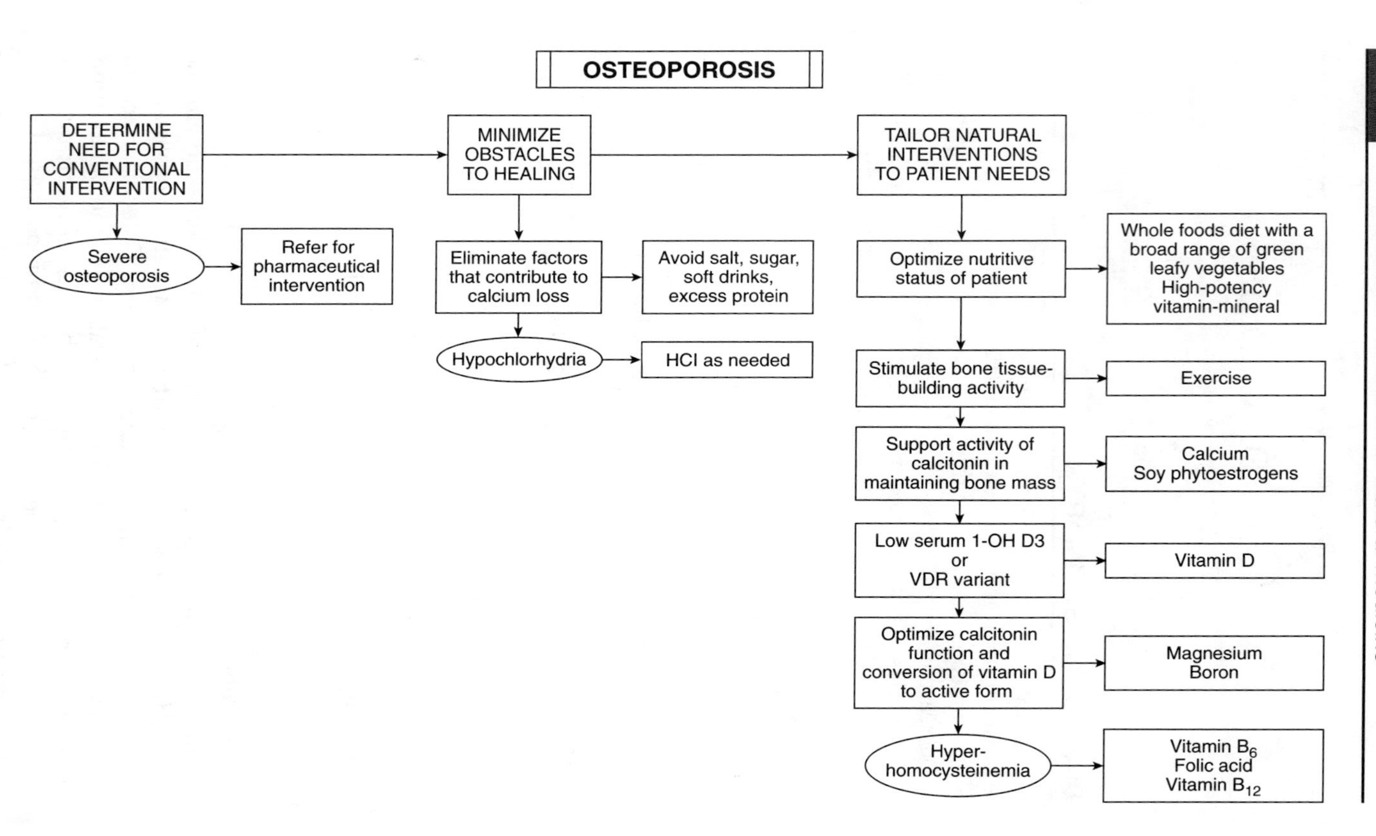
OSTEOPOROSIS
DETERMINE NEED FOR CONVENTIONAL INTERVENTION
Severe osteoporosis
Refer for pharmaceutical intervention
MINIMIZE OBSTACLES TO HEALING
Eliminate factors that contribute to calcium loss
Avoid salt, sugar, soft drinks, excess protein
Hypochlorhydria
HCl as needed
TAILOR NATURAL INTERVENTIONS TO PATIENT NEEDS
Optimize nutritive status of patient
Whole foods diet with a broad range of green leafy vegetables
High-potency vitamin-mineral
Stimulate bone tissue-building activity
Exercise
Support activity of calcitonin in maintaining bone mass
Calcium
Soy phytoestrogens
Low serum 1-OH D3 or VDR variant
Vitamin D
Optimize calcitonin function and conversion of vitamin D to active form
Magnesium
Boron
Hyper-homocysteinemia
Vitamin $B_6$
Folic acid
Vitamin $B_{12}$

- Bone mass rapidly increases in childhood, slows in the late teens, but continues to increase during 20s. In women, the building process is complete by age 17 years. Peak bone mass is at 28 years, then bone mass is slowly lost at a rate of 0.4% per year in the femoral neck. After menopause, the loss accelerates to 2% per year during the first 5 to 10 years. Loss continues in women older than 70 years at much slower rate.

## Risk Factors

- **Genetic factors**: level of peak bone mass is attributable to genetic factors. Young daughters of women with OP fractures and first-degree relatives of women with OP have subnormal bone mass. Black women have greater bone mass compared with white women. Genomic testing is now available to assess the genetic predisposition to a defect in the vitamin D receptor sites (VDR). Women with the VDR defect require substantially greater levels of vitamin D, preferable as 1-OH D3.
- **Lifestyle**: lifestyle, hormonal factors, calcium (Ca) and vitamin D intake, exercise, age of menarche, menstrual regularity, and alcohol and tobacco use have less impact than genetics. Several lifestyle factors affect OP risk after menopause: physical activity, animal protein intake, acid-base homeostasis, Ca and vitamin D intake, heavy smoking and alcohol intake. Requirements for peak bone mass: balanced diet, adequate calories, protein and Ca throughout life. Ca and vitamin D are critical in older women. Ca requirements change with age; menopause increases Ca needs. After age 65 years, women absorb 50% less Ca than do young women. Renal enzymatic activity that produces active vitamin D decreases.
- **Dietary protein**: high intake of animal protein, but not plant protein, is linked to increased risk of forearm fracture. Red meat is acid producing, inducing release of salts from bone to balance acid and maintain acid-base homeostasis. Diets high in fruits and vegetables and plant proteins are alkaline forming.
- **Smoking**: women smokers lose bone more rapidly, have lower bone mass, and have higher fracture rates. Smokers reach menopause up to 2 years earlier. Smoking may interfere with estrogen by an unknown metabolism.
- **Alcohol**: ≥7 oz/week of alcohol increases the risk of falls and hip fractures. Moderate alcohol intake lowers risk of hip fractures in older women; it inhibits bone resorption by increasing estradiol levels and calcitonin excretion.

- **Physical activity**: highly active persons have higher bone mass; prolonged bed rest or confinement to a wheelchair causes rapid, dramatic bone loss. Exercise reduces OP risk by stimulating osteoblasts.

## Hormonal Factors

- Menopause: all women lose bone, but this loss is accelerated in the first 5 years of menopause. Estrogen decline increases rate of bone resorption. The earlier that occurs before the average age of menopause (51 years), the sooner the bones lose the protective effect of endogenous estrogen. Premature menopause (before 40 years), late onset of menarche in adolescence, and periods of amenorrhea or infrequent menses increase risk of OP. Women who missed up to half of their expected menstrual periods have 12% less vertebral bone mass; those who missed more than half had 31% less bone mass than healthy control subjects.
- Ca blood concentration is strictly held within narrow limits. Ca decline triggers increased secretion of parathyroid hormone (PTH) and decreased secretion of calcitonin from the thyroid and parathyroids. Ca excess triggers decreased secretion of PTH and increased secretion of calcitonin.
- PTH increases serum Ca by increasing osteoclast catabolism of bone, decreases excretion of Ca by kidneys, increases absorption of Ca in intestines, and increases kidney conversion of 25-$(OH)D_3$ to 1,25-$(OH)_2D_3$.
- Estrogen deficiency makes osteoclasts more sensitive to PTH, increasing bone breakdown and raising blood Ca. Elevated blood Ca decreases PTH, diminishing active vitamin D and increasing Ca excretion.

## Additional Factors

The more risk factors present, the greater the potential for lower bone mass and risk of fracture. Risk factors alone do not adequately assess low bone mass but can guide clinical assessment risks that contribute to optimal preventive strategies. The individual woman's risk is the most relevant parameter for her future bone health. Diseases and medicines can interrupt normal bone metabolism.

- **Genetic factors**:
  —First-degree relative with low-trauma fracture
  —White or Asian race

—Slender physical frame
—Family history of OP

- **Menstrual status**:
  —Early menopause without hormone replacement therapy or oral contraceptive use
  —History of amenorrhea (from anorexia nervosa, hyperprolactinemia, or exercise-induced amenorrhea), infrequent menses, late menstrual onset, anovulation
  —Premenopausal hypogonadism
- **Diseases**:
  —Kidney disease and kidney stones, rheumatoid arthritis, multiple myeloma, chronic obstructive pulmonary disease, scoliosis, anorexia nervosa, diabetes mellitus, Cushing's disease, hyperthyroidism, primary hyperparathyroidism, hypercalciuria, vitamin D deficiency
  —Gallbladder disease, primary biliary cirrhosis, fat malabsorption, hypochlorhydria, lactose intolerance
  —History of chronic low back pain for more than 15 years
  —History of stress fractures
  —Prolonged bed rest, paralysis, or time in wheelchair
  —History of other fractures after age 45 years
  —Underweight
  —Dental conditions: bone loss in the jaw, dentures before age 60 years, increased tooth loss
  —Nulliparous (never had a full-term pregnancy, that is, no periods of sustained high estrogens)
- **Environmental and lifestyle factors**:
  —Little exposure to sunlight
  —Inadequate Ca and vitamin D intake during pregnancies and nursing
  —Dietary factors: excessive caffeine, high animal protein, high sodium, high phosphate, low dietary Ca
  —Lifestyle factors: sedentary, moderate (or more) alcohol intake, cigarette smoking
- **Medications**:
  —Isoniazid, furosemide, heparin, tetracycline, anticonvulsants, gonadotropin-releasing hormone, cortisone or prednisone, and aluminum-containing antacids, lithium
- **Surgeries**:
  —Total thyroidectomy, removal of part or all of intestines, intestinal bypass surgery for weight control

## DIAGNOSTIC CONSIDERATIONS

- Assess all PM women for risk factors of OP—history, physical examination, diagnostic tests. Goals of evaluation: identify women at risk for OP or fracture; diagnose OP and/or determine severity of OP; rule out secondary causes of bone loss; identify risk factors for falls or injuries.
- Focus history and physical examination on identifying risk factors. Physical signs of OP: loss of height >1.5 inches (measure height annually), excess kyphosis of thoracic spine, dowager's hump, dental caries, tooth loss, receding gums, back pain.
- Radiologic tests of bone mineral density (BMD): BMD testing is optimal to diagnose OP. Gold standard is dual energy x-ray absorptiometry (DEXA). Other methods include computerized tomography (CT) scans, ultrasound of heel, radiographs; none of these tests is optimal for diagnosis and follow-up. The following tests measure BMD and are compared by accuracy.

**Comparison of BMD Tests**

| Method | Site | Accuracy |
|---|---|---|
| Dual-energy x-ray absorptiometry (DEXA) | Hip, spine, total body | 90%-99% |
| Peripheral dual-energy x-ray absorptiometry (PDXA) | Forearm, finger, heel | 90%-99% |
| Single-energy x-ray absorptiometry (SXA) | Heel | 98%-99% |
| Quantitative ultrasound (QUS) | Heel, shin | Not applicable |
| Quantitated computed tomography (QCT) | Spine | 95%-97% |
| Peripheral quantitative computed tomography (PQTC) | Forearm | 92%-98% |

Adapted from Jergas M, Genant HK: Current methods and recent advances in the diagnosis of osteoporosis, *Arthritis Rheum* 36:1649-1662, 1993.

DEXA test requires less radiation exposure than radiographs or CT scans. It can measure both hip and lumbar densities. Hip is the preferred site for BMD testing, especially in patients older than 60 years, because spinal measurements are unreliable because of extraosseous ossification. The spine is useful in early PM women; rates of bone loss are greater because of lower estrogen. Peripheral DEXA sites are accurate but les useful; they may not correlate with fracture risk and BMD at hip and spine. North American Menopause Society guidelines for indications for BMD testing are:

- Secondary causes of bone loss (e.g., steroid use, hyperparathyroidism)
- Radiologic evidence of osteopenia
- All women age 65 years and older
- Younger PM women with fragility fractures since menopause, low body weight, or family history of spine or hip fracture

Many practitioners are increasing their use of BMD testing to aid women in the decision making process about managing menopause symptoms.

Reporting of results of BMD tests: standard deviations of either a Z-score or a T-score. Z-score is based on standard deviation from the mean BMD of women in the same age group. T-score is based on mean peak BMD of normal, young adult women. World Health Organization criteria for diagnosing OP uses T-scores.

**BMD Score Interpretation**

| Status | T-Score | Interpretation |
|---|---|---|
| Normal | Above –1 | BMD within 1 standard deviation of a young normal adult |
| Osteopenia | Between –1 and 12.5 | BMD between 1 and 2.5 standard deviations below a normal young adult |
| OP | Below –2.5 | BMD is ≤2.5 standard deviations below a young normal adult |

## Laboratory Tests of Bone Metabolism

- Biochemical markers of bone turnover
  - —Urine test for breakdown products of bone: cross-linked N-telopeptide of type I collagen or deoxypyridium.
  - —Measure bone turnover correlated with rate of bone loss; not intended to be used for diagnosis of OP or monitoring bone loss.
  - —Use to monitor success (or failure) of therapy; provide quicker feedback compared with DEXA, which can take up to 2 years to detect therapeutic response.
  - —Use DEXA to measure bone density; use urinary bone resorption assessments to measure rate of turnover.

—Reducing urinary markers of breakdown over a 2-year period has produced increases in bone density measurements, but value of markers in clinical practice has yet to be confirmed.

- Additional tests for secondary causes of bone loss: serum Ca, 24-hour urinary Ca, PTH, thyroid-stimulating hormone, free thyroxine, serum albumin, serum alkaline phosphatase, erythrocyte sedimentation rate, complete blood count, and vitamin D levels. Indirect tests of Ca absorption: gastric acid levels, vitamin D levels.

## THERAPEUTIC CONSIDERATIONS

Goals for treating and preventing OP:

- Preserve adequate bone mass
- Preserve bone strength
- Prevent skeletal fragility
- Prevent deterioration of microarchitecture
- Prevent or reduce the risk of fractures

OP is largely preventable. Pharmaceuticals reduce the risk of vertebral and hip fractures by 50%. The North American Menopause Society guidelines and indications for drugs include PM women with:

- Previous vertebral fractures
- BMD T-score values less than –2.5
- BMD T-score less than –2 and previous nonspine fragility fracture, weight <127 lb or family history of hip or spine fracture
- Individuals with secondary causes of bone loss will require individualized management.
- Older PM women with history of previous nontraumatic, nonpathologic vertebral fracture are at very high risk of having another spine fracture or hip fracture. These women particularly are candidates for treatment with proven conventional pharmacologic treatments, no matter what their bone density is.

### Drug Therapy

- **Hormone replacement therapy (HRT)**: both estrogen replacement therapy (ERT) and HRT reduce rate of bone turnover and resorption. ERT can lower resorption rates to that of premenopausal women. ERT and HRT reduce risk by 54%. ERT and HRT are more effective at reducing fracture risk if begun within 5 years of menopause. If used more than 10 years, they produce even greater risk reduction—75% for wrist fractures and 73% for hip fractures. Risks of breast cancer, blood clots, strokes, nonfatal myocardial infarction, cholelithiasis, breast tenderness, fluid retention, uterine bleeding, and headache are increased. Individualize treatment; identify risk/ benefit ratio. ERT and HRT work best during first 5 to 10 years after menopause. The optimal duration and maximal duration have not yet been determined. ERT and HRT are not to be seen as primary long-term treatment except in those who do not tolerate bisphosphonates or who have menopause symptoms that are not responding to other therapies.

- **Bisphosphonates**: inhibit osteoclasts, reducing bone resorption. Examples include alendronate, etidronate, risedronate. They all increase BMD and reduce fracture risk.
- **Other drugs**: selective estrogen receptor modulators, calcitonin, and tibolone (not yet available in the United States).

## Lifestyle Factors

Coffee, alcohol, and smoking cause negative Ca balance and are linked to increased risk of OP; regular exercise reduces risk. Exercise is more critical for maintaining healthy bones than is HRT or ERT.

- **Exercise**: Physical fitness is the major determinant of bone density. One hour of moderate activity three times per week prevents bone loss and increases bone mass in PM women. Immobilization doubles the rate of urinary and fecal Ca excretion, causing negative Ca balance. The most effective practice for strengthening bones is physical activity.

## General Dietary Factors

Dietary factors suggested as causes of OP:

- **Low-Ca, high-phosphorus intake**
- **High-protein diet**
- **High acid-ash diet**
- **High salt intake**
- **Trace mineral deficiencies**
- **Vegetarian diet** (both lacto-ovo and vegan): lowers risk of OP. Bone mass in vegetarians does not differ from omnivores in third, fourth, and fifth decades but does in later decades. Decreased incidence of OP in vegetarians is caused by decreased bone loss

in later years. High-protein and high-phosphate diets increase excretion of Ca in urine. Raising daily protein from 47 to 142 g doubles urine Ca excretion.

- **Gastric acid**: Ca must be ionized in the stomach acid to be absorbed. Poor ionization of Ca is a major problem with Ca carbonate. Decreased gastric acidity occurs in 40% of PM women, but the effects of increased gastric pH only appear when poorly soluble Ca salts such as Ca carbonate are taken after an overnight fast. Fasting patients with insufficient stomach acid only absorb 4% of oral Ca as Ca carbonate, whereas normal stomach acid allows absorption of 22%. Preionized Ca is preferred: Ca citrate, lactate, or gluconate. Forty-five percent of Ca is absorbed from citrate with reduced stomach acid. Yet taken with meals, little difference in Ca absorption is found, even in elderly subjects with atrophic gastritis or those taking $H_2$-receptor antagonists.
- **Sugar**: after refined sugar intake, urinary excretion of Ca increases. The average American consumes 125 g sucrose, 50 g of corn syrup plus other simple sugars, a glass of carbonated beverage loaded with phosphates, and high amount of protein every day.
- **Soft drinks**: are high in phosphates but not Ca. Per capita intake in the United States: 15 oz/day. Soft drink intake in children is a major risk factor for impaired calcification of growing bones. Serum Ca levels are inversely correlated with number of bottles of soft drink consumed each week.
- **Green leafy vegetables**: eating green leafy vegetables (kale, collard greens, parsley, lettuce, etc.) protects against OP. They are rich sources of broad range of vitamins and minerals that maintain healthy bones (Ca, vitamin $K_1$, boron).
- **Vitamin $K_1$**: form of vitamin K in plants. Vitamin $K_1$ converts inactive osteocalcin to its active form. Osteocalcin, the major noncollagen protein in bone, anchors Ca ions into protein matrix. Vitamin K deficiency impairs mineralization of bone because of inadequate active osteocalcin. Very low blood vitamin $K_1$ is found in patients with OP fractures. Fracture severity strongly correlated with level of circulating vitamin K. The lower the level of circulating vitamin K, the lower the bone density. Richest sources of vitamin $K_1$: dark green leafy vegetables, broccoli, lettuce, cabbage, spinach, green tea. Good sources: asparagus, oats, whole wheat, fresh green peas.
- **Boron**: trace mineral protective against OP (*Textbook*, "Boron"). Giving PM women 3 mg/day of boron reduced urinary Ca excre-

tion by 44% and dramatically increased 17-beta-estradiol, the most biologically active estrogen. Boron is required to activate certain hormones, including estrogen and vitamin D. Boron also is required to convert vitamin D to most active form (1,25-$(OH)_2D_3$) in kidneys. Boron deficiency may add to OP and menopausal symptoms. Main sources: fruits and vegetables. Fewer than 10% of Americans meet minimum recommendation of two fruit and three vegetable servings daily; only 51% eat one serving of vegetables per day. Dosage: 3-5 mg boron q.d. Boron mimics some of effects of ERT in PM women.

- **Soy**: has a proestrogen effect on bone. Possible mechanisms of action: binding to estrogen receptors, stimulating formation of sex hormone–binding globulin, and inhibiting tyrosine kinase. Soy inhibits bone loss in ovariectomized animals but not to the same extent as does ERT. Soy phytoestrogen genistein has similar effects maintaining bone. Genistein suppresses osteoclasts, both in vitro and in vivo. Menopausal women had increased mineral levels and density in the lumbar spine after taking 55-90 mg isoflavones for 6 months. Soybean protein diet was effective in preventing bone loss in fourth lumbar vertebra and, to a lesser degree, in the right hip. Soybean protein has more effect on trabecular bone (predominant in spine) than on cortical bone (predominant in hip). Soy effect is not a great as ERT but is encouraging. Among premenopausal, but not perimenopausal, women, those with higher intake of soy isoflavones had higher spine and femoral neck BMD. In PM women, no BMD effect was found in those receiving 56 mg/day of genistein/daidzein; but those receiving 90 mg/day genistein/daidzein had 2% increase in spinal BMD compared with baseline. Some soy products offer as much or more Ca than a serving of dairy products.

### Nutritional Supplements

Bone needs a constant supply of many nutrients. Deficiency of any one adversely affects bone health. In addition to vitamin K and boron (discussed previously), bone needs the following:

- **Calcium**: supplementation was more effective than placebo in reducing rates of bone loss after 2+ years of treatment. Relative risk of fractures of vertebrae dropped 21%, but relative risk for nonvertebral fractures was only 14%. In contrast, dietary sources of Ca (e.g., milk) have failed to show any link with OP unless intake of Ca is extremely low. Clinical studies of the effect of Ca

supplements against OP and hip fracture show no advantage for any one form, especially when given with vitamin D. Differences in absorption are not clinically meaningful. When taken with food, Ca from insoluble salt (e.g., carbonate) is as absorbable as soluble salt (e.g., citrate). Ca carbonate alone significantly prevented bone loss during trials. Ca alone was less effective than Premarin/Ca combination; but Ca supplements have no major health risks. Reserve ERT and HRT for women at high risk for OP. Continued Ca supplementation produces sustained reduction in rate of loss of total BMD in women. Accordingly, incidence of bone fractures was far lower in those taking Ca compared with placebo. Over a 4-year period, Ca-supplemented older PM women (2000 mg q.d.) did not lose bone at hip and ankle. Control subjects (Ca intake, 950 mg q.d.) lost much more bone than the Ca group at all sites of the hip and ankle. No bone loss was seen at the spine, in either group, over the 4-year period. A strong correlation exists between premenopausal bone density and the risk of OP. That being the case, building strong bones should be a lifelong goal, beginning in childhood. However, most women probably are not concerned about OP until a few years before menopause. Fortunately, Ca supplementation does slow bone loss in perimenopausal women. Ca supplementation before menopause is critical to prevention. Oyster shell, dolomite, bone meal, and many other Ca supplements may contain lead. The Food and Drug Administration's tolerable level of lead is 1 μg/800 mg of Ca. Supplements with the greatest range of lead content are unrefined Ca carbonate (source: oyster shells). Total tolerable daily intake of lead for children aged 6 years and under is <6 μg/day. Young children should take refined Ca carbonate or chelated Ca products. Chelated Ca, especially Ca citrate, may be better absorbed than Ca carbonate. Refined Ca carbonate and other refined sources have the lowest lead content. Ca bound to citrate and other Krebs cycle intermediates—fumarate, malate, succinate, aspartate—may be the best form. Krebs cycle intermediates fulfill every requirement for optimum Ca chelating agent:
—Easily ionized
—Almost completely degraded
—Virtually no toxicity
—Increase absorption of other minerals as well.
Ca hydroxyapatite, or purified bone meal, tested at 20% absorption compared with 30% for Ca carbonate and Ca citrate.

**Recommendations for Ca Intake**

| Age | Adequate Intake (Elemental Ca mg/day) |
|---|---|
| 9-18 | 1300 |
| 19-50 | 1000-1200 |

- **Vitamin D**: stimulates absorption of Ca. It is synthesized by action of sunlight on 7-dehydrocholesterol in skin; it may be a hormone. Sunlight changes 7-dehydrocholesterol into vitamin $D_3$ (cholecalciferol). The liver converts it into 25-hydroxycholecalciferol (25-$(OH)D_3$), five times more potent than cholecalciferol ($D_3$). The 25-hydroxycholecalciferol is converted by kidneys to 1,25-dihydroxycholecalciferol (1,25-$(OH)_2D_3$), which is 10 times more potent than D3. Disorders of liver or kidneys impair conversion. Some OP patients have high 25-OH-$D_3$ but low 1,25-$(OH)_2D_3$, signifying kidney impairment. Boron plays a role in kidney conversion. Vitamin $D_3$ at 700 IU/day reduces annual rate of hip fracture by 60%. At 400 IU/day vitamin $D_3$ for 2 years, bone density at hip (femoral neck) increased by 1.9% in the left hip and 2.6% in the right hip. Combined vitamin D and Ca produces slightly better results with 1200 mg/day Ca and 800 IU/day vitamin $D_3$. Vitamin D can be helpful, especially for the elderly in nursing homes, people living away from the equator, and those who do not regularly go outside. Dosage: although earlier research appeared to show that the level of active vitamin $D_3$ does not differ much from 400-800 IU, recent research is showing dosages of 2000 IU/day have substantially better impact. Those with the VDR genetic deficit are being treated with 25,000 IU/D of 1-OH $D_3$. Monitor with serum 1-OH $D_3$.
- **Magnesium (Mg)**: may be as important as Ca supplementation to prevent and treat OP. Women with OP have lower bone Mg than those without OP. Human Mg deficiency is linked to diminished serum levels of most active vitamin D (1,25-$(OH)_2D_3$), also seen in OP. Mechanism: either enzyme responsible for converting 25-$(OH)D_3$ to 1,25-$(OH)_2D_3$ is Mg dependent or Mg mediates PTH and calcitonin secretion. Supplementing at 250-750 mg (as magnesium hydroxide) for 1 year slightly improved BMD.
- **Vitamin $B_6$, folic acid, and vitamin $B_{12}$**: deficiency of these nutrients is common in elderly and may contribute to OP. $B_6$, folate,

and $B_{12}$ act in conversion of methionine to cysteine. Vitamin deficit causes increase in homocysteine, implicated in atherosclerosis and OP (see the chapter on atherosclerosis). Elevated blood homocysteine is seen in PM women and may worsen OP by interfering with collagen cross linking leading to a defective bone matrix. OP entails loss of both organic and inorganic phases of bone; homocysteine theory addresses both factors. Folic acid reduces homocysteine in PM women although none of them were deficient in folic acid according to standard lab criteria. Vitamins $B_6$ and $B_{12}$ help metabolize homocysteine. Combinations of these vitamins produce better results than any one alone.

- **Silicon**: necessary for cross-linking collagen strands, strengthening integrity of connective tissue matrix of bone. Silicon levels are increased at calcification sites in growing bone; recalcification during remodeling may require silicon. In OP patients or when accelerated bone regeneration is desired, silicon requirements may be increased and therefore supplementation may be indicated.
- **Fluoride**: stimulates osteoblastic activity and positive Ca balance. Fluoride is incorporated into crystalline structure of bone as fluorapatite, but bone matrix is poorly formed and weak; long-term excessive exposure makes bones fragile. Therapeutic index for fluoride is quite narrow; at a recommended daily dose of 60-75 mg, sodium fluoride causes side effects in 33%-50% of patients: joint pain, stomach aches, nausea and vomiting—less troublesome if fluoride is taken with meals. Newer preparations such as enteric-coated and timed-release to prevent digestion in stomach give better clinical results with fewer side effects. Fluoride supplementation is not recommended in the treatment of OP.
- **Ipriflavone**: semisynthetic isoflavonoid similar to soy isoflavonoids and approved in Japan, Hungary, and Italy for treatment and prevention of OP. It, has been impressive in clinical studies. Ipriflavone (200 mg t.i.d.) increased BMD measurements by 2% and 5.8% after 6 and 12 months, respectively, in women with OP. Ipriflavone (600 mg/day) produced 6% increase in BMD after 12 months, whereas BMD of control subjects declined by 0.3%. Naturally occurring isoflavonoids like genistein and diadzein in soy may exert similar benefits. Given benefits of soy isoflavonoids against breast cancer, soy foods are encouraged. Mechanism of

action: enhanced calcitonin effects (see above) on Ca metabolism; ipriflavone exerts no estrogenlike effects. Most recent and extensive study has not shown positive results. Ipriflavone may not have an important role in treating OP. It may be more appropriate for women with osteopenia or prevention of OP and not OP treatment. Because of the incidence of decreased lymphocytes and lack of effect, the risk/benefit ratio of ipriflavone must be considered. Ipriflavone may be considered for women for whom other OP treatments are unacceptable, not tolerated, or contraindicated. Monitor BMD to confirm benefit; monitor lymphocyte levels to detect adverse effects.

## THERAPEUTIC APPROACH

OP is a preventable illness if appropriate dietary and lifestyle measures are followed. Building healthy strong bones is lifelong priority. Avoid dietary and lifestyle practices that leach Ca from bone; choose dietary and lifestyle factors that promote bone health.

**Primary goal**: prevention. In severe cases, use recommendations given in this chapter in conjunction with indicated conventional care, including drugs. Bisphosphonates and calcitonin have side effects, but benefits (prevention of hip fracture) often outweigh side effects in severe cases.

- **Exercise**: weight-bearing exercise four times per week plus strength training and/or weight training twice per week.
- **Diet**: avoid dietary factors that promote Ca excretion—salt, sugar, protein, and soft drinks. Increase consumption of green leafy vegetables and soy foods.

### Relative Activities of Vitamin D Forms

| Form | Relative Activity |
|---|---|
| Vitamin $D_3$ | 1 |
| Vitamin $D_2$ | 1 |
| 25-(OH)$D_3$ | 2-5 |
| 25-(OH)$D_2$ | 2-5 |
| 1,25-$(OH)_2D_3$ | 10 |
| 1,25-$(OH)_2D_2$ | 10 |

## Supplements

- **High-potency multiple vitamin/mineral formula**
- **Calcium**: 800-1200 mg q.d. (estimate dietary intake and supplement difference to reach total)
- **Vitamin $D_3$**: 2000-4000 IU q.d.
- **Magnesium**: 400-800 mg q.d.
- **Boron (sodium tetrahydraborate)**: 3-5 mg q.d.

# Otitis Media

## DIAGNOSTIC SUMMARY

### Acute Otitis Media

- Earache or irritability
- History of recent upper respiratory tract infection or allergy
- Red, opaque, bulging eardrum with loss of the normal features
- Fever and chills

### Chronic or Serous Otitis Media

- Painless hearing loss
- Dull, immobile tympanic membrane

## GENERAL CONSIDERATIONS

Otitis media (OM) is inflammation, swelling, or infection of the middle ear. Two types of OM are diagnosed:

- **Acute OM**: usually preceded by upper respiratory tract infection or allergy. Common microorganisms are *Streptococcus pneumoniae* (40%) and *Haemophilus influenzae* (25%).
- **Chronic OM** (also known as serous, secretory, or nonsuppurative OM, chronic OM with effusion; or "glue ear"): constant swelling of middle ear. Acute OM affects two thirds of American children by age 2 years; chronic OM affects two thirds of children younger than 6 years. OM is the most common diagnosis in children and accounts for >50% of all visits to pediatricians. Eight billion dollars are spent annually on medical and surgical treatment.

### Standard Medical Treatment

- Interventions: antibiotics, analgesics (e.g., acetaminophen), and/or antihistamines. If longstanding infection is unresponsive to drugs, surgery is performed that involves placing a tiny plastic myringotomy tube through the eardrum to drain fluid into the throat by the eustachian tube.

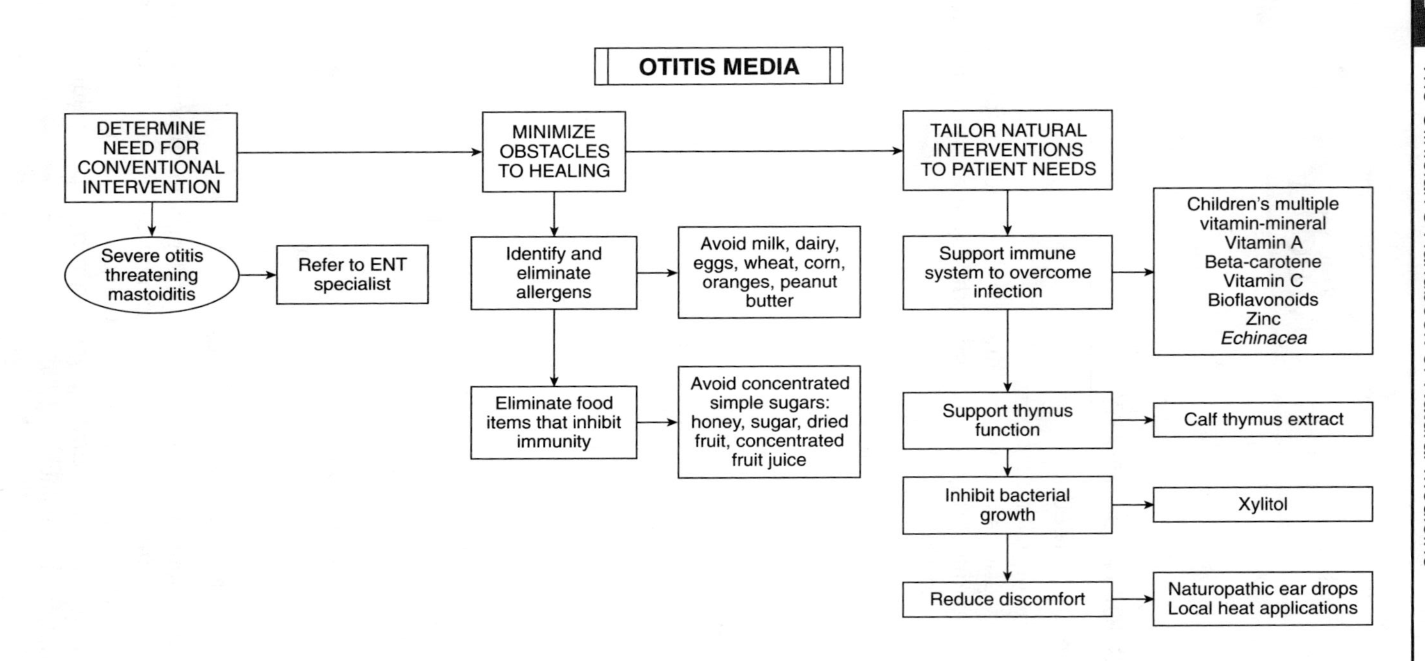
OTITIS MEDIA
DETERMINE NEED FOR CONVENTIONAL INTERVENTION
Severe otitis threatening mastoiditis
Refer to ENT specialist
MINIMIZE OBSTACLES TO HEALING
Identify and eliminate allergens
Avoid milk, dairy, eggs, wheat, corn, oranges, peanut butter
Eliminate food items that inhibit immunity
Avoid concentrated simple sugars: honey, sugar, dried fruit, concentrated fruit juice
TAILOR NATURAL INTERVENTIONS TO PATIENT NEEDS
Support immune system to overcome infection
Children's multiple vitamin-mineral
Vitamin A
Beta-carotene
Vitamin C
Bioflavonoids
Zinc
Echinacea
Support thymus function
Calf thymus extract
Inhibit bacterial growth
Xylitol
Reduce discomfort
Naturopathic ear drops
Local heat applications

- Children with tubes in their ears are more likely to have further problems with OM. Surgery is unnecessary for most children. Only 42% of these surgeries are judged appropriate. No significant differences in clinical course of acute OM have been found between conventional treatments and placebo. No differences have been found between nonantibiotic treatment, ear tubes, ear tubes with antibiotics, and antibiotics alone. Children not receiving antibiotics may have fewer recurrences than those receiving antibiotics because of immune suppression and disturbance of respiratory microflora by antibiotics.
- Results of recent international review: antibiotics are not recommended for OM in most children. Conventional alternative: analgesics (e.g., acetaminophen) and close observation by parent; 80% of children with acute OM respond to placebo within 48 hours. A natural alternative to avoid analgesic toxicity are botanical ear drops (see below).
- Risks of antibiotics: allergic reactions, gastric upset, accelerated bacterial resistance, unfavorable changes in nasopharyngeal bacterial flora. Antibiotics fail to eradicate microbe, may induce middle ear superinfection, and increase return office visits. Concurrent antibiotic and steroid treatment yields poor results.
- Antibiotics induce chronic candidiasis and "superbugs" resistant to antibiotics. They should be used only for underlying systemic infection.
- OM is normally self-limiting. Eighty percent of children's cases spontaneously remit within 2-14 days; children younger than 2 years have a lower spontaneous resolution of 30% after a few days.
- Evaluate each child individually. Follow up: devise physician-family communication before making a decision not to use conventional medicine.
- Special circumstances to prevent hearing loss–induced developmental delays suggest use of ear tubes.
- Pneumococcal and viral vaccines have little benefit because of the multifactorial nature of OM. With risks and complications, vaccinations are warranted at this time for the prevention of otitis media.

## Causes

- Primary risk factors for OM: daycare attendance, wood-burning stoves, parental smoking or exposure to other second-hand smoke, food allergies, not being breastfed, pacifier use.

- Common mechanism is abnormal eustachian tube (ET) function, the underlying cause in virtually all cases of OM.
- ET regulates gas pressure in the middle ear, protects the middle ear from nose and throat secretions and bacteria, and clears fluids from the middle ear. Swallowing opens the ET by action of surrounding muscles. Infants and small children are susceptible to ET problems because of a smaller diameter and more horizontal orientation.
- ET obstruction allows fluid buildup and bacterial infection if immunity is impaired and pathogenic microbes are present. Obstruction results from collapse of tube (weak tissues and/or abnormal opening mechanism), blockage by allergy-induced mucus, mucosal edema, or infection.
- Genetic factors: Monozygotic twins have a higher concordance rate in OM history than do dizygotic twins. No genetic influence has been identified in studies of immunoglobulin markers and human leucocyte antigens.

## THERAPEUTIC CONSIDERATIONS

Treatment goals: ensure ET patency and drainage by identifying and addressing causative factors; support immune system (*Textbook*, "Immune Support"). Bottle feeding: recurrent ear infection is linked to early bottle feeding. Breastfeeding (minimum 3 to 4 months) is protective, possibly because of cow's milk allergy and protective effect of human milk against infection. Bottle feeding while the child is lying on his or her back (bottle propping) leads to regurgitation of bottle contents into the middle ear. Human milk is protective because of its high antibody content inhibiting microbes. Breastfed infants have thymus glands 20 times larger than formula-fed infants.

- **Food allergy**: role of allergy as the major cause of chronic OM has been firmly established in research literature. From 85%-93% of children with OM have allergies: 16% to inhalants only, 14% to food only, 70% to both. Prolonged breastfeeding may prevent OM by avoiding food allergens, particularly if mother avoids sensitizing foods (those to which she is allergic) during pregnancy and lactation. Excluding or limiting foods to which children are commonly allergic (wheat, egg, fowl, dairy), particularly during the first 9 months, also is of value. The child's digestive tract is permeable to antigens, especially during the first 3 months.

Control eating patterns (infrequent repetition of any food, avoid common allergenic foods, and introduce foods in controlled manner—one food at a time, carefully watching for reaction).

- **Allergic reaction**: causes blockage of ET—inflammatory edema of ET mucosa and nasal edema causing Toynbee phenomenon (swallowing with both mouth and nose closed, forcing air and secretions into the middle ear).
- **Chronic OM**: always consider allergy. A total of 93.3% of children tested were allergic to foods, inhalants, or both. Ninety-two percent of children with OM improve when treated with serial dilution titration therapy for inhalants and elimination diet for food allergens. A statistically significant association exists between food allergy and recurrent OM in 78% of patients. Elimination diet ameliorates chronic OM in 86% of patients. Challenge diet with suspected offending food(s) provokes recurrence of serous OM in 94% of patients.
- **Most common food allergens** (in order of frequency): cow's milk, wheat, egg white, peanut, soy, corn, tomato, chicken, apple.
- **Thymus gland extract**: the thymus secretes hormones acting on white blood cells to ensure proper development and function. Oral calf thymus extracts given to children improve immune function, decrease food allergies, and improve resistance to chronic respiratory infections. They may be of particular benefit in chronic OM (*Textbook*, "Food Allergy Testing").
- **Naturopathic herbal ear drops**: otalgia (ear pain) can persist during period of improvement, motivating anxious parents to request unnecessary antibiotics. Naturopathic botanical ear drops are as effective as either antibiotic or anesthetic drops with much less toxicity. Herbal ear drops combination: *Calendula officinalis* flowers (marigold, 28%), *Hypericum perforatum* complete herb (St. John's wort, 30%), and *Verbascum thapsus* flowers (mullein, 25%) in olive oil with essential oils *Allium sativum* (garlic) in 0.05% in olive oil (10%), *Lavandula officinalis* (lavender, 5%), and tocopherol acetate oil (vitamin E, 2%) Dosage: 5 drops t.i.d.
- **Xylitol**: a commonly used sweetener with anticariogenic properties. It is a sugar alcohol derived from birch and other hardwood trees. It inhibits *Streptococcus pneumoniae*. Xylitol reduces acute OM incidence by 40%. It can be given as xylitol (8.4 g/day) chewing gum or lozenge to reduce incidence of OM in daycare centers and schools. Xylitol dosing needs to be four to five times per day, which may decrease compliance and overall efficacy. Side effect is diarrhea.

- **Humidifiers**: are popular treatments for OM and upper respiratory infections in children. Significantly more effusions (fluid in ETs) are observed in lab animals kept in low-humidity environments compared with those kept in more moderate environs. Low humidity may induce nasal swelling and reduce ventilation of ET or may dry ET lining, causing inability to clear fluid and increased secretions. Mast cells of ET mucosa may release histamine and produce edema. Increasing humidity with a humidifier may be an important modality to treat OM with effusion.

## THERAPEUTIC APPROACH

**Goals**: recognize and eliminate allergies, particularly food allergies, and support immune system.

- **Diet**: determining the exact allergen during an acute attack typically is not possible. Eliminate most common allergic foods: milk and dairy, eggs, wheat, corn, oranges, peanut butter. Eliminate concentrated simple carbohydrates (sugar, honey, dried fruit, concentrated fruit juice) that inhibit the immune system.
- **Nutritional supplements**:
  —Children's multiple vitamin/mineral formula
  —Vitamin A: 50,000 IU q.d. for 2 days in children younger than 6 years, and 4 days in children older than 6 years
  —Beta-carotene (natural mixed carotenoids): age in years × 20,000 IU q.d. (up to 200,000 IU q.d.)
  —Vitamin C: age in years × 50 mg every 2 hours
  —Bioflavonoids: age in years × 50 mg every 2 hours
  —Zinc: age in years × 2.5 mg q.d. (up to 30 mg)
  —Thymus extract: equivalent of 120 mg pure polypeptides with molecular weights <10,000 or 500 mg of crude polypeptide fractions daily
- **Botanical medicines**:
  —*Echinacea* spp.: half of adult dosage for children younger than 6 years; full adult dosage for children older than 6 years (*Echinacea* is safe for children); all dosages can be given up to three times daily: dried root (or as tea), 0.5-1 g; freeze-dried plant, 325-650 mg juice of aerial portion of *E. purpurea* stabilized in 22% ethanol: 2-3 mL; tincture (1:5), 2-4 mL; fluid extract (1:1), 2-4 mL; solid (dry powdered) extract (6.5:1 or 3.5% echinacoside), 150-300 mg.

—Xylitol: 8 g/day as either chewing gum chewed throughout day or 10 g of syrup per day in divided doses.

—Naturopathic ear drop formula: 5 drops in affected ear t.i.d.

- **Physical medicine**: local application of heat is often helpful in reducing discomfort; apply as hot pack with warm oil (mullein oil) or by blowing hot air into ear with straw and hair dryer. These tactics help reduce pressure in the middle ear and promote fluid drainage.

# Parkinson's Disease

## DIAGNOSTIC SUMMARY

- Resting tremor (trembling or shaking): usually gets worse when person is at rest and better when person moves. Tremor often begins on one side of the body.
- "Pill rolling" motion of thumb and forefinger.
- Slow movement (bradykinesia) or inability to move (akinesia).
- Difficulty initiating movement.
- Rigid limbs, shuffling gait, stooped posture.
- Reduced or fixed facial expressions ("masked face") and low volume and/or monotone voice.
- Small handwriting (micrographia) that decreases in size toward end of a writing sample.
- Dysphagia may indicate later disease stage.
- Lewy bodies, microscopic protein aggregates, seen only during autopsy, are hallmark of classic Parkinson's disease (PD).

## GENERAL CONSIDERATIONS

- Occurs in 0.3 % of the general population and 1% of the population older than 55 to 60 years. It affects 500,000 people in the United States.
- Progressive neurologic disorder caused by the deterioration of neurons in the brain region that controls muscle movements, causing shortage of neurotransmitter dopamine and leading to movement impairments.
- Features: trembling, muscle rigidity, difficulty walking, problems with balance and coordination.
- Prevalence and incidence rise with age; average age of onset is 60 years; rates are very low in those younger than 40 years and rise in the 70s and 80s.
- Found in many regions of world. True ethnic and/or geographic differences are unclear.

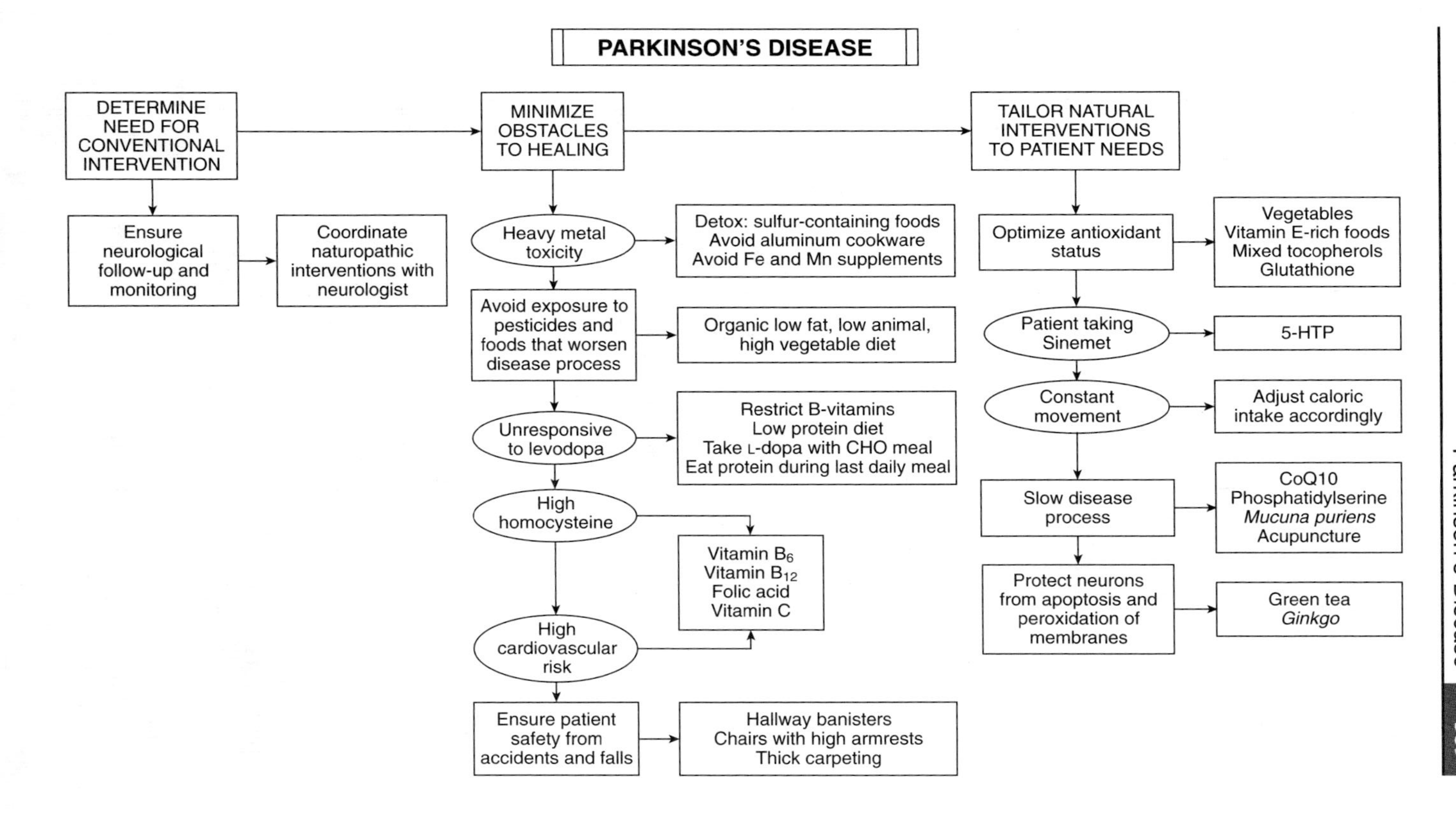
PARKINSON'S DISEASE
DETERMINE NEED FOR CONVENTIONAL INTERVENTION
Ensure neurological follow-up and monitoring
Coordinate naturopathic interventions with neurologist
MINIMIZE OBSTACLES TO HEALING
Heavy metal toxicity
Detox: sulfur-containing foods
Avoid aluminum cookware
Avoid Fe and Mn supplements
Avoid exposure to pesticides and foods that worsen disease process
Organic low fat, low animal, high vegetable diet
Unresponsive to levodopa
Restrict B-vitamins
Low protein diet
Take L-dopa with CHO meal
Eat protein during last daily meal
High homocysteine
High cardiovascular risk
Vitamin $B_6$
Vitamin $B_{12}$
Folic acid
Vitamin C
Ensure patient safety from accidents and falls
Hallway banisters
Chairs with high armrests
Thick carpeting
TAILOR NATURAL INTERVENTIONS TO PATIENT NEEDS
Optimize antioxidant status
Vegetables
Vitamin E-rich foods
Mixed tocopherols
Glutathione
Patient taking Sinemet
5-HTP
Constant movement
Adjust caloric intake accordingly
Slow disease process
CoQ10
Phosphatidylserine
*Mucuna puriens*
Acupuncture
Protect neurons from apoptosis and peroxidation of membranes
Green tea
*Ginkgo*

## Etiology

- Largely unexplained. Suggested pathoses include mitochondrial abnormalities, environmental neurotoxins, selective generation of potential toxins or reduced detoxification capacity, infectious agents, genetic factors.
- Neurons from involved brain regions may be selectively vulnerable because of a heightened propensity to take up endogenous and extrinsic toxins by selective carrier mechanisms—the dopamine transporter.

## Genetics

- Late-onset PD is not linked to genetic susecptibility.
- Onset may involve interaction of genetic and environmental factors.
- Most PD patients do not have family history; only 15% have a first-degree relative with PD.
- Risk of Alzheimer's disease is not increased among relatives of PD patients compared with control subjects.
- Evidence does not support a genetic link between Alzheimer's disease and PD.
- Increased risk for relatives of PD patients: recessive or oligogenic inheritance—interaction of two or more genes is needed.
- Mutations in five genes: alpha-synuclein, parkin, ubiquitin carboxy-terminal hydrolase L1, DJ-1, and NR4A2. Six loci are linked to PD. Most of these genes are linked to early-onset PD—a small percentage of cases.
- Genetic variations do not explain intermittent cases of late-onset PD.
- Genetic mutations in late-onset cases show no clinical correlation with disease states compared with PD patients without mutations.
- Results of twins studies: compared with other complex diseases, genetic effects are low in PD.
- Strategy: prevent and treat environmental factors and lifestyle and nutritional factors.

## Apoptosis

- Loss of brain neurons is a pathologic feature of Parkinson's, Alzheimer's, and Huntington's diseases as well as amyotrophic lateral sclerosis (Lou Gehrig's disease).
- Elevated apoptosis arises from deficits in nerve growth factor and free radical damage.

- Long-term delivery of nerve growth factors can protect against programmed cell death.
- Some natural therapeutics that may decrease programmed cell death—melatonin (see melatonin on p. 598).

## Toxic Exposure

- Implicated in etiology and hasten disease onset of PD: being exposed to pesticides, living in rural areas of industrialized countries, drinking well water.
- Chronic, systemic inhibition of mitochondrial complex I by lipophilic pesticide rotenone can cause highly selective nigrostriatal dopaminergic degeneration, linked behaviorally with hypokinesia and rigidity. Nigral neurons in rotenone-treated rats accumulate fibrillar cytoplasmic inclusions that contain ubiquitin and alpha-synuclein—major constituents of intracellular protein inclusions forming Lewy bodies and Lewy neuritis in dopaminergic neurons of substantia nigra. Long-term rotenone exposure can increase nitric oxide and lipid peroxidation products in the brain cortex and striatum and mimic PD symptoms (akinesia and rigidity) in rats.
- Patients develop parkinsonism after exposure to 1-methyl-4-phenyl-1,2,3,6-tetrahydropyridine (MPTP), a neurotoxic product of pesticide production and contaminant found in synthetic heroin. MPTP crosses the blood-brain barrier, selectively enters dopaminergic cells, and inhibits mitochondrial complex 1 function in the respiratory chain. MPTP is only environmental agent directly linked to development of levodopa-responsive parkinsonism, clinically indistinguishable from classic PD. Other chemicals probably do similar damage.
- Solvents: sustained cumulative exposure is key. No evidence has been found of increased risk for those exposed for shorter periods. Pathogeneis may be worsened by older solvents: trichloroethylene, 1,1,1-trichloroethane, carbon tetrachloride, kerosene, white spirit, and acetone.
- Risk increases with occupational exposure to specific metals: manganese, copper, lead, iron, mercury, zinc, and aluminum. Elevated levels of these metals are in the substantia nigra of patients with PD. Several divalent and trivalent cations accelerate alpha-synuclein fibril formation: aluminum, copper(II), iron(III), cobalt(III), and manganese(II). Long-term mercury inhalation is tied to cortical and cerebellar atrophy, dementia, PD syndrome, and ataxia of lower limbs. Manganese induces damage

in the substantia nigra, globus pallidus, and caudate nucleus, with depletion of dopamine and serotonin. It also is linked to psychiatric changes followed by impaired motor activity with muscle rigidity and tremors.
- Iron buildup: linked to neurologic disorders such as Alzheimer's disease, PD, and type I neurodegeneration with brain iron accumulation. Elevated iron, lipid peroxidation, and decreased glutathione (GSH) and superoxide dismutase (SOD) are present in substantia nigra of patients with PD. Iron may trigger dopaminergic neurodegeneration of PD.

### Oxidative Stress and Glutathione Deficiency

- Oxidative stress adds to the pathogenesis of PD. PD patients have 40% less GSH than normal. Suboptimal GSH also is found in presymptomatic PD (incidental Lewy body disease), but GSH depletion is not primary factor.
- GSH deficiency may be common denominator in all parkinsonism with nigral damage. GSH acts as an antioxidant and a redox regulator. GSH depletion affects mitochondrial function by selective inhibition of mitochondrial complex I activity. Damage from GSH depletion may encourage aggregation of defective proteins, causing death of nigral-striatal dopaminergic neurons.
- GSH depletion may enhance susceptibility of substantia nigra to destruction by toxins. Brain GSH replenishment may be a key to therapeutics for PD.

### Detoxification Dysfunction

- Dysfunction of detoxification may underlie chronic neurologic diseases, such as a defective ability to metabolize sulfur-containing xenobiotics. Altered detoxification may render susceptible persons at higher risk for neurotoxicity when exposed to sulfur-containing compounds.
- Genetics is one factor; nutritional and environmental factors also play a role.

## DIAGNOSTIC CONSIDERATIONS

- No diagnostic test can clearly identify PD. PD is diagnosed by a neurologist evaluating symptoms and severity and applying clinical judgment. A therapeutic trial of dopamine with positive response is suggestive. Brain scans help differentiate true PD from vascular parkinsonism. From 25%-40% of patients with PD develop dementia, making differentiation of PD with Lewy bodies and Alzheimer's disease with parkinsonian characteristics difficult. PD may not exhibit classic resting tremor, but an essential tremor, characterized by unilateral postural tremor, mostly in the upper extremities. Key sign of PD: accompanying bradykinesia and rigidity.

- PD is divided into five stages of the Hoehn and Yahr grading of motor dysfunction:
  —Stage 0 = no signs of disease
  —Stage 1 = unilateral disease
  —Stage 1.5 = unilateral plus axial involvement
  —Stage 2 = bilateral disease without impairment of balance
  —Stage 2.5 = mild bilateral disease with recovery on pull test
  —Stage 3 = mild to moderate bilateral disease; some postural instability; physically independent
  —Stage 4 = severe disability; still able to walk or stand unassisted
  —Stage 5 = wheelchair bound or bedridden unless aided
- Lewy bodies in the substantia nigra are a pathologic hallmark of classic PD. They are acidophilic inclusions of cytoplasm with a dense core and peripheral halo associated with diffuse neuronal loss in substantia nigra linked to deficient dopamine production in nigrostriatal pathway. Lewy bodies cannot be a diagnostic criterion; they are only seen during autopsy. But they also are found in people without PD: 8% of people older than 50 years, 13% of people older than 70 years, and 16% of those older than 80 years.
- Unified PD Disease Rating Scale (UPDRS) grades patients on a number of criteria: behavior, activities, motor function, complications, staging by symptoms, and scale of daily living. Neuroimaging tests aid diagnosis (positron emission tomographic scan with 18-fluourodopa, beta-CIT single-photon emission computed tomography). But UPDRS and neurologic examination are sensitive enough to make a diagnosis.
- Differential diagnosis: normal aging, essential tremor, drug-induced parkinsonism, Parkinson-plus syndromes, vascular parkinsonism, and normal pressure hydrocephalus, dopa-responsive dystonia, juvenile-onset Huntington's disease, and pallidopontonigral degeneration.
- Related diagnoses include the following:
  —**Parkinsonism-plus syndrome**: parkinsonism with other abnormal neurologic symptoms. An example is progressive

supranuclear palsy—early symptoms of PD, then later abnormal eye movements, neck dystonia, dysphagia, decreased response to levodopa.

—**Shy-Drager syndrome (multisystem atrophy)**: parkinsonism with autonomic nervous system abnormalities, cranial nerve abnormalities, peripheral polyneuropathy, spasticity, and/or anterior horn cell dysfunction.

—**Drug-induced parkinsonism**: phenothiazines, butyrophenones, reserpine and related hypertensives, manganese poisoning, carbon monoxide poisoning.

## THERAPEUTIC CONSIDERATIONS

### Conventional Medicine

- No conventional therapy can modify the pathologic progression of the PD neurologic degeneration. But PD is somewhat treatable.
- Levodopa (L-dopa) is a mainstay, synthesized by the enzyme tyrosine hydroxylase from food-derived aromatic amino acid tyrosine. Modern treatment combines levodopa with a peripheral decarboxylase enzyme inhibitor to minimize conversion of levodopa to dopamine outside the nervous system. L-Dopa provides only symptomatic relief without altering disease progression, and it loses efficacy with time. L-Dopa side effects: motor complications (fluctuations and dyskinesias), nausea and vomiting, orthostatic hypotension, sedation, hallucinations, delusions, propensity to gamble, and accelerated growth of malignant melanoma. L-Dopa contributes to decreased slow-wave peristaltic activity and impaired digestion. See newer drugs on p. 604.
- Deep brain stimulation (DBS): involves implanting a brain stimulator in certain areas of the brain. Desired effect is to decrease overactivity of excitatory glutamatergic subthalamo-internal pallidum pathway caused by loss of dopaminergic neurons within the substantia nigra. Stimulation may modulate neuronal activity and thus avoid disease-related abnormal neuronal discharges. Candidates for DBS are selected with strict criteria. DBS may control symptoms so drugs can be reduced.
- Fetal nigral transplantation: to restore lost neuronal tissue. Results are mixed, with a high percentage of postsurgical dyskinesias. Stem cells may offer means to restore dopaminergic circuitry.

### Diet

- Detoxification of heavy metals: high sulfur-containing foods such as garlic and onions and water-soluble fibers such as guar gum, oat bran, pectin, psyllium seed.
- Antioxidants: vegetables and fruits.
- PD patients consume fewer raw vegetables, more carbohydrates, less alcohol and coffee, more meat and equivalent protein and fat compared with control subjects. PD patients may have a higher intake of animal fats.
- Recommendation: higher intake of vegetables, low intake of fat.

### Food Source of Levodopa

- Broad beans: give PD patients improved symptom control. Response to *Vicia faba* (fava beans) may be even greater than to levodopa medication. Fava beans contain levodopa: 100-g serving of *V. faba* pods contains 250 mg levodopa, equal to levodopa in one drug formulation. But unsupervised replacement or coadministration of L-dopa with fava beans is not recommended.

### Ketogenic Diets

- Used for 70+ years to stabilize patients with epilepsy.
- D-beta-hydroxybutyrate (DbetaHB): ketone body produced by hepatocytes and astrocytes during diets that are extremely low in carbohydrates and glucose.
- DbetaHB confers partial protection against dopaminergic neurodegeneration and motor deficits in animals. DbetaHB used for two 6-month-old infants with hyperinsulinemic hypoglycemia at 32 g/day was well tolerated over several months. Long-term effects on cell metabolism and mitochondrial function are unknown.

### Low-Protein Diet

- May be useful for patients taking levodopa.
- A diet of 50 g protein per day for men and 40 g protein per day for women, compared with a high-protein diet of 80 g/day for men and 70 g/day for women improved performance scores, tremor, hand agility, and mobility.
- Levodopa absorption is delayed or diminished by dietary amino acids. Eating a majority of protein in the evening also improved symptoms. Recommendation: take levodopa with a high-

carbohydrate meal and delay protein intake until final meal of the day to optimize efficacy of the drug.

### Detoxification

- Nutritional factors that combat heavy metal poisoning: high-potency multiple vitamin/mineral, minerals (calcium, magnesium, chromium), vitamin C, vitamin B complex, sulfur-containing amino acids (methionine, cysteine, taurine) (*Textbook,* "Metal Toxicity: Assessment of Exposure and Retention" and "Urinary Porphyrins for the Detection of Heavy Metal and Toxic Chemical Exposure").

## NUTRITIONAL CONSIDERATIONS

### 5-Hydroxy-L-Tryptophan

- 5-Hydroxy-L-tryptophan (5-HTP) is beneficial only if used in combination with the drug Sinemet (a combination of L-dopa and decarboxylase inhibitor carbidopa). Brain serotonin is decreased in PD, but reduction in dopamine receptors is more severe. In PD, 5-HTP helps counteract negative effects that L-dopa in Sinemet has on sleep and mood. 5-HTP also improves physical symptoms of PD.
- Nine of 10 people with PD have depression as a reflection of serotonin levels. The lower the level of serotonin, the more severe the depression. Starting 5-HTP at 75 mg and increasing by 25 mg every 3 days until depression was relieved, or up to a maximum of 500 mg/day for 4 months gave impressive results in PD patients on Sinemet. Dosage range for response was only 75 to 125 mg.
- CAUTION: increasing serotonin with 5-HTP in patients not taking Sinemet can worsen symptoms of rigidity.

### Antioxidants

- Prevent damage from oxidation and may reduce risk of PD. They slow progression of PD in patients not yet taking drugs. High dosages are required; increasing antioxidant levels in brain tissue is more difficult.
- Pilot study: 3000 mg/day vitamin C and 3200 IU/day of vitamin E over a 7-year period delayed the need for medication for up to 2-3 years longer than in patients not taking antioxidants.
- Prospective study: health care professionals—76,890 women during 14 years and 47,331 men during 12 years—completed dietary and supplement surveys every 2 to 4 years. Results:

vitamin C and carotenoids did not lower PD risk; vitamin E supplements also were not helpful. Yet vitamin E–rich foods in the diet was protective. Dosages or quality of supplements may have been low, whereas quality of antioxidants in foods may have been higher. Furthermore, alpha-tocopherol is the main form in supplements, but beta-, gamma-, and delta-tocopherol are present in food. Gamma-tocopherol is more effective than alpha-tocopherol at inhibiting peroxynitrite-induced oxidation. Furthermore, supplementing only alpha-tocopherol decreases levels of other forms of vitamin E. Food may be best source, but supplements containing mixed tocopherols would be a better choice than cheaper alpha-tocopherol.

### Glutathione

- Combined intravenous and oral GSH replacement is safe and well tolerated and provides ongoing benefit.
- Precursors N-acetylcysteine and alpha-lipoic acid may also be of use.
- GSH is a systemic antioxidant; repletion may help ameliorate PD-related damage in the heart, liver, muscles.
- High-dose vitamin C provides antioxidant-reducing equivalents that conserve GSH.

### B Vitamins, Folic Acid

- Elevated serum homocysteine is linked to increased risk of coronary heart disease, stroke, and dementia. Increased homocysteine has been linked to PD. Cause: therapy with levodopa. Breakdown of levodopa by catechol-*O*-methyltransferase increases homocysteine formation. Management of PD may increase risk of stroke, heart disease, dementia, and accelerated nigral degeneration.
- Pyridoxine (vitamin $B_6$) helps lower homocysteine. But effects of levodopa may be enhanced by low intake of $B_6$; daily doses of 5+ mg of $B_6$ can reverse drug effect. Patients on levodopa are warned to avoid foods containing high amounts of $B_6$. Lowered $B_6$ should be encouraged in those unresponsive to levodopa. But PD patients with high homocysteine and high risk for cardiac disease who are responding well to medicines may consider increasing B vitamins, with careful monitoring for exacerbated PD symptoms.

### Coenzyme Q10

- Ubiquinone (coenzyme Q10 [CoQ10]) is a cofactor in the electron-transport chain of redox reactions that synthesize

adenosine triphosphate (ATP). Used in cardiovascular diseases, AIDS, and cancer, it may also be helpful in neurodegenerative conditions.
- High-dose CoQ10 may slow symptom progression in early PD. At dosages of 300, 600, and 1200 mg/day over a 6-month period, patients on CoQ10 faired significantly better than did a placebo group, with 1200 mg showing greatest results. At 360 mg for 4 weeks, CoQ10, in treated and stable PD patients, gave mild symptomatic benefit and much better improvement of visual defects compared with placebo.
- High doses (1200, 1800, 2400, and 3000 mg/day) of CoQ10 are safe in the short term (2 weeks). Ubiquinone reaches a blood plateau at 2400 mg/day dosage. Although serum levels of CoQ10 are not necessarily lower in PD patients versus healthy control subjects, doses up to 2400mg may have an added benefit for symptomatic patients. Because of the expense of CoQ10, start at 1200 mg dose and ramp it up if benefits are not seen in the first few months.

### Melatonin

- Hormone manufactured from serotonin and secreted by the pineal gland.
- Powerful antioxidant and treatment option for jet lag, sleep problems, and cancer.
- May be protector of neuronal cells by supporting mitochondrial function and preventing apoptosis.
- Directly scavenges oxidants produced during the normal metabolism and indirectly promotes activity of antioxidant enzymes superoxide dismutase and catalase.
- Increases activities and expression of electron transport chain complexes. Melatonin increases ATP production and promotes GSH homeostasis. It may interact with the mitochondrial genome to enhance production of proteins. Melatonin may help prevent neuronal apoptosis.
- Theoretically, melatonin may actually exacerbate symptoms because of its putative interference with dopamine release. But most studies agree that PD is caused by multiple issues of compromised mitochondrial activity in substantia nigra and loss of GSH, oxidative damage, and increased apoptosis. Clinical studies are needed to evaluate efficacy in PD. If melatonin is used, start with low dose (1-5 mg); gradually increase while carefully monitoring symptoms.

### Reduced Nicotinamide Adenine Dinucleotide

- Coenzyme reduced nicotinamide adenine dinucleotide (NADH) enhances endogenous dopamine production by supplying reducing equivalents to rate-limiting, tyrosine hydroxylase–catalyzed step of dopamine synthesis.
- Both intravenous and intramuscular dosed NADH gave a moderate to very good improvement of disability. Effect of NADH depends on dosage and severity of the case. Optimal dosage: 25-50 mg/day.
- Intravenous dosing seems to work better than intramuscular.
- Homovanillic acid in urine increases; this metabolite indicates stimulation of endogenous L-dopamine biosynthesis.
- One 10-mg treatment over a 30-minute period every day for 7 days, in patients also taking levodopa, improved UPDRS scores and significantly increased plasma levodopa.
- More rigorous studies are needed to confirm benefit and elucidate any side effects.

### Phosphatidylserine

- Major phospholipid in the brain, determining integrity and fluidity of cell membranes.
- Low levels of brain phosphatidylserine (PS) are linked to impaired mental function and depression in the elderly.
- Clinically effective in senile dementia; promising treatment for early Alzheimer's disease. It has greater treatment effects in patients with less-severe cognitive deficits.
- PS accelerates slowed electroencephalography in PD patients with senile dementia of Alzheimer's type. It positively affects anxiety, motivation, and affect.
- Deficient phospholipid metabolism may be caused by toxic insult or oxidative stress. Deficiency of methyl donors—S-adenosylmethionine, folic acid, and vitamin $B_{12}$—or essential fatty acids, the brain may not be able to make sufficient PS. Cosupplementation with docosahexanoic acid is advised when using PS from soy sources.
- PS is well absorbed orally.

### Creatine

- Body-building supplement that acts as a temporal and spatial buffer for cytosolic or mitochondrial pools of cellular energy currency ATP and its regulator, adenosine diphosphate.

- Oral creatine monohydrate enhances memory. It is being studied to treat neurologic and neuromuscular disorders and atherosclerosis.
- Oral intake of creatine significantly increases brain creatine levels but has failed to provide consistent improvement in patients with a variety of neurologic disorders.
- Whether creatine intake will prove beneficial to PD patients in the future is doubtful.

## Botanical Medicines

### *Camellia sinensis* (Green Tea)

- Polyphenols penetrate the blood-brain barrier with antioxidant actions, free radical scavenging, iron-chelating properties, (3)H-dopamine and (3)H-methyl-4-phenylpyridine uptake inhibition, catechol-*O*-methyltransferase activity reduction, protein kinase C or extracellular signal-regulated kinases signal pathway activation, and cell survival/cell cycle gene modulation.
- Green tea polyphenols such as (-)-epigallocatechin-3-gallate (EGCG) are being considered as therapeutic agents to alter brain aging processes and serve as neuroprotective agents.
- Clinical data are limited, but several recent studies suggest green tea polyphenols may protect against PD and other neurodegenerative diseases.
- In animal models of PD, both green tea and oral EGCG prevented loss of tyrosine hydroxylase–positive cells in the substantia nigra and tyrosine hydroxylase activity in striatum and prevented neurotoxin-induced elevations in antioxidant enzymes superoxide dismutase and catalase. These treatments also retained striatal levels of dopamine and its metabolite homovanillic acid and inhibited nitric oxide synthetase in the substantia nigra.

### *Ginkgo biloba*

- *Ginkgo biloba* extract (GBE) effects: stabilizes membranes, is an antioxidant, scavenges free radicals, enhances utilization of oxygen and glucose, is an extremely effective inhibitor of lipid peroxidation of cellular membranes.
- No clinical studies in PD exist, but it is proven beneficial in Alzheimer's disease and useful in animal models of PD, where it is protective in vivo and in vitro.
- Mechanism of action: antioxidation and antiapoptosis. It may also help decrease toxicity of levodopa. Levodopa has a neuro-

toxic effect that GBE may inhibit. Researchers have concluded that combined use of GBE with levodopa is advisable to treat PD and may be better than using levodopa alone.

- Dose-response relation is not yet established for human beings, but 240 mg q.d. GBE shows higher rate of treatment response than does 120 mg q.d.
- Safety: adverse event profile of GBE was not different from placebo. Give GBE consistently for 12+ weeks to determine efficacy.

### *Mucuna pruriens*

- In Ayurveda PD, or "kampavata," is seen as an imbalance of vata dosha.
- *Mucuna puriens*: a legume; rich source of antioxidant vitamin E.
- Rat studies: has an antiparkinson effect, perhaps from components other than levodopa or levodopa-enhancing effect.
- Clinical trial: powdered preparation of this legume is called HP-200; a 7.5-g sachet mixed with water and given orally three to six times per day was given to 26 patients taking synthetic levodopa/carbidopa before treatment and 34 not using medications. Results: statistically significant reductions in Hoehn and Yahr stage and UPDRS scores from baseline to end of 12-week treatment. Adverse effects: mild gastrointestinal upset.

### *Piper methysticum* (Kava Kava)

- No side effects reported with standardized kava extracts at recommended levels in clinical studies.
- CAUTION: isolated reports of kava causing onset of parkinsonian symptoms; case reports that kava may interfere with dopamine and worsen PD. Avoid kava in PD patients or those genetically susceptible.

## OTHER THERAPEUTIC CONSIDERATIONS

### Smoking

- Smoking is linked to lower incidence and delayed onset of PD. Nicotine may enhance striatal stimulation of dopaminergic neurons selectively damaged in PD. Inverse association between smoking and PD has been solidly grounded in multicentered, longstanding research.

- Other nonnicotine chemicals in cigarettes may be neuroprotective by decreasing monoamine oxidase B activity and lowering hydrogen peroxide, a byproduct of dopamine metabolism.
- Other explanations: neuroprotective effect of carbon monoxide in cigarette smoke; carbon monoxide is a free radical scavenger. Or it may reduce dietary intake, conferring an advantage.
- Risk/benefit ratio is quite high with smoking; smoking is not a reasonable prevention for PD.

### Estrogen

- Estrogens may modulate activity of dopamine, act as an antiapoptotic agent, and affect neuronal pathways affected in PD.
- Animal studies: estrogens influence synthesis, release, and metabolism of dopamine and may modulate dopamine receptor expression and function.
- Clinical studies: conflicting findings whether PD symptoms may worsen after menopause and whether hormone replacement therapy can be protective. Several variables—age, dose and formulation, timing and length of dosing period—may determine effect. Monitor menstrual pattern correlations to symptoms to make best patient-specific choices for hormone replacement therapy.

### Weak Electromagnetic Fields

- Extracranial treatment with low frequency pico-Tesla magnetic fields may be an effective, safe, and revolutionary modality to manage symptoms.
- Theory: intermittent-pulsed pico-Tesla electromagnetic fields (EMFs) may induce in PD reactivation of reticular-limbic-pineal systems; nondopaminergic systems might be positively affected by weak EMFs.
- Case studies: decreased need for medicines, decreased micrographic symptoms, and return of absent dream recall, all associated with right hemispheric dysfunction.
- Drawback: only one researcher is involved and no follow-up during decade since original work.

### Hypnosis

- Mindset affects severity of most movement disorders, including PD. Symptoms improve with relaxation and are exacerbated by anxiety.

- Case study: hypnosis while monitoring patient with polygraphic electroencephalogram-electromyogram revealed direct correlation between degree of trance and tremor cessation. Effect only lasted a few hours after each session, but clinical gains manifested over 6 months with repeated practice of guided imagery.
- Techniques used during trance: role-play time distortion was most effective in halting tremors.

## THERAPEUTIC APPROACH

Diagnosis: besides standard neurologic rating scales and imaging, serum iron, ferritin, and total iron binding identify iron overload. Rule out blood homocysteine. Careful history and testing for heavy metal and pesticide toxicities.

### Dietary Recommendations

- Eat a low-fat, low-animal, and high-fiber vegetable diet.
- Eat vitamin E–rich foods: sunflower seeds, almonds, chard, mustard greens, broccoli, olives, kale, turnip greens, and papaya.
- Avoid foods high in pesticides and attempt to eat organic foods exclusively.
- To detoxify heavy metals, eat high sulfur–containing foods—garlic, onions, and eggs—plus water-soluble fibers: guar gum, oat bran, pectin, and psyllium seed.
- Patients taking levodopa: lower protein intake (50 g q.d. for men and 40 g q.d. for women); take medication with a high-carbohydrate meal and delay protein intake until the final meal of the day to optimize therapeutic efficacy of medication.
- Because of constant movement, weight loss may be an issue; adjust caloric intake to specific patient needs.

### Lifestyle Recommendations

- Avoid cooking in aluminum pots.
- Banisters along walls and chairs with higher arms ease the ability to walk through halls and sit.
- Thick carpeting may be helpful to avoid falls.

### Nutritional Supplementation

- Avoid iron and maganese supplements.
- 5-HTP: 75 to 125 mg q.d. in patients taking Sinemet (levodopa plus carbidopa). Those not on this drug should avoid 5-HTP.

- Vitamin C: 3000 mg q.d.
- Vitamin E: 1000 IU q.d. mixed tocopherols. Avoid supplements that are solely alpha-tocopherol.
- Glutathione: orally and/or intravenously.
- Restrict B vitamins in patients who are levodopa unresponsive to see if drug treatment efficacy improves. B vitamins and folic acid may be increased in patients with high homocysteine levels and those at greater cardiac risk along with careful monitoring of PD symptoms.
- CoQ10: 1200-2400 mg q.d.
- Phosphatidylserine: 100 mg t.i.d.

## Botanical Medicines

- **Green tea**: 3 cups q.d. or 3 g of soluble components providing 240-320 mg polyphenols. For green tea extract standardized for 80% total polyphenol and 55% epigallocatechin gallate content: 300-400 mg q.d.
- ***Ginkgo biloba* extract**: 240 mg q.d. for 12+ weeks.
- ***Mucuna pruriens***: 7.5 g mixed with water and given orally three to six times per day.

## Conventional Medications

- **Sinemet**: is a combination of L-dopa and carbidopa.
- **Amantadine (Symmetrel)**: modulates motor fluctuations; is a dopamine receptor agonist.
  —Other dopamine receptor agonists: bromocriptine, pergolide, pramipexole, ropinirole.
- **Tolcapone (Tasmar) or entacapone (Comtan)**: inhibit dopamine breakdown.
- **Anticholinergic drugs**: for resting tremor.
- **Clozapine**: for levadopa-induced dyskinesias.

(Note: All these medications can produce hallucinations and daytime somnolence.)

# Pelvic Inflammatory Disease

## DIAGNOSTIC SUMMARY

- Dyspareunia.
- Mucopurulent cervical discharge.
- Pelvic pain; bilateral adnexal tenderness.
- Palpable adnexal mass.
- Elevated temperature (>101° F).
- Cervical motion tenderness.
- White blood cell count 20,000/µL, with marked leukocytosis and/or elevated sedimentation rate
- *Neisseria gonorrhea* and *Chlamydia trachomatis* most common, followed by *Ureaplasma urealyticum, Mycoplasma hominis, Streptococcus* spp., *Escherichia coli, Haemophilus influenzae, Peptostreptococcus,* and *Peptococcus*.*
- Transvaginal ultrasound showing thickened, fluid-filled tubes or tubo-ovarian mass.
- Acute and chronic endometritis on endometrial biopsy.
- Laparoscopy is the gold standard.
- New Centers for Disease Control and Prevention (CDC) recommendations are that all sexually active adolescents undergo routine screening for *Chlamydia* during annual pelvic examinations.
- CDC also recommends that routine screening of asymptomatic women between ages 20 and 24 years should be considered, particularly if she has a new male sexual partner, has more than one male sexual partner, or does not use barrier contraception.

---

*Testing methods for *Neisseria gonorrhea* and *Chlamydia* include cell culture (gold standard), direct fluorescent antibody testing, enzyme immunoassay antigen detection technique, nucleic acid hybridization tests (DNA probes), nucleic acid amplification (polymerase chain reaction or ligase chain reaction), and the newer ThinPrep Pap collection system (Cytyc Corporation, Marlborough, Mass.).

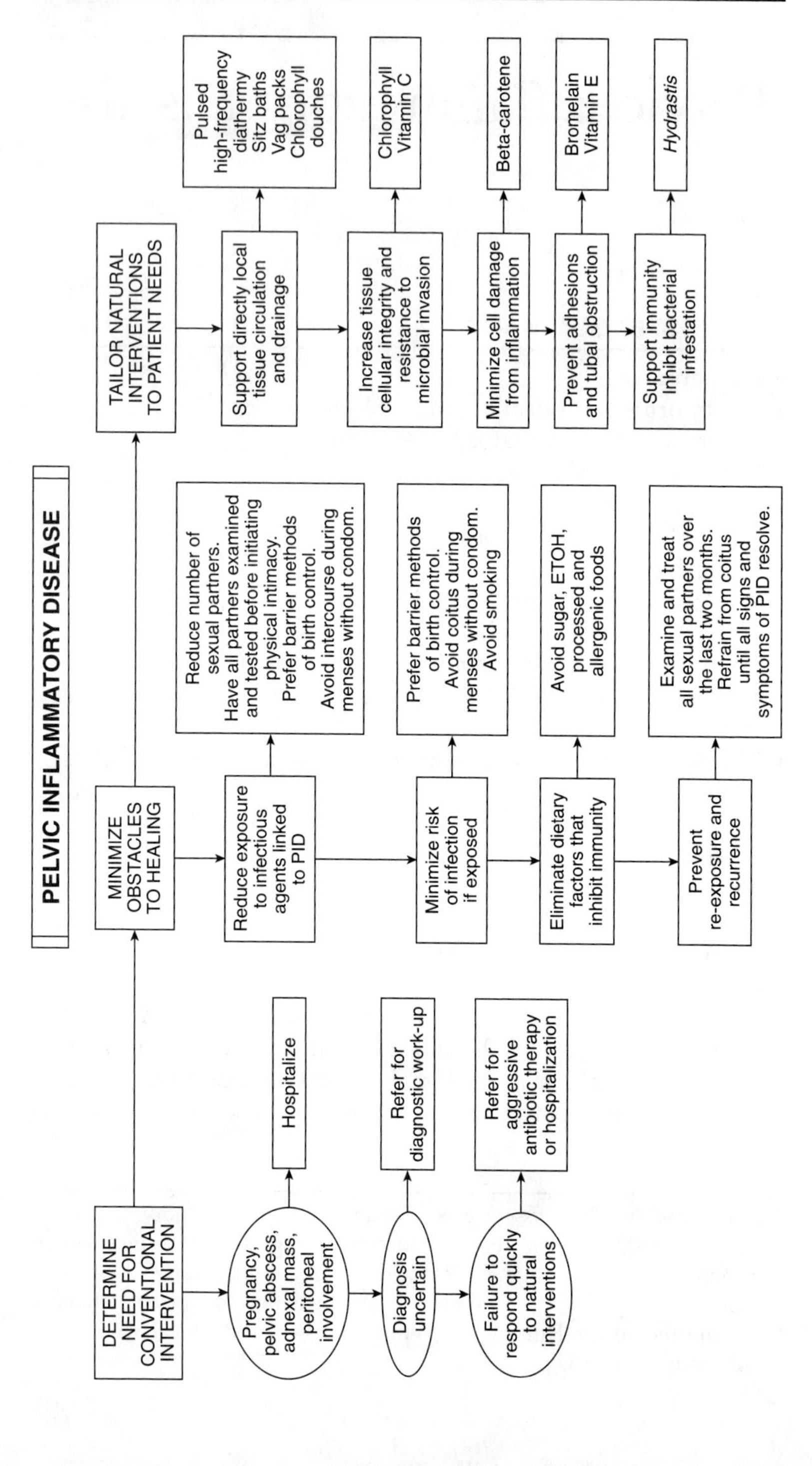
PELVIC INFLAMMATORY DISEASE
DETERMINE NEED FOR CONVENTIONAL INTERVENTION
Pregnancy, pelvic abscess, adnexal mass, peritoneal involvement
Hospitalize
Diagnosis uncertain
Refer for diagnostic work-up
Failure to respond quickly to natural interventions
Refer for aggressive antibiotic therapy or hospitalization
MINIMIZE OBSTACLES TO HEALING
Reduce exposure to infectious agents linked to PID
Reduce number of sexual partners. Have all partners examined and tested before initiating physical intimacy. Prefer barrier methods of birth control. Avoid intercourse during menses without condom.
Minimize risk of infection if exposed
Prefer barrier methods of birth control. Avoid coitus during menses without condom. Avoid smoking
Eliminate dietary factors that inhibit immunity
Avoid sugar, ETOH, processed and allergenic foods
Prevent re-exposure and recurrence
Examine and treat all sexual partners over the last two months. Refrain from coitus until all signs and symptoms of PID resolve.
TAILOR NATURAL INTERVENTIONS TO PATIENT NEEDS
Support directly local tissue circulation and drainage
Pulsed high-frequency diathermy
Sitz baths
Vag packs
Chlorophyll douches
Increase tissue cellular integrity and resistance to microbial invasion
Chlorophyll
Vitamin C
Minimize cell damage from inflammation
Beta-carotene
Prevent adhesions and tubal obstruction
Bromelain
Vitamin E
Support immunity
Inhibit bacterial infestation
Hydrastis

## GENERAL CONSIDERATIONS

Pelvic inflammatory disease (PID) is a categorical name for a range of pelvic infections and inflammations. The CDC defines PID as abdominal and adnexal tenderness and cervical motion tenderness in the absence of another definable cause of symptoms. Diagnosis does not require elevated white blood cell (WBC) count, erythrocyte sedimentation rate (ESR), or fever. Salpingitis is a particular condition under PID (adnexa always involved by definition); noninfectious states (pelvic adhesions and chronic salpingitis) also are included. PID leads to 2.5 million outpatient visits annually in the United States. Twenty-five percent of patients have serious long-term sequelae with risk of recurrence. Risk of ectopic pregnancy increases sixfold after one episode of PID. PID carries a 13% risk of infertility after one infection and a 70% risk after three.

### Etiology

Organisms listed above are implicated in the etiology of PID; *Neisseria gonorrhoeae* and *Chlamydia trachomatis* are the most common. Asymptomatic chlamydial infections are a major cause of PID. A higher proportion of PID cases are ascribed to *C. trachomatis* than to *N. gonorrhea*.

- ***N. gonorrhea*** **(GC)**: a delicate and fastidious species with high infectivity, preferring human columnar and transitional epithelia. In less than 1 hour after intercourse GC can establish itself on the urethral mucosa, resisting the flow of urine. Favored sites in the lower female genital tract are Bartholin's and Skene's glands, urethra, and endocervical canal. Spreading occurs from the endocervix across endometrium to tubal mucosa or by migration through subendothelial vascular and lymphatic channels. The most common method of spreading is vector; GC attached to spermatozoa are physically carried to the fallopian tubes. Retrograde menstruation or uterine contractions during intercourse are other modes of dissemination. Acute state: GC and polymorphonuclear leukocytes accumulate in subepithelial connective tissue, causing patchy destruction of overlying mucosa. Consequent mucosal thinning may facilitate GC penetration into deeper tissue; GC survive only a short time in the fallopian tubes. Descent of the microbe beyond surfaces being examined makes it difficult to detect. Concomitant infections occur; the primary role of GC is paving the way for secondary invaders from normal vaginal flora. *C. trachomatis* and anaerobic bacteria superinfections are possible.

- ***C. trachomatis* (CT)**: 20%-30% of PID cases are caused by CT; acute chlamydial PID may be subclinical or silent in 66%-75% of cases. Lab diagnosis is difficult. It is frequently asymptomatic.
- **Anaerobes**: most commonly isolated from fallopian tubes or cul-de-sacs of PID patients. They are probably not the chief causative agents, but opportunists commonly found in immunocompromised hosts. They generally are of endogenous origin; cervixes and vaginas of normal healthy women contain anaerobes and aerobes. Anaerobic infections are more common in older patients and women with a history of prior PID.
- **Other organisms**: facultative aerobic organisms in tuboperitoneal fluids from women with salpingitis include coliforms, *Haemophilus influenzae*, streptococci, and *Mycoplasma hominis*. *M. hominis* is a common agent of polymicrobial milieu of PID, present in 81% of female patients with GC and 64% of those without.

## Complications

Sequelae of PID are abdominal pain, infertility, ectopic pregnancy, dyspareunia. Dyspareunia often is not investigated but is frequently found in the post-PID sufferer.

- Death from salpingitis is rare and generally from rupture of tubo-ovarian abscess with subsequent peritonitis, with mortality rate of 5.2%-5.9% for tubo-ovarian abscesses.
- Fitz-Hugh–Curtis syndrome: perihepatitis complicating primary PID. It has characteristic violin-string adhesions attaching liver to abdominal wall. Adhesions are from local peritonitis involving the anterior liver surface and adjacent abdominal wall. CT is a more frequent cause than GC.
- Infertility: PID puts women at risk for recurrence. After fallopian tubes are damaged by infection, normal defense mechanisms are impaired. Reinfection is the most important cause of infertility after PID.
- Ectopic pregnancy: sevenfold to tenfold increased risk.

## Risk Factors

These include sexual contact, age, use or history of use of intrauterine device (IUD), previous history of PID, earlier "sexual debut," especially with multiple sexual partners.

- Risk in sexually active 15-year-olds is 1 in 8; in average 24-year-olds, the risk is 1 in 80. Cervical mucus in younger women may be estrogen dominated, creating an environment more accessible to pathogens.

- Women with multiple partners have a 4.6-fold greater risk than do monogamous women.
- IUDs increase risk. Oral contraceptive (OC) users have less risk of GC but more risk for CT invasion. Barrier methods of birth control decrease PID risk (women with vasectomized partners may have less risk).
- Iatrogenic: the following invasive procedures may introduce pathogens or disturb tract flora and induce PID: cervical dilation, abortion, curettage, tubal insufflation, hysterosalpingography, insertion of IUD. PID may not strictly be a sexually transmitted disease (STD).

### Pathogen Access to Upper Female Tract

Menstruation, sperm, and trichomonads help transport pathogens into the salpinx.

- Infections occurring around menses tend to be GC rather than CT. Menstrual regurgitation may carry sloughed endometrium with attached GC or intracellular CT that proliferate in tubal epithelium or on peritoneal surfaces.
- Human sperm: bacteriospermia is a cause of infertility in men; 66%-75% of men who tested positive for GC were asymptomatic. Sperm are vectors. Cervical mucus is an effective mechanical and immunologic barrier between flora of the vagina and upper tract. Yet organisms attached to sperm can easily traverse mucus column. Sperm migrate through menstrual plasma but not during the luteal phase or through cervical mucus of pregnancy. Sperm is intimately associated with cytomegalovirus, *Toxoplasma, Ureoplasma urealyticum,* and *Chlamydia.*
- Motile trichomonads are another transporter, ascending from the vagina to the fallopian tubes, carrying additional invaders. Key observation: trichomonads are never isolated from human beings when heavy bacterial contamination is absent.

## DIAGNOSIS

Pelvic or lower abdominal pain is the most dependable symptom of PID, but it is not specific. Rebound tenderness is not reliable; cervical motion tenderness and adnexal tenderness are much more common. Clinical picture is misleading; many patients with PID have atypical signs and symptoms. Some have no signs and symptoms at all.

### Common Signs and Symptoms in Acute PID

| Symptom | Incidence (%) |
|---|---|
| Lower abdominal pain | 90 |
| Adnexal tenderness on palpation | 90 |
| Pain on movement of the cervix | 90 |
| Vaginal discharge | 55 |
| Adnexal mass or swelling | 50 |
| Fever or chills | 40 |
| Irregular vaginal bleeding | 35 |
| Anorexia, nausea, and vomiting | 25 |

- Patients with GC may appear more toxic and febrile with leukocytosis. CT PID may give elevated ESR. Most GC PID occurs at or shortly after menses. GC PID has a more severe clinical picture, but tissue damage and long-term sequelae can be more severe in CT. Many infections are mixed.
- Putrid discharge yields anaerobes; an offensive odor is diagnostic of anaerobic infection and indicative of well-developed PID, with opportunistic anaerobes following primary invaders.

### Differential Diagnosis of PID

- Acute appendicitis
- Acute cholecystitis
- Acute pyelonephritis
- Ectopic pregnancy
- Endometriosis
- Hemorrhagic ovarian cysts
- Intrauterine pregnancy
- Mesenteric lymphadenitis
- Ovarian cyst with torsion
- Ovarian tumor
- Pelvic thrombophlebitis
- Septic abortion

NOTE: Potentially lethal conditions: ectopic pregnancy, tubo-ovarian abscess, ovarian cyst rupture with hemorrhage, appendicitis.

- Fitz-Hugh–Curtis syndrome: symptoms from upper right quadrant in sexually active women may be an indirect sign of genital infection. Pain has sudden onset, overshadowing underlying PID.
- Rupture of tubo-ovarian abscess: sudden severe exacerbation of pain. Pain is referred to side of rupture, followed by generalized peritonitis and collapse. Shoulder pain is possible. Pulse is elevated out of proportion to fever, up to 170 beats/min. Surgery within 12 hours is required or death is probable.
- Careful history: STDs, birth control methods, sexual activity, recent medical procedures, and nature and onset of symptoms. Evaluate source, severity, and characteristics of pelvic and abdominal pain. Look for mucopurulent cervicitis. Culture cervix for GC and CT.

## Laboratory Diagnosis

Lab findings during active PID are inconsistent. Organisms found in different sectors of the female genitourinary tract are poorly correlated. Pathogens in the cervix often are not found in adnexa. GC from peritoneum is not found in the upper tract. PID results from infection of endometrium and fallopian tubes by a wide array of bacteria, often in synergistic combination; inaccessible site of infection makes microbiologic confirmation difficult. Use conservative search.

- Invasive sampling of exudate and tissue only warranted as last resort; diagnostic laparoscopies have death rate of 5.2/100,000 and major complications in 4.6/1000 procedures.
- Upper tract culture by cervical entrance with a double-lumen, catheter-protected brush is the most recent and least invasive technique, but it is poorly correlated and frequently compromised by lower tract contamination.
- Complete blood count and ESR are essential. ESR in pregnancy is elevated from increased plasma fibrinogen and globulin. ESR is increased in anemia because of a higher plasma/erythrocyte ratio. Suspect infection with ESR >35 in the absence of pregnancy and anemia.
- C-reactive protein (CRP): local inflammatory reaction follows cell death in internal organs, inducing increased synthesis of series of plasma proteins. C-reactive protein is an acute-phase reactant that increases 1-2 days after any tissue injury affecting more than epithelial layer. Increased CRP is quantitatively matched with

degree of tissue injury. This nonspecific test does not stand alone; it must be evaluated by WBC count and ESR.

- Endocervical smears and cultures are potentially misleading.
- Culture of endocervical sampling is preferred when diagnosis is problematic and in cases of suspected sexual assault. Main advantage: highly specific, and organisms can be preserved for additional testing.
- Urinalysis helps with differential diagnosis.
- Serum human chorionic gonadotropin: to rule out pregnancy.
- Abdominal and/or transvaginal ultrasound: to rule out ectopic pregnancy.
- Other tests:
  —Enzyme immunoassay
  —Direct fluorescent antibody
  —Nucleic acid probes
  —Nucleic acid amplification techniques (polymerase chain reaction and ligase chain reaction)
  —Liver enzymes not elevated with chlamydial perihepatitis; the parenchyma are not involved.
  —Infections are polymicrobial. Mixed infections are common; isolation of particular microbe from the cervix does not prove it is the sole etiologic agent. Isolation does not rule out other organisms.

## THERAPEUTIC CONSIDERATIONS

- Hospitalization is recommended for surgical emergency or suspected sepsis, pregnancy, failure to respond to oral antibiotics, suspicion of tubo-ovarian abscess, adnexal masses, or peritoneal involvement. Refer if diagnosis is uncertain or surgical emergency threatens. Give antibiotic therapy plus supportive therapies if patient's clinical and lab status can be reassessed in 48-72 hours. Lab values and objective patient criteria should direct all acute-phase treatment. CDC guidelines: "Most experts encourage hospitalization and treatment with intravenous antibiotics."
- Antibiotics: broad-spectrum regimens tailored to clinical severity and lab findings, patient compliance, cost and availability of medicines. CDC outpatient recommendations (August 2000) are:
  —Ceftriaxone 500 mg intramuscularly plus doxycycline 100 mg orally b.i.d. for 14 days or ofloxacin 400 mg orally b.i.d. for 14 days.

—Consider adding metronidazole to either regimen for better anaerobic coverage. Always add metronidazole for women with bacterial vaginosis and for immunosuppressed women. Reexamine patient in 72 hours to ascertain improvement.

Antibiotics are not always curative. Antibiotic resistance is increasing rapidly; 15% of women with PID do not respond to primary antimicrobial treatment, 20% have at least one recurrence, and 15% are rendered infertile. Fundamental approach of combining immune enhancement and nontoxic therapies is more sound. But no evidence-based therapies exclusively using natural therapies for the treatment of PID are available. Antibiotics, herbal or pharmaceutical, can help in the first phase of treatment but are insufficient intervention for devastating sequelae.

## Physical Medicine

- **Diathermy**: pulsed high-frequency diathermy is quite beneficial in PID. Pulsing electric energy of short duration (65 μs every 1600 ms) at a high intensity achieves desired therapeutic result without hyperpyrexia associated with diathermy. Local recovery is enhanced, reticuloendothelial system is stimulated, and gamma-globulin fractions are increased.
- **Sitz baths**: contrast sitz bath increases pelvic circulation and drainage, stimulates influx of macrophages, and decongests pelvic inflammatory reaction (*Textbook,* "Hydrotherapy").

## Nutritional Supplements

- **Chlorophyll derivatives**: these are cell-stimulating agents that regenerate tissues. They enhance production of hemoglobin and red blood cells and are nontoxic. They increase resistance of cells so that enzymatic digestion of cell membranes by invading bacteria or their toxins is checked. They are theorized to break down carbon dioxide, resulting in liberation of oxygen that inhibits anaerobic bacteria. Careful vaginal douching with chlorophyll is recommended in every case of PID to forestall or diminish anaerobes and encourage cervical and possibly upper tract healing. These tissues must be healed to reduce risk of infertility or ectopic pregnancy. Discharge from several leukorrhea cases was cleared up in almost every instance with a few applications of chlorophyll.
- **Vitamin C**: antiinflammatory effects help decrease tissue destruction. Vitamin C supports collagen tissue repair that helps prevent

spread of infection (important in GC spread through subepithelial connective tissue, disorganizing collagen matrix). Fibrinolytic activity helps prevent pelvic scarring.

- **Beta-carotene**: the normal ovary has high beta-carotene. Maintain optimal carotene to optimize defense against nearby inflammation. It potentiates beneficial effects of interferon and enhances antibody response and WBC activity. It is an antioxidant, limiting cell damage from inflammation (*Textbook,* "Beta-carotene and Other Carotenoids").
- **Bromelain**: adnexal exudate in PID frequently suppurates to form abscesses. Alleviating tissue irritation during initial stages allows resorption of exudate with fewer adhesions. Adhesions form as exudate lingers because structures are overwhelmed by inflammation. Agglutination of villous fold in lumen of the tube may cause scarring and tubal occlusion. Bromelain activates fibrinolysis, diminishing sequelae of exudates. It has antimicrobial properties and penetrates the salpinx (*Textbook,* "Bromelain).

## Botanical Medicines

- **Vaginal depletion packs**: recommended to promote drainage of exudate from involved tissues. They may also stimulate immune cells within the vagina to provide first line of defense (*Textbook,* "Vaginal Depletion Pack").
- ***Hydrastis canadensis* (goldenseal)**: immune-potentiating. It has specific antichlamydial properties. The general antibacterial nature of goldenseal justifies its use in PID. It is trophorestorative to mucous membranes; use throughout the rehabilitation period (*Textbook, "Hydrastis canadensis* [Goldenseal] and Other Berberine-Containing Botanicals").
- ***Symphytum officinale* (comfrey)**: a soothing demulcent best used in the second phase of treatment. The allantoin content encourages cell regeneration. (Note: Only preparations from the aerial portion should be used.)

## Prevention

Woman with no history of PID need to be concerned about asymptomatic male carriers of STDs. Choice of birth control method is pivotal. Barrier methods of contraception reduce risk of PID.

- **OCs**: inhibit GC. Some researchers suggest OC use after first episode of PID to prevent recurrence. Estrogens create thicker cervical plug and protective against GC. OCs decrease length and volume of menstrual flow, thus decreasing exposure of GC to this culture medium. OCs may give higher risk of CT. Progesterone induces hyperplasia and hypersecretion, producing cervical eversion, exposing endocervical columnar epithelium, a target tissue of CT. Estradiol may suppress endocervical antibodies necessary to resolve CT. Estrogen-treated individuals may have higher number of infected cervical cells and longer duration of infection. Because women are not selectively exposed to GC versus CT, OCs are not recommended.

- **IUDs**: are associated with a small increased risk of PID, especially in the first four months of use. IUDs are an STD disaster; they allow bacterial colonization on the surface while reducing local immunologic capacity. If a woman with suspected PID has an IUD, it needs to be removed 12-24 hours after initiation of antibiotic therapy to prevent spread of infection during its removal. IUDs are not recommended.
- **Barrier methods**: excellent choices to prevent PID. Condom is preferred to cervical protectors; sperm reach the vaginal vault more rarely.
- **Douching**: avoid haphazard douching; it disturbs vaginal flora. All forms of douching increase risk of PID and cause organisms to ascend into the upper genital tract. Use with caution; PID has been correlated to frequency of douching; those who douched 3+ times per month were 3.6 times more likely to get PID than those who douched less than once per month.

## Intercourse During Menses

- Intercourse during menses is not recommended unless a condom is used. GC risk is increased by the loss of the protective cervical mucus plug and the prevalence of blood, a medium of choice for GC. The endometrium also is thought to offer local protection against bacterial invasion, and this layer is being sloughed off during menses.
- Smoking: current and former smokers, compared with those who have never smoked, have increased risk of PID. Women who smoke 10+ cigarettes daily have a higher risk than those who smoke less.
- Patient education: review signs and symptoms of PID with all sexually active women. Encourage early intervention if clinical picture of PID appears.

## THERAPEUTIC APPROACH

Two phases of treatment: (1) eliminate all pathogens and normalize adnexal microflora, and (2) rehabilitate damaged tissues. Avoid intercourse until all signs and symptoms have resolved and male partners have been examined and treated. All partners during 2 months before illness must be examined and treated. Increase bed rest. These therapies are adjunctive to appropriate antibiotic treatment and immune support. CAUTION: referral for aggressive antibiotic treatment or hospitalization is mandatory if patient does not respond quickly.

- **Diet**: limit all dietary inhibitors of immunity (sugar, alcohol, processed and allergenic foods) during both phases of treatment.
- **Supplements**:
  - —Beta-carotene: 100,000 IU q.d. for 2+ months
  - —Vitamin E: 400 IU q.d. for 3 months
  - —Vitamin C: 500 mg q.i.d. during first week of treatment, then decrease over a 3-day period to 250 mg t.i.d.
  - —Chlorophyll: 10 mg of fat/oil soluble q.i.d. for 1 month
  - —Bromelain: 250 mg (potency 1800 milk clotting units [MCU]) q.i.d. for first week and t.i.d. for 6 weeks
- **Botanical medicines**:
  - —*Symphytum officinale* (aerial portion only and after the acute phase): 500 mg freeze-dried herb t.i.d.; 1:1 fluid extract, 30 drops b.i.d.
  - —*Hydrastis canadensis*: 400 mg solid extract t.i.d. during acute phase; 200 mg t.i.d. during recovery
  - —Chlorophyll: douches alternating with vaginal packs
  - —Vaginal packs: daily during acute phase until adequate clinical and lab response; after acute phase, vaginal packs three times per week, alternating with chlorophyll douches for 3 weeks.
- **Physical medicine**:
  - —Diathermy: pulsed, high-intensity diathermy for 10 minutes over suprapubic area, 10 minutes over liver, and 10 minutes in area of left adrenal (the right being presumably stimulated with the liver).
  - —Sitz baths: one to two times per day throughout acute phase; contrast sitz baths are given in groups of three alterations of hot to cold; two separate tubs are necessary to facilitate this process. The hot should be 105°-115° F, the cold 55°-85° F, with the temperatures dependent on the strength of the

patient. Standard treatment is 3 minutes hot and 30 seconds cold; the water level in the hot tub is set 2.5 cm higher than in the cold. Adequate draping is necessary to prevent chilling. As with all hydrotherapy treatments, always finish with the cold.

# Peptic Ulcers

## DIAGNOSTIC SUMMARY

- Epigastric distress 45-60 minutes after meals or nocturnal pain; both are relieved by food, antacids, or vomiting.
- Epigastric tenderness and guarding.
- Symptoms chronic and periodic.
- Gastric analysis shows acid in all cases, with hypersecretion in approximately half the patients with duodenal ulcers.
- Ulcer crater or deformity usually occurring at the duodenal bulb (duodenal ulcer) or pylorus (gastric ulcer) on radiograph or fiberoptic examination.
- Positive test for occult blood in stool.

## GENERAL CONSIDERATIONS

Peptic ulcers (PUs) occur in the stomach (gastric) and first portion of the small intestine (duodenal). Duodenal ulcers are more common; the prevalence is 6%-12% in the United States. Ten percent of the U.S. population has clinical evidence of duodenal ulcer during their lifetimes. PU is four times more common in men than women and four to five times more common than benign gastric ulcer.

- Most PUs are associated with abdominal discomfort 45-60 minutes after meals or during the night described as gnawing, burning, cramplike, aching, or heartburn. Eating or antacids usually give great relief. In the elderly, presentation may be subtle and atypical compared with younger patients, leading to a delay in diagnosis.
- Duodenal ulcer (DU) and gastric ulcer (GU) result from similar mechanisms—specifically, some influence damaging protective factors lining the stomach and duodenum.
- Gastric acid is corrosive with a pH of 1-3. Lining of the stomach and small intestine is protected by a layer of mucin; constant

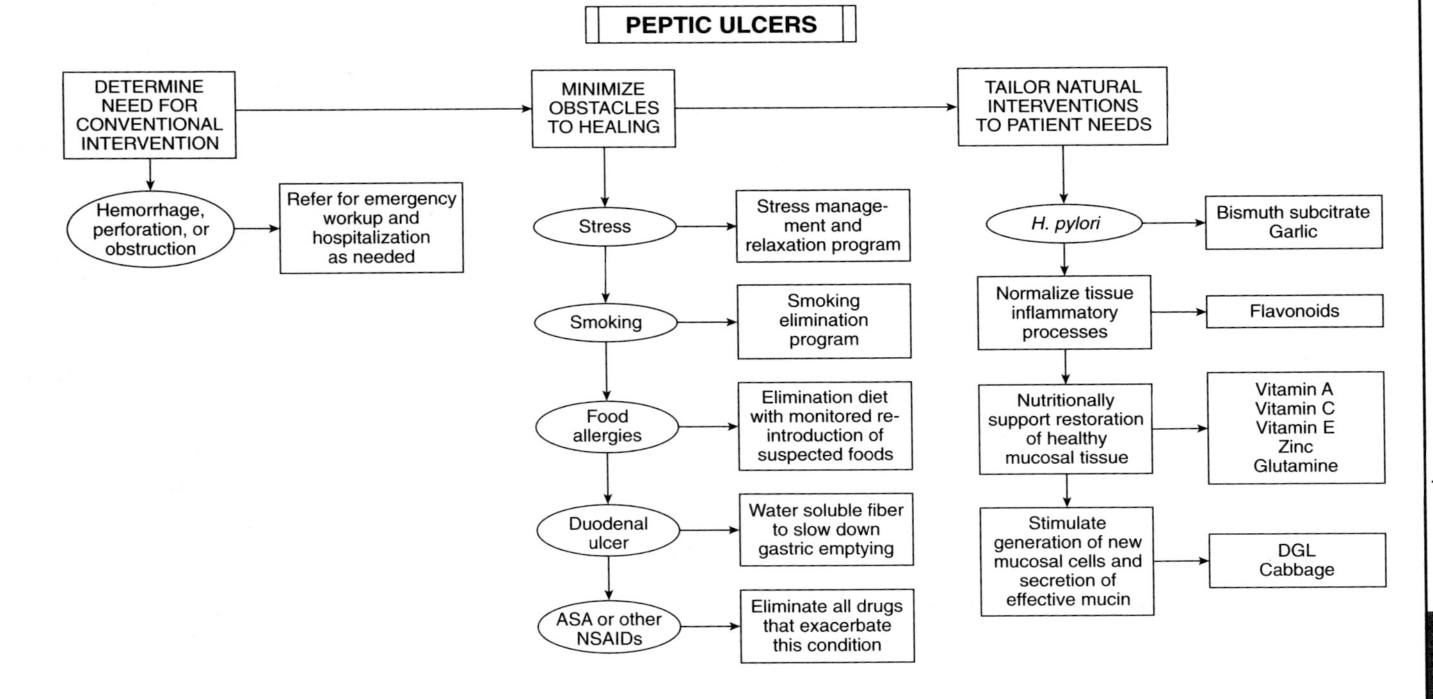
PEPTIC ULCERS
DETERMINE NEED FOR CONVENTIONAL INTERVENTION
Hemorrhage, perforation, or obstruction
Refer for emergency workup and hospitalization as needed
MINIMIZE OBSTACLES TO HEALING
Stress
Stress management and relaxation program
Smoking
Smoking elimination program
Food allergies
Elimination diet with monitored re-introduction of suspected foods
Duodenal ulcer
Water soluble fiber to slow down gastric emptying
ASA or other NSAIDs
Eliminate all drugs that exacerbate this condition
TAILOR NATURAL INTERVENTIONS TO PATIENT NEEDS
H. pylori
Bismuth subcitrate Garlic
Normalize tissue inflammatory processes
Flavonoids
Nutritionally support restoration of healthy mucosal tissue
Vitamin A Vitamin C Vitamin E Zinc Glutamine
Stimulate generation of new mucosal cells and secretion of effective mucin
DGL Cabbage

renewing of intestinal cells and secretion of factors neutralizing acid on contact with the mucosa are also protective.

- GUs are linked to acid output that is normal or reduced; half of patients with DUs have increased gastric acid output. That increase may be attributable to an increased number of parietal cells; patients with DUs have twice as many parietal cells as do normal control subjects. This is problematic only when integrity of protective factors is impaired.
- Loss of integrity can be linked to *Helicobacter pylori*, nonsteroidal antiinflammatory drugs (NSAIDs), alcohol, nutrient deficiency, stress. *H. pylori* and NSAID use are most significant.
- Chronic diseases associated with increased risk of PUs: Crohn's disease, chronic renal failure, liver cirrhosis, cystic fibrosis, chronic obstructive pulmonary disease, systemic mastocytosis (condition of too many immune mast cells in body), and myeloproliferative disorders (polycythemia vera, chronic myelogenous leukemia, agnogenic myeloid metaplasia, and essential thrombocythemia).
- *H. pylori*: 90%-100% of patients with DUs, 70% with GUs, and 50% of people older than 50 years test positive for *H. pylori*. Yet 80% of *H. Pylori*–infected people never develop ulcers. Tests: antibodies to *H. pylori* in blood or saliva, culturing material collected during endoscopy, measure of breath for urea. Low gastric output and low antioxidant content in gastrointestinal (GI) mucosa may predispose to *H. pylori* colonization, which in turn increases gastric pH, setting up positive feedback and increasing the risk for colonization of other organisms.
- Aspirin (ASA) and other NSAIDs: are linked to significant risk of PU; NSAIDs plus smoking is a harmful combination. Increased risk of GI bleeding is present with PU at all dosages; 75 mg q.d. ASA is associated with 40% less bleeding than 300 mg q.d. and 30% less bleeding than 150 mg q.d. Thus conventional prophylactic ASA regimen is not free of risk of PU. NSAID ulcers have declined by replacing these drugs with selective cyclooxygenase-2 inhibitors (Rofecoxib, Celecoxib) for arthritides, but the problem remains an ongoing issue because of the increased use of ASA for cardioprotection.

## THERAPEUTIC CONSIDERATIONS

PU complications are hemorrhage, perforation, and obstruction. These are **medical emergencies** requiring immediate hospitalization. Identify causes and eliminate them.

## Lifestyle Factors

- **Stress and emotions**: men and women with PUs have distinctly different psychological profiles. The number of stressful life events is not significantly different in patients with PU compared with ulcer-free control subjects. Patient's response to stress is a significant factor. People who perceive stress in their lives are at increased risk of developing peptic ulcers (*Textbook,* "Peptic Ulcer—Duodenal and Gastric"). Psychological factors are important in some patients but not in others. Ulcer patients tend to repress emotions; encourage discovery of enjoyable outlets of self-expression and emotions.
- **Smoking**: increased frequency, decreased response to PU therapy, and increased mortality rate are linked to smoking. Three postulated mechanisms are (1) decreased pancreatic bicarbonate secretion, (2) increased reflux of bile salts into the stomach, and (3) acceleration of gastric emptying into the duodenum. Bile salts are quite irritating to the stomach and first portions of the duodenum. Bile salt reflux induced by smoking is the most likely factor. But psychological aspects of smoking also are important; chronic anxiety and psychological stress linked to smoking worsen ulceration.

## Nutritional Factors

- **Food allergy**: this is the prime etiological factor. PU lesions are histologically similar to Arthus reaction (local inflammatory response caused by deposition of immune complexes in tissues). Ninety-eight percent of patients with PU had coexisting lower and upper respiratory tract allergic disease. Elimination diet is successful in treating and preventing recurrent ulcers. Food allergy is consistent with high recurrence rate of PUs. Milk should be avoided; the higher the milk consumption, the greater the likelihood of ulcer. Milk significantly increases stomach acid production.
- **Fiber**: a diet rich in fiber is linked to a reduced rate of DUs compared with a low-fiber diet. A high-fiber diet in patients with recently healed DUs reduced recurrence rate by half. Fiber delays gastric emptying of liquid phase, counteracting rapid movement into duodenum. Supplemental fibers used: pectin, guar gum, psyllium; diet rich in plant foods is best.
- **Cabbage**: raw cabbage juice is effective in treating PUs. A dosage of 1 L/day. fresh juice in divided doses has induced total ulcer healing in only 10 days. High glutamine content of cabbage juice

is a healing factor. A dosage of 1.6 g q.d. glutamine is more effective than conventional treatment; almost all patients tested showed complete relief and healing within 4 weeks. Glutamine is involved in biosynthesis of hexosamine moiety in certain mucoproteins.

- **Bismuth subcitrate**: bismuth is a naturally occurring mineral antacid and inhibitor of *H. pylori*. Bismuth subsalicylate (Pepto-Bismol) is the most popular form, but bismuth subcitrate produces the best results against *H. pylori* and treating PUs. Bismuth subcitrate is available through compounding pharmacies (International Academy of Compounding Pharmacists, 800-927-4227). The advantage of bismuth over standard antibiotics is the risk of developing bacterial resistance to antibiotics that is unlikely relative to bismuth. Dosage for bismuth subcitrate is 240 mg b.i.d. before meals. For bismuth subsalicylate, dosage is 500 mg q.i.d.. Bismuth preparations are extremely safe at these dosages. Bismuth subcitrate may cause temporary and harmless darkening of the tongue and/or stool. Avoid bismuth subsalicylate in children recovering from the flu, chickenpox, or other viral infection because it may mask nausea and vomiting of Reye's syndrome, a rare but serious illness.
- **Flavonoids**: counteract production and secretion of histamine (a factor in ulcer formation). Antiallergy compounds are indicated as a result of probable allergic etiology. Catechin inhibits histidine decarboxylase. Catechin displays significant antiulcer activity in various models. A dosage of 1000 mg catechin five times per day reduces histamine in gastric tissue of normal patients and those with GUs and DUs and acute gastritis. Several flavonoids inhibit *H. pylori* in a concentration-dependent manner. They augment natural defense factors that prevent ulcer formation. Flavone (most potent flavonoid studied in this context) has an effect similar to bismuth subcitrate.

## Miscellaneous

- **Vitamins A and E**: inhibit development of stress ulcers in rats and help maintain integrity of mucosal barrier.
- **Zinc**: increases mucin production in vitro and has a protective effect on PUs in animals and curative effect in human beings.
- **Melatonin**: pineal hormone used to treat jet lag and insomnia-like conditions. It also has antioxidant properties. Melatonin mitigates gastric lining breakdown and ulcer formation. Research

has focused on hypersecretion situations; therefore melatonin may be most applicable for DUs, entailing acid hypersecretion.

## Botanical Medicines

- ***Glycyrrhiza glabra* (licorice)**: used historically for PUs. The aldosterone-like side effects of glycyrrhizinic acid (GA) are avoided by removal of GA from licorice to form deglycyrrhizinated licorice (DGL).
  —DGL is an antiulcer agent with no known side effects (*Textbook, "Glycyrrhiza glabra* [Licorice]"). DGL stimulates differentiation to glandular cells plus mucus formation and secretion. No significant differences exist in recurrence rates between cimitidine and DGL. It prevents ASA-induced ulceration and gastric bleeding.
  —DGL is composed of several flavonoids that inhibit *H. pylori.*
  —DGL must mix with saliva to be effective; this may promote release of salivary compounds that stimulate growth and regeneration of stomach and intestinal cells. DGL in capsule form has not been shown to be effective
  —Dosage: 2-4 380-mg chewable DGL tablets between meals or 20 minutes before meals; continue at least 8-16 weeks after full therapeutic and symptomatic response.
- ***Rheum spp.* (rhubarb)**: in cases of active intestinal bleeding, rhubarb is extremely effective. Alcohol-extracted rhubarb tablets (*Rheum officinale Baill, Rheum palmatum L., Rheum tanguticum Maxim ex Balf*) have been more than 90% effective in clinical trials with bleeding GUs and DUs. Time taken for stool occult blood test to change from positive to negative was 53-57 hours. Benefits are from astringent anthraquinones and flavonoids.
- **Plantain banana**: dried extract of unripe plantain banana is antiulcerogenic against a variety of experimentally induced ulcers in rats. The effect is similar to that of DGL—stimulation of mucosal cell growth rather than inhibition of gastric acid secretion.
- ***Zingiber officinale* (ginger root)**: used traditionally for GI ailments—indigestion, motion sickness, and nausea associated with pregnancy. A methanol extract of ginger root effectively inhibited 19 strains of *H. pylori.* Given ginger's safety profile and reasonable cost, it is worth trying.
- ***Artemisia douglasiana***: located on Western slopes of the Rocky Mountains, this folk remedy has been used in Argentina to treat gastric ulcers and skin lesions for decades. *Artemisia* and its

active constituent dehydroleucodine act as antioxidants and, similar to DGL and plantain, confer gastric lining protection by enhancing mucus secretion.

- ***Allium sativum* (garlic)**: high intake of garlic and onions reduces the risk of stomach cancer. Garlic inhibits growth of *H. pylori.* Garlic is useful for antibiotic-resistant strains as well. Human clinical trials are needed to verify efficacy.

## THERAPEUTIC APPROACH

PU disease refers to a heterogeneous group of disorders with a common final pathway leading to ulcerative lesion in gastric or duodenal mucosa. Determine which factors are most relevant. A more general approach may be easier to implement:

- Identify and eliminate or reduce all factors implicated in etiology: food allergy, cigarette smoking, stress, drugs (especially ASA and other NSAIDs).
- Inhibit exacerbating factors (e.g., reducing excess acid secretion if present) and promote tissue resistance.
- Follow proper diet and lifestyle to prevent recurrence.
- **Complications**: hemorrhage, perforation, and obstruction are emergencies requiring immediate hospitalization.
- **Psychological**: stress reduction program to eliminate or control stressors, plus a regular relaxation plan.
- **Diet**: eliminate allergenic foods, emphasize high-fiber foods, encourage cabbage family vegetables.
- **Supplements**:
  —Vitamin A: 20,000 IU t.i.d.
  —Vitamin C: 500 mg t.i.d.
  —Vitamin E (mixed tocopherols): 100 IU t.i.d.
  —Flavonoids: 500 mg t.i.d.
  —Zinc: 20 mg q.d.
  —L-Glutamine: 500 mg t.i.d.
  —Bismuth subcitrate: 240 mg b.i.d. before meals
- **Botanical medicine**:
  —DGL: 380-760 mg dissolved in mouth 20 minutes before meals t.i.d.

# Periodontal Disease

## DIAGNOSTIC SUMMARY

- Gingivitis: inflammation of the gingiva characterized by erythema, contour changes, and bleeding.
- Periodontitis: localized pain, loose teeth, demonstration of dental pockets, erythema, swelling and/or suppuration; radiographs may reveal alveolar bone destruction.

## GENERAL CONSIDERATIONS

Periodontal disease (PD) is an inclusive term for the inflammatory condition of gingiva (gingivitis) and/or periodontium (periodontitis). The disease process progresses from gingivitis to periodontitis. It may be a manifestation of a systemic condition (diabetes mellitus, collagen diseases, leukemia or other disorders of leukocyte function, anemia, or vitamin deficiency). It is linked to atherosclerosis by an increased level of serum C-reactive protein, a marker for inflammation and risk factor for coronary artery disease.

- Alveolar bone loss may be noninflammatory; definition of periodontal disease excludes processes causing only tooth loss (mainly from osteoporosis or endocrine imbalances). These conditions reflect systemic disease.
- Focus on the underlying condition rather than PD. Noninflammatory alveolar bone loss is a separate entity that involves a different etiology (see the chapter on osteoporasis).
- Focus of this chapter is nutrition and lifestyle improvement as adjuncts to the control and prevention of causes of inflammatory PD.
- Best treated with combined expertise of a dentist or periodontist and nutritionally minded physician. Oral hygiene is paramount but insufficient in many cases; host defense must be normalized; nutritional status determines status of host defense factors.

Prevalence and epidemiology: prevalence increases directly with age: 15% at age 10 years, 38% at 20 years, 46% at 35 years, and 54%

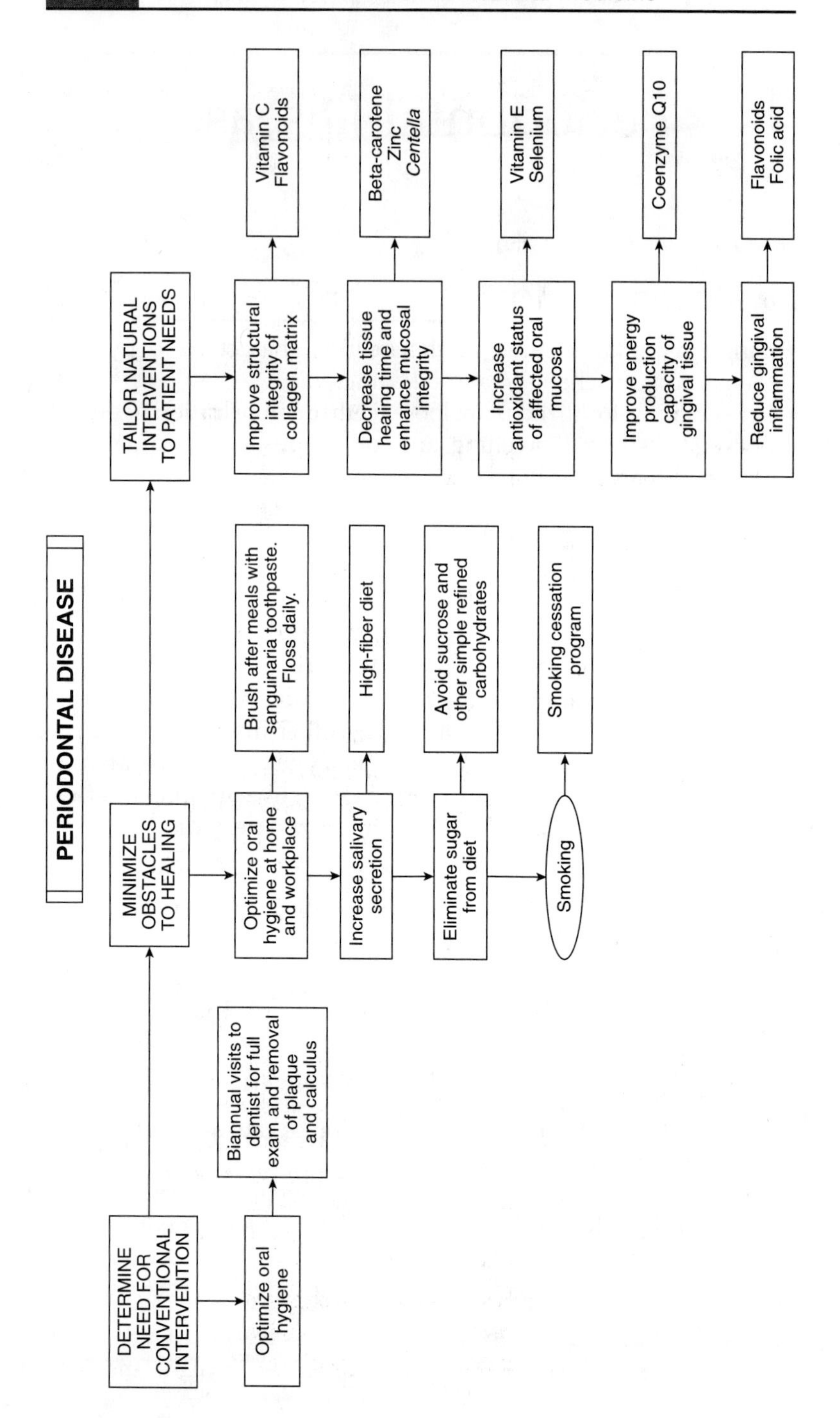
PERIODONTAL DISEASE
DETERMINE NEED FOR CONVENTIONAL INTERVENTION
Optimize oral hygiene
Biannual visits to dentist for full exam and removal of plaque and calculus
MINIMIZE OBSTACLES TO HEALING
Optimize oral hygiene at home and workplace
Brush after meals with sanguinaria toothpaste. Floss daily.
Increase salivary secretion
High-fiber diet
Eliminate sugar from diet
Avoid sucrose and other simple refined carbohydrates
Smoking
Smoking cessation program
TAILOR NATURAL INTERVENTIONS TO PATIENT NEEDS
Improve structural integrity of collagen matrix
Vitamin C
Flavonoids
Decrease tissue healing time and enhance mucosal integrity
Beta-carotene
Zinc
*Centella*
Increase antioxidant status of affected oral mucosa
Vitamin E
Selenium
Improve energy production capacity of gingival tissue
Coenzyme Q10
Reduce gingival inflammation
Flavonoids
Folic acid

at 50 years. Men have a higher prevalence and severity than women. Prevalence is inversely related to increasing levels of education and income. Rural inhabitants have higher severity and prevalence than their urban counterparts.

## Pathophysiology

Factors involved in host resistance include:

- **Gingival sulcus**: V-shaped crevice that surrounds each tooth, bounded by tooth on one side and epithelium lining free margin of gingiva on the other. Sulcus is ideal for bacteria; it is resistant to the cleaning action of saliva. Gingival fluid (sulcular fluid) is a rich nutrient source for microorganisms. Depth of gingival sulcus is a diagnostic parameter. Patients with PD should be monitored biannually by a dentist.
- **Bacterial factors**: bacterial plaque is the etiologic agent in PD. Bacteria secrete compounds detrimental to host defenses: endotoxins and exotoxins, free radicals and collagen-destroying enzymes, leukotoxins, bacterial antigens, waste products, and toxic compounds.
- **Polymorphonuclear leukocytes**: neutrophils (PMNs) are the first line of defense against microbes. PMN functional defects are catastrophic to the periodontium. PMNs are depressed in the elderly and those with diabetes, Crohn's disease, Chédiak-Higashi syndrome, Down's syndrome, and juvenile periodontitis—establishing an extremely high risk for rapidly progressing periodontal disease. Transient neutropenia and PMN function defects may cause alternating quiescence and exacerbation in PD. PMNs release numerous free radicals, collagenases, hyaluronidases, inflammatory mediators, and an osteoclast stimulator.
- **Macrophages and monocytes**: increased numbers in PD. They phagocytize bacteria and debris. They are the primary source of prostaglandins in diseased gingiva, and they release abundant enzymes involved in collagen destruction.
- **Lymphocytes**: produce lymphokines. Their role is overshadowed by other immune components. They promote PMN and monocyte chemotaxis, fibroblast destruction, and osteoclast activation.
- **Complement system**: 22 proteins (>10% of total serum globulin) whose activation initiates cascade (classic or alternative pathway) triggering immunologic and nonspecific resistance to infection

and pathogenesis of tissue injury. Products of complement activation regulate the release of mediators from mast cells; promotion of smooth muscle contraction; chemotaxis of PMNs, monocytes, and eosinophils; and phagocytosis by immune adherence. Net effect is increased gingival permeability, increased penetration of bacteria and byproducts, and initiation of positive feedback cycle. Other effects include solubilization of immune complexes, cell membrane lysis, neutralization of viruses, and killing of bacteria. In PD, activation of complement by an alternative pathway in the periodontal pocket is a major factor in tissue destruction.

- **Mast cells and immunoglobulin (Ig) E**: mast cell degranulation releases inflammatory mediators (histamine, prostaglandins, leukotrienes, kinins, serotonin, heparin, serine proteases). It is initiated by IgE complexes, complement components, mechanical trauma, endotoxins, and free radicals. Increased IgE in gingiva of PD patients suggests allergic factor in progression of PD in some patients.
- **Amalgam restorations**: faulty dental restorations and prostheses are common causes of gingival inflammation and periodontal destruction. Overhanging margins are ideal for plaque and bacteria. Silver amalgam decreases activities of antioxidant enzymes. Mercury accumulation depletes free radical–scavenging enzymes, glutathione peroxidase, superoxide dismutase, and catalase. Proteoglycans and glycosaminoglycans (GAGs) of collagen are sensitive to free radicals.
- **Miscellaneous local factors**: food impaction, unreplaced missing teeth, malocclusion, tongue thrusting, bruxism, toothbrush trauma, mouth breathing, tobacco.
- **Tobacco**: smoking is linked to increased susceptibility to severe PD and tooth loss. The harmful effects are free radical damage to epithelial cells. Smoking greatly reduces ascorbate, potentiating damaging effects. Carotenes and flavonoids greatly reduce toxic effects of smoking.
- **Structure and integrity of collagen matrix**: collagen of periodontal membrane serves as periosteum to alveolar bone. This allows dissipation of tremendous pressure exerted during mastication. Collagen matrix of periodontium (specifically extracellular proteoglycans of gingival epithelium) determines rate of diffusion and permeability of inflammatory mediators, bacteria and byproducts, and destructive enzymes. Because of the high rate of protein turnover in periodontal collagen, integrity of collagen

is vulnerable to atrophy when cofactors needed for collagen synthesis (protein; vitamins C, $B_6$, and A; zinc and copper) are absent or deficient. Collagen of periodontium is rich in GAGs: heparin sulfate, dermatan sulfate, and chondroitin 4-sulfate. Stabilizing collagen is the major treatment goal.

## THERAPEUTIC CONSIDERATIONS

Therapeutic goals in treating PD from nutritional perspective:

- Decrease wound healing time
- Improve membrane and collagen integrity
- Decrease inflammation and free radical damage
- Enhance immune status.

**Vitamin C (ascorbic acid)**: plays a major role in preventing PD. Classic symptom of gingivitis in scurvy shows ascorbate maintains membrane and collagen integrity and immunocompetence. Deficiency is linked to defective collagen, ground substance, and intercellular cement substance in mesenchymal tissue. Deficiency effects on bone are retardation or cessation of osteoid formation, impaired osteoblastic activity, and osteoporosis. Subclinical deficiency also delays wound healing. Decreased vitamin C is linked to increased permeability of oral mucosa to endotoxin and bacterial byproducts and impaired leukocyte functions (PMNs). It increases chemotaxis and phagocytosis by PMNs; enhances lymphoproliferative response to mitogens; and increases interferon levels, antibody response, immunoglobulin levels, and secretion of thymic hormones. Vitamin C has antioxidant and antiinflammatory properties and decreases wound healing time.

**Sucrose**: sugar increases plaque accumulation. It decreases PMN chemotaxis and phagocytosis because of osmotic effects and competition with vitamin C. The average American consumes 175 g sucrose q.d. and other refined carbohydrates; this habit increases risk for PD.

**Vitamin A**: deficiency predisposes to PD. Deficiency is linked to:

- Keratinizing metaplasia of gingival epithelium
- Early karyolysis of gingival epithelial cells
- Inflammatory infiltration and degeneration
- Periodontal pocket formation
- Gingival calculus formation

- Increased susceptibility to infection
- Abnormal alveolar bone formation

Vitamin A supports collagen synthesis and wound healing, maintains integrity of epithelial and mucosal surfaces and their secretions, and enhances immune function. Beta-carotene may be better because of its affinity for epithelial tissue and potent antioxidant activity.

**Zinc (Zn) and copper (Cu)**: Zn is synergist with vitamin A. Severity of PD is linked to increased Cu/Zn ratio—consistent with other causes of inflammation—and signifies activation of metallothionein, which increases ceruloplasmin formation while increasing Zn sequestration in response to inflammation. Zn functions in gingiva and periodontium include:

- Stabilization of membranes
- Inhibition of calcium influxes
- Antioxidant activity
- Metallocomponent in 40 enzymes, including enzymes for DNA, RNA, and collagen synthesis
- Inhibition of plaque growth
- Inhibition of mast cell degranulation
- Numerous immune activities, including increased PMN chemotaxis and phagocytosis

Zn reduces wound healing time. It is active in calcium- and calmodulin-mediated processes (mast cell degranulation, tissue damage induced by endotoxin, and increased vascular permeability). Twice-daily use of mouthwash with 5% Zn solution inhibits plaque growth.

**Vitamin E and selenium (Se)**: function synergistically in antioxidant mechanisms that deter PD. They potentiate each other's effects. Vitamin E decreases wound healing time. Antioxidant effects of vitamin E are needed for silver amalgam to prevent toxic effects of mercury on antioxidant enzymes. Se and vitamin E prevent free radicals from damaging gingival proteoglycans and GAGs, deterring periodontal disease. Mercury depletes the tissues of the antioxidant enzymes superoxide dismutase, glutathione peroxidase, and catalase. In animal studies, this toxic effect of mercury is prevented by supplementation with vitamin E.

**Coenzyme Q10**: ubiquinone is a coenzyme in mitochondrial oxidative phosphorylation and an antioxidant; 70% of patients with PD studied responded favorably to supplementation; it was superior to placebo in a double-blind study.

**Flavonoids**: these are the most important components of an anti-PD program; they reduce inflammation and stabilize collagen by the following:

- Decreasing membrane permeability, thereby decreasing load of inflammatory mediators and bacterial products
- Preventing free radical damage by potent antioxidant properties
- Inhibiting enzymatic cleavage by hyaluronidases and collagenases
- Inhibiting mast cell degranulation
- Cross-linking with collagen fibers directly

Supplement quercetin, catechin, anthocyanidins/proanthocyanidins; rutin has little collagen-stabilizing effect. 3-0-methyl-(+)-catechin retards plaque growth and alveolar bone resorption in animal models.

**Folic acid**: most common deficiency in the world; given either topically or systemically, it reduces gingival inflammation by reducing color changes, bleeding tendency, exudate flow, and plaque scores. Folate mouthwash (0.1% folic acid) is much more effective than oral supplement at 2 or 5 mg q.d., suggesting a local mechanism; binds plaque-derived endotoxin. Folate mouthwash is particularly indicated for pregnant women and oral contraceptive users and in exaggerated gingival inflammatory response or folate antimetabolites (phenytoin, methotrexate).

- Epithelium of cervix and oral mucosa suffer from end-organ folate deficiency under hormonal influences of pregnancy and oral contraceptives; cervical dysplasia of oral contraception also responds to pharmacologic dose of folate (8-30 mg q.d.); sera and leukocytes of pregnant women and oral contraceptive users contain macromolecule that binds folate, a major factor for end-organ folate deficiency.

## Botanical Medicines

- ***Sanguinaria canadensis* (bloodroot)**: contains benzophenanthridine alkaloids—sanguinarine in commercial toothpastes and mouth rinses. Sanguinarine is antimicrobial and antiinflammatory; it inhibits bacterial adherence. Bacteria aggregate and

become morphologically irregular. It is less effective than chlorhexidine mouthwash but effective in many cases and is a natural compound versus a synthetic.
- ***Centella asiatica* (gotu kola)**: triterpenoids demonstrate impressive wound healing; useful in severe PD or if surgery required. It speeds up recovery after laser surgery for severe PD.

## THERAPEUTIC APPROACH

Control all relevant factors; general approach is recommended. Smoking greatly decreases the success of any therapy for PD.

- **Hygiene**: periodic visits to the dentist to eliminate plaque and calculus; brush after meals and floss daily.
- **Diet**: high in dietary fiber, which is protective from increased salivary secretion; avoid sucrose and all refined carbohydrates.
- **Supplements**:
  —Vitamin C: 3-5 g q.d. in divided doses
  —Vitamin E (mixed tocopherols): 400-800 IU q.d.
  —Beta-carotenes: 250,000 IU q.d. (higher doses if indicated) for up to 6 months (instead of vitamin A because of similar effects and greater safety)
  —Se: 400 mg q.d.
  —Zn: 30 mg q.d. of Zn picolinate (60 mg q.d. if another form); wash mouth with 15 mL of 5% solution b.i.d.
  —Folic acid: 2 mg q.d.; wash mouth with 15 mL of 0.1% solution b.i.d.
  —Quercetin: 500 mg t.i.d.
- **Botanical medicines**: high flavonoid–containing extracts, such as those from bilberry (*Vaccinium myrtillus*), hawthorn (*Crataegus spp.*), grapeseed (*Vitis vinifera*), or green tea (*Camellia sinensis*); green tea extract or liberal consumption of green tea is most cost effective; green tea extract with 50% polyphenols with a dosage of 200-300 mg b.i.d.
- ***Sanguinaria canadensis***: use toothpaste containing extract.
- ***Centella asiatica* triterpenoids**: 30 mg b.i.d. of pure triterpenoids.

# Pneumonia: Bacterial, Mycoplasmal, and Viral

## GENERAL CONSIDERATIONS

Acute pneumonia is the seventh leading cause of death in the United States. It is particularly dangerous in the elderly. It usually occurs in immunocompromised persons, especially drug and/or alcohol abusers. In healthy people, pneumonia follows an insult to host defenses such as viral infection (influenza), cigarette smoke and noxious fumes, impaired consciousness (which depresses gag reflex, allowing aspiration), neoplasms, and hospitalization. In immunocompetent, nonelderly adults, cigarette smoking is the strongest independent risk factor for invasive pneumococcal disease.

- Airway distal to the larynx is normally sterile; mucus-covered ciliated epithelium propels sputum to larger bronchi and trachea, evoking a cough reflex. Respiratory secretions contain substances with nonspecific antimicrobial actions: alpha-1-antitrypsin, lysozyme, and lactoferrin. Alveolar defenses are alveolar macrophages, a rich vasculature to deploy lymphocytes and granulocytes rapidly, and an efficient lymphatic drainage network.

### Immunoglobulin Respiratory System Defenses

- Immunoglobulin (Ig) A: abundant in secretions of the upper respiratory tract. It protects against viruses. In the lower tract, IgA helps:
  —Agglutinate bacteria
  —Neutralize microbial toxins
  —Reduce bacterial attachment to mucosal surfaces
  —Activate alternative complement pathway when complexed with an antigen
- IgG is present in the lower respiratory tract; it:
  —Serum agglutinates and opsonizes bacteria
  —Activates complement
  —Promotes chemotaxis of granulocytes and macrophages

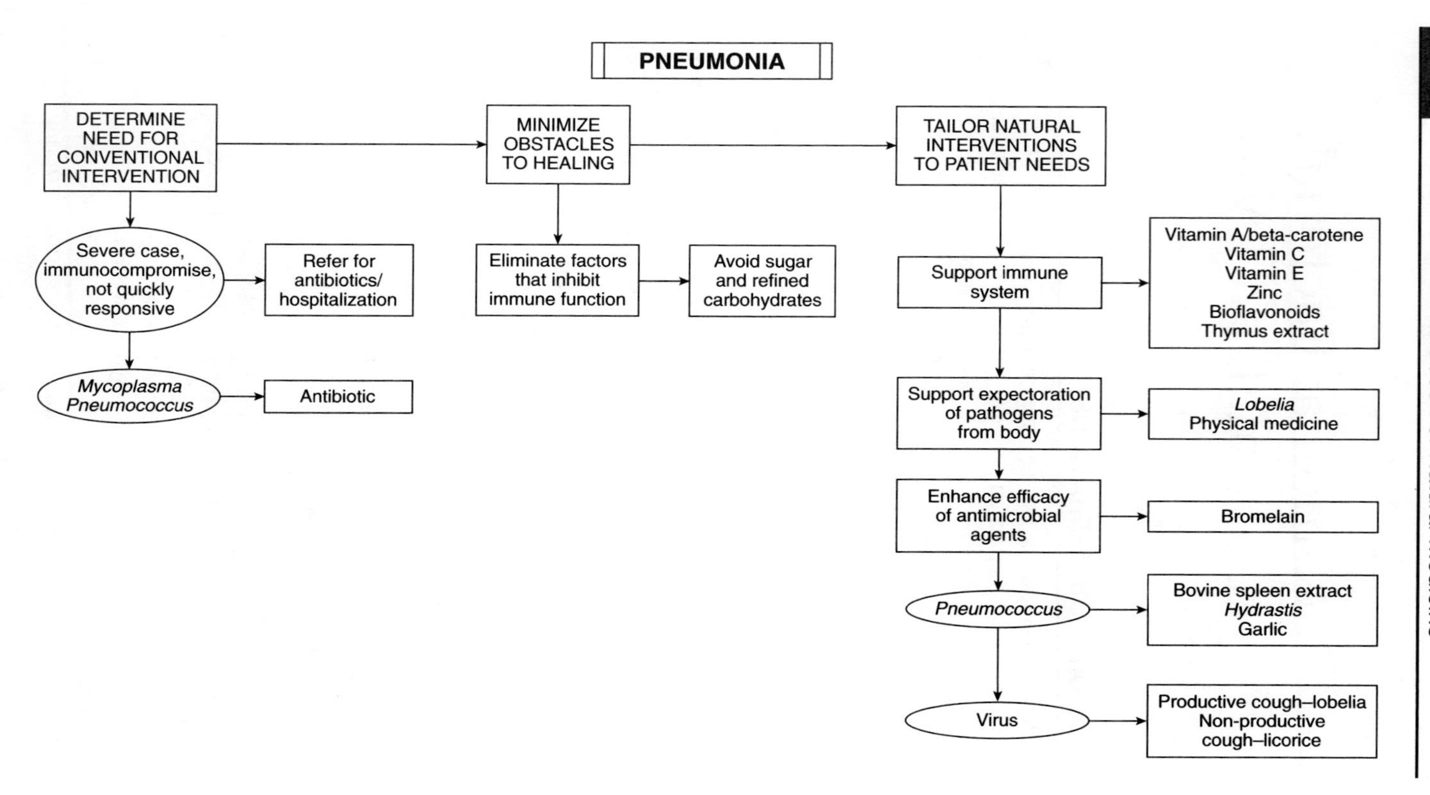
PNEUMONIA
DETERMINE NEED FOR CONVENTIONAL INTERVENTION
Severe case, immunocompromise, not quickly responsive
Refer for antibiotics/ hospitalization
*Mycoplasma Pneumococcus*
Antibiotic
MINIMIZE OBSTACLES TO HEALING
Eliminate factors that inhibit immune function
Avoid sugar and refined carbohydrates
TAILOR NATURAL INTERVENTIONS TO PATIENT NEEDS
Support immune system
Vitamin A/beta-carotene
Vitamin C
Vitamin E
Zinc
Bioflavonoids
Thymus extract
Support expectoration of pathogens from body
*Lobelia*
Physical medicine
Enhance efficacy of antimicrobial agents
Bromelain
*Pneumococcus*
Bovine spleen extract
*Hydrastis*
Garlic
Virus
Productive cough–lobelia
Non-productive cough–licorice

—Neutralizes bacterial toxins and viruses
—Lyses gram-negative bacteria

## THERAPEUTIC CONSIDERATIONS: ALL TYPES OF PNEUMONIA

- **Expectorants (botanical)**: impaired cough reflexes are theorized to play a role in recurrent pneumonia; these botanicals help this condition and prevent recurrences. Botanical expectorants increase quantity, decrease viscosity, and promote expulsion of secretions of the respiratory mucosa. Many have antibacterial and/or antiviral activity. Some are antitussives. *Lobelia inflata* helps promote cough reflex; it is much more effective in clearing the lungs than the antitussive *Glycyrrhiza glabra* (licorice).
  —Productive cough: use lobelia
  —Nonproductive cough: use licorice
- **Other useful expectorants**: balsam of Peru, senega root, grindelia, wild cherry bark, horehound
- **Bromelain**: a mucolytic (discussed under pneumococcal pneumonia later).
- **Vitamin C**: effective in large doses only when started on the first or second day of infection. If started later, it only lessens severity. In pneumonia, white blood cells (WBCs) uptake large amounts of vitamin C. In elderly patients vitamin C increased tissue vitamin C, even during acute respiratory infection. Patients fared much better than those on placebo. The most obvious benefit is in patients with most severe illness.
- **Vitamin A**: valuable in pneumonia, especially in children with measles because of the increased rate of excretion of vitamin A during severe infection. Study subjects with fever excreted much more retinol than did those without fever. A dosage of 400,000 IU (120 mg retinyl palmitate, half on admission and half a day later) given to children with measles reduced the death rate by >50% and duration of pneumonia, diarrhea, and hospital stay by 33%. Positive associations have been noted with vitamin A and concurrent zinc supplements. In children aged 6 months to 3 years, those given initial high doses of vitamin A followed by 4 months of elemental zinc (10 mg/day for infants and 20 mg/day for children older than 1 year) had reduced incidence of pneumonia that was not present in the group given only vitamin A.

- **Vitamin E**: influenza complicated by pneumonia induces a sharp rise in lipid peroxides. Alpha-tocopherol decreases lipid peroxides and improves clinical response.
- **Bromelain**: a useful adjunct therapy with fibrinolytic, antiinflammatory, and mucolytic actions. It enhances antibiotic absorption. Mucolysis is responsible for its efficacy in respiratory tract diseases such as pneumonia, bronchitis, sinusitis.
- **Bottle blowing**: reduced length of hospitalization for community-acquired pneumonia. Patient instructions: sit up and blow bubbles in a bottle containing 10 cm water through a plastic tube 20 times on 10 occasions daily. This exercise also reduces the number of days with fever. Early mobilization itself decreases hospital stays in patients with pneumonia. Despite positive clinical results, C-reactive protein, peak expiratory flow, and vital capacity are not significantly affected. Respiratory pressure changes induced by this exercise may improve bacterial clearance. This technique decreases pulmonary function impairment and increases total lung capacity in patients after coronary artery bypass. To decrease the frequency of respiratory infections such as pneumonia and limit their duration, consider this or similar activity, such as playing a wind instrument.

## THERAPEUTIC APPROACH: ALL TYPES OF PNEUMONIA

Enhance immune system (*Textbook*, "Immune Support"); support respiratory tract drainage with local heat, massage, and expectorants. Multivitamin supplement, including full complement of micronutrients, is advised for all persons older than 50 years to strengthen the immune system and reduce the risk of respiratory infection.

- **Supplements**:
  —Vitamin A: 50,000 IU q.d. for 1 week *or* beta-carotene: 200,000 IU q.d. (avoid vitamin A in menstruating women because of teratogenic effect)
  —Vitamin C: 500 mg every 2 hours
  —Vitamin E (mixed tocopherols): 200 IU q.d.
  —Bioflavonoids: 1000 mg q.d.
  —Zinc: 30 mg q.d.
  —Thymus extract: 120 mg pure polypeptides with molecular weights <10,000 *or* 500 mg crude polypeptide fraction
- **Botanicals**:
  —*Lobelia inflata*: dried herb, 0.2-0.6 g t.i.d.; tincture, 15-30 drops t.i.d.; fluid extract, 8-10 drops t.i.d.

—*Echinacea* spp.: dried root (or as tea), 0.5-1 g; freeze-dried plant, 325-650 mg; juice of aerial portion of *Echinacea purpurea* stabilized in 22% ethanol, 2-3 mL; tincture (1:5), 2-4 mL; fluid extract (1:1), 2-4 mL; solid (dry powdered) extract (6.5:1 or 3.5% echinacoside), 150-300 mg

- **Physical therapy**:
  —Diathermy to chest and back: 30 min/day
  —Mustard poultice: once per day
  —Lymphatic massage: t.i.d.
  —Postural drainage: t.i.d.
  —Bottle blowing therapy: blow bubbles into bottle containing 10 cm water through plastic tube 20 times on 10 occasions daily

For best results, use diathermy, then lymphatic massage, and finally postural drainage.

## MYCOPLASMAL PNEUMONIA

### Diagnostic Summary

- Most commonly occurs in children or young adults.
- Insidious onset over several days.
- Nonproductive cough, minimal physical findings, temperature generally less than 102° F.
- Headache and malaise are common early symptoms.
- WBC count is normal or slightly elevated.
- Radiographic pattern patchy or inhomogeneous.

## THERAPEUTIC CONSIDERATIONS

Mycoplasma are bacteria that lack cell walls. *Mycoplasma pneumoniae* is the most frequent cause of community-acquired, nonpyogenic pneumonia. Tracheobronchitis is more common than pneumonia. It often occurs with pharyngitis in children. It entails a slow recovery, but the course is variable. No specific natural medicine recommendations are available for mycoplasmal infections. Antibiotics (erythromycin 250-500 mg q.i.d.) are indicated; enhancement of general immunity is recommended.

## PNEUMOCOCCAL (STREPTOCOCCAL) PNEUMONIA

### Diagnostic Summary

- Pneumonia usually preceded by upper respiratory infection.
- Sudden onset of shaking, chills, fever, and chest pain.

- Sputum pinkish or blood-specked at first, rusty at height of infection, and yellow and mucopurulent during resolution.
- Gram-positive diplococci present in the sputum smear.
- Initially chest excursion diminished on the involved side; breath sounds are suppressed; fine inspiratory rales audible.
- Later classic signs of consolidation (bronchial breathing, crepitant rales, dullness).
- Leukocytosis.
- Radiograph shows lobar or segmental consolidation.

## THERAPEUTIC CONSIDERATIONS

Pneumococcal pneumonia (*Streptococcus pneumoniae*) is the most common bacterial pneumonia and most common cause of pneumonia requiring hospitalization; use careful clinical judgment to determine disease severity and patient's immune status. Antibiotics and hospitalization may be needed, especially for elderly or immunocompromised patients. Unfortunately, resistance rates to antibiotics and proportion of highly resistant strains are on the rise. Consider natural therapeutics in cases resistant to antibiotics or as an adjunct to strengthen immune response and increase therapeutic effect. Blood culture is more accurate than sputum culture; the nasopharynx is the natural habitat of pneumococci.

- **Bovine spleen extracts**: most specific natural medicine for pneumococcal pneumonia (*Textbook,* "Homeopathy"). Postsplenectomy syndrome includes increased risk of pneumococcal pneumonia (2.5% of splenectomized patients die from pneumococcal pneumonia within 5 years). Spleen extracts rich in tuftsin may be an effective natural alternative to vaccines and prophylactic antibiotics in these patients. Spleen extracts increase WBCs in patients with extreme WBC deficiencies and are beneficial in malaria and typhoid fever.
- ***Hydrastis canadensis*** **(goldenseal)**: berberine-containing botanicals are very important. Berberine has documented antibiotic activity against pathogenic streptococci but it spares normal gastrointestinal microflora.
- ***Allium sativum*** **(garlic)**: broad spectrum of antibiotic activity against gram-positive and gram-negative bacteria. It is an effective antibacterial agent in vivo against *Streptococcus pneumoniae.* Consider it in cases of antibiotic resistance or as an adjunct to antibiotics.

- **Antibiotics**: conventional antibiotics, typically penicillin G or V, are quite beneficial. An appropriately prescribed course of antibiotics gives substantial clinical improvement within a few days.

## ADDITIONAL THERAPIES

- **Supplements**:
  —Bovine spleen extracts: hydrolyzed (predigested) concentrated for tuftsin and splenopentin content preferred: 50 mg q.d. tuftsin and splenopentin or roughly 1.5 g q.d. of total spleen peptides.
  —Bromelain (1200-1800 MCU): 500-750 mg t.i.d. between meals.
- **Botanical medicines**:
  —*Hydrastis canadensis*: dosage based on berberine content; standardized extracts in doses three times daily are preferred: dried root or as infusion (tea), 2-4 g; tincture (1:5), 6-12 mL (1.5-3 tsp); fluid extract (1:1), 2-4 mL (0.5-1 tsp); solid (powdered dry) extract (4:1 or 8%-12% alkaloid content), 250-500 mg.
  —Garlic: commercial product providing daily dose equal to at least 4000 mg of fresh garlic, which translates to at least 10 mg allicin or total allicin potential of 4000 μg (*Textbook, "Allium sativum* [Garlic]").
- **Antibiotic**: penicillin V, 500 mg q.i.d. for uncomplicated cases.

## VIRAL PNEUMONIA

### Diagnostic Summary

- Onset typical of influenza: fever, myalgia, and headache.
- Other symptoms, signs, and X-ray findings are similar to mycoplasmal pneumonia.

## THERAPEUTIC CONSIDERATIONS

Apply treatment recommendations given under general discussion of pneumonia. *Glycyrrhiza glabra* (licorice) is an antiviral, immune-enhancing expectorant (*Textbook, "Glycyrrhiza glabra* [Licorice]") but it also has an antitussive an effect. For an unproductive cough, use licorice; for a productive cough, use lobelia.

- ***Glycyrrhiza glabra* (licorice)**: powdered root, 1-2 g; fluid extract (1:1), 2-4 mL; solid (dry powdered) extract (4:1), 250-500 mg.

# Porphyrias

## DIAGNOSTIC SUMMARY

- Unexplained abdominal pain, possibly including nausea and vomiting
- Acute peripheral or central nervous system dysfunction
- Mental abnormalities ranging from confusion to acute psychosis
- Urinary porphobilinogen during attack
- Majority of carriers are asymptomatic, except when exposed to drugs or chemicals that exacerbate condition

## GENERAL CONSIDERATIONS

- Once considered rare, the prevalence now may be higher. Allopathic medicine has some therapies, but naturopathy has an array of effective modalities for therapy and prevention.
- Classic triad: abdominal pain, constipation (or diarrhea), and vomiting.
- Acute intermittent porphyria has periods of exacerbation and remission.
- Genetic deficits of porphyria affect all tissues but primarily the hematopoietic tissues of bone marrow and the cytochrome P-450 system in the liver because of the greater number of porphyrin precursors required. The liver is the major site where inherited or acquired deficits in heme synthesis manifest.

### Classifications of Porphyria

- Hepatic or erythropoietic origin. Both classes are characterized by overproduction of porphyrin or precursors.
- Biosynthesis of heme is controlled differently in the liver and bone marrow. Rate-limiting enzyme in the liver is aminolevulinic acid (ALA) synthase. In bone marrow, it is partly regulated by uptake of iron.

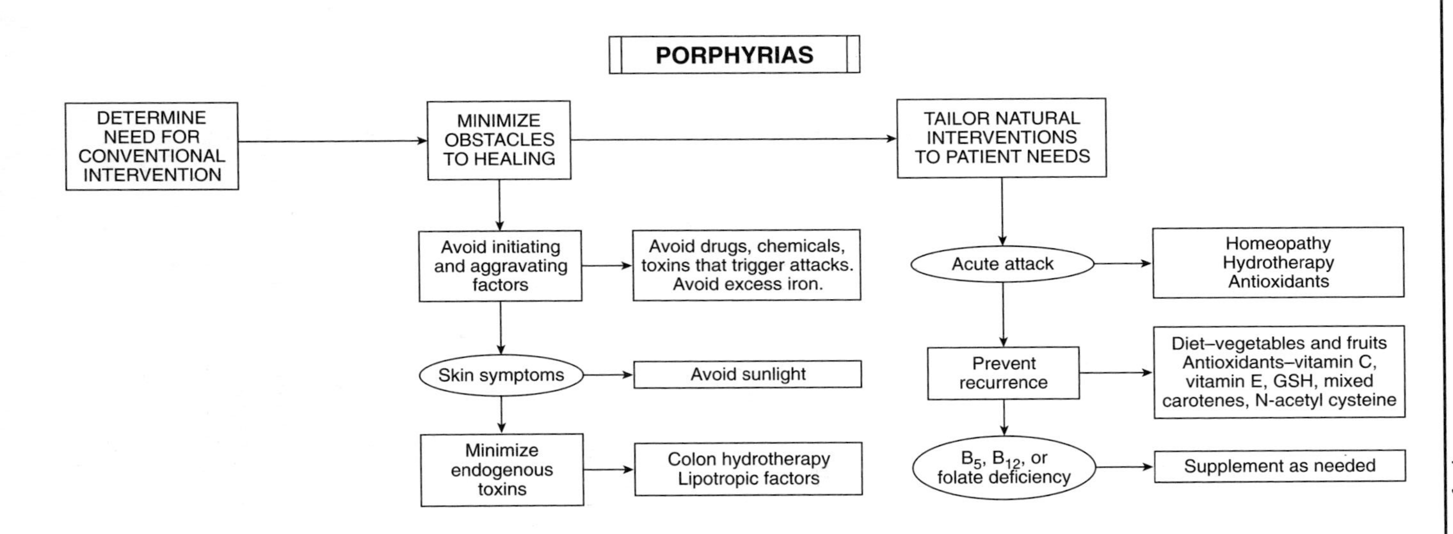
PORPHYRIAS
DETERMINE NEED FOR CONVENTIONAL INTERVENTION
MINIMIZE OBSTACLES TO HEALING
TAILOR NATURAL INTERVENTIONS TO PATIENT NEEDS
Avoid initiating and aggravating factors
Avoid drugs, chemicals, toxins that trigger attacks. Avoid excess iron.
Skin symptoms
Avoid sunlight
Minimize endogenous toxins
Colon hydrotherapy Lipotropic factors
Acute attack
Homeopathy Hydrotherapy Antioxidants
Prevent recurrence
Diet–vegetables and fruits Antioxidants–vitamin C, vitamin E, GSH, mixed carotenes, N-acetyl cysteine
$B_5$, $B_{12}$, or folate deficiency
Supplement as needed

- Acute hepatic porphyries: rapid onset of symptoms, largely neurologic; erythropoietic variety manifests primarily in skin as cutaneous photosensitivity.

**Primary Porphyrias**

| | |
|---|---|
| Hepatic porphyrias | ALA-dehydrase-deficiency porphyria |
| | Acute intermittent porphyria |
| | Porphyria cutanea tarda |
| | Hereditary coproporphyria |
| | Variegate porphyria |
| Erythropoietic porphyrias | X-linked sideroblastic anemia |
| | Congenital erythropoietic porphyria |
| | Erythrocytic protoporphyria |

## Signs and Symptoms of Hepatic Porphyrias

- Acute attacks: wide variety of symptoms ranging from skin lesions to abdominal pain to neurologic symptoms of varying degrees of intensity.
- Abdominal, back, or extremity pains increase over a 24- to 48-hour period (mimics appendicitis or an acute abdomen). Rebound tenderness usually is not present.
- Nausea and vomiting.
- Anxiety and restlessness.
- Constipation that worsens as condition develops.
- Tachycardia, suggesting infectious process or bowel toxicity.
- Severity of symptoms out of proportion to presenting signs. Bowel symptoms are caused by a neurologic disturbance.
- Mental abnormalities: confusion to acute psychosis can be the first presentation.
- Prolonged attacks impair sensory and motor function, causing respiratory paralysis and death.
- Many patients have been misdiagnosed with schizophrenia and confined to mental institutions.
- Majority of carriers are asymptomatic except when exposed to drugs or chemicals that exacerbate the condition.
- Neurologic symptoms and sequelae of acute and/or prolonged attack can take months to clear, but eventual recovery occurs in the majority of cases.

## Biochemistry

- Biosynthesis of heme is the main purpose for porphyrogenic pathway. Heme is a member of a group of compounds including cytochromes (oxidation and reduction reactions), chlorophyll (photosynthesis), and vitamin $B_{12}$. It is formed from succinyl coenzyme A and combined with globin chains synthesized on ribosomes in plasma of developing red blood cells (RBCs). In the liver heme is used to make detoxifying cytochrome P-450. Heme synthesis begins and ends in mitochondrion, with part occurring in cytoplasm. All tissues form heme, but primary sites are bone marrow and the liver.
- Rate-limiting enzyme for heme synthesis is ALA synthase, which is the initial enzyme in the cascade. It is regulated by a feedback response to tissue demand for heme. With the formation of uroporphyrinogen, branching generates porphyrin isomers. Isomer III results in the formation of uroporphyrinogen III, modified to be more lipophilic for excretion from the body. The majority of the pathway favors heme production.

## Heme Formation

- Regulated by action of ferrochelatase in mitochondria. Reducing substances are required: ascorbic acid, cysteine, or glutathione. Iron must be in ferrous rather than ferric form. Ferrochelatase is inhibited by high levels of heme, which also inhibit ALA synthase.
- Multiple control systems regulate the metabolic pathway.
- RBC incorporation of heme, iron, and glycine occurs in maturing reticulocytes but is lost as the cell ages. Hypoxia and erythropoietin stimulate ALA synthase in RBCs but not the liver; drugs and chemicals affect the liver but not erythropoietic tissues.

## Manifestation

- Genetic or acquired deficits limit flow of heme precursors through a cascade that forms hemoglobin. Deficiency manifests from increased demand; certain drugs, chemicals, steroids, estrogens, oral contraceptives, progesterone, or testosterone that burdens cytochrome P-450 can precipitate an acute attack.
- This results from partial removal of feedback on delta-ALA synthase (ALA-S). Depending on enzyme deficit, heme precursors follow different pathways and accumulate in tissues—skin and nervous system—causing signs and symptoms.
- Attacks are more frequently in women than in men, especially premenstrually. Expression of porphyria increases with age from

increased exposures to toxins and the aging body's decreasing ability to adapt.
- Skin symptoms: some porphyric precursors absorb light at 400 nm, raising the potential energy of the molecule to an excited state of highly reactive oxygen species. Histamine and proteolytic enzyme release induce oxidative damage. Beta-carotene protects against these injuries.
- Neuropsychiatric changes occur in hepatic porphyrias (ALA-dehydrase-deficiency porphyria, acute intermittent porphyria, porphyria cutanea tarda, hereditary coproporphyria, and variegate porphyria) with excess production of ALA and porphobilinogen (PBG). Exact mechanism of how porphyrins affect the central nervous system is unknown.
- Familial porphyria cutanea tarda: occurs at a younger age than spontaneous porphyria cutanea tarda despite no difference in biochemical features. Reason: either genetic predisposition to sequestering ferritin in the liver or increased sensitivity to alcohol ingestion. Even manifestations among family members vary.

## Etiologic Agents

- Prescription medicines, estrogens, some herbal medicines, heavy metals, organophosphates, burdens on cytochrome P-450.
- Exogenous estrogens: oral contraceptives, estrogen patches, or estrogen replacement therapy or hormone replacement therapy. Estrogens enhance porphyrin-inducing activities of other agents; women are more vulnerable to environmental exposures than are men.
- Herbicides decrease activity of enzymes of porphyric pathway and increase porphyrins in nerve tissue.
- Theory: unexplained chemical-associated illnesses, such as multiple chemical sensitivity (MCS) syndrome, may be mild chronic porphyria or acquired abnormalities in heme synthesis. Exposures to porphyrogenic substances or severe infection overpower the deficient enzyme system, causing accumulation of specific porphyrins. Symptoms arise from increased porphyrinogen and not accumulation of the toxin itself.
- Expediting the distinction between "real" porphyria and secondary porphyrinopathies: porphyria diagnosis is based on urinary and/or fecal porphyrin excretions twice to 20 times the upper limit of normal. This excludes persons with lesser degrees of porphyrogenic activity, some whose conditions are in remission or not subject to environmental exposures.

- Intensity of symptoms varies widely. Ten percent have acute, severe attacks; 25% have chronic symptoms of varying degrees; 65% have no symptoms but become susceptible under the right circumstances.
- Alternative theory: Patients with MCS may, at times, have modest increases in urinary coproporphyrin, commonly found in asymptomatic subjects or those with diverse other conditions (e.g., diabetes mellitus, heavy alcohol use, liver disease, anemias). Secondary coproporphyrinuria does not indicate coproporphyria.
- Modern exposures to offending agents will increase unmasking of underlying deficits.

## Laboratory Diagnosis

- Small amounts of porphyrins (coproporphyrin) are excreted in normal human urine. Coproporphyrin also is in bile and feces. ALA, PBG, and uroporphyrin are excreted in urine; coproporphyrin is preferentially and protoporphyrin exclusively excreted in bile and feces.
- Fecal excretion is affected by diet and bowel flora; arriving at "normal" values is difficult. PBG in urine of healthy persons is <1.5 mg q.d. and undetectable by conventional testing. Watson-Schwartz qualitative test for PBG is positive in acute intermittent porphyria in acute attacks and variegate porphyria and hereditary coproporphyria in latent periods. High rate of false-negatives are attributable to its subjective nature. A substance present in yeast tablets can induce false-positive Watson-Schwartz test result.
- Cost-effective strategy for acute symptoms: for neurovisceral features suggesting acute porphyric syndrome, use rapid screening test for urinary PBG. For solar urticaria and acute photosensitivity (protoporphyria), test for increased RBC porphyrins. For vesiculobullous formation (porphyria cutanea tarda, hereditary coproporphyria, or variegate porphyria), test for urinary porphyrins. Confirm positive screening test results with targeted quantitative testing.
- Enzymatic assays and DNA-based testing usually are not needed for acute disease. They are useful for evaluation and genetic counseling. Isolating specific DNA encoding heme biosynthetic pathway enzymes provides precise heterozygote identification and prenatal diagnosis in families with known defects.
- Cell markers to identify porphyria in the absence of symptoms: WBC manganese, calcium, iron, and zinc, plus RBC calcium

differing in concentration between groups classified as acute intermittent porphyria gene carriers. Manganese is the most discriminative of all variables. Increased cellular manganese by factor of 4 suggests an increased likelihood of developing acute intermittent porphyria.

- Specific deficit must be determined; successful treatment outcomes depend on correct diagnosis (*Textbook,* "Urinary Porphyrins for the Detection of Heavy Metal and Toxic Chemical Exposure").

## THERAPEUTIC CONSIDERATIONS

- Identify patients predisposed or susceptible to porphyric episodes: medical history of periodic psychotic episodes, nervous breakdowns, unexplained abdominal pains, unusual symptoms. Prevention is the first option because porphyric episodes are difficult to control.
- Treatment of acute episodes is demanding because of severity and a changing clinical picture. Presentations differ depending on the degree of toxicity, genetic component, and patient response to therapy.
- Homeopathy has been successful; medicines depend on the clinical picture. Constitutional prescribing does not work as well during the acute state; several prescriptions may be needed to stabilize the patient. Prescriptions may need to be frequently changed as disease stages progress. Frequent follow-up, perhaps daily, is needed to assess clinical state.
- Patient education: helps overcome disbelief and denial. Delineate which symptoms go with each condition. Inform other physicians that patient is seeking to keep prescription drugs to a minimum. Course of therapy to reach state of insusceptibility to toxins is long, with exacerbations and remissions. Help patient understand this.
- Identify and limit offending agents. Take a complete history of environmental and work exposures. Often simply changing work environment eliminates attacks.

### Toxins Known to Cause or Exacerbate Porphyria

Intoxications:

- **Alcoholism**
- **Foreign and environmental chemicals** such as hexachlorobenzene, polyhalogenated biphenyls, dioxins, vinyl chloride, carbon tetrachloride, benzene, chloroform

- **Heavy metals** such as lead, arsenic, mercury
- **Drugs**
- **Adverse effect of drugs**:
  —Analgesics
  —Sedatives
  —Hypnotics
  —Anesthetics
  —Sex hormones
  —Sulfa antibiotics

## Drugs Known to Cause or Exacerbate Porphyria*

- Amidopyrine
- Aminoglutethimide
- Antipyrine
- Barbiturates
- Captopril
- Carbamazepine
- Carbromal
- Chloral hydrate
- Chloramphenicol
- Chlordiazepoxide
- Chlorpropamide
- Danazol
- Dapsone
- Diazepam
- Diclofenac
- Diltiazem
- Diphenhydramine
- Diphenylhydantoin
- Doxycycline
- Ergot preparations
- Erythromycin
- Estrogen
- Ethanol (acute)
- Ethchlorvynol
- Ethinamate
- Furosemide
- Glutethimide
- Griseofulvin
- Hydralazine
- Hydrochlorothiazide
- Imipramine
- Isopropyl meprobamate
- Lidocaine
- Mephenytoin
- Meprobamate
- Methyldopa
- Methyprylon
- Metoclopramide
- Metronidazole
- N-butylscopolammonium bromide
- Nifedipine
- Nitrous oxide
- Novobiocin
- Oral contraceptives
- Orphenadrine
- Oxycodone
- Pentazocine
- Phenobarbital
- Phenylbutazone
- Phenytoin
- Piroxicam
- Pivampicillin
- Primidone
- Progesterone
- Pyrazinamide
- Pyrazolone preparations
- Sodium valproate
- Succinimides
- Sulfonamide antibiotics
- Sulfonethylmethane
- Sulfonmethane
- Synthetic estrogens, progestins
- Terfenadine
- Tetracyclines
- Theophylline
- Tolazamide
- Tolbutamide
- Trimethadione
- Valproic acid
- Verapamil

*This list includes many drugs that can exacerbate porphyria, but it is not complete.

## Nutritional Therapies

- **Diet**: during acute intermittent porphyria attacks, increasing complex carbohydrates helps alleviate symptoms. Often the patient is ingesting high amounts of carbohydrates when first seen and weight gain follows. Intravenous glucose (300 g/day) can be given. A more complete parenteral nutritional regimen is preferable. Avoid fasting or rapid weight loss that can precipitate acute intermittent porphyria. High-fiber fruits and vegetables improve several porphyria measures. In a study of porphyria cutanea tarda (PCT), 500 kcal/day of fruits and vegetables decreased body mass index, serum alanine aminotransferase (ALT) from 122.0 to 75.6 U/L, serum aspartate aminotransferase (AST) from 91.8 to 55.2 U/L, serum iron from 188.6 to 140.2 mg/dL, and serum ferritin from 574 to 499 ng/mL. Diet also improved skin lesions and decreased urinary coproporphyrin and uroporphyrins.
- **Antioxidants**: along with homeopathy, antioxidants are the mainstay of case management during acute porphyric episodes. Once stabilized, an ongoing regimen of antioxidants—vitamin C, vitamin E, GSH, beta-carotene, N-acetyl cysteine—should prevent recurrence. Vitamin C is low in patients with PCT. High-dose vitamin E (1 g/d alpha-tocopherol) in PCT decreases urinary uroporphyrins (50% of C8 carboxyls) with clinical improvement. Effect lasts only as long as vitamin E is supplemented.
- **Vitamin B complex**: pantothenic acid (vitamin $B_5$) facilitates formation of succinyl coenzyme A (CoA) (by the tricarboxylic acid cycle) and glycine, precursors to ALA; supplementation is helpful. Transformation of succinyl CoA involves vitamin $B_{12}$–dependent enzyme; check $B_{12}$ and folic acid status. The initial reaction is oxygen dependent; therefore oxygen therapy may be contraindicated in delta-ALA porphyria. ALA formation needs pyridoxal-5′-phosphate (P5P); any substance that inhibits enzyme systems is countered in part by P5P. But P5P may not play an important role.
- **Carotenes**: all cutaneous porphyrias are alleviated by avoiding sunlight. Treating erythropoietic protoporphyria with large doses of beta-carotene is effective and may improve tolerance to sunlight. Mixed carotenoids (alpha-carotene, beta-carotene, and lycopene) are effective in cell cultures, but single carotenes are ineffective.

- **Iron (Fe)**: excessive Fe stores and intake aggravate several porphyrias. Avoid Fe unless clearly indicated by low Fe stores.
- **Detoxification**: liver and colon detoxification eliminates toxins that may exacerbate the condition. Methods: colon hydrotherapy, constitutional hydrotherapy, sauna, antioxidants, or oxygen therapy (ozone). Lipotropic factors that enhance the liver cytochrome P-450 system are contraindicated during acute attacks but are useful when patient is in a quiet, stable period. Lipotropics and antioxidants help decrease acute attacks. Chelation with ethylenediamine tetra-acetic acid (EDTA) and ethanol extracts of botanicals is contraindicated in patients predisposed to porphyria.
- **Constitutional hydrotherapy**: quite effective during acute flare-up, normalizing liver function and neurologic symptoms. Daily sessions may be needed.
- **Ozone therapy**: indicated for deficit of coproporphyrinogen oxidase causing deficit of coproporphyrinogen in hereditary coproporphyria. It is contraindicated in deficit of ALA synthase; oxygen enhances the pathway, resulting in exacerbation of symptoms.

## THERAPEUTIC APPROACH

- **Identify condition early**: avoid initiating and aggravating factors. Limit sun exposure in cutaneous manifestations.
- **Diet**: rich in fruits and vegetables, low in iron.
- **Supplements**:
  —Vitamin E (mixed tocopherols): 400-1000 IU q.d.
  —Mixed carotenes: 25-50 mg q.d.

# Premenstrual Syndrome

## DIAGNOSTIC SUMMARY

- Recurrent signs and symptoms that develop during the late luteal phase of the menstrual cycle and disappear by end of full flow of menses.
- Typical symptoms: decreased energy, tension, irritability, depression, headache, altered sex drive, breast pain, backache, abdominal bloating, edema of fingers and ankles.

## GENERAL CONSIDERATIONS

- Premenstrual syndrome (PMS) is cyclic constellation of symptoms appearing during the late luteal phase of the menstrual cycle and disappearing by the end of full flow of menses; they do not appear during the follicular phase.
- Most common symptoms: decreased energy, tension, irritability, anger, food cravings, depression, headache, altered sex drive, breast pain, muscle aches, abdominal bloating, edema of fingers and ankles.
- Affects 30% to 40% of menstruating women; 80% of women have emotional or physical changes without much difficulty. From 2.5%-5% of women have severe symptoms that jeopardize home life and work. Peak occurrence is during the 30s and 40s.
- Premenstrual dysphoric disorder (PMDD) is a separate DSM diagnostic category of severe PMS with depression, irritability, and severe mood swings.
- Etiology theory: interaction of cyclic changes in the ovarian steroids estrogen and progesterone cause changes in brain neurotransmitters, inducing emotional and physical symptoms. Why sensitivity to ovarian steroid–induced neurotransmitter changes differ among women is not known. Serotonin is most implicated. Whether PMS and PMDD are related to absolute serotonin levels, reduced blood levels, or serotonin transport remains unclear.
- Other neurotransmitter systems include opioid and gamma-aminobutyric acid.

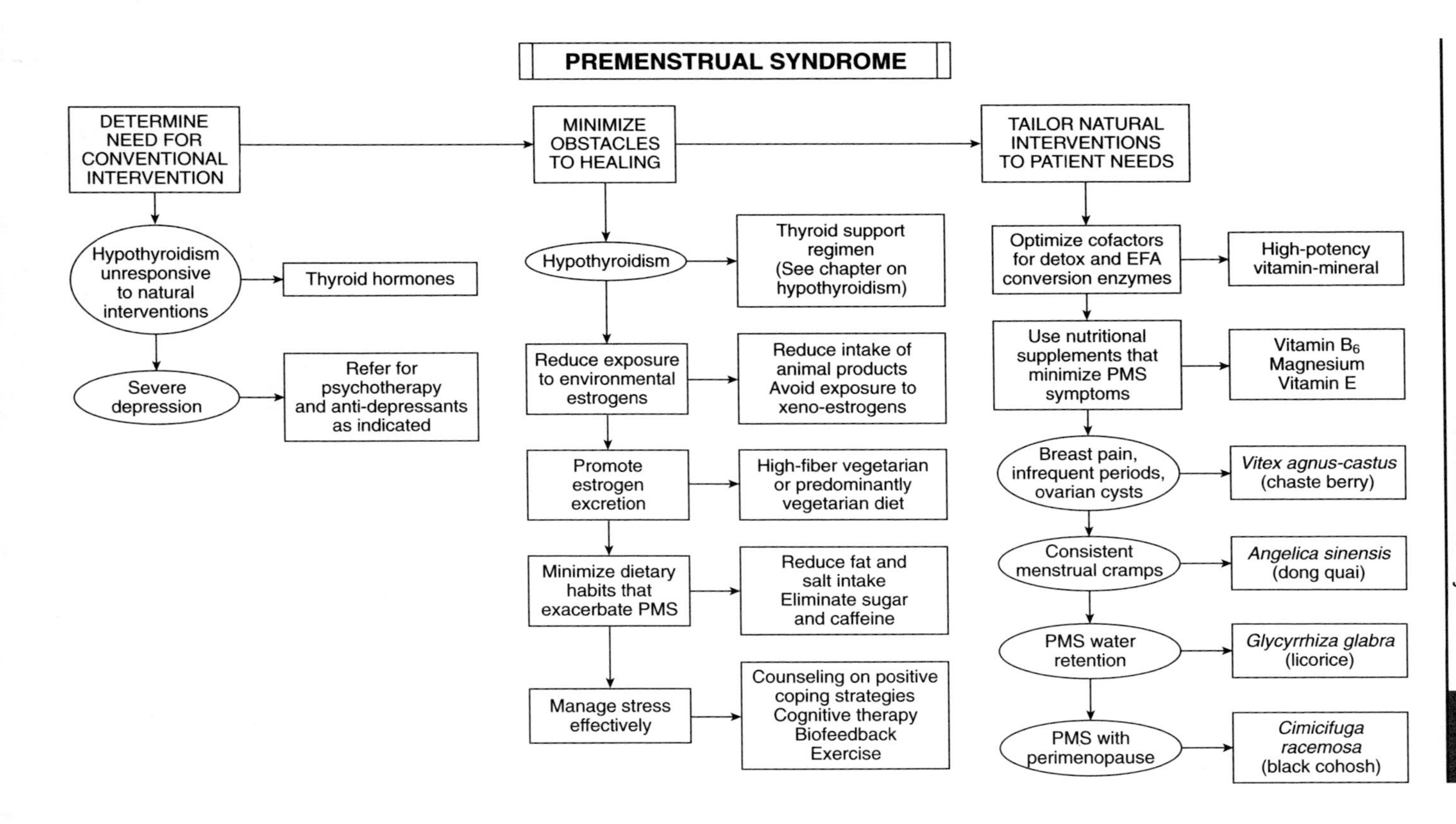
PREMENSTRUAL SYNDROME
DETERMINE NEED FOR CONVENTIONAL INTERVENTION
Hypothyroidism unresponsive to natural interventions
Thyroid hormones
Severe depression
Refer for psychotherapy and anti-depressants as indicated
MINIMIZE OBSTACLES TO HEALING
Hypothyroidism
Thyroid support regimen (See chapter on hypothyroidism)
Reduce exposure to environmental estrogens
Reduce intake of animal products Avoid exposure to xeno-estrogens
Promote estrogen excretion
High-fiber vegetarian or predominantly vegetarian diet
Minimize dietary habits that exacerbate PMS
Reduce fat and salt intake Eliminate sugar and caffeine
Manage stress effectively
Counseling on positive coping strategies Cognitive therapy Biofeedback Exercise
TAILOR NATURAL INTERVENTIONS TO PATIENT NEEDS
Optimize cofactors for detox and EFA conversion enzymes
High-potency vitamin-mineral
Use nutritional supplements that minimize PMS symptoms
Vitamin B6 Magnesium Vitamin E
Breast pain, infrequent periods, ovarian cysts
Vitex agnus-castus (chaste berry)
Consistent menstrual cramps
Angelica sinensis (dong quai)
PMS water retention
Glycyrrhiza glabra (licorice)
PMS with perimenopause
Cimicifuga racemosa (black cohosh)

- Serotonin agents can alleviate psychological and physical symptoms in most patients with PMDD. Fluoxetine, sertraline, paroxetine, fluvoxamine, citalopram, and venlafaxine are more effective than placebo for PMDD.

### Diagnosis and Classifications

- **Diagnosis**: connecting symptoms attributed to PMS and occurrence during luteal phase of menstrual cycle.
- **Tools**: symptom questionnaire and menstrual symptom diary.
- **Key defining feature of both PMS and PMDD**: timing of symptoms; they appear only during the luteal phase and disappear before or during menstrual flow.
- **Rule out other disorders**: medical or psychiatric history (many mental and physical disorders mimic PMS and many coexist).
- Only one of the following is required for diagnosis of PMS: mild psychological discomfort, bloating and weight gain, breast tenderness, swelling of hands and feet, various aches and pains, poor concentration, sleep disturbance, and change in appetite.
- Diagnosis of PMDD requires at least five of the symptoms below, with at least one being a core symptom and occurring during the luteal phase and remitting with menses or a few days after onset of menses for at least two cycles:
  —Depressed mood or dysphoria (core symptom)
  —Anxiety or tension (core symptom)
  —Affective lability (core symptom)
  —Irritability (core symptom)
  —Decreased interest in activities
  —Poor concentration
  —Lack of energy
  —Change in appetite, overeating, or food cravings
  —Hypersomnia or insomnia
  —Feeling overwhelmed
  —Additional physical symptoms (breast tenderness, bloating, headache, joint or muscle pain)

## THERAPEUTIC CONSIDERATIONS

### Estrogen Metabolism

- Estrogen excess produces cholestasis—diminished bile flow or stasis of bile ("sluggish liver"). But indicators of liver status (alkaline phosphatase, aspartate aminotransferase, alanine aminotransferase, gamma-glutamyl transpeptidase) are normal.

- Causes of cholestasis: estrogen excess or oral contraceptives, pregnancy, presence of gallstones, alcohol, endotoxins, hereditary disorders such as Gilbert's syndrome, anabolic steroids, various chemicals or drugs, nutritional deficiencies.
- Cholestasis reduces estrogen detoxification and clearance. A positive feedback scenario is produced.
- Estrogen excess during the luteal phase negatively affects endorphin levels. When the estrogen/progesterone ratio is increased, endorphins decline. Low endorphins during the luteal phase are common in women with PMS. Endorphins are lowered by stress and raised by exercise.

### Estrogen Impairs Vitamin $B_6$

Estrogens negatively affect vitamin $B_6$ function. $B_6$ is low in depressed patients, especially women taking estrogens (oral contraceptives or Premarin). $B_6$ supplementation positively affects all PMS symptoms (particularly depression) in many women. Improvement arises from reducing mid-luteal estrogen and increasing mid-luteal progesterone.

### Gut Microecology

- The liver detoxifies by attaching glucuronic acid to toxins and excreting them in bile. Bacterial enzyme beta-glucuronidase uncouples (breaks) bond between excreted toxins and glucuronic acid. Excess beta-glucuronidase activity is linked to increased estrogen-dependent breast cancer and PMS.
- Activity of this enzyme is reduced by restoring healthy bacterial flora. Dietary guidelines and probiotics (*Lactobacillus acidophilus* and *Bifidobacterium bifidum*) help normalize intestinal flora.
- Dosing: based on number of live organisms; 1-10 billion viable *L. acidophilus* or *B. bifidum* cells daily is sufficient.

### Liver Detoxification

- Diet: low in saturated and trans fats; high in plant foods—vegetables, fruits, legumes, whole grains, nuts and seeds; low in sugar and white flour products.
- Lipotropic factors hasten removal or decrease deposition of fat and bile in the liver through their interaction with fat metabolism. They "decongest" the liver and improve liver function and fat metabolism. Lipotropic agents include choline, methionine, betaine, folic acid, and vitamin $B_{12}$. Use with herbal cholagogues

and choleretics. Daily dosage: 1000 mg choline and 500 mg methionine and/or cysteine.

### Environmental Estrogens (Xenoestrogens)

- Halogenated hydrocarbons: toxic pesticides dichlorodiphenyltrichloroethane (DDT), dichlorodiphenyldichloroethylene (DDE), polychlorinated biphenyl (PCB), dieldrin, and chlordane.
- Hard to break down; stored in fat cells.
- Mimic estrogen in body; major factor in estrogen-related health problems such as PMS, breast cancer, and low sperm counts.

### Dietary Considerations

Guy Abraham, MD, stated that compared with symptom-free women, PMS patients consume:

- 62% more refined carbohydrates
- 275% more refined sugar
- 79% more dairy products
- 78% more sodium
- 53% less iron
- 77% less manganese
- 52% less zinc.

Seven most important dietary recommendations for PMS:

- Vegetarian or predominantly vegetarian diet
- Reduce fat intake
- Eliminate sugar
- Reduce exposure to environmental estrogens
- Increase intake of soy foods
- Eliminate caffeine
- Keep salt intake low

#### Vegetarian Diet and Estrogen Metabolism

- Vegetarian women excrete two to three times more estrogen in their feces; have 50% lower blood levels of free estrogen; and have a lower incidence of breast cancer, heart disease, and menopausal symptoms compared with omnivores because of their lower fat and higher fiber intake.
- Reduce saturated fat and cholesterol (animal products) and increase fiber-rich plant foods (fruits, vegetables, grains, legumes).
- Limit animal protein to no more than 110-170 mg/day; recommend fish, skinless poultry, lean cuts of meat.

- Fiber promotes excretion of estrogens by favorable bacterial flora with less beta-glucuronidase activity.

### Fat Intake and Estrogen Metabolism

- Decreasing fat intake, especially saturated fat, reduces circulating estrogen by 36%. Low-fat diet improves PMS symptoms and reduces the risk of cancer, heart disease, and stroke. Keep fat intake to <30% of calories.
- Easiest way is to eat less animal products and more plant foods.

### Sugar

- Simple sugars increase insulin secretion and disturb glycemic control in hypoglycemics and diabetics. Sugar combined with caffeine has a detrimental effect on PMS and mood.
- Chocolate is the most significant symptom-producing food in PMS.
- Sugar impairs estrogen metabolism. PMS is more common in women eating a high-sugar diet. High sugar intake is associated with higher estrogen levels.
- Teach patients to read food labels carefully for clues about sugar content.

### Caffeine

- Avoid caffeine, especially if anxiety or depression or breast tenderness and fibrocystic breast disease are major symptoms.
- Caffeine intake is linked to severity of PMS: anxiety, irritability, insomnia, depression.

### Salt

- Excessive salt and diminished potassium stress the kidney's ability to maintain fluid volume.
- Salt sensitivity: high sodium intake increases blood pressure and/or water retention. Patients with water retention during mid-luteal phase may be sensitive to salt.
- Potassium intake must be concurrently increased with high-potassium foods (fruits and vegetables). Decrease high-sodium foods (processed foods). Keep total daily sodium intake <1800 mg.

## Hormone Therapy

### Progesterone Therapy

- Reservations: controlled clinical trials have failed to demonstrate consistent superiority of progesterone therapy over placebo. Positive studies used dosages that far exceed normal levels for progesterone (200-400 mg b.i.d. as a vaginal or rectal suppository from 14 days before expected onset of menstruation until onset of vaginal bleeding). Side effects include irregularity of menstruation, vaginal itching, and headache.
- Philosophy: address underlying causative factors—reduced detoxification or clearance of estrogen; reduced corpus luteum function.
- Progesterone creams are not recommended as a first step for treating PMS, but only as an option in difficult cases and when other nonhormonal methods have failed.

### Thyroid Function

- Hypothyroidism affects a large percentage of women with PMS.
- Many women with PMS and confirmed hypothyroidism given thyroid hormone have complete relief of symptoms (see the chapter on hypothyroidism).

## Stress, Endorphins, and Exercise

- Extreme, unusual, or long-lasting stress triggers brain changes by altered adrenal function and endorphin secretion or action. Domino effect alters normal physiology.

### Exercise

- Women who exercise regularly do not have PMS as often as do sedentary women. Regular exercisers get lower scores on impaired concentration, negative mood, behavior change, and pain.
- High exercisers have greater positive mood scores and the least depression and anxiety. Differences are most apparent during premenstrual and menstrual phases. Women who frequently exercise (but who are not competitive athletes) are protected from PMS. Exercise elevates endorphins and lowers cortisol.

### Coping Style

- Patients with PMS tend to use negative coping styles: feelings of helplessness, overeating, too much television, emotional outbursts, overspending, excessive behavior, dependence on chemicals, legal and illicit drugs, alcohol, smoking.

### Psychotherapy

- Biofeedback or short-term individual counseling (especially cognitive therapy) are clinically efficacious.
- Cognitive therapy can produce excellent results that are maintained over time.

### Depression and Low Serotonin

- Depression is common feature of PMS. Symptoms are more severe in depressed women. Eighty percent of 12 million Americans on Prozac are women ages 25 to 50 years.
- Cause: decrease in brain neurotransmitters, especially serotonin and gamma-aminobutyric acid.

## Nutritional Supplements

### Vitamin $B_6$

- Although PMS has multiple causes, $B_6$ supplementation alone benefits most patients.
- Some women cannot convert $B_6$ to its active form, pyridoxal-5-phosphate (P5P), because of a deficiency in another nutrient (e.g., vitamin $B_2$ or magnesium [Mg]). Use a broader-spectrum nutritional supplement or injectable P5P.
- Therapeutic dosage of $B_6$: 50-100 mg q.d. Divide dosages >50 mg into 50-mg doses throughout the day; 50 mg oral $B_6$ is all the liver can handle at once.
- Toxicity: one-time doses >2000 mg/day can produce nerve toxicity (tingling sensations in feet, loss of muscle coordination, and degeneration of nerve tissue). Long-term dosing >500 mg q.d. can be toxic if taken daily for many months or years. Rare reports suggest toxicity of long-term dosing as low as 150 mg/day. Supplemental $B_6$ overwhelms the liver's ability to add a phosphate group to produce the active form of P5P.
- Vitamin $B_6$ and Mg work together in many enzyme systems. $B_6$ may improve PMS by increasing accumulation of Mg within cells.

### Magnesium

- Mg deficiency is a causative factor in PMS, accounting for a wide range of symptoms. Mg deficiency and PMS share many common features; Mg supplementation can effectively treat PMS.
- Study findings: plasma Mg does not differ between PMS patients and control subjects. Menstrual cycle does not affect plasma Mg. Patients with PMS have lower cell Mg levels consistent across the menstrual cycle compared with control subjects. Mg measures do not correlate with severity of mood symptoms.
- Women with PMS have "vulnerability to luteal phase mood state destabilization." Chronic, enduring intracellular Mg depletion is a predisposing factor toward destabilization.
- Mg deficiency in PMS induces excessive nervous sensitivity with generalized aches and pains and lower premenstrual pain threshold.
- Better results are achieved by combining $B_6$ and other nutrients.
- Optimal intake for Mg: 6 mg/kg body weight. This is difficult to achieve by diet alone; supplementation is recommended. PMS dosage: 12 mg/kg body weight.
- Mg bound to aspartate or Krebs cycle intermediates (malate, succinate, fumarate, or citrate) is preferred over oxide, gluconate, sulfate, and chloride for better absorption and fewer side effects (laxative effects).

### Calcium

- Calcium (Ca) is a double-edged sword in PMS. High Ca intake from high milk consumption may be a causative factor; Ca, vitamin D, and phosphorus in milk may reduce the absorption of Mg.
- Ca supplementation (1000-1336 mg) can improve PMS symptoms. Ca and manganese supplementation (1336 and 5.6 mg, respectively) can improve mood, concentration, and behavior; 1000 mg/day can improve mood and water retention.
- Theory: Ca improves altered hormonal patterns, neurotransmitter levels, and smooth muscle responsiveness in PMS.
- Women with PMS have reduced bone mineral density (by dual-photon absorptiometry).

### Zinc

- Zinc (Zn) levels are low in women with PMS.
- Zn serves as a control factor for prolactin secretion. When Zn levels are low, prolactin release increases; high Zn levels

inhibit this release. In high-prolactin states, zinc is quite useful.
- Dosage for elevated prolactin in women: 30-45 mg picolinate form.

### Vitamin E

- Vitamin E has reduced breast tenderness, nervous tension, headache, fatigue, depression, and insomnia of PMS after 3 months of use. It also increased energy levels and reduced headaches and cravings for sweets.
- Dose: 400 IU q.d.

### Essential Fatty Acids

- Women with PMS have decreased gamma-linolenic acid (GLA), which is derived from linoleic acid. This conversion requires $B_6$, Mg, and Zn as cofactors in the key conversion enzyme, delta-6-desaturase.
- Evening primrose, blackcurrant, and borage oils contain GLA, with typical levels being 9, 12, and 22%, respectively.
- Meta-analysis of clinical trials of evening primrose oil for PMS found little value in management of PMS. A better approach is to provide nutrients required for proper essential fatty acid metabolism plus adequate essential fatty acids and GLA.

### Multiple Vitamin/Mineral Supplements

- Nutritional deficiency is common among women with PMS.
- High-potency multiple vitamin/mineral formulations produce significant benefits in PMS.
- Patients with PMS given a multivitamin/mineral supplement with high doses of Mg and $B_6$ have reductions (70%+ reduction) in both premenopausal and postmenstrual symptoms.

## Botanical Medicines

Herbs traditionally used have a tonic effect on the female glandular system because of phytoestrogens or other compounds that improve hormonal balance of the female system and improve blood flow to female organs. Phytoestrogen activity is only 2% as strong as estrogen; thus phytoestrogens have a balancing action on estrogen effects. If estrogen levels are low, phytoestrogens will increase estrogen effect. If estrogen levels are high, phytoestrogens compete with estrogen, decreasing estrogen effects.

Often the same plant is recommended for PMS, menopause, and irregular menses. Many are termed uterine tonics because they nourish and tone female glandular and organ system. This nonspecific mode of action makes many herbs useful in a broad range of female conditions.

### *Angelica sinensis* (Dong Quai)

- Used in Asia for menopausal symptoms (hot flashes), dysmenorrhea (painful menstruation), amenorrhea (absence of menstruation), and metrorrhagia (abnormal menstruation) and to ensure a healthy pregnancy and easy delivery.
- Uterine tonic, causing initial increase in uterine contraction followed by relaxation. It increases uterine weight and glucose utilization by the liver and uterus.
- Dosage schedule: start on day 14; continue until menses begins unless patient typically has dysmenorrhea, in which case continue until menses cease.

### *Glycyrrhiza glabra* (Licorice)

- Lowers estrogen while simultaneously raising progesterone. It raises progesterone by inhibiting enzyme that breaks it down.
- Reduces water retention by blocking aldosterone. Glycyrrhetinic acid binds to aldosterone receptors, but its activity is only 25% as strong as aldosterone. If aldosterone levels are normal, long-term ingestion of licorice in large doses may cause symptoms of hyperaldosterone-induced hypertension caused by sodium and water retention.
- Preventing side effects: high-potassium, low-sodium diet. Avoid in patients with a history of hypertension, renal failure, or current use of digitalis.
- Dosage schedule: begin on day 14 of cycle and continue until menstruation.

### *Cimicifuga racemosa* (Black Cohosh)

- Used by American Indians and colonists for menstrual cramps and menopause.
- Remefemin, an extract of black cohosh standardized to contain 1 mg of triterpenes calculated as 27-deoxyacteine per tablet and used in Germany for 40+ years, is a safe and effective natural alternative to hormone replacement therapy for menopause and PMS.

- Remefemin "performed very well" in PMS; it reduced depression, anxiety, tension, mood swings.

### *Vitex agnus castus* (Chaste Tree)

- Used traditionally to suppress libido.
- Single most important herb for PMS. Graded as good or very good by physicians in the treatment of PMS. Thirty-three percent of women achieve complete resolution of symptoms; another 57% have significant improvement.
- Alters gonadotropin-releasing hormone (GnRH) and follicle-stimulating hormone–releasing hormone (FSH-RH), normalizing secretion of other hormones, reducing prolactin, and reducing estrogen/progesterone ratio.
- Reduces irritability, mood changes, anger, headache, and breast tenderness. Bloating is only symptom that does not change significantly with *Vitex*.
- Dosage: *Vitex* standardized extract (20-mg tablet standardized for casticin) daily.

### *Ginkgo biloba*

- Effective against congestive symptoms of PMS: breast pain or tenderness and vascular congestion.
- Dosage: ginkgo extract of 25% ginkgo flavonglycosides at 80 mg b.i.d. from day 16 to day 5 of cycle.

### *Hypericum perforatum* (St. John's Wort)

- Dosage: 300 mg St. John's wort standardized to 900 μg hypericin.
- Reduces emotional symptoms of PMS overall by 51%, with 67% of women tested having at least a 50% decrease in severity of symptoms—crying, depression, confusion, feeling out of control, nervous tension, anxiety, and insomnia.

## THERAPEUTIC APPROACH

Seven key steps to consider:

1. Evaluate PMS symptoms by having patient complete a questionnaire.
2. Rule out psychiatric or other medical condition.
3. Implement dietary recommendations for PMS:
   a. Vegetarian or predominantly vegetarian diet

   b. Reduce fat
   c. Eliminate sugar
   d. Reduce exposure to environmental estrogens
   e. Eliminate caffeine
   f. Keep salt intake low
4. Follow guidelines for nutritional supplementation given below.
5. Select appropriate herbal support:
   a. PMS-associated breast pain, infrequent periods, or history of ovarian cysts: *Vitex agnus castus*
   b. Menstrual cramps: *Angelica sinensis*
   c. PMS water retention: *Glycyrrhiza glabra*
   d. Perimenopause symptoms as well as PMS: *Cimicifuga racemosa*
6. Establish a program for stress reduction; recommend regular exercise.
7. If after at least three complete periods the patient does not have significant improvement or complete resolution of symptoms, identify additional causative factors as detailed above or change treatment program.

## Nutritional Supplements

- Multivitamin/mineral supplement
- Vitamin $B_6$: 100 mg q.d.
- Mg: 500 mg q.d.
- Vitamin E (mixed tocopherols): 400 IU q.d.

## Botanical Medicines

- *Angelica sinensis*: t.i.d.
  —Powdered root or as tea: 1-2 g
  —Tincture (1:5): 4 mL (1 tsp)
  —Fluid extract: 1 mL (¼ tsp)
- *Glycyrrhiza glabra*: t.i.d.
  —Powdered root or as tea: 1-2 g
  —Fluid extract (1:1): 4 mL (1 tsp)
  —Solid (dry powdered) extract (4:1): 250-500 mg
- *Cimicifuga racemosa*
  —Standardized extract (4 mg 27-deoxyacteine): 1 tablet q.d. or b.i.d.
- *Vitex agnus castus*: q.d.
  —Standardized extract (0.5% agnuside): 175-225 mg daily or 20 mg standardized to casticin
  —Liquid extract: 2 mL

- *Ginkgo biloba*
  —80 mg standardized extract b.i.d.
- *Hypericum perforatum*
  —300 mg standardized extract (900 μg hypericin ) q.d. to t.i.d.

## Signs and Symptoms of Premenstrual Syndrome

- Behavioral
  —Nervousness, anxiety, and irritability
  —Mood swings and mild to severe personality change
  —Fatigue, lethargy, and depression
- Gastrointestinal
  —Abdominal bloating
  —Diarrhea and/or constipation
  —Change in appetite (usually craving of sugar)
- Female
  —Tender and enlarged breasts
  —Uterine cramping
  —Altered libido
- General
  —Headache
  —Backache
  —Acne
  —Edema of fingers and ankles

## Primary Causes of Premenstrual Syndrome

- Estrogen excess
- Progesterone deficiency
- Elevated prolactin levels
- Hypothyroidism
- Stress, endogenous opioid deficiency, and adrenal dysfunction
- Depression
- Nutritional abnormalities
- Macronutrient disturbances or excesses
- Micronutrient deficiency

## Physiologic Effects of an Increased Estrogen to Progesterone Ratio

- Impaired liver function
- Reduced manufacture of serotonin
- Decreased action of vitamin $B_6$
- Increased aldosterone secretion
- Increased prolactin secretion

# Proctologic Conditions

## ANORECTAL ANATOMY

- Anorectal region:
  - —Anus: extends from 3 to 4 cm above anal verge and merges with rectum
  - —Rectum: 12 to 18 cm in length
  - —Anal verge: demarcation point from perianal skin to anal skin
- Anal canal:
  - —Dentate line: demarcation between ectoderm of external squamous epithelium and rectal entodermal mucosa. Anal canal does not contain sebaceous or sweat glands; it is innervated by somatic nerves up to and slightly beyond dentate line; it is sensitive to pain. Above the dentate line, rectal mucosa is relatively insensitive to pain but registers distention and inflammation as diffuse visceral pain.
  - —Anorectal line: point above which rectum expands outward into pelvic bowl.
- Rectal columns, anal valves, anal glands, and anal crypts: occupy area between dentate and anorectal lines. Anal glands provide mucus to lubricate passage of stool and empty into anal crypts. This area is the locus of anal fistula or perirectal abscess if crypt becomes impacted, unable to discharge mucus. Anal fissures lie below the dentate line. Midway between dentate and anorectal lines lies the white line of Hilton, or pectinate line, the location of the intersphincteric groove, the region that lies between internal and external sphincters. The internal sphincter is controlled by the autonomic nervous system; the external sphincter is under somatic or voluntary control.
- Vascular supply: inferior mesenteric artery and internal iliac artery; superior, middle and inferior rectal arteries; anastomosis between these branches. Venous return: superior and middle hemorrhoid veins that empty into inferior mesenteric veins and,

*Text continued on p. 671*

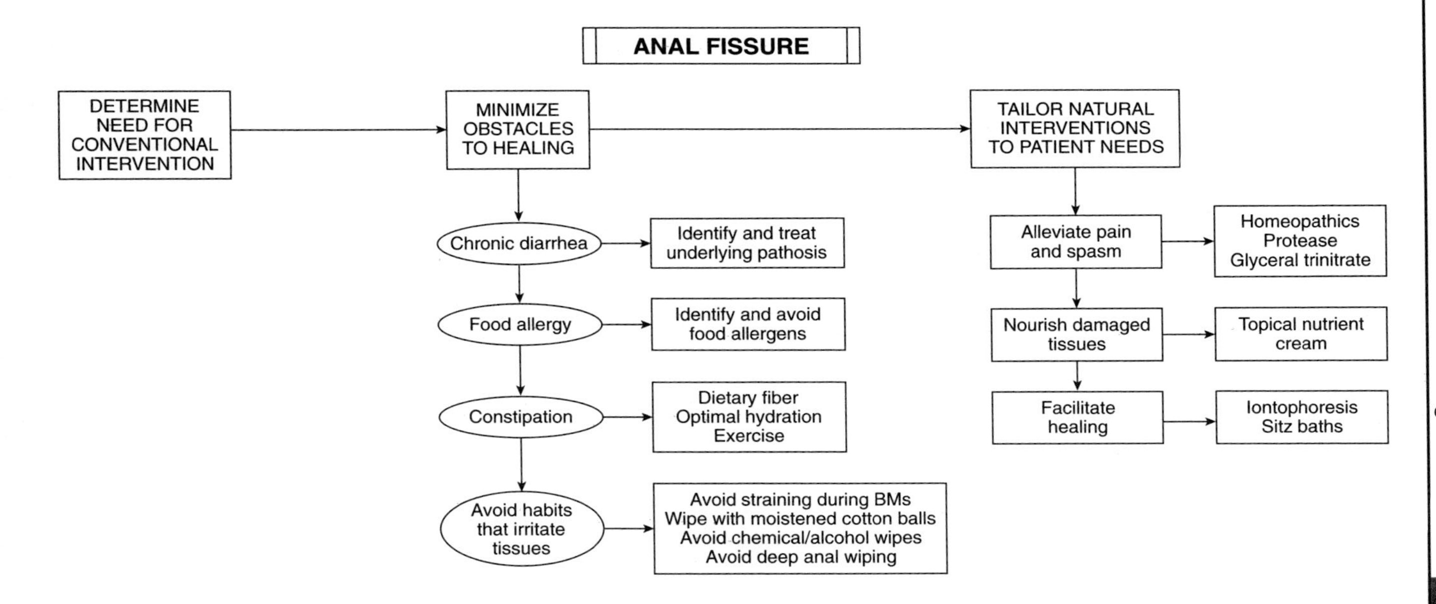
ANAL FISSURE
DETERMINE NEED FOR CONVENTIONAL INTERVENTION
MINIMIZE OBSTACLES TO HEALING
Chronic diarrhea
Identify and treat underlying pathosis
Food allergy
Identify and avoid food allergens
Constipation
Dietary fiber
Optimal hydration
Exercise
Avoid habits that irritate tissues
Avoid straining during BMs
Wipe with moistened cotton balls
Avoid chemical/alcohol wipes
Avoid deep anal wiping
TAILOR NATURAL INTERVENTIONS TO PATIENT NEEDS
Alleviate pain and spasm
Homeopathics
Protease
Glyceral trinitrate
Nourish damaged tissues
Topical nutrient cream
Facilitate healing
Iontophoresis
Sitz baths

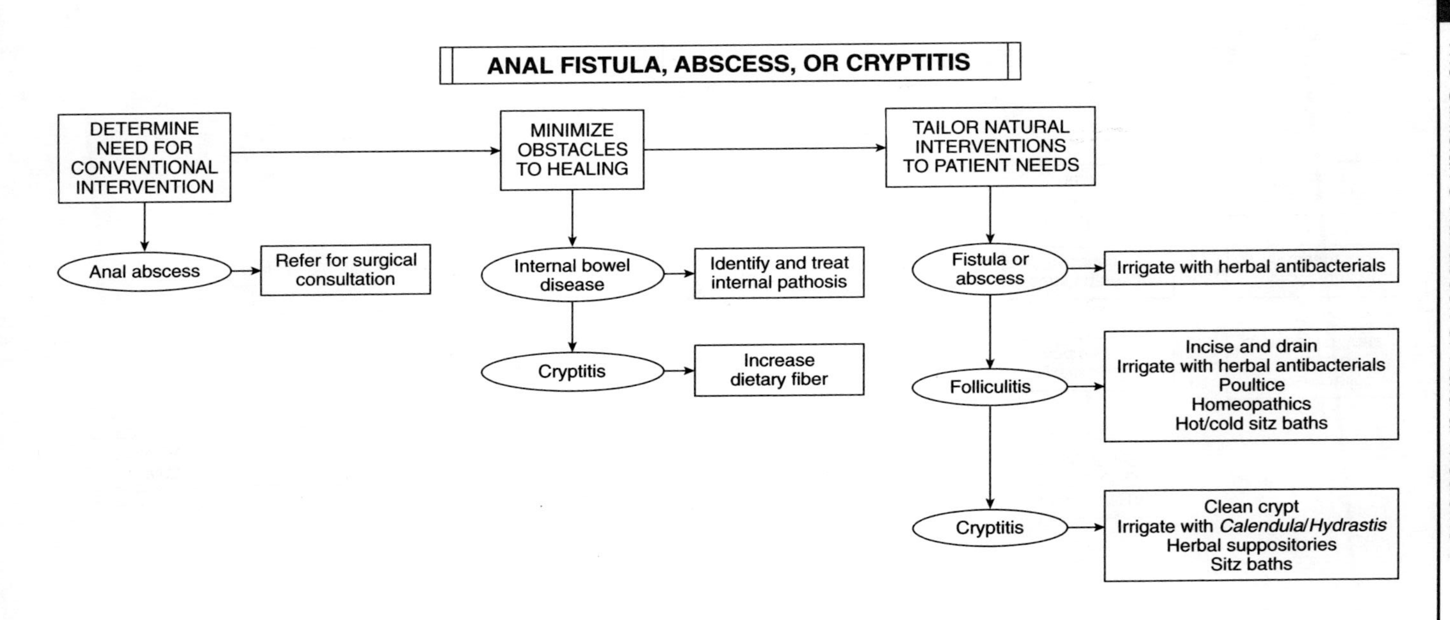
ANAL FISTULA, ABSCESS, OR CRYPTITIS
DETERMINE NEED FOR CONVENTIONAL INTERVENTION
Anal abscess
Refer for surgical consultation
MINIMIZE OBSTACLES TO HEALING
Internal bowel disease
Identify and treat internal pathosis
Cryptitis
Increase dietary fiber
TAILOR NATURAL INTERVENTIONS TO PATIENT NEEDS
Fistula or abscess
Irrigate with herbal antibacterials
Folliculitis
Incise and drain
Irrigate with herbal antibacterials
Poultice
Homeopathics
Hot/cold sitz baths
Cryptitis
Clean crypt
Irrigate with *Calendula*/*Hydrastis*
Herbal suppositories
Sitz baths

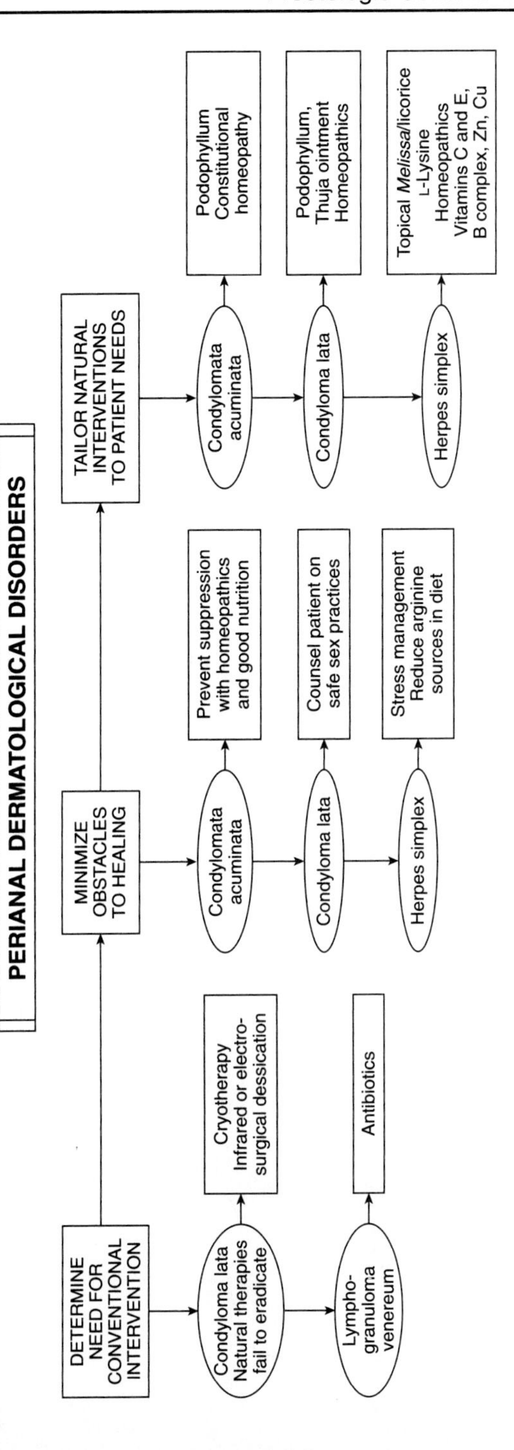
PERIANAL DERMATOLOGICAL DISORDERS
DETERMINE NEED FOR CONVENTIONAL INTERVENTION
Condyloma lata Natural therapies fail to eradicate
Cryotherapy Infrared or electro-surgical dessication
Lympho-granuloma venereum
Antibiotics
MINIMIZE OBSTACLES TO HEALING
Condylomata acuminata
Prevent suppression with homeopathics and good nutrition
Condyloma lata
Counsel patient on safe sex practices
Herpes simplex
Stress management Reduce arginine sources in diet
TAILOR NATURAL INTERVENTIONS TO PATIENT NEEDS
Condylomata acuminata
Podophyllum Constitutional homeopathy
Condyloma lata
Podophyllum, Thuja ointment Homeopathics
Herpes simplex
Topical Melissa/licorice L-Lysine Homeopathics Vitamins C and E, B complex, Zn, Cu

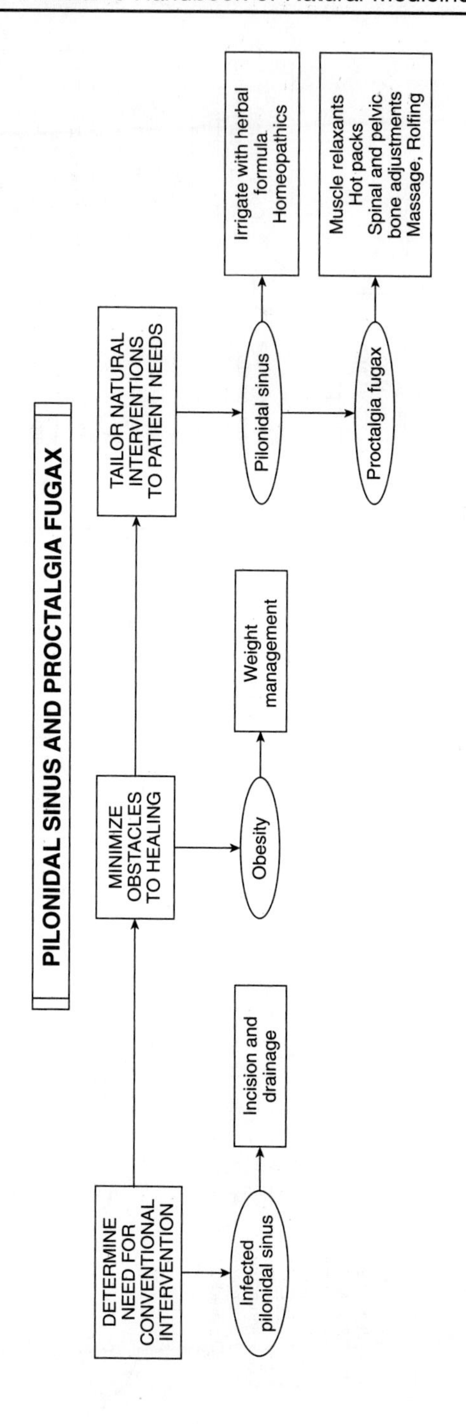
PILONIDAL SINUS AND PROCTALGIA FUGAX
DETERMINE NEED FOR CONVENTIONAL INTERVENTION
Infected pilonidal sinus
Incision and drainage
MINIMIZE OBSTACLES TO HEALING
Obesity
Weight management
TAILOR NATURAL INTERVENTIONS TO PATIENT NEEDS
Pilonidal sinus
Irrigate with herbal formula
Homeopathics
Proctalgia fugax
Muscle relaxants
Hot packs
Spinal and pelvic bone adjustments
Massage, Rolfing

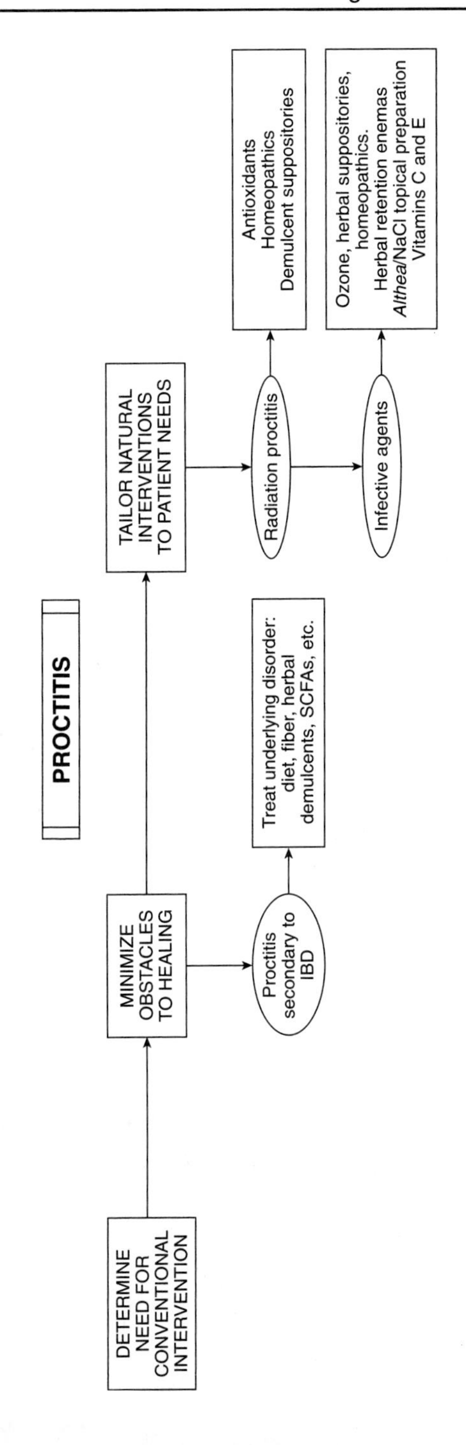
PROCTITIS
DETERMINE NEED FOR CONVENTIONAL INTERVENTION
MINIMIZE OBSTACLES TO HEALING
Proctitis secondary to IBD
Treat underlying disorder: diet, fiber, herbal demulcents, SCFAs, etc.
TAILOR NATURAL INTERVENTIONS TO PATIENT NEEDS
Radiation proctitis
Antioxidants
Homeopathics
Demulcent suppositories
Infective agents
Ozone, herbal suppositories, homeopathics.
Herbal retention enemas
*Althea*/NaCl topical preparation
Vitamins C and E

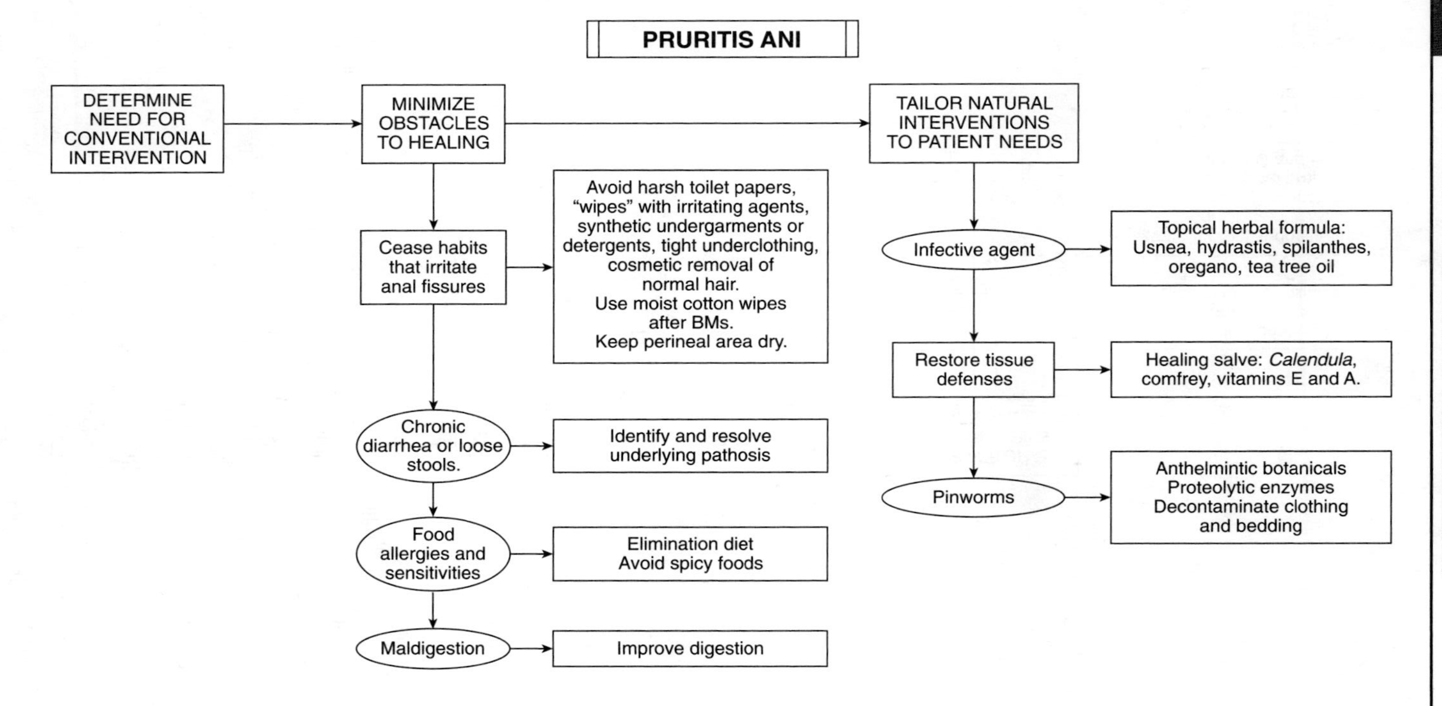
PRURITIS ANI
DETERMINE NEED FOR CONVENTIONAL INTERVENTION
MINIMIZE OBSTACLES TO HEALING
Cease habits that irritate anal fissures
Avoid harsh toilet papers, "wipes" with irritating agents, synthetic undergarments or detergents, tight underclothing, cosmetic removal of normal hair.
Use moist cotton wipes after BMs.
Keep perineal area dry.
Chronic diarrhea or loose stools.
Identify and resolve underlying pathosis
Food allergies and sensitivities
Elimination diet
Avoid spicy foods
Maldigestion
Improve digestion
TAILOR NATURAL INTERVENTIONS TO PATIENT NEEDS
Infective agent
Topical herbal formula: Usnea, hydrastis, spilanthes, oregano, tea tree oil
Restore tissue defenses
Healing salve: Calendula, comfrey, vitamins E and A.
Pinworms
Anthelmintic botanicals
Proteolytic enzymes
Decontaminate clothing and bedding

subsequently, portal vein and internal iliac vein, vena cava, bypassing liver.

- Muscles: levator ani muscle forms the floor of the pelvis and helps form the puborectalis sling. The puborectalis sling causes the bowel to change direction as it penetrates the pelvic floor, making passage of stool easier. The sphincter mechanism controls continence.
- Innervation of anal canal: pudendal nerves originating from S2, S3, and S4.
- Presenting symptoms: pain, tenderness, rectal spasm, bleeding, itching, protrusions, eruptions, discharges, constipation, diarrhea, changes in stool pattern, sacral backache, shooting pains down limbs, cramping and painful menses, urinary disturbances, anemia, prostatitis, restlessness (in children), foreign bodies. Seemingly unrelated symptoms may have their origin in the anorectal tract.

## ANAL DISEASES

### Anal Fistula and Anal Abscess

- Result of infection of an anal crypt whose distal end lies near the dentate line. Anal glands become infected because of impacted feces. Infection progresses into intersphincteric space but generally does not penetrate beyond the external sphincter. Most anal glands lie posteriorly; thus most abscesses drain from a line posterior to the ischial tuberosities; anterior ones drain radially from points of origin. Rectal fistula or abscess may indicate internal bowel disease: diverticulitis, trauma to area, or immune system incompetence such as HIV.
- Weak points of highly vascularized rectal mucosa are anal glands impacted with feces. Surrounding tissue is swollen, red, and painful to touch. If infection remains in the intersphincteric space, rectal pain is seemingly without specific findings. Eliciting pain with pressure on examination provides a clue regarding the source. The patient may have a fever of unknown origin.
- Adjacent ischiorectal fossae have fatty tissue that allows distension of the rectum. An abscess can progress in many directions. In true perianal abscess, incision and drainage are contraindicated; bulk of lesion is untouched because of the invasion of underlying tissues and caverns of pus. Unlike other abscesses, do not allow perianal abscesses to come to a head and rupture to avoid excess necrosis of the anal sphincter.

- Obtain surgical consult for rectal abscess. Surgery opens the tract, allowing healing by second intention. Localized treatment helps abscess drain if it has ruptured or if patient presents acutely and referral is not immediately possible. Irrigate with herbal antibacterial agents: *Hydrastis, Usnea,* and *Calendula succus* in 0.9% saline will help drainage.
- Folliculitis with abscess: incise and drain. They do not involve anal canal or ischiorectal fossa. Homeopathics: *Calcarea sulphurica, Silicea, Hepar sulphuris, Myristica.* Poultices of onion, garlic, or potatoes have drawing action. Also use alternating hot and cold sitz baths. After abscess breaks open or is incised and drained, irrigate with these herbal solutions.

## Anal Cryptitis

- Anal crypts are pockets between grooves formed by rectal columns at their distal point ending at the dentate line. Anal cryptitis, as separate from fistula, is debatable and rare. Symptom: pain worsened by bowel movement (BM). Signs: localized tenderness and redness at dentate line; rectal spasm. Rule out rectal fissure. Chronic cases suggest bacterial infection of gonorrhea.
- Treatment: herbal suppository, sitz baths, increased dietary fiber, local anesthesia as needed. Clean crypt with crypt hook if needed; irrigate with solution of *Calendula succus* and *Hydrastis* in normal saline.

## Anal Fissure

- Anal fissure: slitlike separation of anal mucosa that lies below the dentate line. Majority (70%-80%) are in the posterior midline region; anterior midline lesions (10%-20%) are more common in women. Oval anal sphincter (rather than round), coming to a Y or narrow point at posterior midline, predisposes to fissure. Anal fissure also occurs in children with chronic diarrhea or hard stool. Fissure may also arise from congenital anal deformity. Lesions in anteroposterior vertical axis suggest internal bowel disease—Crohn's disease, squamous cell or adenocarcinoma of rectum, syphilitic fissure, and ulceration of tuberculosis (TB).
- Very painful from the somatic innervation of spasm of the anal sphincter induced by stretching during BM. Anal fissure triggers vicious cycle—pain causing sphincter spasm with tightening of sphincter and increased pain with BM. Symptoms: severe pain during and after BM and bleeding. As lesion enlarges it may ulcerate and become infected. Conventional treatment: rectal

dilation, internal sphincterotomy, electrodessication, or surgical excision.

- Causes: passage of large, hard stools; childbirth trauma; chronic diarrhea; trauma; food allergy; prolonged straining to pass stool. High risk: Infants and young children ingesting large amounts of cow's milk, with chronic constipation, especially if breastfed only a short time. Personality traits: intense, compulsive. Predisposing factors: previous anal or rectal operation, syphilis, Crohn's disease.
- Examination: difficult because of pain and spasm; anoscopic examination requires anesthesia. Local injection of 1% or 2% lidocaine into rectal sphincter at the 3 o'clock and 9 o'clock positions relaxes it enough for examination. Fissures are visible without anoscope; pull back anal skin and examine tissue. Sentinel pile or enlarged papillae suggest chronic anal fissure. Anal stenosis and fibrosis indicate chronic state.
- Differential diagnosis: Crohn's disease, especially if patient is younger, has history of periodic or chronic diarrhea, and fissure lies in anteroposterior vertical axis; squamous cell carcinoma; syphilitic ulcers; rarely TB. Spasm of levator ani muscle has no lesion.
- Treatment is challenging. Surgery removes the lesion and alleviates pain, but lesion will return if underlying cause is unresolved. Surgery predisposes to fecal incontinence later in life. Educate patient that healing will have exacerbations and remissions.
- Initial treatment: alleviate pain and spasm. Homeopathics: promptly relieve if simillimum is found; aid healing process. Remedies: *Chamomilla*, graphite, nitric acid, *Ratanhia, Sepia, Silicea thuja*. Dose frequently. Protease 2500 μU, 2 capsules t.i.d. between meals and before bed, alleviates pain. Use preparation of 0.2% glycerol trinitrate topically to relieve rectal spasm and 5% lidocaine cream for local pain. Glycerol trinitrate relieves rectal spasm and increases blood flow to sphincter. (Decreased sphincter blood flow may be a precipitating mechanism of fissure.)
- Topical cream of vitamins A and E, panthenol, calendula, and comfrey enhances healing by nourishing tissues. Some of the commercial preparations contain boric acid for a styptic effect. Apply cream topically after every BM and at bedtime. As healing occurs, twice-daily administration suffices until lesion resolves.
- Iontophoresis: use zinc electrode and apply positive current to facilitate healing by hardening underlying fissure, decreasing

bleeding, and relieving pain. Patient lies on negative dispersing pad and current is applied for 10 minutes at 10 mA.
- Patient should avoid straining during BM and use cotton balls moistened with water, rather than toilet paper or chemical or alcohol wipes; avoid wiping deep into anal canal.
- Sitz baths increase blood flow. Alternative: spray hot and cold water on perineal area.
- Increase dietary fiber if condition is caused by chronic constipation. If chronic diarrhea, identify cause. Diet changes are mandatory in irritable bowel syndrome, Crohn's disease, and so forth. Higher rates of hemorrhoids and Crohn's disease occur with blood group O because of food intolerance.
- Frequent follow-up: assess healing; reassure patient. After healing, maintain proper bowel function and good dietary habits.

## Hemorrhoids

### Internal Hemorrhoids

- Begin to develop during the 20s; symptoms manifest in the 30s. Fifty percent of persons older than 50 years have symptomatic hemorrhoids; one third of total U.S. population have hemorrhoids to some degree.
- Causes: genetics, excessive venous pressure, pregnancy, long periods of standing or sitting, straining at stool, heavy lifting, portal vein lacking valves. Factors increasing venous congestion in perianal region can precipitate hemorrhoids: increasing intraabdominal pressure (e.g., defecation, pregnancy, coughing, sneezing, vomiting, physical exertion, and portal hypertension from cirrhosis), straining during BM, and standing or sitting for prolonged periods.
- Presenting symptoms: itching, burning, irritation with BM, swelling of anus and perianal region, blood on toilet paper or in bowl, seepage of mucus. Rarely are internal hemorrhoids painful or itchy. Hallmark of hemorrhoids: bleeding or protrusion after passing stool. Pain of internal hemorrhoids occurs with strangulation from prolapse and thrombosis. Other pain is from a coexisting lesion, such as a fissure. Itching is rare with internal hemorrhoids except with excess mucus.
- Originate above anorectal line in the right anterior, right posterior, and left lateral quadrants. Other areas have secondary hemorrhoids. Occasionally internal hemorrhoid enlarges enough to prolapse below anal sphincter.

- Classified by symptoms and examination findings. Stage I: bleed but do not protrude. Stage II: protrude after BM; spontaneously reduce. Stage III: protrude with BM; must be manually reduced. Stage IV: protrude; not reducible. Stages II, III, and IV may or may not bleed. Stage IV: possible strangulation with decreased blood flow and thrombosis.
- Internal-external, or mixed hemorrhoids: combination of contiguous external and internal hemorrhoids that appear as baggy swellings. Treating internal hemorrhoid may resolve external portion. If patient has external hemorrhoids, internal ones are probably present.
- Hemorrhoids are rare in cultures with high-fiber, unrefined diets. Low-fiber diet leads to strain during BMs because of smaller, harder stools. Straining increases abdominal pressure, obstructing venous return, increasing pelvic congestion, and weakening veins.

### Treatment

- High-fiber diet rich in vegetables, fruits, legumes, and whole grains promotes peristalsis and keeps feces soft, bulky, easy to pass, with less straining.
- Natural bulking compounds: psyllium seeds and guar gum attract water to form a gelatinous mass. They are less irritating than wheat bran and other cellulose fibers. They reduce symptoms (bleeding, pain, pruritus, prolapse) and improve bowel habits within 6 weeks.
- Breakfast: 7.5-fold increase in odds of hemorrhoids or anal fissures in persons who do not eat breakfast.
- Flavonoids: rutin and hydroxyethyl rutoside (HER) prevent and treat hemorrhoids by strengthening venous tissues. HER (1000 mg q.d. for 4 weeks) relieves hemorrhoidal signs and symptoms in pregnant women. Micronized flavonoid combination (diosmin 90% and hesperidin 10%) for 8 weeks before delivery and 4 weeks after delivery also helps pregnant women. Treatment is well accepted and does not affect pregnancy, fetal development, birth weight, infant growth, or feeding.
- Topical treatments: suppositories, ointments, and anorectal pads only provide temporary relief. Natural ingredients: witch hazel (*Hamamelis*), cocoa butter, Peruvian balsam, zinc oxide, allantoin, homeopathics. Hydrocortisone cream relieves itching. Prolonged use can aggravate pruritus ani.

- Botanical medicines: used topically, as suppositories, or taken internally. Rectal suppositories after galvanic, infrared, or laser therapy facilitate healing and decrease bleeding.
- Hydrotherapy: warm sitz bath for uncomplicated acute flare-up; alternate hot and cold sitz baths for chronic conditions.
- Surgery: stage I and II are managed medically, especially if acute. Herbal suppositories and indicated homeopathics can calm flare-ups. Uncomplicated asymptomatic stage I and II: treatment not recommended; increase dietary fiber and improve diet choices. Injection of sclerosing agents: useful in stage I and II but contraindicated with anal fissure, inflammatory bowel disease, Crohn's disease, leukemia, portal hypertension. Sclerosing therapy is not usually effective in stage III and IV. Rubber band ligation: office procedure to remove redundant tissue and cause scarring replaced by new tissue. It induces sense of fullness and pressure; pain occurs if band is too close to pectinate line. Complications: bleeding; sometimes septicemia and death. Used for stage I, II, and occasionally stage III hemorrhoids; success is based on physician's skill in placing band.
- Cryosurgery: liquid nitrogen or nitrous oxide applied to hemorrhoid to destroy venous plexus, triggering scarring and tissue replacement. Used for stage II and III and condyloma but contraindicated for stage IV, chronic ulcers, and acutely thrombosed hemorrhoids. Sequelae: pain, swelling, and bleeding.
- Hemorrhoidectomy, the removal of redundant tissue, is the most invasive; requires outpatient surgical setting. Complications: pain and rectal sphincter instability.
- Monopolar direct current technique (inverse galvanism) of Keesey: treatment of choice in the United States; painless, effective, and safe outpatient treatment of all grades of hemorrhoids. It also relieves chronic anal fissures associated with internal hemorrhoids. Relief of chronic pain can occur after two treatments; anal fissures can heal in 4 weeks. This office procedure requires no anesthetic except locally for hypersensitive or nervous patients. Use 2% procaine solution injected directly into hemorrhoid. Chemicophysiologic action causes absorption and destruction of vein and permanent cure. Mechanism of action: introduced into interior of hemorrhoid, the negative pole of galvanic current generates $H_2$ gas and $OH^-$ ions at contact with water of blood and tissues. Hydroxide destroys hemorrhoid and capillaries, producing hydrolysis and then hardening of hemorrhoid. Resolution: either absorption or rupture, with discharge of

thrombosed elements into rectum, then contraction of residual tissues. Patient is freely ambulant after procedure. Hemorrhoid disappears 7 to 10 days after treatment. Treat each separate hemorrhoid; larger hemorrhoids may need more than one treatment. Treat only one or two hemorrhoids at one time to minimize bleeding and allow healing.

- Infrared coagulation (IRC): for stage I and II and combined with Keesey treatment for stage III and IV. Burst of intense heat is generated internally and shot through blue anodized sapphire tip to surface of hemorrhoid. IRC "coagulates" redundant tissue to a depth depending on the amount of time of light burst, 1 to 1.5 seconds. A 7- to 10-day period of healing is needed between treatments. Keesey treatment plus IRC usually reduces number of treatments needed per hemorrhoid. Compared with rubber band, laser, or cryotherapy, IRC gives better results and has less morbidity.
- Prevention: reduce straining during BM and sitting or standing for prolonged periods; address underlying liver disease. Eat a high-fiber diet for proper bowel activity, including nutrients and botanicals that enhance integrity of venous structures, proanthocyanidin- and anthocyanidin-rich foods (blackberries, cherries, blueberries, etc.) to strengthen vein structures. Supplements: vitamins A and B complex, antioxidant vitamins C and E, and zinc maintain vascular integrity and facilitate healing.

### External Hemorrhoids

- External hemorrhoids arise from dilation of external rectal plexus or thrombosis constipation, diarrhea, heavy lifting, or Valsalva from sneezing, coughing, or childbirth.
- Symptoms: often-painful perianal lump with bleeding; mild to little discomfort; resolve on their own if homeostasis is restored. External anal skin tags are remnants of previous external hemorrhoids. Thrombosis and increasing distension trigger cycle of acute edema and pain, worsened by BM or prolonged sitting, and bleeding after stool.
- Differential diagnosis: prolapsed internal hemorrhoid, perianal abscess, rectal fissure with sentinel pile, hypertrophied anal papillae, irritated skin tag, and condyloma latum or acuminata.
- Treatment: unless thrombosed or excessively painful, manage medically. Relieve pressure and dissolve thrombosis. Long-term management: patient education, dietary changes, enhanced

vascular integrity. Initial treatment: enzyme protease 2400 μU 2 capsules between meals t.i.d. and 2 capsules at bedtime reduce thrombosis and decrease pain. Alternating sitz baths relieve pain and increase blood flow. Homeopathics: *Aesculus, Aloe, Hamamelis,* muriatic acid, *Ratanhia,* and *Sepia* relieve pain and speed healing.

- Long-term management: dietary changes to eliminate offending foods; increase dietary fiber with fruits and vegetables or over-the-counter fiber supplement. Herbal medicines: *Aesculus, Collinsonia, Hamamelis, Althea,* and *Ulmus* restore venous sufficiency and soothe inflamed tissues. Regulating bowel function with herbal laxatives may help normalize intestinal and colon function.
- Acute thrombosed external hemorrhoid: prompt surgical excision or incision is in order. Anesthesia before evacuation of clot is needed. Excision leaves wound that should not be sutured but allowed to heal, but this leads to increased postoperative pain. Incision and debridement of clot reduce pain but may close too early, reforming thrombus. Consult text on minor or rectal surgery.
- Herbal anodynes *Piscidia* and *Belladonna* for pain of rectal spasm; *Hyoscyamus niger* facilitates postoperative management. Topicals: *Arnica, Hypericum,* and *Calendula succus.*
- Alternating sitz baths with ½ ounce of Betadine enhances healing and decreases chance of infection. Protease 2400 μU can give pain relief. Homeopathic *Arnica, Calendula,* and *Staphisagria* also give pain relief.

## PERIANAL DERMATOLOGIC DISORDERS

### Condylomata Acuminata

- Symptoms: sticking or foreign body sensation perianally. Large lesion interferes with defecation; hygiene is problematic. Lesion is soft, moist, reddish pink, pedunculated. Differentiation: condylomata lata of secondary syphilis. Rapid plasma reagin test with reflexive fluorescent treponemal antibodies is warranted. Diagnosis of condylomata acuminata is made by biopsy.
- Treatment: solution of 25% podophyllum applied topically 6 to 8 hours before patient washes it off. Several applications may be necessary. Infrared coagulation after injection of subcutaneous 1% or 2% lidocaine. Proper homeopathics coupled with good nutritional program can prevent suppression of lesions

contributing to deepening of the disease process. A number of homeopathics cover genital warts. Administering constitutional homeopathic medicine eradicates lesion and decreases susceptibility to reoccurrence.

### Condyloma Lata

- Anogenital warts: caused by human papilloma viruses (HPV) types 6, 11, 16, 18, 31, 33, and 35; transmitted by sexual contact. Appearance: soft, moist, pink to gray, flat to pedunculated excresences, often in clusters. Location: warm, moist regions of anogenital region, often clustered around anus in homosexual men and women who practice receptive anal intercourse.
- Differential diagnosis: flat lesion of condyloma lata of secondary syphilis; squamous cell carcinoma if lesion does not respond to therapy or by biopsy.
- Treatment: 25% podophyllum, thuja ointment, homeopathics, cryotherapy, infrared or electrosurgical desiccation.

### Lymphogranuloma Venereum

- Infective agent: serotype of *Chlamydia trachomatis*.
- Appearance: papule lesion that ulcerates and heals rapidly. If in rectal mucosa, signs and symptoms of proctitis are present. Extremely painful inguinal adenitis or buboes subsequently arise. Later stages: fistulation, ulceration, fibrosis, rectal or anal stenosis, lymphedema of legs and genitalia. Non–lymphogranuloma venereum *Chlamydia* serotypes can also be implicated in proctitis but without severity of symptoms.
- WBC counts may reach 20,000/mL if lymphatic involvement; anemia is possible. Culture of chlamydial serotype from infected lesion is diagnostic, but complement fixation and immunofluorescent antibody tests are available.
- If treated promptly, prognosis is good. Cellular changes worsen prognosis. Allopathic treatment: antibiotics such as doxycycline, erythromycin, sulfisoxazole are effective. Homeopathic and herbals: see treatments under proctitis.

### Herpes

- Most frequently encountered perianal lesion. Symptoms and signs: burning, searing pain; confused with rectal fissure. Examination: vesicles on erythematous base erode and form ulcers. With HIV or other immunocompromised condition, lesions can form deep ulcers of prolonged duration. Diagnosis: by Tzanck smear or viral culture.

- Treatment: address current eruption. Topicals: licorice root and *Melissa officinalis* extracts alleviate burning and pain and facilitate healing; zinc sulfate 2% is useful. Homeopathics address pain and eruptions and decrease susceptibility to outbreaks. Stress reduction: herpes eruptions often occur during excessive stress or other illness.
- Long-term strategies: decrease arginine-containing foods such as nuts, peanuts, chocolate. Increasing lysine at 500 to 1000 mg/day reduces outbreaks. Vitamins C, E, and B complex and zinc and copper are beneficial.

## Pilonidal Sinus

- Definition: rare congenital tract that runs from coccyx or sacrum to perineum with constant drainage. Congenital and acquired factors contribute. Symptom: chronic discharge.
- Prevalence: most common in young white adults; rare in Africans; almost never seen in Asians. Predisposing factors: congenital postanal dimples, obesity, deep intergluteal cleft, excess body hair.
- Differentiated from anal fistula and furunculosis by its midline orientation and by passing probe through sinus noting passage toward sacrum rather than anus.
- Treatment: if sinus is infected, incision and drainage may be needed but irrigation with herbal formula mentioned for abscess may help. Weight reduction and removal of excess regional hair reduces risk of infection and symptoms. Homeopathics *Silicea, Calcarea sulphuricum, Hepar sulphuris* are useful. Homeopathic thuja as intercurrent treatment has resolved obstinate cases.

## Proctalgia Fugax

- Proctalgia fugax, or levator spasm syndrome: more common in men than women. Symptoms: searing pain near coccyx or rectum lasting brief but intense period of time; usually resolves on its own; awakes patient from sleep but may occur anytime.
- Cause: spasm of levator ani or pubococcygeal muscle, with deep-seated often heavy, aching or searing pain; feels localized in rectum and/or prostate in men.
- Signs: tense, tight levator ani muscle, tender with pressure, often drawn up above anal sphincter.
- Mechanisms: poor posture, chronic anxiety, mental fixation on rectal area, misalignment of coccyx or other bones comprising pelvic bowl.

- Differential diagnosis: lumbar disk disease, coccygodynia, prostatitis, presacral tumor, developing ischiorectal abscess, spinal cord tumor, rectal lesion.
- Treatment: reassure patient of etiology. Try muscle relaxants; hot packs; spinal and pelvic bone adjustments; massage to lower abdomen, lumbo-sacral spine, and perineum. Chronic cases respond to deep tissue work (Rolfing).

## Proctitis

- Symptoms: rectal pain, tenesmus, rectal discharge, blood in stool.
- Signs: WBCs in large numbers seen on wet prep, Gram or Wright's stain. Conduct anoscopic examination for inflammation, mucopurulent discharge, mucosal friability, bleeding, and ulceration. Severe ulceration and bleeding suggest Lymphogranuloma venereum chlamydial serotype.
- Causative agents: *Chlamydia* (genital and LGV immunotypes), yeast, bacteria (gonorrhea), parasites, trauma, lectins, excessive fiber in diet, external radiation, syphilis, trichomonas, Crohn's disease. Higher risk of ulcerative proctitis exists in smokers and persons who have had appendectomy.
- Treatment: based on etiology. If caused by external-beam radiation for colon cancer or radium seed implants for prostate cancer, commence therapy before treatment and continue during and for several weeks after treatment has ceased. Radiation proctitis benefits from antioxidants. No ill effects on radiation occur when combined with antioxidants. Concurrent homeopathic *Radium bromatum* 200 C potency before and after radiotherapy decreases skin burning. Other homeopathics: X-ray, sol, cadmium metallicum. Demulcent rectal suppositories soothe inflamed rectal mucosa and decrease pain.
- Proctitis secondary to inflammatory bowel disease: treat underlying disease with diet, fiber, herbal demulcents, enteric-coated peppermint oil. Short chain fatty acids administered rectally alleviate symptoms of proctocolitis.
- Infective agents: bacteria, chlamydia, yeast, fungi, trichomonas, and parasites. Treatment: injection of ozone; herbal suppositories; homeopathics; retention enema consisting of *Hydrastis, Usnea, Echinacea, Yarrow* if trichomonas is agent; *Althea* in a base of 0.9% NaCl is effective. Apply this combination topically during initial examination to begin treatment. Vitamins C and E facilitate healing.

- Continue treatment for 10 to 14 days before reexamination and assessment. In ulcerative disease, treatment may be longer for complete healing.

## Pruritus Ani

- Symptoms: chronic itching of perianal skin; excoriation from scratching; eventual thickening of chronically affected areas; scratching at night during sleep or awakened from sleep by itching; intermittent to constant itching, burning, and soreness. Topical ointments give temporary relief. Signs: varying degrees of erythema, swelling, excoriation, thickening, and fissuring from scratching.
- Causes: excessive wiping with harsh toilet papers; "wipes" impregnated with drying alcohol, dyes, and antibacterial or fungal agents; synthetic undergarments or detergents, tight underclothing that decreases air circulation; chronic diarrhea or loose stools. Cosmetic removal of normal hair disrupts normal bacterial flora.
- Infective agents: pinworms and candida. Perianal itching, largely at night, suggests *Enterobius vermicularis* (pinworms), common in children and communicable to members of family. Wet prep reveals candida; adhesive tape preparation reveals pinworms.
- Periodic and chronic diarrhea: itching caused by acidic stool and aggressive cleaning of area. Compulsive cleaners can use cotton wipes, bath or shower cleansers, or moist towels.
- Soaps, detergents, bleaches, dyes, perfumes: recent onset may be caused by a change in product. Aggravating foods: peanuts, coffee, colas, beer, spicy foods, acidic foods, food allergens.
- Diseases: psoriasis, contact dermatitis, precancerous or cancerous lesions, Bowen's disease (intraepithelial epithelioma), keratoacanthoma, melanoma, squamous cell carcinoma, basal cell carcinoma.
- Lab tests: culture and sensitivity if bacterial infection is suspected; KOH and/or wet prep for yeast or fungi; Woods lamp examination for *Tinea cruris;* punch biopsy of suspicious lesions.
- Treatments: eliminate spicy or offending foods, food allergens; improve patient's digestion. Infective agent identified: topical therapy for yeast, fungi, or bacteria. Initially wash with 3% $H_2O_2$, then apply topical herbal formula of *Usnea, Hydrastis, Spilanthes,* oregano, and tea tree oil; allow to dry. Reestablish skin defensive barrier: apply healing salve containing calendula, comfrey,

vitamins E and A. Resolution occurs within 7 to 10 days if underlying cause is removed.
- Pinworms: wash all clothing and bedding in warm to hot water to eliminate eggs laid outside rectum at night.
- Use moist cotton wipes after stool and eliminate excess moisture in the perineal area to break the cycle. Zinc oxide topically also has proven effective in the treatment of pruritus ani.

## Botanicals for Anorectal Diseases

- *Aesculus hippocastanum*: tonic, astringent, febrifuge, narcotic and antiseptic, high in tannic acid and aesculin. Indications: pain relief of internal viscera, hemorrhoids, rectal irritation with marked congestion and sense of spasmodic closing of rectum as if foreign body were present; itching, sensation of heat, aching, or rectal pains; rectal neuralgia and proctitis.
- *Achillea millefolium* (yarrow): slightly astringent; alterative and diuretic; tonic on mucus membranes to stem mild hemorrhage. Indications: bleeding hemorrhoids with mucoid discharges.
- *Althea officinalis* (marshmallow): high in mucilage; restores electrical charge to inflamed rectal mucosa. In rectal suppositories it decreases swelling, irritation, and inflammation.
- *Cinnamomum*: used in herbal rectal suppositories to stem hemorrhage.
- *Collinsonia canadensis* (stone root): alterative, tonic, stimulant, and diuretic. Indications: tones venous vascular tissue; hemorrhoids from chronic constipation and venous insufficiency; sense of constriction, weight, and heat in rectum with very dry stools; proctitis, anal fistulas, and rectal ulcer.
- *Hamamelis virginiana* (witch hazel): tonic and astringent; restores vascular integrity. Indications: varicose veins, hemorrhages, hemorrhoids; venous tissues that are pale and flaccid; deep redness because of vascular engorgement and stagnation of blood; hemorrhoids are very painful and may ulcerate.
- *Hydrastis canadensis* (goldenseal): antibacterial; contains hydrastine, berberine, canadine, and acrid resins. Actions: affects ulcerations on mucus membranes, controls mild hemorrhages; astringent effect on hemorrhoids. Indications: hemorrhoids from constipation with sinking feeling in stomach and dull headache; painful anal fissures with severe burning before, during, and after stool.
- *Ruscus aculeatus* (butcher's broom): reduces venous swelling; vasoconstrictive action reduces bleeding.

# Psoriasis

## DIAGNOSTIC SUMMARY

- Sharply bordered reddened rash or plaques covered with overlapping silvery scales.
- Characteristically involves the scalp, the extensor surfaces (backside of the wrists, elbows, knees, buttocks, and ankles), and sites of repeated trauma.
- Family history in 50% of cases.
- Nail involvement results in characteristic "oil drop" stippling.
- Possible arthritis.

## GENERAL CONSIDERATIONS

Psoriasis is an extremely common skin disorder. The rate of occurrence in the United States is 2%-4%. It affects few blacks in the tropics but is more common among blacks in temperate zones. It is common among the Japanese and rare in American Indians. It affects men and women equally. Mean onset age is 27.8 years, but 2% have onset by age 2 years.

- Classic hyperproliferative skin disorder: rate of cell division is very high (1000 times greater than normal skin), exceeding rate in squamous cell carcinoma. Even in uninvolved skin, number of proliferating cells is 2.5 times greater than in nonpsoriatics.
- Basic defect is within skin cells. Incidence is increased in human leukocyte antigen (HLA) $B_{13}$, HLA-$B_{16}$, and HLA-$B_{17}$—genetic error in mitotic control. Thirty-six percent of patients have family members with psoriasis. Cell division rate is controlled by delicate balance between cyclic adenosine monophosphate (cAMP) and cyclic guanosine monophosphate (cGMP); increased cGMP is linked to increased proliferation; increased cAMP is linked to enhanced cell maturation and decreased proliferation. Decreased cAMP and increased cGMP have been measured in skin of psoriatics.

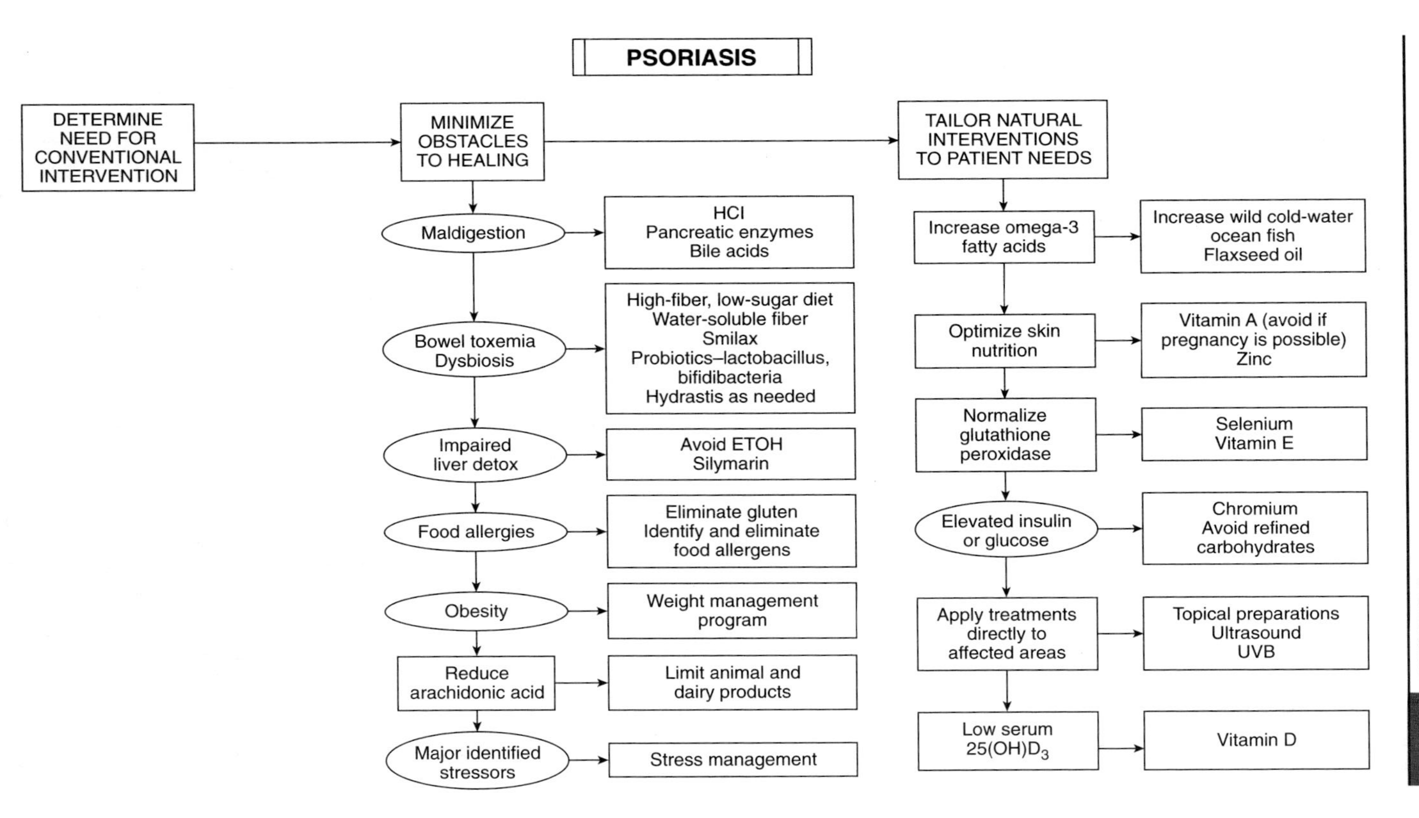
PSORIASIS
DETERMINE NEED FOR CONVENTIONAL INTERVENTION
MINIMIZE OBSTACLES TO HEALING
TAILOR NATURAL INTERVENTIONS TO PATIENT NEEDS
Maldigestion
HCl
Pancreatic enzymes
Bile acids
Bowel toxemia
Dysbiosis
High-fiber, low-sugar diet
Water-soluble fiber
Smilax
Probiotics–lactobacillus, bifidibacteria
Hydrastis as needed
Impaired liver detox
Avoid ETOH
Silymarin
Food allergies
Eliminate gluten
Identify and eliminate food allergens
Obesity
Weight management program
Reduce arachidonic acid
Limit animal and dairy products
Major identified stressors
Stress management
Increase omega-3 fatty acids
Increase wild cold-water ocean fish
Flaxseed oil
Optimize skin nutrition
Vitamin A (avoid if pregnancy is possible)
Zinc
Normalize glutathione peroxidase
Selenium
Vitamin E
Elevated insulin or glucose
Chromium
Avoid refined carbohydrates
Apply treatments directly to affected areas
Topical preparations
Ultrasound
UVB
Low serum 25(OH)D3
Vitamin D

- Abnormal immune stimulation: immune system may play a role in psoriasis. Activation of T-lymphocytes leading to release of cytokines results in proliferation of keratinocytes. This is initiated by unidentified antigens causing maturation of epidermal antigen-presenting cells (Langerhans cells), which migrate to regional lymph nodes. Antigen-presenting cells interact with naive T-cells, causing T-cell activation. Activated immune cells enter circulation, then extravasate through blood vessels to skin sites of inflammation as part of cytokine cascade in psoriatic lesions. Unidentified antigens are at the root of cascade.
- Psoriasis is linked to celiac disease and Crohn's disease. Bowel mucosa of psoriatics without bowel symptoms has microscopic lesions and increased permeability. Factors leading to poor intestinal function encourage increased intestinal permeability and inflammation, allowing antigenic and endotoxic compounds to exit intestines, travel in bloodstream, and initiate activated immune cascades in susceptible tissues.

## THERAPEUTIC CONSIDERATIONS

Decreasing sources of blood-borne antigenic immune activators and rebalancing cAMP/cGMP ratio are achievable by natural medicine. Controllable factors contributing to psoriasis are described later.

### Gastrointestinal Function

#### Incomplete Protein Digestion

Incomplete digestion or poor absorption increases amino acids and polypeptides in bowel, where they are metabolized by bowel bacteria into toxins. Toxic metabolites of arginine and ornithine are polyamines (putrescine, spermidine, cadaverine) and are increased in psoriatics. Polyamines inhibit formation of cAMP, inducing excess cell proliferation. Lowered skin and urinary polyamines are linked to clinical improvement. Natural compounds inhibit formation of polyamines; vitamin A and berberine alkaloids of *Hydrastis canadensis* (goldenseal) inhibit bacterial decarboxylase enzyme, which converts amino acids into polyamines. Evaluate digestive function with Heidelburg gastric analysis and/or comprehensive digestive stool analysis. Reinforce digestion (hydrochloric acid, pancreatic enzymes).

### Bowel Toxemia

Gut-derived toxins are implicated: endotoxins (compounds from cell walls of gram-negative bacteria), streptococci, *Candida albicans*, yeast, and immunoglobulin (Ig) E and IgA immune complexes). They increase cGMP in skin cells, promoting proliferation. Chronic candidiasis may play a role in many cases.

- Low-fiber diet is linked to increased gut-derived toxins. Fiber of fruits, vegetables, whole grains, and legumes bind toxins and promote their excretion.
- Aqueous extract of *Smilax sarsaparilla* is effective in psoriasis, particularly chronic, large plaque-forming variety. It improved psoriasis in 62% of patients and completely cleared another 18% (80% benefited). Benefit is from sarsaparilla components binding and excretion of endotoxins. Severity and response correlate well with level of circulating endotoxins. Control of gut-derived toxins is critical. Support fecal excretion and proper handling of absorbed endotoxins by liver.

### Liver Function

Correcting abnormal liver function is beneficial. The liver filters and detoxifies portal blood from the bowel. Structurally, hepatic architecture may be altered in psoriatics. If the liver is overwhelmed by excess bowel toxins or if the liver's detoxification ability is decreased, systemic toxin level increases and psoriasis worsens. Alcohol worsens psoriasis; it increases toxin absorption by damaging gut mucosa and impairs liver function. Eliminate alcohol. Silymarin, a flavonoid of *Silybum marianum*, is valuable in treating psoriasis by improving liver function, inhibiting inflammation, and reducing excess cellular proliferation.

### Bile Deficiencies

- Bile acids normally present in intestines detoxify bacterial endotoxins. Bile acid deficiency allows endotoxins to translocate into bloodstream, inducing release of inflammatory cytokines that aggravate psoriasis.
- Hungarian study: Oral bile acid (dehydrocholic acid) supplementation for 1 to 6 weeks plus diet high in vegetables and fruits and devoid of hot spices, alcohol, raw onion, garlic, and carbonated soft drinks alleviated symptoms in 78.8% of patients, whereas only 24.9% of those on conventional therapies recovered during treatment period. Bile acids effects were more pronounced

in acute form of psoriasis; 95.1% of patients became asymptomatic. A total of 57.9% were asymptomatic 2 years later compared with 6.0% on conventional treatment. Product and dosage: 2 to 3 Supra Chol sugar-coated pills q.d. or dehydrocholic acid powder (acidum dehydrocholicum pulvis) at two to three doses of 0.25 g q.d.

- Theoretical risk of malignancy with sluggish intestinal function and long-term bile acid therapy causes researchers to recommend supplementing only after fatty meals after initial treatment period. Ursodeoxycholic acid may have protective effect on colon mucosa; it reduces risk of colon cancer, even in ulcerative colitis and primary sclerosing cholangitis. Consider bile acids for short-term treatment of psoriasis; monitor colon before and after treatment in patients at high risk for colon cancer.

## Nutrition

Omega-3 fatty acids: serum free fatty acids are abnormal in psoriatics. Fish oil at 10-12 g (providing 1.8 g eicosapentaenoic acid [EPA] and 1.2 g docosahexaenoic acid [DHA]) improves symptoms. Equivalent amount of EPA is available in 150 g of salmon, mackerel, or herring. Wild cold-water fish plus 1 tbsp flaxseed oil daily may be advantageous because of the lipid peroxides in many fish oil products.

EPA improves psoriasis because of competition for arachidonic acid binding sites, inhibiting synthesis of inflammatory leukotrienes from arachidonic acid, which are many times greater than normal in psoriatics. Leukotrienes promote guanylate cyclase activity.

- Cellular free arachidonic acid and 12-hydroxyeicosatetraenoic acid (HETE) (product of lipoxygenase metabolism of arachidonic acid) are 250 and 810 times greater, respectively, than uninvolved epidermal tissue. A tissue-intrinsic unidentified inhibitor of cyclooxygenase is involved.
- Trauma releases free arachidonic acid. Plaques arise at sites of repeated trauma. Increased 12-HETE stimulates 5-lipoxygenase, promoting leukotriene formation. This pathway is inhibited by EPA and glutathione peroxidase; selenium deficiency may contribute (see later in the section on individual nutrients).
- Cyclooxygenase inhibitors (aspirin, nonsteroidal antiinflammatory drugs) may exacerbate psoriasis. Lipoxygenase inhibitors (benoxaprofen) may improve psoriasis. Natural substances (quer-

cetin, ubiquitous plant flavonoid), vitamin E, onion, and garlic inhibit lipoxygenase.

- Arachidonic acid is found only in animal tissues; limit intake of animal fats and dairy. Diet, fasting, and food allergy control: psoriasis is positively linked to body mass index and inversely related to intake of carrots, tomatoes, fresh fruits, and index of beta-carotene intake. Fasting and vegetarian regimens help psoriatics, probably because of decreased gut-derived toxins and polyamines. Gluten-free and elimination diets are beneficial.

### Individual Nutrients

- Decreased vitamin A and zinc, which are critical to skin health, are common in psoriasis.
- Chromium is indicated to increase insulin receptor sensitivity; psoriatics have increased serum insulin and glucose.
- Glutathione peroxidase (GP) is low in psoriatics, possibly because of alcohol abuse, malnutrition, and excess skin loss of hyperproliferation. GP is normalized with oral selenium (Se) and vitamin E. Low concentrations in whole blood Se are common in psoriasis. Lowest levels of whole blood Se are found in male patients with widespread disease of long duration requiring methotrexate and retinoids.
- Active vitamin D (1,25-dihydroxycholecalciferol) plays a role in controlling keratinocyte proliferation and differentiation. Vitamin D encourages shift toward T-helper 2 cytokine expression, with increase in interleukin (IL) 10 and decrease in IL-8, which may improve psoriasis. Topical active vitamin D and oral 1 alpha(OH)$D_3$ may be helpful. Patients with severe psoriasis have very low serum vitamin D, which normalizes with oral 1 alpha(OH)$D_3$. Clinical use of vitamin D was limited by hypercalcemia; synthetic vitamin D analogues have less effect on calcium homeostasis. If ultraviolet light therapy is used, apply topical vitamin D after phototherapy to avoid degradation of active compound in ointment.
- Fumaric acid: oral dimethyl fumaric acid (240 mg q.d.) or monoethyl fumaric acid (720 mg q.d.) and topical 1%-3% monoethyl fumaric acid are useful, but side effects (flushing of skin, nausea, diarrhea, malaise, gastric pain, mild liver and kidney disturbances) can occur. Use only if other natural therapies fail.

### Psychological Aspects

Thirty nine percent of psoriatics report specific stressful event within 1 month before initial episode. Such patients have better prognosis. Correlation occurs mostly in patients with repeated stressors of four times or more in 1 year. A few cases are successfully treated with hypnosis and biofeedback alone.

### Physical Therapeutics

Sunlight (ultraviolet light) is extremely beneficial. Outdoor 4-week heliotherapy promotes significant clearance of symptoms in 84% of subjects. Nonprescription commercial tanning beds have improved psoriasis severity and health-related quality of life. Combining retinoid acitretin (vitamin A derivative) with a 4- to 5-day per week tanning regimen induced complete or near complete recovery in 83% of 23 subjects. Specific UV exposure induces vitamin D synthesis in skin. The standard medical treatment is the drug psoralen plus ultraviolet A (PUVA) therapy at 320-340 nm. Ultraviolet B (UVB, 280-320 nm) alone inhibits cell proliferation and is as effective as PUVA with fewer side effects. UVB is the dominant light at the Dead Sea, where 80%-85% of psoriatics clear in 4 weeks. More study is needed to clarify risks, benefits, and specific UV therapy for varying presentations of psoriasis. UV deactivates vitamin D topicals; apply topicals only after UV treatment. Monitor light therapy carefully, especially in those at risk for skin cancer.

Induction of elevation of temperature (42°-45° C) to affected area by ultrasound and heating pads can be effective. Researchers have used hypotonic sulphate water (Leopoldine water) in a baleotherapeutic manner, yielding favorable immunohistologic profiles of affected tissues: decreased numbers of T-lymphocytes, Langerhans cells, and markers of keratinocyte inflammation.

### Topical Treatments

Botanical alternatives to hydrocortisone: glycyrrhetinic acid from licorice *(Glycyrrhiza glabra)*, chamomile *(Matricaria chamomilla)*, and capsaicin from cayenne pepper *(Capsicum frutescens)*.

- *Glycyrrhiza glabra* (licorice root): glycyrrhetinic acid effect is similar to topical hydrocortisone for psoriasis and eczema; it is superior to topical cortisone in chronic cases. It can potentiate effects of topical hydrocortisone by inhibiting 11-beta-hydroxy-steroid dehydrogenase, which catalyzes conversion of hydrocortisone to inactive form.
- *Matricaria chamomilla* (chamomile): used widely in Europe for psoriasis, eczema, and dry, flaky, irritated skin. Flavonoid

and essential oil components are antiinflammatory and antiallergic.

- *Capsicum frutescens* (cayenne pepper): capsaicin is the active component of cayenne pepper. Topically applied, capsaicin stimulates and then blocks small-diameter pain fibers by depleting pain neurotransmitter substance P, which is elevated in the skin of psoriatics and activates inflammatory mediators in psoriasis. Topical 0.025% or 0.075% capsaicin, applied four times per day for 6 weeks, is effective in improving psoriasis; it reduces scaling, thickness, erythema, and pruritus.. Burning, stinging, itching, and skin redness were noted by half of patients initially, but diminished or vanished with continued application. It is proven superior to placebo.
- *Aloe vera*: topical extract in hydrophilic cream, applied three times daily, is highly effective in psoriasis vulgaris. It was well tolerated by all patients studied over 4-12 months of treatment, with no adverse drug-related symptoms and no dropouts.

### Other Possible Therapies

In vitro preliminary discoveries of keratinocytic antiproliferative activity among botanicals: *Mahonia aquifolium*, *Centella asiatica*, *Zanthoxylum* spp., *Tabebuia impetiginosa* (lapacho), *Chelidonium majus*, curcumin, pine bark, and Sicilian botanicals such as *Verbena*. Which of these may prove effective in future clinical trials is not known.

## THERAPEUTIC APPROACH

Decrease bowel toxemia; rebalance fatty acid and inflammatory processes in skin; use therapeutic regimen to further balance abnormal cell proliferation.

- **Diet**: Limit sugar, meat, animal fats, and alcohol. Increase dietary fiber and cold-water fish. Normalize weight. Eliminate gluten. Identify and address food allergies.
- **Supplements**:
  —High-potency multiple vitamin/mineral formula
  —Flaxseed oil: 1 tbsp q.d.
  —Vitamin A: 50,000 IU q.d. (avoid in pregnant women or those who may become pregnant)
  —Vitamin D: 2000 IU q.d.
  —Vitamin E (mixed tocopherols): 400 IU q.d.
  —Chromium: 400 mg q.d.

—Selenium: 200 mg q.d.
—Zinc: 30 mg q.d.

- **Consider digestive enzymes and/or bile acids with meals.**
  —Water-soluble fiber (psyllium, pectin, guar gum): 5 g at bedtime.
- **Botanical medicines**:
  —*Hydrastis canadensis* (goldenseal): dosage based on berberine content; standardized extracts three times daily are preferred: dried root or as infusion (tea), 2-4 g; fluid extract (1:1), 2-4 mL (0.5-1 tsp); solid (powdered dry) extract (4:1 or 8%-12% alkaloid content), 250-500 mg
  —*Smilax sarsaparilla* (three times daily): dried root or by decoction, 1-4 g; liquid extract (1:1), 8-16 mL (2-4 tsp); solid extract (4:1), 250-500 mg;
  —*Silybum marianum* (milk thistle): silymarin, 70-210 mg t.i.d.
- **Psychological**: evaluate stress levels and use stress reduction techniques as appropriate.
- **Physical medicine**:
  —Ultrasound: 42°-45° C, 20 minutes, three times per week
  —UVB: 295-305 nm, 2 mW/cm$^2$, 3 minutes, three times per week
- **Topical treatment**: preparations containing one or more of the ingredients described above; apply to affected areas of skin two to three times daily.

# Rheumatoid Arthritis

## DIAGNOSTIC SUMMARY

- Fatigue, low-grade fever, weakness, weight loss, joint stiffness, and vague joint pain preceding painful, swollen joints by several weeks.
- Severe joint pain with inflammation beginning insidiously in small joints and progressing to all joints.
- Radiographic findings: soft tissue swelling, erosion of cartilage, and joint space narrowing.
- Rheumatoid factor (RF) in serum.
- Extraarticular manifestations: vasculitis, muscle atrophy, subcutaneous and systemic granulomas, pleurisy, pericarditis, pulmonary fibrosis, lymphadenopathy, splenomegaly, anemia, and leukopenia.

## GENERAL CONSIDERATIONS

Rheumatoid arthritis (RA) is a chronic inflammatory condition affecting the entire body but especially synovial membranes of joints. Joints involved include the hands, feet, wrists, ankles, and knees. RA affects 0.3%-1.0% of the population. Women outnumber men by 3:1. Age of onset is 20-40 years, but it may begin at any age. Onset is gradual but occasionally quite abrupt. Several joints usually are involved at onset in a symmetric pattern (both hands, wrists, or ankles). In one third of cases, RA initially is confined to one or a few joints. Affected joints are warm, tender, and swollen. Overlying skin has a ruddy, purplish hue. Disease progression results in joint deformities in the hands and feet ("swan neck," "boutonnière," and "cock-up toes").

### Pathogenesis

An autoimmune reaction is the cause—antibodies against components of joint tissues. T-helper cell balance and production of tumor necrosis factor-alpha (TNF-alpha), a proinflammatory cytokine,

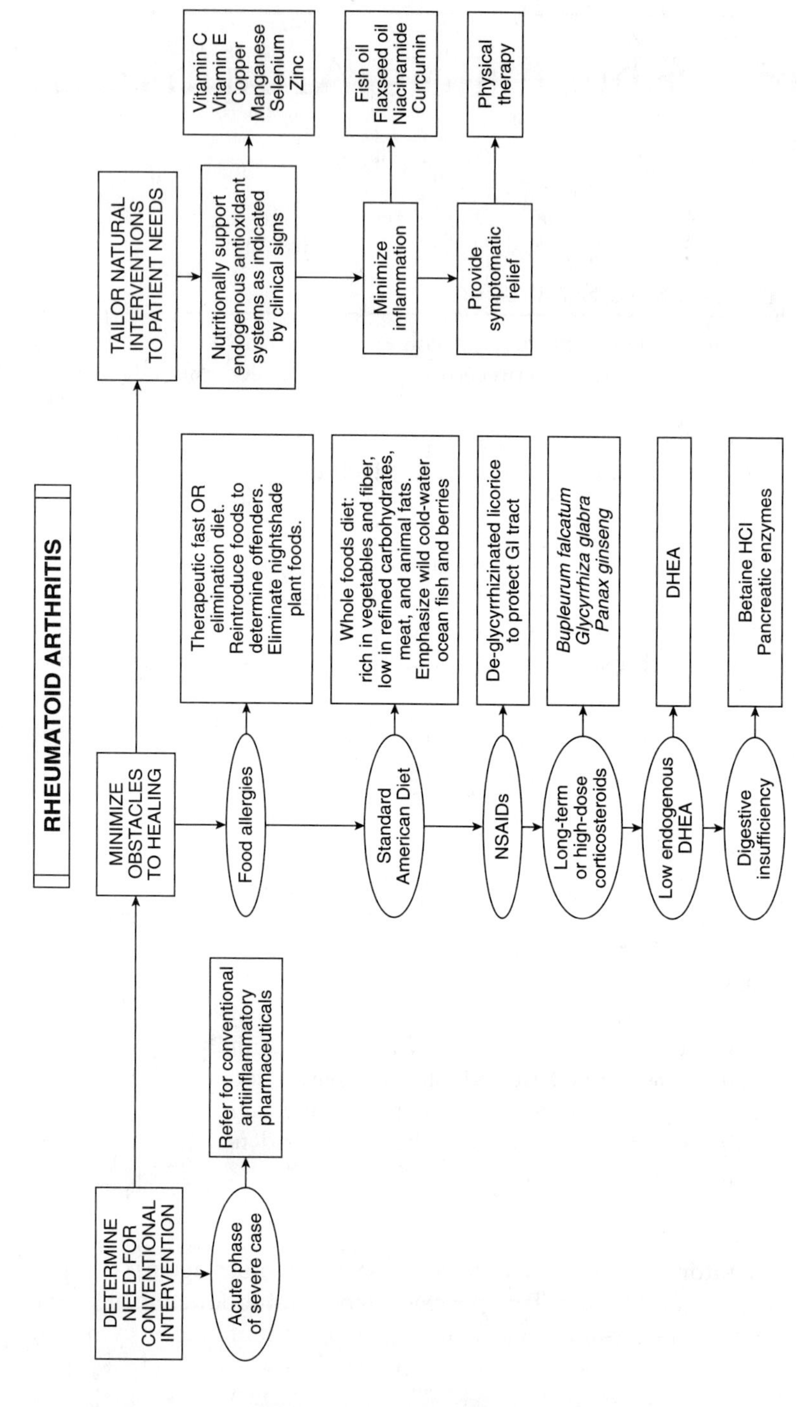
RHEUMATOID ARTHRITIS
DETERMINE NEED FOR CONVENTIONAL INTERVENTION
Acute phase of severe case
Refer for conventional antiinflammatory pharmaceuticals
MINIMIZE OBSTACLES TO HEALING
Food allergies
Therapeutic fast OR elimination diet. Reintroduce foods to determine offenders. Eliminate nightshade plant foods.
Standard American Diet
Whole foods diet: rich in vegetables and fiber, low in refined carbohydrates, meat, and animal fats. Emphasize wild cold-water ocean fish and berries
NSAIDs
De-glycyrrhizinated licorice to protect GI tract
Long-term or high-dose corticosteroids
Bupleurum falcatum Glycyrrhiza glabra Panax ginseng
Low endogenous DHEA
DHEA
Digestive insufficiency
Betaine HCl Pancreatic enzymes
TAILOR NATURAL INTERVENTIONS TO PATIENT NEEDS
Nutritionally support endogenous antioxidant systems as indicated by clinical signs
Vitamin C Vitamin E Copper Manganese Selenium Zinc
Minimize inflammation
Fish oil Flaxseed oil Niacinamide Curcumin
Provide symptomatic relief
Physical therapy

may play a key role. Triggering mechanism is unknown. Factors are genetic susceptibility, abnormal bowel permeability, lifestyle and nutritional factors, food allergies, and microorganisms. RA is classic multifactorial disease involving genetic and environmental factors.

- **Genetic factors**: human leukocyte antigen (HLA) region on 6p21 is implicated. Severe RA also is found at four times the expected rate in first-degree relatives of probands with seropositive disease. Environmental factors—low economic status, smoking, poor diet, and psychological factors—are major factors in development of RA and may affect levels of pain and disability. This is demonstrated in monozygotic twins.
- **Abnormal bowel permeability**: RA patients have increased intestinal permeability to dietary and bacterial antigens plus alterations in bowel flora. Food allergies may contribute to increased permeability. Nonsteroidal antiinflammatory drugs (NSAIDs) are implicated. Permeability to gut-derived antigens increases endotoxins (lipopolysaccharide components of cell walls of gram-negative bacteria) and immune complexes characteristic of RA. Permeability and inappropriate bacterial flora can increase absorption of antigens similar to antigens in joint tissues. Antibodies to microbial antigens may cross-react with joint tissue antigens; antibodies to *Campylobacter, Salmonella,* and *Shigella* cross-react with collagen, whereas antibodies to *Klebsiella pneumoniae, Proteus vulgaris,* and *Yersinia enterocolitica* cross-react with other joint tissues.
- **Dysbiosis and small intestinal bacterial overgrowth**: many RA patients exhibit altered microbial flora and small intestinal bacterial overgrowth (SIBO). Degree of SIBO is linked to severity of symptoms and disease activity (*Textbook,* "Bacterial Overgrowth of the Small Intestine Breath Test").
- **Abnormal antibodies and immune complexes**: serum and joint fluid of nearly all RA patients contain rheumatoid factor (RF), antibodies against Fc fragment of immunoglobulin (Ig) G. RF antibodies belong to IgM, IgG, and IgA classes, but only IgM RF is readily measured by latex agglutination, bentonite flocculation, and sensitized sheep or human red blood cell (RBC) test. Most of RF is formed locally in affected joints by infiltration of activated B-cells and plasma cells. Serum titer of RF correlates with severity of symptoms. Circulating immune complexes contribute to pathogenesis; cell-mediated, humoral, and nonspecific immune responses to immune complexes lead to proliferative

inflammation. Abnormalities are similar to Arthus reaction and serum sickness, immune complex–induced reactions dependent on neutrophils, and complement activation. Amount of circulating immune complexes is not correlated with disease activity, but immune complexes and abnormal antibodies plus sequelae are major factors in RA.

- **Microbial hypotheses**: not in themselves comprehensive enough to explain all events observed in RA. Variety of suggested microbes: Epstein-Barr virus, rubella virus, amebic organisms, and *Mycoplasma*. No microbial agent is consistently isolated in RA patients. Attempts to isolate whole organisms from synovial fluids and antibodies to viable, whole organisms, and failure to isolate offending organisms, are suggestive to some researchers of atypical viral-like agent(s). Microbial factors (immune complexes) contribute, but a single causative microbe is unlikely.
- **Decreased dehydroepiandrosterone (DHEA) levels**: defective androgen synthesis is proposed as a predisposing factor. Androgens are immune suppressive where DHEA inhibits cytokines because of nuclear factor-kappa B inhibition. Chronically low levels of DHEA are found in RA. DHEA sulfate levels are lower in postmenopausal women (aged 45-65 years) with RA than in postmenopausal control subjects. Adrenocortical hormones (e.g., DHEA and testosterone) are decreased in early stages of RA. Supplemental DHEA (200 mg q.d.) is beneficial in systemic lupus erythematosus (SLE). It may be beneficial for RA despite absence of double-blind clinical studies. It can be used conservatively to correct physiologic deficit. Use 24-hour urinary test. It can be used aggressively to affect RA; dosage required is >50 mg q.d. Major side effect is mild to severe acne and possibly increased androgenization in women.

## DIAGNOSIS

Easily recognized in advanced and characteristic form. Early diagnosis is more difficult.

**Classic RA**: diagnosis requires seven of the following criteria. Criteria 1-5: joint signs or symptoms must be continuous for 6 weeks. Any one of the exclusionary features excludes patient from this and other categories:

- Morning stiffness
- Pain on motion or tenderness in at least one joint

- Swelling (soft tissue thickening or fluid, not bony overgrowth alone) in at least one joint
- Swelling of at least one other joint; any interval free of joint symptoms between joint involvement may not be more than 3 months
- Bilateral joint swelling—proximal interphalangeal, metacarpophalangeal, or metatarsophalangeal joints—is acceptable without absolute symmetry; terminal phalangeal joint involvement does not fulfill this criterion
- Subcutaneous nodules over bony prominences, on extensor surfaces, or in juxtaarticular regions
- Radiographic changes: bony decalcification localized to, or most marked adjacent to, involved joints and not simply degenerative changes (which do not exclude patients from any RA group)
- Positive agglutination test: RF tested by acceptable method
- Poor mucin precipitate from synovial fluid or inflammatory synovial effusion with 2000+ white blood cells (WBCs)/$mm^3$ and without crystals
- Histologic changes in synovium with three or more of the following: marked villous hypertrophy, proliferation of superficial synovial cells often with pallisading, marked infiltration of chronic inflammatory cells with tendency to form lymphoid nodules, deposition of compact fibrin either on surface or interstitially, foci of necrosis
- Histologic changes in nodules: granulomatous foci with central zones of cell necrosis, surrounded by a palisade of proliferated mononuclear and peripheral fibrosis and chronic inflammatory cell infiltration

**Definite RA**: requires five of the above criteria; criteria 1-5: joint signs must be continuous for 6+ weeks.

**Probable RA**: requires three of the above criteria; in at least one of criteria 1-5, joint signs and symptoms continuous for 6+ weeks.

**Possible RA**: requires two of the following criteria, and total duration of joint symptoms must be 3+ months:

- Morning stiffness
- Tenderness or pain on motion with history of recurrence or persistence of 3 weeks
- History or observation of joint swelling
- Elevated sedimentation rate or C-reactive protein (CRP)
- Iritis

## Laboratory and Radiographic Findings

- **Rheumatoid factor**: nonrheumatoid diseases elevate RF; diseases share common feature of chronic inflammation with persistent antigenic challenge and include other connective tissue diseases (SLE, Sjögren's syndrome, polymyositis, and scleroderma) and infectious diseases (tuberculosis, leprosy, syphilis, viral hepatitis, bacterial infections, infectious mononucleosis, and influenza). Positive results occur in idiopathic pulmonary fibrosis, sarcoidosis, chronic active hepatitis and cirrhosis, lymphomas, cryoglobulinemia, and repeated blood transfusions. RF is transiently elevated after immunizations and other assaults to immune system. Overall prevalence is 4%; persons older than 60 years show prevalence >40%. RF titers in elderly healthy persons are typically low (<1:80).
- **Antinuclear antibodies (ANAs)**: found in 20%-60% of RA patients. Titers specific for native DNA typically are normal. Titers to single-stranded or denatured DNA usually are elevated. ANA titers typically are lower in RA than in SLE.
- **Epstein-Barr virus antibodies**: identified by immunodiffusion or by immunofluorescence in serum of most RA patients. They are called antirheumatoid arthritis precipitin (anti-RAP) and antirheumatoid arthritis nuclear antigen (anti-RANA). The significance is undetermined.
- **Other lab abnormalities**: anemia is common—normocytic and normochromic or hypochromic. Decreased erythropoiesis is common in chronic inflammatory conditions. Serum iron (Fe) level and total Fe-binding capacity usually are low, but Fe supplements are of no value and may actually promote free radical damage. Fe supplement is not indicated unless anemia is caused by blood loss. Serum ferritin levels are useful in determining appropriateness of Fe therapy; ferritin is elevated during acute inflammation and correlates with other indicators of disease activity (erythrocyte sedimentation rate [ESR] and CRP). ESR commonly is elevated and useful as a rough estimator of disease activity in patient monitoring, but occasionally it does not accurately reflect disease activity.
- **Synovial fluid**: reflects degree of inflammation. High fibrinogen may lead to spontaneous clotting of fluid. It should not be confused with mucin clot. Adding 1% acetic acid will dissolve fibrin. In RA, mucin clot is poor because of smaller-than-normal polymers of hyaluronic acid. Neutrophils are primary cells in fluid, with a range of 10,000-50,000/$mm^3$. Complement generally is

low and neutrophils contain cytoplasmic inclusion bodies with ingested immune complexes.

- **Radiographic findings**: soft tissue swelling, erosion of cartilage, and subtle joint space narrowing early in disease process. As disease progresses, erosion of joint spaces is more pronounced, as is diffuse osteoporosis.

## THERAPEUTIC CONSIDERATIONS

Study of therapeutic efficacy requires 20 years of follow-up. In a study of RA patients after 20 years of aggressive conventional treatment, only 18% were able to lead normal lives. Most patients (54%) were either dead (35%) or severely disabled (19%). Most deaths were directly related to RA. RA is a multifactorial condition requiring a comprehensive approach focused on reducing contributing factors (gut permeability, circulating immune complexes, free radicals, immune dysfunction), controlling inflammation, and promoting joint regeneration. Foremost in the natural approach is to use diet to control inflammation.

### Diet

Diet is strongly implicated in RA as both a cause and a cure. RA is not found in societies that eat a primitive diet. It is found at a relatively high rate in societies consuming a Western diet. A diet rich in whole foods, vegetables, and fiber and low in sugar, meat, refined carbohydrates, and saturated fat, is protective against RA. Eliminate food allergens. Follow vegetarian diet. Change dietary fats and oils. Increase antioxidant nutrients.

- **Food allergy**: eliminating allergic foods is quite beneficial to some RA patients. Any food can aggravate RA. Most common offending foods are wheat, corn, milk and dairy, beef, and nightshade (tomato, potato, eggplant, peppers, and tobacco) plus food additives. Short-term fasting (vegetable broth and juices) followed by a vegetarian diet substantially reduces disease activity in many patients because it eliminates food allergens, improves dietary fatty acids, and increases colon flora.
- **Colon microflora**: altered flora are linked to RA and other autoimmune diseases. More than 400 different species are found in the colon. Intestinal flora is significantly altered when patients change from an omnivorous to a vegetarian diet. Positive changes

in colon flora correlate with improvements in RA. The total surface area of the gastrointestinal system is 300-400 $m^2$. Only a single epithelial layer separates the host from enormous amounts of dietary and microbial antigens. Gut-associated lymphoid tissue (largest lymphoid organ) is protective. Alterations in intestinal flora change antigenic challenge, with significant impact on disease activity. Gas-liquid chromatography of fatty acids in stool samples may be a relatively quick and easy method of forecasting clinical improvement in RA.

- **Digestion**: incompletely digested food molecules can be inappropriately absorbed. Many patients with RA are deficient in hydrochloric acid and pancreatic enzymes; incomplete digestion may be a major factor. Digestive aids are warranted. Pancreatic enzymes offer additional benefits; proteases in pancreatin reduce circulating levels of immune complexes in autoimmune diseases (RA, SLE, periarteritis nodosa, scleroderma, ulcerative colitis, Crohn's disease, multiple sclerosis, AIDS). As clinical improvement corresponds with decreased immune complexes (use ESR as rough indicator), pancreatin or bromelain supplements are often warranted.
- **Dietary fats**: fatty acids are precursors of inflammatory prostaglandins, thromboxanes, and leukotrienes. Altering dietary fatty acids can increase or decrease inflammation depending on preponderant type ingested. Goals are to reduce arachidonic acid (AA) and increase dihomo-gamma-linolenic acid (DHGLA) and eicosapentaenoic acid (EPA). Vegetarian diets are beneficial, in part, by decreasing AA and conversion to inflammatory eicosanoids while supplying linoleic and linolenic acids. Wild cold-water fish (mackerel, herring, sardines, and salmon) are rich sources of EPA, which competes with AA for prostaglandin and leukotriene production. The net effect is reduced inflammatory and allergic response. Consumption of broiled or baked fish correlates with decreased risk of RA; a dose-dependent response was noted—two or more servings per week are more protective than one serving per week. The best diet for RA is a vegetarian diet with the exception of cold-water ocean fish; flaxseed oil also is useful.

## Psychological Aspects

- Major factors: psychological makeup, coping style, social support, belief systems, and patient-physician relationship.

- Pessimistic patients with passive coping strategies (e.g., staying in bed) have increased depression and worse physical functioning. Optimistic RA patients report better psychosocial and physical functioning.
- Patients confident in their ability to decrease pain with spiritual and religious coping methods have reduced joint pain and greater general social support. Positive support of spouse and/or family is inversely related to depression and quality of life.
- Common concepts among RA patients: eight major themes to keep in mind by physician—severe pain, self-esteem, negative feelings, reflections of the past, concentration on recovery from disease, a comfortable mind in pain, support of family and others, and new life. Explore these issues with RA patients to facilitate self-expression and control of their lives.
- Physician-patient relationship: physicians have frustration with patients lacking social support and with histories of abuse, somatization disorders, and obsessive-compulsive disorders. Key issue: unmarried status and loss of control over illness. Such patients rely on provider for social support, which is "frustrating" to physician. In addition, patient needs to be seen as individual, not as a mere diagnosis, and to be believed about subjective suffering and acknowledged. RA patients view quick dispersal of antidepressants as sign of physician disinterest. RA patient needs validation and understanding from physician.

## Nutritional Supplements

- **Gamma linolenic acid (GLA)**: Evening primrose (EPO), black currant, and borage oil contain GLA, an omega-6 fatty acid and precursor to antiinflammatory prostaglandins of 1-series. Although quite popular, research on GLA in RA is controversial and not as strong as research on omega-3 oils. Long-term GLA supplementation increases tissue AA and decreases tissue EPA, contrary to treatment goal. Key factor is whether subjects are allowed to take antiinflammatory drugs; drugs inhibit formation of inflammatory prostaglandins, masking negative effects of altered tissue fatty acid profile produced by GLA. Dosage of 1.4 g q.d. EPO is 9% GLA: 31-500 mg caps EPO required daily at cost of $100/month. Omega-3 oils are a better choice. GLA can be formed from linoleic acid; whether effects are from GLA versus linoleic acid is difficult to determine. Most sources of GLA are much richer in linoleic acid than GLA (EPO contains 9% GLA, but 72% linoleic acid).

- **Omega-3 fatty acids**: fish oil EPA studies consistently show less morning stiffness and tender joints. It reduces production of inflammatory compounds secreted by WBCs. Many, but not all, commercially available fish oils have high levels of lipid peroxides. Use wild cold-water fish and flaxseed oil or lab-certified fish oil. Flaxseed oil is not as effective in increasing tissue EPA and lowering tissue AA as fish oils. For flaxseed oil to be effective, patients must minimize dietary omega-6 fatty acids (other vegetable oils) while supplementing with 13 g (1 tbsp) flaxseed oil q.d. Flax can inhibit autoimmune reaction as well as EPA. Conversion of alpha-linolenic acid to EPA requires adequate zinc nutriture. Zinc deficiency is common in RA.
- **Dietary antioxidants**: fresh fruits and vegetables are the best sources of dietary antioxidants. Vitamin C, beta-carotene, vitamin E, selenium, and zinc are well recognized as antioxidants. Flavonoids neutralize inflammation and support collagen structures. Risk of RA is highest in people with lowest levels of nutrient antioxidants (serum alpha-tocopherol, beta-carotene, and vitamin C).
- **Selenium (Se) and vitamin E**: Se levels are low in RA patients. Se is an antioxidant and cofactor in the free radical scavenging enzyme glutathione peroxidase, which reduces inflammatory prostaglandins and leukotrienes. Se and vitamin E have a positive effect. Food sources: Brazil nuts, fish, and whole grains. The amount of Se in grains and other plant foods is related to amount of Se in soil.
- **Zinc (Zn)**: antioxidant and cofactor in antioxidant enzyme superoxide dismutase (copper-zinc SOD). Zn has slight therapeutic effect alone. Zn picolinate, monomethionine, or citrate forms are preferred. Foods rich in Zn are oysters, whole grains, nuts, and seeds.
- **Manganese (Mn) and SOD**: Mn functions in a different form of SOD. Mn-SOD is deficient in RA patients. Injectable form of enzyme (available in Europe) is effective in treating RA. Whether oral SOD escapes digestion in the gastrointestinal tract to exert therapeutic effect is not clear. Mn supplements increase SOD activity. No clinical studies have been conducted to determine efficacy of Mn in RA. RA patients are low in Mn. Dietary sources are nuts, whole grains, dried fruits, and green leafy vegetables. Meats, dairy, poultry, and seafood are poor sources of Mn.

- **Vitamin C**: antioxidant. WBC and plasma ascorbate are significantly decreased in RA patients. Vitamin C supplements increased SOD activity and decreased histamine levels and provide some antiinflammatory effects. Food sources are broccoli, Brussels sprouts, cabbage, citrus fruits, tomatoes, and berries.
- **Pantothenic acid**: whole blood pantothenic acid is lower in RA patients than in normal control subjects. Disease activity is inversely correlated with pantothenic acid levels. Correcting low pantothenic acid levels to normal improves duration of morning stiffness, degree of disability, and severity of pain. Dietary sources: whole grains and legumes.
- **Pyridoxine (vitamin $B_6$)**: Low levels of blood pyridoxal 5′-phosphate (P5P) are linked to inflammatory indicators of RA. Plasma $B_6$ levels are higher in patients with lower ESR, lower CRP, fewer disabilities, less pain and fatigue, and fewer swollen joints. Low $B_6$ is caused by ongoing chronic inflammatory processes. Homocysteine is increased in these $B_6$-deficient patients, increasing risk of cardiovascular disease. RA patients have increased risk for comorbidity and death from cardiovascular disease—left ventricular diastolic dysfunction, pulmonary hypertension, and first-time myocardial infarction.
- **Copper (Cu)**: Cu aspirinate (salicylate) yields better results in reducing pain and inflammation than standard aspirin. Wearing of CU bracelets is a long-time folk remedy. Cu is absorbed through the skin and is chelated to another compound able to exert antiinflammatory action. Cu is a component (with zinc) in one type of SOD (copper-zinc SOD). Deficiency may increase susceptibility to free radical damage. Excess intake of Cu is detrimental because of its ability to combine with peroxides and damage joint tissues.
- **Sulfur**: sulfur (cysteine) content in fingernails of arthritics is lower than in healthy control subjects. Intragluteal colloidal sulfur alleviates pain and swelling. Increased consumption of sulfur-rich foods (legumes, garlic, onions, Brussels sprouts, and cabbage) or supplements may be beneficial.
- **Niacinamide**: Kaufman and Hoffer treatment of RA and osteoarthritis (OA) uses high-dose niacinamide (900-4000 mg in divided doses q.d.). This is confirmed in OA (*Textbook*, "Osteoarthritis") but not fully evaluated in clinical studies of RA. Niacinamide affects the autoimmune process involved in insulin-dependent diabetes mellitus (*Textbook*, "Diabetes Mellitus").

## Botanical Medicines

- ***Curcuma longa* (turmeric)**: curcumin is a yellow pigment of *Curcuma longa*, which exerts excellent antiinflammatory and antioxidant effects. Curcumin is as effective as cortisone or phenylbutazone in models of acute inflammation but without side effects. It inhibits formation of leukotrienes and other mediators of inflammation. In models of chronic inflammation, curcumin is much less active in adrenalectomized animals, suggesting that it enhances the body's own antiinflammatory mechanisms. Its beneficial effects in human studies are comparable to standard drugs but without side effects at recommended doses. In postoperative inflammation model for NSAIDs, curcumin has comparable antiinflammatory action to phenylbutazone. It does not possess direct analgesic action. Turmeric or curcumin is beneficial in acute exacerbations of RA. Dosage for curcumin: 400-600 mg t.i.d.; turmeric dosage: 8000-60,000 mg. Curcumin is formulated with bromelain to enhance absorption. Bromelain also is antiinflammatory. Curcumin-bromelain combination is taken on an empty stomach 20 minutes before meals or between meals. A lipid base (lecithin, fish oils, or essential fatty acids) may increase absorption.
- **Bromelain**: mixture of enzymes in pineapple. It reduces inflammation in RA. Mechanisms: it inhibits proinflammatory compounds and activates compounds that break down fibrin. Fibrin forms a matrix that isolates the area of inflammation. This results in blockage of blood vessels and inadequate tissue drainage and edema. Bromelain blocks inflammatory production of kinin compounds that increase swelling and pain.
- ***Zingiber officinalis* (ginger)**: has antioxidant effects. It inhibits prostaglandin, thromboxane, and leukotriene synthesis. Fresh ginger may be more effective in RA than dried preparations; fresh contains protease with antiinflammatory action similar to bromelain. It substantially improves RA symptoms—pain relief, joint mobility, and decreased swelling and morning stiffness. Recommended dosage: 500-1000 mg q.d. Some patients have taken three to four times this amount with quicker and better relief. Forms: 1 g of dry powdered ginger root. Average daily dietary dose: 8-10 g in India; fresh (or freeze-dried) ginger root at equivalent dosage may be better because of a higher gingerol level and active protease. Daily dosage of 2-4 g of dry powdered ginger may be effective; it is equivalent to 20 g (⅔ oz) fresh ginger root (0.5-inch slice). Incorporate it into fresh

fruit and vegetable juices. No side effects are apparent at these levels.

- ***Bupleuri falcatum*** **(Chinese thoroughwax), licorice, and** ***Panax***: *Bupleuri* root is a component in Chinese traditional formulas for inflammatory conditions. It is now used in combination with corticosteroid drugs (prednisone). It enhances the activity of cortisone. Active constituents are steroid-like saikosaponins. Antiinflammatory action: increase adrenal release of cortisone and other corticosteroids and potentiate their effects, prevent adrenal atrophy caused by corticosteroids. *Bupleuri* is recommended for patients on corticosteroids to protect adrenals. *Glycyrrhiza glabra* (licorice) and *Panax ginseng* enhance action of *Bupleuri*. Licorice and ginseng have antiinflammatory constituents and improve adrenal function. Licorice inhibits breakdown of adrenal hormones by the liver. Together *Bupleuri* and licorice increase corticosteroids in circulation. These plants are used to restore adrenal function in patients with a history of long-term or high-dosage corticosteroid use.

## Physical Medicine

- Has a major role in managing RA. It is not curative, but it does improve comfort and preserve joint and muscle function. Heat relieves stiffness and pain, relaxes muscles, and increases range of motion (ROM). Moist heat (moist packs and hot baths) is more effective than dry heat (heating pad). Paraffin baths are used if skin irritation from water immersion develops. Cold packs are valuable during acute flare-ups. Strengthening and ROM exercises preserve joint function. For well-developed disease and inflammation, begin with progressive, passive ROM and isometrics. As inflammation subsides, add active ROM and isotonics exercises.
- High-intensity, long-term exercise in RA: Over a 2-year period, intensive exercise did not increase radiographic damage of large joints, except possibly in patients with considerable baseline damage. High-intensity exercise improved functionality and created better mood and sense of well-being.
- Balneotherapy: therapeutic mineral baths and mud packs are a European tradition. Israeli studies of Dead Sea spa therapy have been confirmed in conditions of high barometric pressures, low humidity, high temperatures, paucity of rainfall, and absence of air pollution. Modalities are mud packs, sulfur baths, and bathing in the Dead Sea. It provides significant improvement in duration

of morning stiffness, 15-m walk time, grip strength, activities of daily living assessment, patient's assessment of disease activity, number of active joints, and Ritchie articular index. Improvement is noted with Dead Sea bathing being superior to regular hot baths with table salt. Trace elements (zinc and copper—components of SOD—plus boron, selenium, rubidium) may be absorbed through the skin. No side effects or aggravation of disease has been noted.

## THERAPEUTIC APPROACH

Effective treatment requires controlling as many contributing factors as possible. Foremost are dietary measures to reduce causes and ameliorate symptoms. Give symptom relief through conventional physical therapy (exercise, heat, cold, massage, diathermy, lasers, and paraffin baths), antiinflammatory botanicals and nutrients and, as appropriate, bowel detoxification. In severe cases, NSAIDs may be necessary in the acute phase. Natural measures enhance efficacy of drugs; lower dosages are required. When drugs are given, prescribe deglycyrrhizinated licorice (DGL) to protect against peptic ulcers.

- **Diet**: therapeutic fast or elimination diet followed by careful reintroduction of foods to detect those that initiate symptoms. Any food can aggravate RA. Most common offenders are wheat, corn, milk and other dairy, beef, nightshade (*Solanum* family) foods (tomato, potato, eggplants, peppers, and tobacco). After isolating and eliminating allergens, eat healthy diet rich in whole foods, vegetables, and fiber and low in sugar, meat, refined carbohydrates, and animal fats. Particularly beneficial are wild cold-water fish (mackerel, herring, sardines, and salmon) and flavonoid-rich berries (cherries, hawthorn berries, blueberries, blackberries) and their extracts.
- **Supplements**:
  —DHEA: 50-200 mg q.d.
  —EPA: 1.8 g q.d. (or flaxseed oil: 1 tbsp q.d.)
  —Niacinamide: 500 mg q.i.d. (monitor liver enzymes)
  —Pantothenic acid: 500 mg q.d.
  —Quercetin: 250 mg between meals t.i.d.
  —Vitamin A: 5000 IU q.d.
  —Vitamin C: 1-3 g q.d. in divided doses
  —Vitamin E (mixed tocopherols): 400 IU q.d.

—Cu: 1 mg q.d.
—Mn: 15 mg q.d.
—Se: 200 mg q.d.
—Zn: 45 mg q.d.
—Betaine HCl: 5-70 grains with meals (*Textbook,* "Hydrochloric Acid Supplementation: Patient Instructions")
—Pancreatin (10X USP): 350-750 mg between meals t.i.d. *or* bromelain: 250-750 mg (1800-2000 MCU) between meals t.i.d.
—Fish oil supplement: if wild cold-water fish are not available; minimal daily dose: 3 g combined EPA/DHA; use a high-quality lab-tested product

- **Botanical medicines**: used alone or in combination. Severe inflammation and joint destruction require more aggressive therapy. Patients with a history of corticosteroid use and those weaning off corticosteroids, use *Bupleuri falcatum, Glycyrrhiza glabra,* and *Panax ginseng* to prevent and/or reverse adrenal atrophy:
  —Curcumin: 400 mg t.i.d. (or ginger: incorporate 8-10 g fresh ginger into diet daily or ginger extracts standardized to 20% gingerol and shogaol at dosage = 100-200 mg t.i.d.)
  —*Bupleuri falcatum*: dried root, 2-4 g; tincture (1:5), 5-10 mL; fluid extract (1:1), 2-4 mL; solid extract (4:1), 200-400 mg
  —*Panax ginseng*: crude herb, 4.5-6 g q.d.; standardized extract (5% ginsenosides), 100 mg q.d. to t.i.d.
  —*Glycyrrhiza glabra*: dried root, 2-4 g; tincture (1:5), 10-20 mL; fluid extract (1:1), 4-6 mL; solid extract (4:1), 250-500 mg
- **Physical medicine**:
  —Heat (moist packs, hot baths): 20-30 min q.d. to t.i.d.
  —Cold packs for acute flare-ups
  —Paraffin baths (if hot water causes skin irritation)
  —Active (or in severe cases, passive) ROM exercises: 3-10 repetitions q.d. to b.i.d.
  —Progressive isometric (and isotonic as joints improve) exercise: 3-10 repetitions several times per day with generous periods of rest
  —Massage: one to three times per week

# Rosacea

## DIAGNOSTIC SUMMARY

- Chronic acneiform eruption on the face of middle-aged and older adults associated with facial flushing and telangiectasia.
- The acneiform component is characterized by papules, pustules, and seborrhea; the vascular component by erythema and telangiectasia; and the glandular component by hyperplasia of the soft tissue of the nose (rhinophyma).
- The primary involvement occurs over the flush areas of the cheeks and nose.

## GENERAL CONSIDERATIONS

- Rosacea is a chronic skin disorder; the nose and cheeks are abnormally red and may be covered with pimples similar to acne (see the chapter on acne). It was originally called acne rosacea because inflammatory papules and pustules closely mimic acne vulgaris. Rosacea inflammation is vascular, occurs between ages 25 and 70 years, and is more common in people with fair complexions. It is more common in women (3:1) but more severe in men. Thirteen million Americans are affected.
- Rosacea is divided into three stages:
  —Stage I. Erythematotelangiectatic rosacea: erythema triggered by hot beverages, spicy foods, and alcohol may persist for hours; telangiectasia is noticeable on central third of face; and burning, stinging, and itching occur after application of cosmetics, fragrances, and sunscreens.
  —Stage II. Inflammatory papules and pustules, or papulopustular rosacea: flushing, telangiectasia, and seborrhea increase; facial pore enlargement is minimal.
  —Stage III. Phymatous rosacea: deep inflammatory nodules, large telangiectatic vessels, markedly dilated facial pores, and sebaceous gland hyperplasia and tissue hyperplasia, especially of nose (rhinophyma). Only a small number progress to this stage.

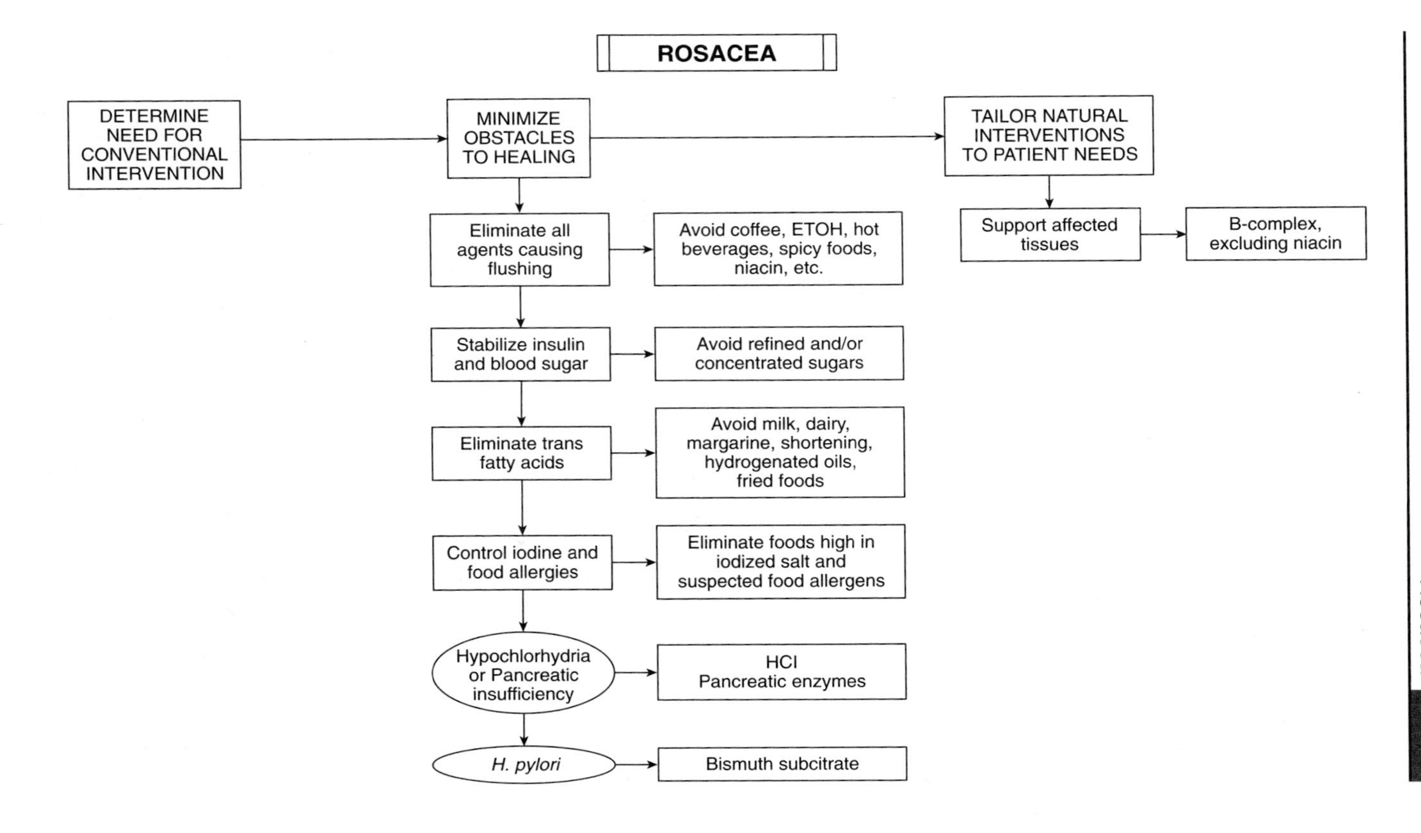
ROSACEA
DETERMINE NEED FOR CONVENTIONAL INTERVENTION
MINIMIZE OBSTACLES TO HEALING
TAILOR NATURAL INTERVENTIONS TO PATIENT NEEDS
Support affected tissues
B-complex, excluding niacin
Eliminate all agents causing flushing
Avoid coffee, ETOH, hot beverages, spicy foods, niacin, etc.
Stabilize insulin and blood sugar
Avoid refined and/or concentrated sugars
Eliminate trans fatty acids
Avoid milk, dairy, margarine, shortening, hydrogenated oils, fried foods
Control iodine and food allergies
Eliminate foods high in iodized salt and suspected food allergens
Hypochlorhydria or Pancreatic insufficiency
HCl
Pancreatic enzymes
H. pylori
Bismuth subcitrate

- Ocular rosacea: spectrum of eye findings associated with skin problems. The eyes have a watery or bloodshot appearance, with sensation of foreign body, burning or stinging, dryness, itching, light sensitivity, or other signs and symptoms. Sties are a common sign of rosacea ocular disease. Some may have decreased visual acuity because of corneal complications.

### Etiology

The cause of rosacea is poorly understood despite numerous theories. Causative factors suspected include the following:

- The mite *Demodex folliculorum*
- Alcoholism
- Menopausal flushing
- Vasomotor neurosis
- Seborrheic diathesis
- Local infection
- Food allergies
- B vitamin deficiencies
- Gastrointestinal disorders

Most cases display moderate to severe seborrhea, but sebum production is not increased in many. Vasomotor lability is prevalent; migraine headaches are three times more common than in matched control subjects.

## THERAPEUTIC CONSIDERATIONS

- Avoid stimuli that exacerbate rosacea—exposure to extremes of heat and cold, excessive sunlight, ingestion of hot liquids, alcohol, spicy foods.
- Conventional treatment: oral tetracycline, especially for papular or pustular lesions; however, this treatment usually only controls rather than eradicates. Topical antibiotics or synthetic retinoids are less successful. Topical corticosteroids initially improve, but long-term therapy may actually lead to rosacea. Chronic skin changes and severe rhinophyma may require laser or surgical intervention, respectively.
- Natural approach: identify and eliminate contributing factors. Key factors: hypochlorhydria, eradication of *Helicobacter pylori*, elimination of food allergies, optimal intake of B vitamins.
  —Hypochlorhydria: gastric analysis of rosacea patients indicates hypochlorhydria. Psychological factors (worry,

depression, stress) reduce gastric acidity. Hydrochloric acid supplements improve patients with achlorhydria or hypochlorhydria. Secretion of lipase also is decreased (bicarbonate and chymotrypsin are normal). Pancreatic supplements benefit.

—*H. pylori*: high incidence of gastric *H. pylori* is found in rosacea patients. Flushing reaction in rosacea may be caused by gastrin or vasoactive intestinal peptides. Some histologically positive patients are serologically negative. Clinical success in treating rosacea with metronidazole and abatement of *H. pylori* isolates and serology after treatment provide evidence connecting rosacea with *H. pylori*. Yet *H. pylori* may be associated with rosacea and not be causative; rosacea patients may have similar rates of *H. pylori* as do healthy subjects. Rosacea patients report "indigestion" more often and use more antacids than does the general population. Many studies confirm a strong link between *H. pylori* and rosacea and correlation between severity of rosacea and level of infection.

—Food allergy: migraine headaches accompanying rosacea point to food intolerance, as does reflex flushing by vasodilator substances. Rosacea may be a hypersensitivity disorder; dietary factors could exacerbate skin flushing.

—B vitamins: large doses of B vitamins are quite effective, with riboflavin (vitamin $B_2$) as key factor.

- Mite *Demodex folliculorum* is considered a factor, but it is a normal inhabitant of follicles. It may account for more granulomatous response of some patients (researchers were able to infect skin of $B_2$-deficient rats with *Demodex*, but not skin of normal rats). Delayed hypersensitivity reaction in follicles is triggered by *D. folliculorum* antigens and stimulates progression of affection to papulopustular stage.
- Some patients' rosacea may be aggravated by large doses of these nutrients. Inflammation and exacerbations of acne related to vitamins $B_2$, $B_6$, and $B_{12}$ are reported in European literature.

## THERAPEUTIC APPROACH

Cause(s) are undetermined, but adequate treatment is possible for most patients. Eradicate *H. pylori* infection (when present). Control hypochlorhydria and food intolerance. Support with vitamin B complex and avoid vasodilating foods.

- General recommendations: see the chapter on acne.
- Treat *H. Pylori* infection, if present. See the chapter on peptic ulcers.
- Diet: avoid coffee, alcohol, hot beverages, spicy foods, and any other food or drink causing flush. Eliminate refined and/or concentrated sugars, trans fatty acids (milk, milk products, margarine, shortening, synthetically hydrogenated vegetable oils, fried foods). Avoid foods high in iodized salt.
- Supplements:
  —Vitamin B complex: 100 mg q.d. (avoid niacin)
  —Pancreas extract (8×-10× USP): 350-500 mg before meals
  —Hydrochloric acid (*Textbook,* "Hydrochloric Acid Supplementation: Patient Instructions")

# Seborrheic Dermatitis

## DIAGNOSTIC SUMMARY

- Superficial erythematous papules and scaly eruptions on scalp, cheeks, and intertrigo of axilla, groin, and neck.
- Usually nonpruritic.
- Seasonal, worse in winter.

## GENERAL CONSIDERATIONS

- Seborrheic dermatitis (SD) is a common papulosquamous condition with an appearance similar to eczema. It may be associated with excessive oiliness (seborrhea) and dandruff. Scale is yellowish and either dry or greasy. Erythematous, follicular, scaly papules may coalesce into large plaques or circinate patches. Flexural involvement often is complicated with *Candida* infection.
- Occurs in infancy (between 2 and 12 weeks of age) and in the middle-aged and elderly.
- Prognosis: lifelong recurrence.
- Cause is unknown. Genetic predisposition, emotional stress, diet, hormones, and infection with yeastlike organisms are implicated.
- Common manifestation of AIDS, affecting 83%; gives increased credence to the infection theory of SD.

## THERAPEUTIC CONSIDERATIONS

### Nutrition

**Food allergy**: SD begins as cradle cap. It is not primarily an allergic disease, but it is linked to food allergy (67% have some form of allergy by age 10 years).

**Biotin**: underlying factor in infants is biotin deficiency. Syndrome is clinically similar to SD induced in rats fed a diet high in raw egg white (high in avidin, a glycoprotein that binds biotin, making it biounavailable).

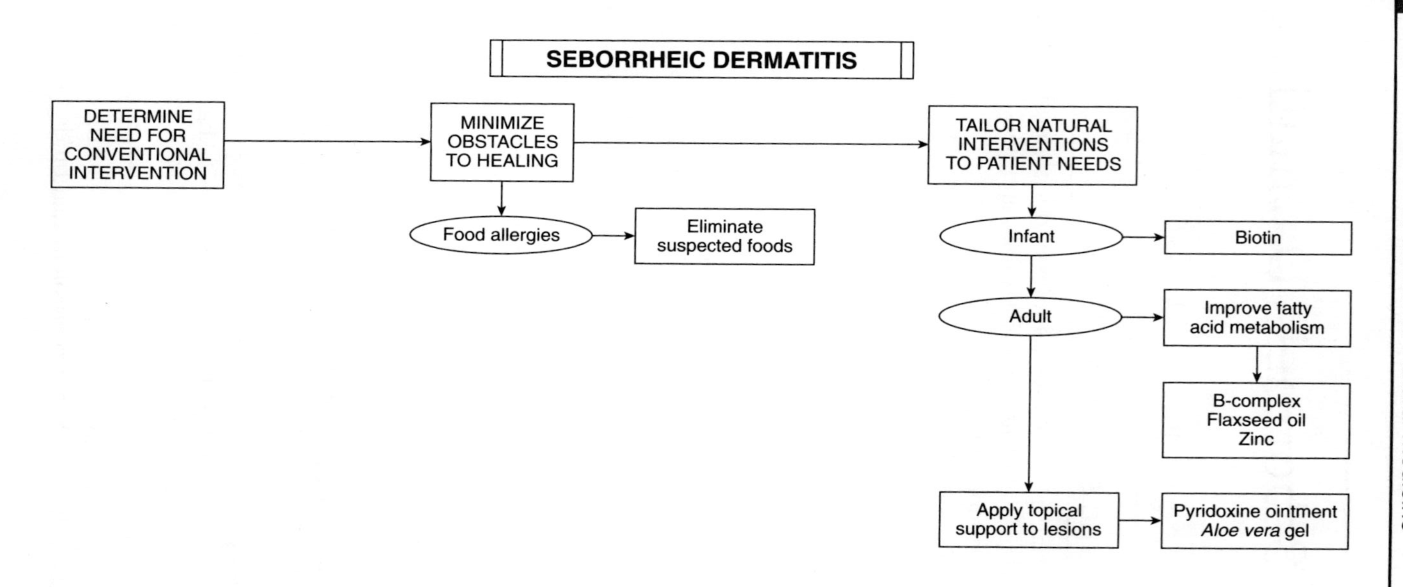
SEBORRHEIC DERMATITIS
DETERMINE NEED FOR CONVENTIONAL INTERVENTION
MINIMIZE OBSTACLES TO HEALING
Food allergies
Eliminate suspected foods
TAILOR NATURAL INTERVENTIONS TO PATIENT NEEDS
Infant
Biotin
Adult
Improve fatty acid metabolism
B-complex
Flaxseed oil
Zinc
Apply topical support to lesions
Pyridoxine ointment
Aloe vera gel

- Large portion of human biotin supply is provided by intestinal bacteria. Dysbiosis may cause biotin deficiency in infants. SD is successfully treated with biotin in nursing mothers and infants.
- In adults, biotin alone is ineffective. Long-chain fatty acid synthesis may be impaired in SD lesions. B vitamins (biotin, pyridoxine, pantothenic acid, niacin, thiamin, and lipotropics) are vital for fatty acid metabolism.
- Pyridoxine: $B_6$ deficiency in human beings and rats causes lesions indistinguishable from SD.
- Treatment with oral and parenteral $B_6$ has been unsuccessful.
- In the sicca form of disorder (involving scalp [dandruff], brow, nasolabial folds, and bearded area with varying degrees of greasy, adherent scales on erythematous base), all patients cleared completely within 10 days with a local water-soluble ointment containing 50 mg/g pyridoxine. Other types of SD (flexural and infected) are unresponsive.
- In patients with elevated urinary xanthurenic acid, oral, parenteral, and local $B_6$ all normalized excretion levels, implying transcutaneous absorption of $B_6$. But improvement from topical $B_6$ may be caused by reducing sebaceous secretion rate from the ointment itself; adding $B_6$ had no effect.
- Check patient for exposure to $B_6$ antimetabolites: hydrazine dyes (FD&C yellow #5) and drugs (isoniazid and hydralazine), dopamine, penicillamine, oral contraceptives, and excessive protein intake.

**Folic acid**: oral folic acid is only moderately successful (tetrahydro form showed dramatic results for one patient unresponsive to folic acid after childbirth). Sicca form is unresponsive. Parenteral injections of vitamin $B_{12}$ (synthetic and liver extracted) are quite effective in many cases. Vitamin $B_{12}$ is a cofactor (with choline) in 5-methyl-tetrahydrofolate methyltransferase, which regenerates tetrahydrofolate. Folate may become trapped as 5-methyltetrahydrofolate by lack of $B_{12}$ and/or choline.

**Miscellaneous factors**: other B vitamins may be involved in SD. Experimentally induced ariboflavinosis produces sicca form of SD.

## Botanical Medicine

- ***Aloe vera* gel**: can be helpful topically. Thirty percent crude aloe emulsion cream twice daily for 4 to 6 weeks improved scaling and itching in 62% of subjects compared with only 25% using placebo.

## THERAPEUTIC APPROACH

Optimal approach is unclear. Effective therapy, however, is available for most patients:

- Infants: alleviate biotin deficiency, control food allergies.
- Adults: correct impaired long-chain fatty acid synthesis with large doses of vitamin B complex.

Maximize therapeutic results with a broad-spectrum approach.

The following dosages are for adults; modify children's doses according to weight.

- **Diet**: detect and treat food allergies; in nursing infants, consider food allergies of mother.
- **Supplements**:
  —Biotin: 3 mg b.i.d.
  —Vitamin B complex: 50 mg b.i.d.
  —Zinc: 25 mg q.d. (picolinate)
  —Flaxseed oil: 1 tbsp q.d.
- **Topical treatment**:
  —Pyridoxine ointment: 50 mg/g (in water-soluble base)
  —*Aloe vera* gel

# Senile (Aging-Related) Cataracts

## DIAGNOSTIC SUMMARY

- Clouding or opacity in the crystalline lens of the eye.
- Absence or altered red reflex (small cataracts stand out as dark defects).
- Gradual loss of vision.

## GENERAL CONSIDERATIONS

- Leading cause of impaired vision and blindness in the United States; 4 million people have vision-impairing cataract, and 40,000 people in the country are blind because of cataracts. Cataract surgery is the most common major surgical procedure in the United States.
- Classified by location and appearance of lens opacities, cause or significant contributing factor, and age of onset.
- Causes and contributing factors: ocular disease, injury, surgery, systemic diseases (diabetes mellitus, galactosemia), toxin, ultraviolet and near-ultraviolet light, radiation exposure, and hereditary disease.
- Transparency of lens decreases with age. Most elderly people have some degree of cataract formation, including progressive increase in size, weight, and density of lens throughout life.
- Histopathology of cataract:
  - —Fibrous metaplasia of epithelium
  - —Liquefaction of fibers resulting in Morgagnian globule formation (drops of fluid beneath capsule and between lens fibers)
  - —Sclerosis (melding of fibers)
  - —Posterior migration and swelling of epithelium
- Topoanatomic classification of cataracts:
  - —Anterior subcapsular cataract: fibrous metaplasia of lens epithelium (after iritis and adherence of iris to lens [posterior synechia])

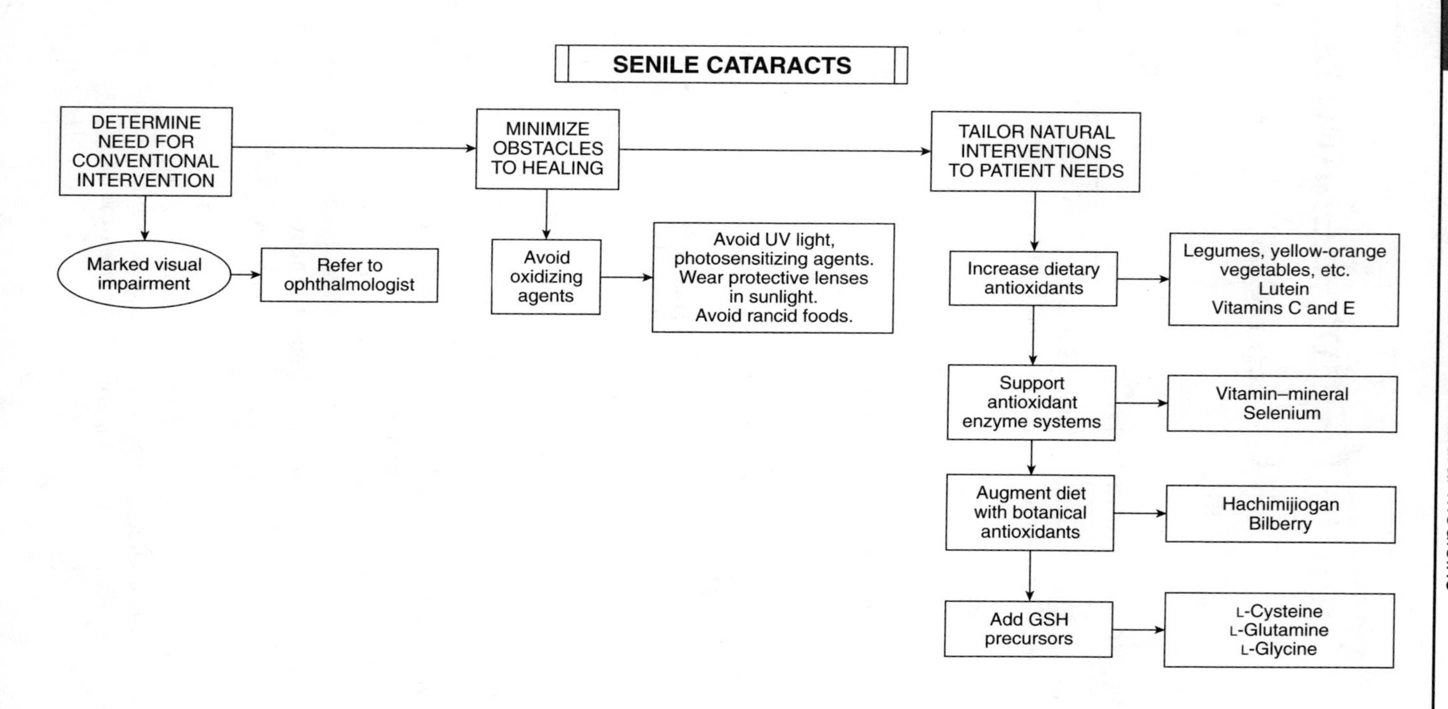
SENILE CATARACTS
DETERMINE NEED FOR CONVENTIONAL INTERVENTION
Marked visual impairment
Refer to ophthalmologist
MINIMIZE OBSTACLES TO HEALING
Avoid oxidizing agents
Avoid UV light, photosensitizing agents. Wear protective lenses in sunlight. Avoid rancid foods.
TAILOR NATURAL INTERVENTIONS TO PATIENT NEEDS
Increase dietary antioxidants
Legumes, yellow-orange vegetables, etc. Lutein Vitamins C and E
Support antioxidant enzyme systems
Vitamin–mineral Selenium
Augment diet with botanical antioxidants
Hachimijiogan Bilberry
Add GSH precursors
L-Cysteine L-Glutamine L-Glycine

—Anterior cortical cataract: liquefaction of lens fibers and Morgagnian globules in cortex anteriorly
—Nuclear cataract: exaggeration of normal, aging-related, melding of fibers in nucleus
—Posterior cortical cataract: liquefaction and globular degeneration of posterior lens cortex
—Posterior subcapsular cataract: epithelial cells migrate posteriorly under capsule and form large, irregular nucleated cells

Seventy-five percent of senile cataracts are cortical; 25% are nuclear. Cortical cataracts take three forms:

- Spoke wheel, beginning in periphery and coursing anteriorly and posteriorly to nucleus
- Perinuclear punctate opacities
- Granular opacities under posterior capsule (subcapsular cataracts)

## THERAPEUTIC CONSIDERATIONS

- Etiology of cataract: inability to maintain normal homeostatic concentrations of sodium ($Na^+$), potassium ($K^+$), and calcium ($Ca^{2+}$) within lens, the result of decreased $Na^+$, $K^+$ adenosine triphosphatase (ATPase) activity—a defect from free radical damage to sulfhydryl proteins in the lens, including $Na^+$, $K^+$-ATPase that contains a sulfhydryl component.
- Normal protective mechanisms are unable to prevent free radical damage; the lens depends on superoxide dismutase (SOD), catalase, glutathione (GSH), and accessory antioxidants vitamins E and C and selenium (Se) to prevent free radical damage.
- People with higher intake of vitamins C and E, Se, and carotenes have a much lower risk for cataracts.
- Nutritional supplements—such as multiple vitamin/mineral formulas, vitamins C and E, B vitamins ($B_{12}$, folic acid), vitamin A—also offer significant protection against nuclear and cortical cataracts.

### Antioxidants

- **Lutein**: yellow-orange carotene that protects against macular degeneration and cataract formation. Like the macula, the lens concentrates lutein. Spinach (high in lutein) consumption is inversely related to cataract extraction. Intake of lutein is inversely associated with cataract extraction (20%-50% risk reduction). Lutein (15 mg) given three times per week for up to 2 years to patients with age-related cataracts improved visual acuity and glare sensitivity.

- **Vitamin C**: high intake of vitamin C from dietary sources or supplements protects against cataract formation. Supplements can halt cataract progression and, in some cases, improve vision. Supplements reduced cataract development and number of surgeries required among cataract patients over a period of 11 years. Dosage necessary to increase vitamin C content of lens: 1000 mg. Vitamin C in blood is 0.5 mg/dL, but in adrenal and pituitary glands the level is 100 times this and in the liver, spleen, and lens of eye it is 20 times higher. Enormous amounts of energy are required to pull vitamin C out of blood against a tremendous gradient. Keeping blood vitamin C elevated with high dosing reduces the gradient.
- **Glutathione (GSH)**: GSH is a tripeptide composed of glycine, glutamic acid, and cysteine. It is in very high concentrations in lens. GSH is a key protective factor against intralenticular and extralenticular toxins and is an antioxidant. It maintains reduced sulfhydryl bonds within lens proteins. It is a coenzyme of various enzyme systems. GSH participates in amino acid transport with gamma-glutamyl transpeptidase. It also is involved in cation transport. GSH is diminished in virtually all forms of cataracts.
- **Ascorbic acid (AA) and GSH interactions**: work in close conjunction as the most important host protective factor against induction of cataracts.
- **Selenium and vitamin E**: antioxidants that function synergistically. GSH peroxidase is Se dependent. Se content in lens with cataract is 15% of normal. Se in serum and aqueous humor is much lower in cataract patients than in control subjects, but Se in the lens itself did not differ much in cataract patients and normal subjects. Decreased Se in aqueous humor is a major finding. Excess $H_2O_2$ (25 times normal) is in the aqueous humor of cataract patients and is associated with increased lipid peroxidation and altered lens permeability from damaged sodium-potassium pump. The lens is left unprotected against free radical and sun damage. Se-dependent GSH peroxidase breaks down $H_2O_2$. Vitamin E supplementation alone (500 IU q.d.) does not retard progression of cataracts. Vitamin E (400 IU) plus vitamin C (500 mg) and beta-carotene (15 mg) failed to

affect the development or progression of cataracts in a 7-year trial.

- **Superoxide dismutase (SOD)**: activity in human lens is lower than in other tissues because of increased ascorbate and GSH. Progressive SOD decrease parallels cataract progression. Oral SOD supplements do not affect tissue SOD activity. Trace mineral cofactors of SOD that are greatly reduced in cataractous lens are preferred (copper, 90%; manganese, 50%; zinc, 90%).
- **Catalase**: concentrated in epithelial portion of lens (anterior surface); very low levels are in the rest of lens. Primary function is to reduce (to water and oxygen) hydrogen peroxide formed from oxidation of ascorbate.
- **Tetrahydrobiopterin ($BH_4$)**: pteridine compounds protect against cataract formation by preventing oxidation and damage by ultraviolet light. They prevent formation of high-molecular-weight proteins in lens. Tetrahydrobiopterin is a coenzyme in hydroxylation of monoamines (phenylalanine hydroxylase, tyrosine hydroxylase, tryptophan hydroxylase). Decreased pteridine-synthesizing enzymes and tetrahydrobiopterin are found in senile cataracts. Supplemental folic acid may help compensate.

## Other Nutritional Factors

- **Riboflavin**: lenticular GSH requires flavin adenine dinucleotide (FAD) as coenzyme for GSH reductase. Vitamin $B_2$ is a precursor of FAD. Vitamin $B_2$ deficiency may enhance cataract formation by depressed GSH reductase activity. Vitamin $B_2$ deficiency is common in the elderly (33%). Riboflavin status can be determined by red blood cell GSH reductase activity before and after FAD stimulation. Correction of the deficiency is warranted, but no more than 10 mg q.d. Vitamin $B_2$ should be prescribed for cataract patients because of a photosensitizing effect—superoxide radicals generated by interaction of light, ambient oxygen, and riboflavin/FAD. Vitamin $B_2$ and light (at physiologic levels) were used experimentally to induce cataracts. Excess vitamin $B_2$ does more harm than good in cataract patients.
- **Amino acids**: methionine is a component of lens antioxidant enzyme methionine sulfoxide reductase. It is a precursor of cysteine, a component of GSH. Cysteine and other amino acid precursors of GSH are helpful in cataract treatment.

- **Zinc, vitamin A, and beta-carotene**: antioxidants are vital for normal epithelial integrity. Beta-carotene may act as a filter, protecting against light-induced damage to fiber portion of lens. Beta-carotene is the most significant singlet oxygen free radical scavenger and is used to treat photosensitive disorders.
- **Melatonin**: efficient free radical scavenger and antioxidant. It neutralizes hydroxyl and peroxyl radicals; enhances endogenous and exogenous antioxidant efficiency; and inhibits DNA damage, lipid peroxidation, and cataract formation in animals. It is present at significant levels in the cell nucleus, aqueous cytosol, and lipid-rich cell membranes.

## Diet

Protective action is derived from some vegetables, fruit, calcium, folic acid, and vitamin E. Increased incidence arises with elevated salt and fat intake.

- **Dairy products**: cataracts often develop in infants with homozygous deficiency of either galactokinase or galactose-1-phosphate uridyl transferase. They also occur in lab animals fed a high-galactose diet. Abnormalities of galactose metabolism are identified by measuring activity of these enzymes in red blood cells. This is an important mechanism in 30% of cataract patients, but only diabetic cataracts. It is probably not relevant to senile cataracts (see the chapter on diabetes mellitus).

## Heavy Metals

Increased concentrations are found in aging lens and cataractous lens; levels are higher in cataracts, but significance is unknown.

- Cadmium (Cd): concentration in cataractous lens is two to three times higher than control subjects. Cd displaces Zn from binding in enyzmes by binding to sulfhydryl groups. Cd contributes to deactivation of free radical quenching and other protective and repair mechanisms.
- Other elevated elements of unknown significance include bromine, cobalt, iridium, and nickel.

## Botanical Medicines

- **Flavonoid-rich extracts**: *Vaccinium myrtillus* (bilberry), *Vitis vinifera* (grapeseed), *Pinus maritima* (pine bark), and curcumin from

*Curcuma longa* (turmeric). Flavonoid components in well-defined diets may be protective. Bilberry anthocyanosides may offer the greatest protection; bilberry plus vitamin E stopped progression of cataract in 97% of patients with senile cortical cataracts.

- **Hachimijiogan**: ancient Chinese formula that increases antioxidant level of lens. It has been used in treating cataracts for hundreds of years. Therapeutic effect is impressive in early stages; 60% of subjects noted significant improvement, 20% showed no progression, and only 20% displayed progression of cataract. It contains the following eight herbs (per 24 g dose):
  —*Rehmannia glutinosa*: 6000 mg
  —*Poria cocos sclerotium*: 3000 mg
  —*Dioscorea opposita*: 3000 mg
  —*Cornus officinalis*: 3000 mg
  —*Epimedium grandiflorum*: 3000 mg
  —*Alisma plantago*: 3000 mg
  —*Astragalus membranaceus*: 2000 mg
  —*Cinnamomum cassia*: 1000 mg

## THERAPEUTIC APPROACH

Marked vision improvement is gained from cataract removal and lens implant. Prevention or treatment at an early stage is most effective. Free radical damage is the primary inducing factor; avoid oxidizing agents and promote free radical scavenging. Avoid direct ultraviolet light, bright light, and photosensitizing substances. Wear protective lenses outdoors. Greatly increase antioxidant nutrients. Progression can be stopped and early lesions can be reversed. Significant reversal of well-developed cataracts is unlikely. The elderly are especially susceptible to nutrient deficiencies; ensure they are ingesting and assimilating adequate macronutrients and micronutrients.

- **Diet**: avoid rancid foods and other sources of free radicals. Increase legumes (sulfur-containing amino acids methionine and cysteine), yellow vegetables (carotenes), and foods rich in vitamins C and E.
- **Supplements**:
  —High-potency multiple vitamin/mineral formula
  —Lutein: 5-15 mg q.d.
  —Vitamin C: 1 g t.i.d.
  —Vitamin E: 600-800 IU q.d. (mixed tocopherols)

—Selenium: 400 mg q.d.
—L-Cysteine: 400 mg q.d.
—L-Glutamine: 200 mg q.d.
—L-Glycine: 200 mg q.d.

- **Botanical medicines**:
  —Bilberry extract (25% anthocyanidin): 80 mg t.i.d.
  —Hachimijiogan formula: 150 mg t.i.d.

# Streptococcal Pharyngitis

## DIAGNOSTIC SUMMARY

- Abrupt onset of sore throat, fever, malaise, nausea, and headache.
- Throat red and edematous, with or without exudation.
- Tender cervical lymph nodes.
- Positive rapid detection of streptococcal antigen.
- Group A streptococci on throat culture.

## GENERAL CONSIDERATIONS

Throat cultures yield group A beta-hemolytic streptococci in <20% of patients with sore throat. Signs and symptoms of "strep throat" resemble viral pharyngitis, requiring culture for definitive diagnosis. 10%-25% of general, asymptomatic population are carriers for group A *Streptococcus*.

- Rapid strep screens detect group A strep antigens. Definitive positive culture takes 2 days. Antibiotics during this period lead to unnecessary development of antibiotic-resistant organisms and patient exposure to antibiotics. Second-generation rapid strep screens (Strep A OIA test) have excellent sensitivity and specificity that will someday replace throat culture as the diagnostic gold standard.
- Even if positive for strep, antibiotics may not be necessary; strep throat usually is self-limiting. Clinical recovery is similar in cases treated with antibiotics and those that were not.
- Concern with not using antibiotics: "nonsuppurative poststreptococcal syndromes" (rheumatic fever, poststreptococcal glomerulonephritis). But antibiotics do not significantly reduce incidence of sequelae. Most cases of sequelae are the result of the patient not consulting a physician. The dogma is that acute rheumatic fever can only be caused by group A streptococcal infection of the upper respiratory tract, but *Streptococcal pyoderma* is major cause in Aboriginal people of northern Australia and perhaps other high-incidence communities. In settings where rheumatic

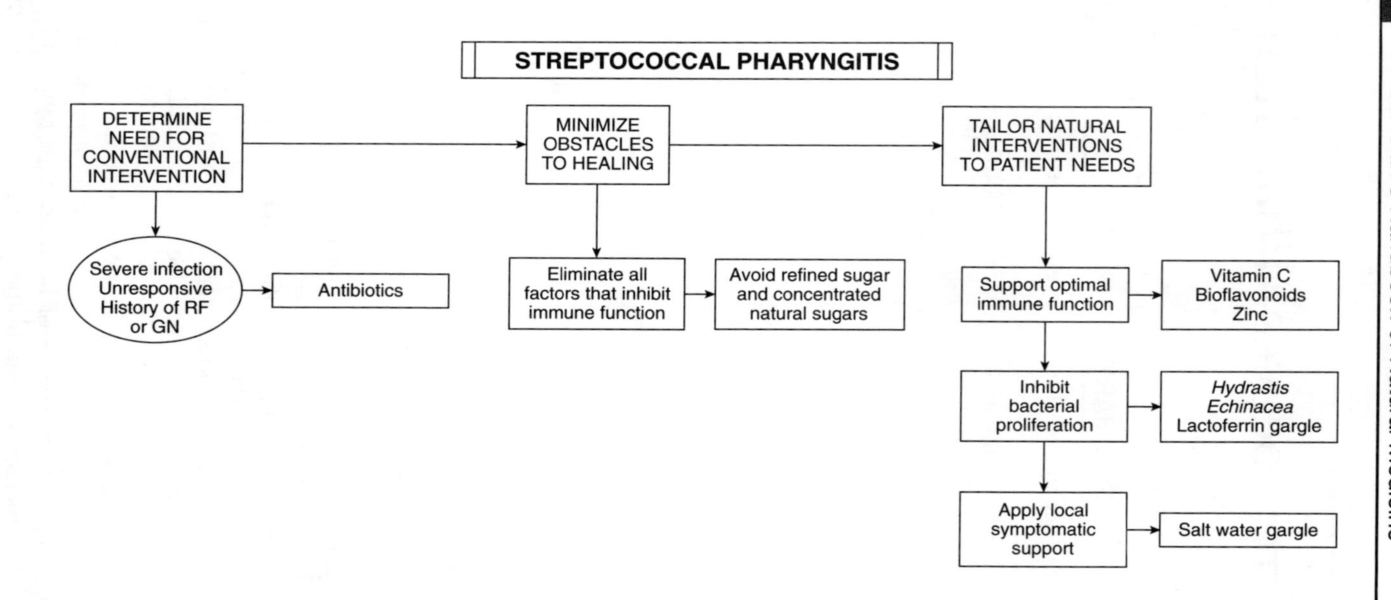
STREPTOCOCCAL PHARYNGITIS
DETERMINE NEED FOR CONVENTIONAL INTERVENTION
Severe infection
Unresponsive
History of RF or GN
Antibiotics
MINIMIZE OBSTACLES TO HEALING
Eliminate all factors that inhibit immune function
Avoid refined sugar and concentrated natural sugars
TAILOR NATURAL INTERVENTIONS TO PATIENT NEEDS
Support optimal immune function
Vitamin C
Bioflavonoids
Zinc
Inhibit bacterial proliferation
Hydrastis
Echinacea
Lactoferrin gargle
Apply local symptomatic support
Salt water gargle

fever is rare, Group A streptococcal strains causing pharyngitis have lower virulence in causing rheumatic fever.

- Reserve antibiotics for patients with severe infection who are unresponsive to therapy (unresponsive after 1 week of immune support) and those with history of rheumatic fever (RF) or glomerulonephritis (GN). Even then, antibiotics such as penicillin fail to eradicate strep in more than 20% of patients; beta-lactase–positive organisms (*Staphylococcus aureus* and *Bacteroides* spp.) deactivate penicillin. Stronger antibiotics (e.g., celphasporin) may be required.
- Dramatic decrease in incidence of RF began before advent of antibiotics. Improved socioeconomic, hygienic, and nutritional conditions are more important. Present attack rates after strep infection are 0.4%-2.8% for RF and 0.2%-20% for GN.

## THERAPEUTIC CONSIDERATIONS

Primary therapeutic consideration is status of patient's immune system. If immune function is good, illness is short lived. Enhance immune function (*Textbook,* "Immune Support") to shorten course. If immune function is poor, make every effort to strengthen immune system.

- **Vitamin C**: vitamin C deficiency correlates with strep sequelae. RF is virtually nonexistent in tropics, where vitamin C intake is higher. Eighteen percent of children in high-risk groups have subnormal serum vitamin C, which is preventive against RF in animals. Highly positive results arise when children are given orange juice supplementation. Promising research was dropped because of the advent of supposedly effective antibiotics.
- ***Hydrastis canadensis* (goldenseal) and *Echinacea angustifolia***: berberine alkaloids of Hydrastis exert antibiotic activity against strep and inhibit attachment of group A strep to pharyngeal epithelial cells. Streptococci secrete hyaluronidase to colonize tissue; this enzyme is inhibited by *Echinacea* and bioflavonoids. *Echinacea* promotes increased phagocytosis, natural killer cell activity, and properdin levels (*Textbook, "Echinacea* Species" [Narrow-Leafed Purple Coneflower]" and "*Hydrastis canadensis* [Goldenseal] and Other Berberine-Containing Botanicals").
- **Bacteriotherapy**: colonizing throat with group A non–beta-hemolytic strep may prevent recurrent group A beta-hemolytic streptococci pharyngitis. Spray was used for at least 5 days; no side effects were reported.

- **Lactoferrin**: low concentrations of bovine lactoferrin hinder in vitro invasion of cultured epithelial cells by group A streptococci from patients with pharyngitis. In tonsil specimens from children treated for 15 days before tonsillectomy with both oral erythromycin (500 mg t.i.d.) and lactoferrin gargles (100 mg t.i.d.), a lower number of intracellular group A streptococci was found compared with children treated with erythromycin alone (500 mg t.i.d.).

## THERAPEUTIC APPROACH

If antibiotics are used, follow recommendations for *Lactobacillus acidophilus* (*Textbook,* "Probiotics").

- **Supplements**:
  —Vitamin C: 500 mg every 2 hours
  —Bioflavonoids: 1000 mg q.d.
  —Zinc: 30 mg q.d.
- **Botanical medicines**:
  —*Echinacea* spp. (t.i.d.): dried root (or as tea), 0.5-1 g; freeze-dried plant: 325-650 mg; juice of aerial portion of *E. purpurea* stabilized in 22% ethanol, 2-3 mL; tincture (1:5), 2-4 mL; fluid extract (1:1), 2-4 mL; solid (dry powdered) extract (6.5:1 or 3.5% echinacoside), 150-300 mg.
  —*Hydrastis canadensis* (goldenseal) (dosage based on berberine content; standardized extracts are preferred) (t.i.d.): dried root or as infusion (tea), 2-4 g; tincture (1:5), 6-12 mL (1.5-3 tsp); fluid extract (1:1), 2-4 mL (0.5-1 tsp); solid (powdered dry) extract (4:1 or 8%-12% alkaloid content), 250-500 mg.
- Local treatment: gargle with lactoferrin (100 mg) dissolved in water three times daily. Alternatively, gargle with salt water twice per day as 1 tbsp salt/240 mL of warm water.

# Trichomoniasis

## DIAGNOSTIC SUMMARY

- Profuse, malodorous, white to green discharge from vagina.
- Discharge usually has a pH greater than 4.5, a weak amine odor, and large numbers of white blood cells and trichomonads on wet mount.
- Vulvovaginal pruritus, burning, and/or irritation.
- Vulva and introitus usually show erythema.
- Cervix may or may not have a mottled erythema "strawberry cervix" (less than 5%).
- Dysuria and/or dyspareunia may be present.
- Rule out trichomoniasis in men exhibiting signs of prostatitis, urethritis, or epididymitis.

## GENERAL CONSIDERATIONS

Trichomoniasis (trich) is a common disease affecting one in five women in the United States during their lifetime. Five million cases appear each year. It is present in 3%-15% of asymptomatic women treated at obstetric/gynecologic clinics and 20%-50% of women treated at sexually transmitted disease clinics.

- Gonorrhea (GC) and trich commonly coexist; 40% of women with trich have GC and vice versa.
- Trich frequently causes cervical erosion (90%), a factor in malignancy.
- Trich may complicate interpretation of Pap smears, increasing number of false-positive results.
- Trich increases sterility in women (salpingitis) and men (toxins decrease motility of spermatozoa).
- Increased postpartum fever and discharge in women with *Trichomonas vaginalis* at delivery.
- Neonates infected from passage through the birth canal may manifest serious illness (rare).
- Prostatitis and epididymitis are common in infected men.

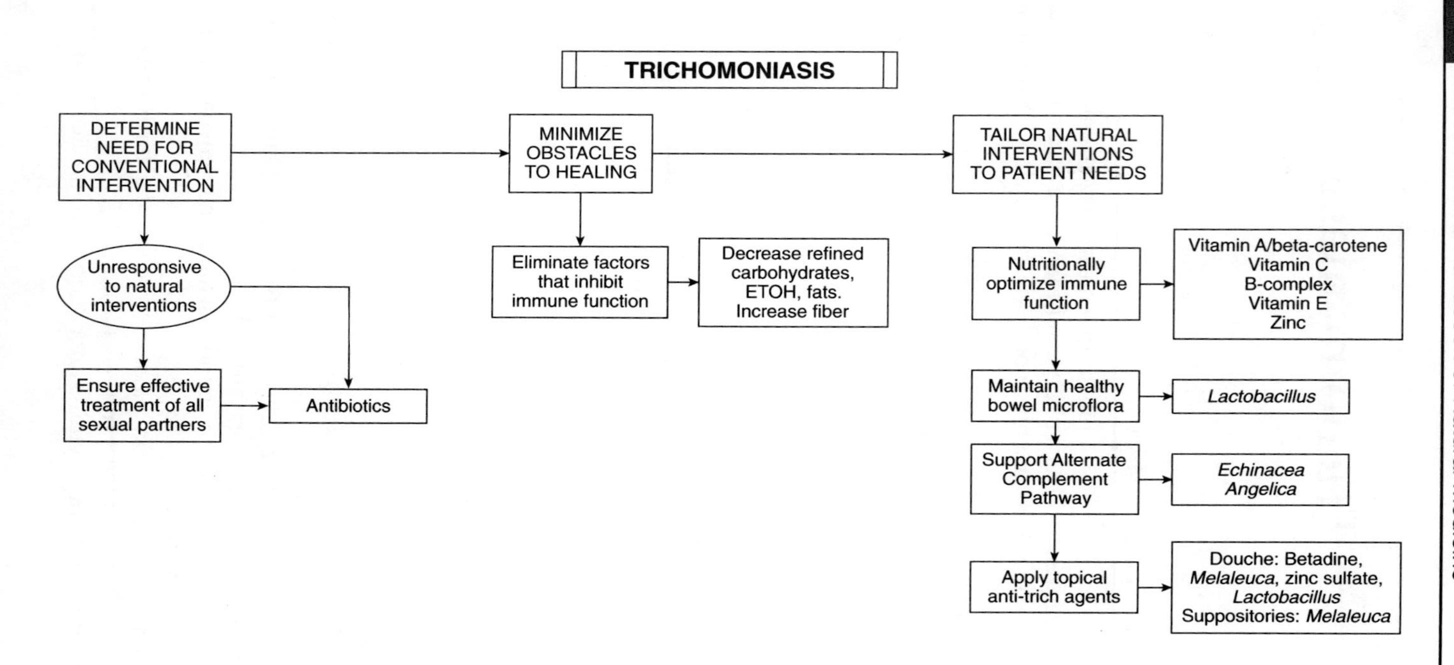

TRICHOMONIASIS
DETERMINE NEED FOR CONVENTIONAL INTERVENTION
Unresponsive to natural interventions
Ensure effective treatment of all sexual partners
Antibiotics
MINIMIZE OBSTACLES TO HEALING
Eliminate factors that inhibit immune function
Decrease refined carbohydrates, ETOH, fats. Increase fiber
TAILOR NATURAL INTERVENTIONS TO PATIENT NEEDS
Nutritionally optimize immune function
Vitamin A/beta-carotene
Vitamin C
B-complex
Vitamin E
Zinc
Maintain healthy bowel microflora
Lactobacillus
Support Alternate Complement Pathway
Echinacea
Angelica
Apply topical anti-trich agents
Douche: Betadine, Melaleuca, zinc sulfate, Lactobacillus
Suppositories: Melaleuca

- Infection may confuse and/or complicate other genitourinary tract problems.
- Metronidazole (Flagyl) (most common anti-trich agent) is carcinogenic and teratogenic in rodents.
- Trich increases HIV transmission and infectivity where HIV seropositive men with concomitant trichomoniasis may have sixfold higher concentration of HIV RNA in seminal plasma.

## DIAGNOSIS

*Trichomonas vaginalis* is a flagellate 15-18 mm long, shaped like a turnip, with three to four anterior and one posterior flagella mounted in undulating membrane. Transmission is through sexual intercourse; men and women are reservoirs. Diagnosis is by signs and symptoms (above), saline wet mount, and culture. Trich cultures (Feinberg *Trichomonas* medium) increase diagnostic sensitivity. Fifty percent of women with *Trichomonas* (defined by positive culture) have the organism identified by microscopic wet mount. Although microscopic wet mount is commonly used and a quick method to identify trich compared with culture, sensitivity of wet mount ranges from only 45%-60%. In men a reliable culture site has not been established, and cultures from urine and seminal samples give low yield. The organism can be cultured from vagina and paraurethral glands in 98%, the urethra in 82%, and endocervix in 13%. In only 56%-65% is *T. vaginalis* seen on Pap smear; thus Pap smear is an unreliable form of diagnosis. DNA-based test called Affirm VP system uses synthetic oligonucleotide probes for detection of *T. vaginalis*, *Gardnerella vaginalis*, and *Candida* spp. from a single vaginal swab, with sensitivity of 92% and specificity of 98% compared with wet mount and sensitivity of 92% and specificity of 99% compared with culture. Newer diagnostics such as polymerase chain reaction (PCR) can increase identification in men and women. Unfortunately, PCR is restricted to research settings because of technical complexity and cost.

### Trichomonal Vaginitis

- Sexual transmission is the route of infection. Prevalence is highest among women with multiple partners and women with other sexually transmitted infections. Transmission rates are high from men to women; an 80%-100% prevalence exists in female partners of infected men.

- In women, *T. vaginalis* infests the vagina and urethra and may involve the endocervix, Bartholin's glands, Skene's glands, and bladder.
  —Vagina is a good reservoir; estrogen causes walls to be glycogenated. Prepubescent and postmenopausal women seldom have trich symptoms.
  —Elevated pH increases susceptibility. Normal adult vaginal pH is 3.5-4.5 because of *Lactobacillus acidophilus* converting free glucose into lactic acid. Decreased lactobacilli increase pH. *Trichomonas* grow optimally at a pH of 5.5-5.8. Other conditions increasing vaginal pH are progesterone (latter half of menstrual cycle and during pregnancy), excess intravaginal secretions (cervical mucus), and bacterial overgrowth (*Streptococcus, Proteus*).

### *Trichomonas* in the Male

Incidence is lower in men, but 5%-15% of nongonococcal urethritis cases are caused by *Trichomonas*. Transmission rate of 70% exists among men having sexual contact with infected women in the previous 48 hours. Trich often is asymptomatic but mild urethritis, prostatitis, and epididymitis are reported. Trich is a factor in male infertility, identified in semen, urethral discharge, and urine in addition to prostatic fluid, prostatic secretions, and semen of 23% of men with chronic non-GC prostatitis. It persists in the male genitourinary tract; reinfection of sexually active treated women is well documented. Sexual partners must be treated. Among both women and men, *T. vaginalis* is linked to enhanced HIV acquisition and transmission.

## THERAPEUTIC CONSIDERATIONS

- **Conventional therapy**: metronidazole and tinidazole, a second-generation nitroimidazole used for metronidazole-resistant infection. Paromomycin is used for difficult cases of nitroimidazole-resistant *T. vaginitis*, but severe local side effects are common. Metronidazole cure rates are >90% dosed at 500 mg b.i.d. for 7 days or as a single 2-g dose. To reduce recurrence, sexual partners should be treated concurrently. Side effects of metronidazole include nausea and vomiting, metallic taste, and gastrointestinal upset. Patients must avoid alcohol during therapy. As a long-term high-dose use for resistant trich, metronidazole rarely causes peripheral neuropathy—<1% in more than 35 years of use.

- **Diet**: affects body defenses. The "fertility of the soil," not the pathogenicity of the microbe, allows trich to flourish. Implement a well-balanced diet high in natural fiber (vegetable, fruits), and low in fat, sugar, and refined carbohydrates.
- **Lifestyle**: depression and anxiety are linked to exacerbations of trich infections. Reduce stress with exercise and meditation. Safe sex or abstinence (while infected) lowers incidence of infection and reinfection. Sixty-six percent of prostitutes not practicing safe sex have trich infection.

## Nutritional Supplements

- **Vitamin E**: doses twofold to tenfold greater than the recommended daily allowance enhance antibody responses, accelerate clearance of particulate matter by reticuloendothelial system, and enhance host resistance. Megadose vitamin E in healthy volunteer inhibits multiple immune functions.
- **Calcium (Ca) and magnesium (Mg)**: bivalent cations regulate external membrane functions of body cells. Ca and Mg ions also help activate complement pathway; *Trichomonas* activate alternate complement pathway (ACP), leading to parasite lysis. Unlike classic complement pathway (requiring both Ca and Mg), ACP requires only Mg.
- **Zinc**: has broad antimicrobial spectrum against genitourinary pathogens: gram-positive and -negative bacteria, *T. vaginalis, Candida albicans, Chlamydia trachomatis,* viruses. Trichomonads are readily killed by Zn at concentration of 0.042% (6.4 mmol/L); Zn concentration in prostatic fluid ranges from 0.015%-0.10% (2.3-15.3 mmol/L), suggesting persistent trichomonal infections in men may be caused by Zn deficiency. Zn sulfate (220 mg b.i.d. for 3 weeks) is a possible treatment for trich infections refractory to metronidazole. For women with drug-resistant trich, Zn douches plus metronidazole may relieve.
- **Iron (Fe)**: deficiency too small to lower hemoglobin values can cause immune dysfunctions. Fe-deficient human beings have defective macrophage and neutrophil functions. Fe excess increases growth of the pathogen.

## Botanical Medicines

*Trichomonas* activates ACP that lyses *T. vaginalis*. Botanicals that activate ACP are *Angelica* spp. and *Echinacea purpurea*. *Angelica* spp.

contain coumarin compounds, which activate both classic and alternate pathways (*Textbook, "Angelica* Species"). Inulin (a constituent of *Echinacea*) activates complement and promotes chemotaxis of neutrophils, monocytes, and eosinophils (*Textbook, "Echinacea* Species [Narrow-Leafed Purple Coneflower]").

### Topical Trichomonacides

- **Betadine (povidone-iodine)**: iodine is a potent trichomonacide. Povidone-iodine (PVP) is a broad-spectrum antimicrobial for vaginal pathogens. PVP (iodine absorbed into polyvinyl pyrrolidone) has advantages over iodine—little sensitizing potential, does not sting, water soluble, washes out of clothing. Success rate is 98.1% in intractable trichomonal, monolial, nonspecific, and mixed vaginitis with 2-week regimen with Betadine preparations. A 28-day course of Betadine pessaries is indicated if patient is using oral contraceptives.
- **Propolis**: ethanol extract of propolis (150 mg/mL) is 100% lethal in vitro on protozoans *T. vaginalis* and *Toxoplasma gondii* after 24 hours of contact. It decreases the inflammation associated with trichomonal vaginitis.
- **Essential oils**: diverse antimicrobial action of essential oils has been demonstrated. Strong antitrichomonal properties, found in *Mentha piperita* (peppermint) and *Lavandula angustifolia* (lavender) have the fastest killing effects (15-20 minutes).
- ***Melaleuca alternifolia* (tea tree) oil**: powerful topical antimicrobial agent (*Textbook, "Melaleuca alternifolia* [Tea Tree]"). A 40% solution is very effective with no irritation, burning, or other side effects. Daily douches (0.4% solution *Melaleuca* oil in 1 L water) also are effective.
- **Berberine botanicals**: contain the plant alkaloid berberine sulphate. They inhibit in vitro several protozoa: *Entamoeba histolytica, Giardia lamblia,* and *T. vaginalis.* No clinical trials have been reported in trichomoniasis (*Textbook, "Hydrastis canadensis* [Goldenseal] and Other Berberine-Containing Botanicals").

## THERAPEUTIC APPROACH

- Given the risk of serious sequelae of trichomoniasis and the high success of pharmaceuticals, systemic metronidazole should be carefully considered as a possible first-line treatment, with simultaneous and subsequent naturopathic therapies to decrease risk of recurrence and treat underlying suspectibilities. Naturopathic therapies may be used as first-line therapy in cases of allergy to metronidazole or pregnancy. But metronidazole does not increase teratogenic risk, according to studies.

- *Trichomonas* is a sexually transmitted disease; treatment of the sexual partner(s) is necessary to prevent reinfection. During treatment, avoid sexual intercourse. Use condom otherwise.
- **Diet**: decrease refined carbohydrates, alcohol, and fats; increase fiber.
- **Nutritional supplements**:
  —Vitamin A: 25,000 IU q.d. (or beta-carotene: 200,000 IU q.d.)
  —Vitamin C: 500-1000 mg q4h
  —Vitamin B complex: 20-50 mg q.d.
  —Zinc (picolinate): 10-15 mg q.d.
  —Vitamin E (mixed tocopherols): 200 IU q.d.
  —*Lactobacillus acidophilus*: 2 caps q.d.
  If effective, *L. acidophilus* changes the quantity and quality of stool. If this change does not occur, check quality of product (*Textbook,* "Probiotics").
- **Botanical medicines (t.i.d.)**:
  —*Hydrastis canadensis*: dried root, 0.5-1.0 g; tincture (1:10), 6-2 mL; fluid extract (1:1), 1-2 mL; solid extract (4:1), 250 mg
  —*Echinacea angustifolia*: dried root, 1-2 g; tincture (1:10), 8-12 mL; fluid extract, 1.5-3.0 mL; solid extract (6.5:1), 250 mg
  —*Angelica* spp.: dried root or rhizome, 1-2 g; tincture (1:5), 3-5 mL; fluid extract (1:1), 0.5-2 mL
- **Topical treatment**:
  —Betadine douche, pessary, or saturated tampon b.i.d. for 14 days
  —*Melaleuca alternifolia* oil (40% solution): swab on affected area b.i.d. or douche, 1 L of a 0.4% solution b.i.d.; suppository, one at night
  —Zn sulfate douche: 1% solution b.i.d.
  —*Lactobacillus* culture yogurt douches daily, preferably in the morning

# Urticaria

## DIAGNOSTIC SUMMARY

- **Urticaria (hives)**: well-circumscribed erythematous wheals with raised serpiginous borders and blanched centers that may coalesce to become giant wheals. Limited to the superficial portion of the dermis.
- **Angioedema**: similar eruptions to urticaria but with larger, well-demarcated edematous areas that involve subcutaneous structures as well as the dermis.
- **Chronic versus acute**: recurrent episodes of urticaria and/or angioedema of less than 6 weeks' duration are considered acute, whereas attacks persisting beyond this period are designated chronic.
- **Special forms**: special forms have characteristic features—dermographism, cholinergic urticaria, solar urticaria, cold urticaria.

Urticaria are experienced by 14%-25% of the general population. Young adults (postadolescence through third decade) are most often affected. At least 40% of patients with idiopathic chronic urticaria have clinically relevant functional autoantibodies to high-affinity immunoglobulin E (IgE) receptor on basophils and mast cells. The term autoimmune urticaria is used for this subgroup of patients presenting with continuous ordinary urticaria.

## PATHOPHYSIOLOGY

Urticaria are named for the stinging nettle plant (*Urtica dioica*), which contains histaminic acid. Mechanism is the release of inflammatory mediators from mast cells or basophilic leukocytes. Mechanisms involve agents other than IgE–anti-IgE complexes. The incidence of IgE-mediated urticaria is probably low compared with nonimmunologic urticaria. Signs and symptoms are consistent despite diverse etiologic and initiating factors, yet pathogenesis is not ascribed to any one mechanism. Mast cells and mast cell–dependent mediators play the most prominent role.

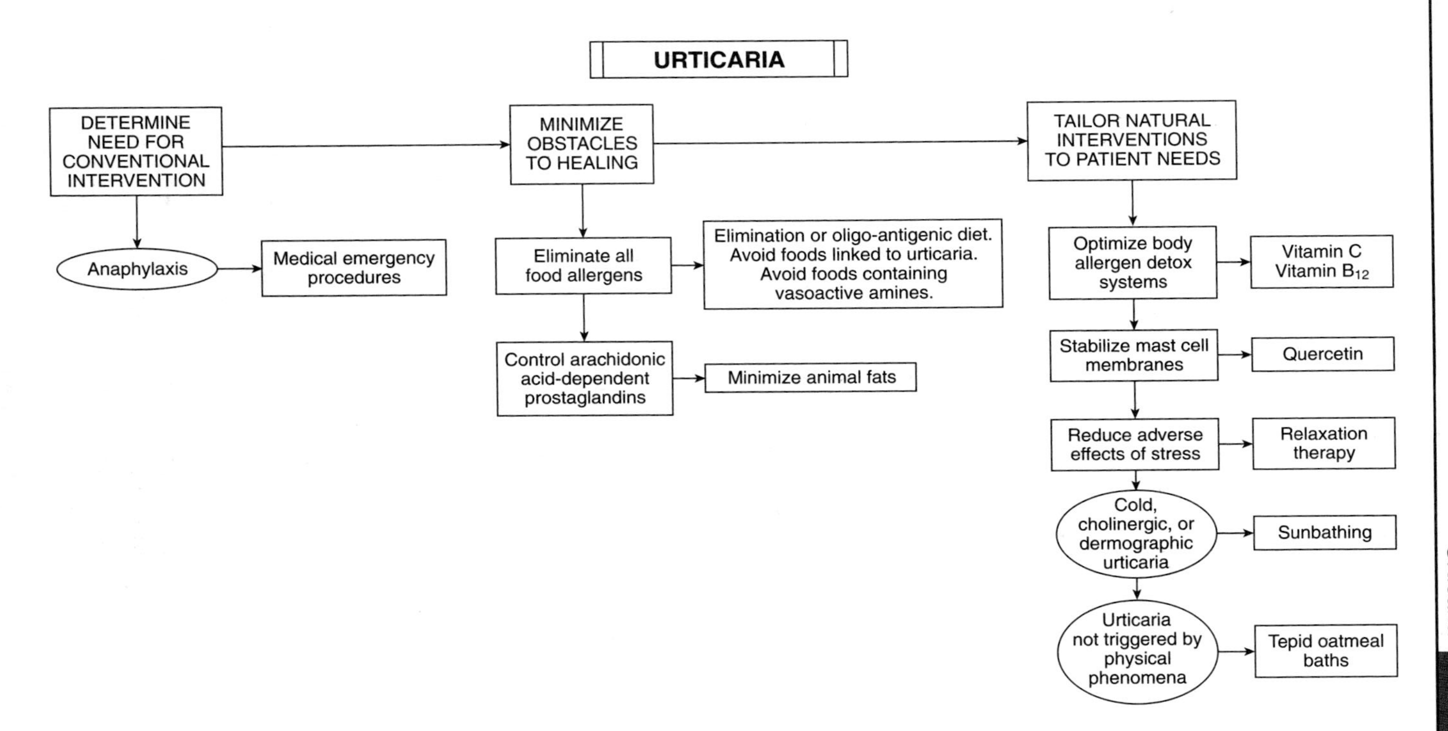
URTICARIA
DETERMINE NEED FOR CONVENTIONAL INTERVENTION
Anaphylaxis
Medical emergency procedures
MINIMIZE OBSTACLES TO HEALING
Eliminate all food allergens
Elimination or oligo-antigenic diet. Avoid foods linked to urticaria. Avoid foods containing vasoactive amines.
Control arachidonic acid-dependent prostaglandins
Minimize animal fats
TAILOR NATURAL INTERVENTIONS TO PATIENT NEEDS
Optimize body allergen detox systems
Vitamin C
Vitamin B12
Stabilize mast cell membranes
Quercetin
Reduce adverse effects of stress
Relaxation therapy
Cold, cholinergic, or dermographic urticaria
Sunbathing
Urticaria not triggered by physical phenomena
Tepid oatmeal baths

- Three distinct sources of mediators:
  - **Preformed mediators**: contained in granules and released immediately
  - **Secondarily formed mediators**: generated immediately or within minutes by interaction of primary mediators and nearby cells and tissues
  - **Granule matrix–derived mediators**: preformed but slowly dissociate from granule after discharge and remain in tissues for hours
- Most common immunologic mechanism is mediated by IgE.
- Early vascular changes arise from mast cells—histamine and end products of arachidonic acid. Wheal and flare occur within minutes of initiation and last 30-60 minutes.
- Prolonged and delayed reactions represent leukocytic infiltration in response to mast cell chemotactic factors. They develop over time—erythema, edema, and induration beginning within 2 hours and lasting 12-24 hours. Leukocyte infiltration may induce second wave of mast cell activation or release toxic lysosomal enzymes and mediators.
- Events triggered by mediators depend on type of mediator and tissues where they are released.

## CAUSES OF URTICARIA

### Physical

Urticaria can result from reactions to physical stimuli. Most common forms of physical urticarias are dermographic, cholinergic, and cold urticarias. Less-common types of physical urticaria or angioedema are contact, solar, pressure, heat contact, aquagenic, vibratory, and exercise induced.

**Dermographism**: defined as readily elicited whealing of skin evolving rapidly after moderate pressure. Simple contact with furniture, garters, bracelets, watch bands, towels, or bedding can cause urticaria. Incidence of dermographism is 1.5%-5%. This is the most frequent physical urticaria. Female/male ratio is 2:1. Average age of onset is in the third decade. Incidence is much greater among obese persons wearing tight clothing.

- **Lesions start within 1-2 minutes of contact**: erythema, replaced within 3-5 minutes by edema and surrounding reflex urticaria. Maximal edema occurs within 10-15 minutes. Erythema regresses within an hour; edema persists up to 3 hours.

- **Associated with other diseases**: parasitosis, insect bites, neuropsychiatric disorders, hormonal changes, thyroid disorders, pregnancy, menopause, diabetes, immunologic alterations, other urticarias, during or after drug therapy, *Candida albicans,* angioedema, hypereosinophilia.
- **Cholinergic urticaria**: heat reflex urticaria is the second most frequent physical urticaria. These lesions involve stimulation of sweat glands by cholinergic afferent fibers. Lesions are pinpoint wheals surrounded by reflex erythema. Wheals arise at or between follicles, preferentially on upper trunk and arms.
- **Three basic types of stimuli**: passive overheating, physical exercise, and emotional stress.
- **Eliciting activities**: physical exercise, warm bath or sauna, eating hot spices, drinking alcohol.
- **Lesions**: arise within 2-10 minutes and last 30-50 minutes.
- **Systemic symptoms**: suggest generalized mast cell release beyond skin—headache, periorbital edema, lacrimation and burning of eyes, nausea and vomiting, abdominal cramps, diarrhea, dizziness, hypotension, and asthmatic attacks.
- **Cold urticaria**: urticarial and/or angioedematous reaction of skin making contact with cold objects, water, or air. Lesions are restricted to area of exposure. Develop within a few seconds to minutes after removal of cold object and rewarming of skin. The colder the object or element, the faster the reaction. Widespread local exposure and generalized urticaria are accompanied by flushing, headache, chills, dizziness, tachycardia, abdominal pain, nausea, vomiting, myalgia, shortness of breath, wheezing, unconsciousness.
  —Cold urticaria accompanies a variety of clinical conditions, including viral infections, parasitic infestations, syphilis, multiple insect bites, penicillin injections, dietary changes, stress. Children with cold urticaria have higher risk of anaphylaxis, especially triggered by swimming.
  —Associated with infectious mononucleosis, cryoglobulinemia, and myeloma, in which cold urticaria may precede diagnosis by several years.

## Autoimmune Urticaria

- A minority of cases of chronic urticaria have an autoimmune basis, involving autoantibodies to IgE or the FcεRIα subunit of high-affinity IgE mast cell receptor. Autoimmune antibodies are found in 24%-76% of patients with chronic urticaria. They have a more severe, prolonged course of disease. Middle-aged women have higher rates of urticaria and autoimmunity, particularly for thyroid disease. Thyroid autoantibodies are found more frequently in patients with IgE-receptor autoantibodies (see thyroid section below).

- Autoimmunity is linked to bowel permeabilities. Subclinical impairments of small bowel red blood cell function may induce higher sensitivity to histamine in the gastrointestinal tract. Naturopathic approach treats overt and subclinical gastrointestinal permeability to decrease systemic inflammatory responses to endotoxins.

## Drugs

- Leading cause of urticaria in adults. In children, attributable to foods, food additives, or infections. Most drugs are small molecules incapable of inducing antigenic or allergenic activity by themselves. Typically they act as haptens binding to endogenous macromolecules, inducing hapten-specific antibodies. Alternatively, they interact directly with mast cells, inducing degranulation. Many drugs produce urticaria, most commonly penicillin and aspirin.
- **Penicillin**: antibiotics are most common cause of drug-induced urticaria. Population rate of allergenicity of penicillin is 10%, with 25% of these displaying urticaria, angioedema, or anaphylaxis. Penicillin cannot be destroyed by boiling or steam distillation and is undetected in foods. Penicillin in milk is more allergenic than in meat; penicillin can be degraded into more allergenic compounds in the presence of carbohydrate and metals.
- **Aspirin (ASA) and nonsteroidal antiinflammatory drugs (NSAIDs)**: Urticaria is a more common indicator of ASA sensitivity than asthma (*Textbook,* "Asthma"). Incidence of ASA sensitivity in patients with chronic urticaria is 20 times greater than normal control subjects. From 2%-67% of patients with chronic urticaria are sensitive to ASA. Aspirin inhibits cyclooxygenase by shunting eicosanoids towards leukotriene synthesis and increasing smooth muscle contraction and vascular permeability. ASA and other NSAIDs increase gut permeability and may alter normal handling of antigens. Dosage of 650 mg ASA q.d. for 3 weeks may desensitize patients and reduce responsiveness to foods that typically cause a reaction. Effect also occurs in patients with asthma but disappears within 9 days after stopping treat-

ment from a loss of effect or possible placebo response. NSAIDs are associated with prolonged and more pronounced autoreactivity in urticaria.

## Food Allergy

IgE-mediated urticaria occurs on ingestion of a specific reaginic antigen. Most common are milk, fish, meat, eggs, beans, and nuts, citrus, kiwis, peanuts, and apples. An atopic patient experiences urticaria triggered by IgE mechanisms, although pseudoallergic reactions can occur in which direct mast cell histamine release is involved. Basic requirement for food allergy is absorption of an allergen through the intestinal mucosa. Aromatic volatile ingredients in tomatoes, wine, and culinary herbs (basil, fenugreek, cumin, dill, ginger, coriander, caraway, curcuma, parsley, pepper, rosemary, and thyme) may be initiating factors in some non-IgE events.

- Factors increasing gut permeability: vasoactive amines in foods or produced by bacterial action on amino acids, alcohol, NSAIDs, and food additives (*Textbook,* "Intestinal Permeability Assessment").
- Food allergies may induce increased gut permeability in urticaria. Gut permeability is linked to autoimmunity. Chronic urticaria are partially related to autoimmune processes (see autoimmune urticaria on p. 739); therefore, depending on genetic susceptibility, bowel permeability may play a key role instigating and prolonging immune activity leading to chronic urticaria.
- Alterations occur in gastric acidity, intestinal motility, and function of the small intestine and biliary tract in 85% of patients with chronic urticaria, including selective IgA deficiency, gastroenteritis, hypochlorhydria, and achlorhydria. These changes may alter barrier and immune function of the gut wall.
- IgG reactions may cause the most adverse food reactions (*Textbook,* "Food Allergy Testing"). IgG antigen–antibody complexes can promote complement activation and anaphylatoxins triggering mast cell degranulation.

## Food Additives

- **Food colorants**: food additives are a major factor in chronic urticaria in children. Colorants (azo dyes), flavorings (salicylates, aspartame), preservatives (benzoates, nitrites, sorbic acid), antioxidants (hydroxytoluene, sulfite, gallate), and emulsifiers and stabilizers (polysorbates, vegetable gums) produce urticaria in sensitive people.

- **Tartrazine (azo dye FD&C yellow #5)**: first food dye reported to induce urticaria. Of the average daily per-capita consumption of certified dyes in the United States (15 mg), 85% is tartrazine. Children consume much more. Tartrazine sensitivity is in 0.1% of the population and 20%-50% in persons sensitive to ASA. Tartrazine is a cyclooxygenase inhibitor and inducer of asthma and urticaria in children. Tartrazine, benzoate, and ASA increase lymphokine leukocyte inhibitory factor, increasing perivascular mast cells and mononuclear cells; 95% of urticaria patients have increased perivascular mast cells and mononuclear cells. Eliminating food dyes from the diet is very beneficial.

## Food Flavorings

- **Salicylates**: Salicylic acid esters are used to flavor foods—cake mixes, puddings, ice cream, chewing gum, and soft drinks. Mechanism of action is similar to ASA. Daily salicylate intake from foods is 10-200 mg; level of salicylate used in clinical testing is 300 mg. Dietary sources are fruit (berries, dried fruits); raisins and prunes have the highest amounts. Also implicated are licorice and peppermint candies. Moderate levels are in nuts and seeds. Salicylate is very high in some herbs and condiments such as curry powder, paprika, thyme, dill, oregano, and turmeric.
- **Other flavoring agents**: cinnamon, vanilla, menthol, and other volatile compounds may produce urticaria. Artificial sweetener aspartame can as well.

## Food Preservatives

- **Benzoates**: benzoic acid and benzoates are the most common food preservatives. Incidence of adverse reactions overall is <1%, but positive challenges in patients with chronic urticaria vary from 4%-44%. Fish and shrimp may have very high levels of benzoates, triggering common adverse reactions to these foods in patients with urticaria.
- **Butylated hydroxytoluene (BHT) and butylated hydroxyanisole**: primary antioxidants in prepared and packaged foods. Fifteen percent of patients with chronic urticaria test positive to oral challenge with BHT.
- **Sulfites**: induce asthma, urticaria, and angioedema in sensitive persons. They are ubiquitous in foods and drugs. They prevent microbial spoilage, browning, and color change. They are sprayed on fresh foods (shrimp, fruits, vegetables) and used as

antioxidants and preservatives in pharmaceuticals. Average per-capita intake is 2-3 mg/day. Wine and beer drinkers ingest up to 10 mg/day. Persons relying on restaurant meals ingest up to 150 mg/day. Enzyme sulfite oxidase metabolizes sulfites to safer sulfates excreted in urine. Those with poorly functioning sulfoxidation system have increased urine sulfite/sulfate ratio. Sulfite oxidase depends on the trace mineral molybdenum.

- **Food emulsifiers and stabilizers**: most foods containing these also contain antioxidants, preservatives, and dyes. Polysorbate in ice cream can induce urticaria. Vegetable gums (e.g., acacia, gum arabic, tragacanth, quince, and carrgeenan) induce urticaria in susceptible individuals.

## Infections

Infections are a major cause of urticaria in children. In adults, immune tolerance occurs to many microbes from repeated exposure.

- **Bacterial infections**: contribute to urticaria in two settings
  —Acute *Streptococcus* tonsillitis in children: acute urticaria predominate
  —Chronic dental infections in adults: chronic urticaria predominate
- **Viruses**: hepatitis B is the most frequent cause of viral-induced urticaria. One study showed 15.3% of patients with chronic urticaria had anti–hepatitis B surface antibodies. Urticaria are also linked to infectious mononucleosis (5%) and may develop several weeks before clinical manifestation.
- ***Candida albicans***: 19%-81% of patients with chronic urticaria react positively to immediate skin test with *Candida* antigens. Sensitivity to *Candida* is an important factor in 25% of patients with chronic urticaria. Seventy percent of patients with a positive skin reaction also react to oral provocation with foods prepared with yeasts. Elimination of organism can cure some individuals with positive skin tests, but more patients responded to a yeast-free diet than to elimination of organism. Yeast-free diet excludes bread, buns, sausage, wine, beer, cider, grapes, sultanas, Marmite, Bovril, vinegar, tomato, catsup, pickles, and prepared foods containing food yeasts. Use diet plus eliminate yeast with nystatin. Desensitizing patients to *Candida* by yeast cell wall extract is helpful in some, but treatment also included increasing gastrointestinal fermentation and acidity plus elimination of yeast.

## THERAPEUTIC CONSIDERATIONS

- **Psychological factors (stress)**: the most frequent primary cause in chronic urticaria. Stress decreases intestinal secretory IgA. Relaxation therapy and hypnosis may be beneficial for some patients.
- **Ultraviolet light therapy**: some benefit in chronic urticaria. Both ultraviolet A and B have been used. Cold, cholinergic, and dermographic urticaria respond most favorably.
- **Thyroid**: association of thyroid disease and autoimmunity with urticaria is well established. Prevalence of antithyroid antibodies in normal population is 3%-6% and is commonly found with other autoimmune conditions (e.g., pernicious anemia and vitiligo). Subset of patients with chronic urticaria is best helped by suppressing glandular inflammation, by thyroid hormone therapy (as described below), surgery, or antithyroid medication.
  —Some patients with presumed idiopathic chronic urticaria and angioedema also have thyroid autoimmunity. L-Thyroxine therapy has induced remission within 4 weeks in some. Thyroid hormone replacement therapy has dramatically improved chronic urticaria in patients with normal thyroid function but also thyroid autoimmunity. Antithyroid antibodies did not correlate with clinical response. Resolution of chronic urticaria associated with thyrotoxicosis has occurred in patients treated with antithyroid medication or radioactive iodine. With a fully diagnosed thyroid condition, do not treat presumptively with suppressive thyroid medication. Utility of thyroid hormone therapy in euthyroid patients with chronic urticaria has not been proven in controlled trials, but looking for thyroid autoimmunity is warranted in cases refractory to other therapies.

## DIAGNOSIS

### Physical Evaluation and History

- **Careful history**: identify all medicines, supplements, and botanicals; travel, recent infection, occupational exposure; timing and onset of lesions; morphology; associated symptoms; family medical history, preexisting allergies.
- **Contact sensitivities**: latex and exposure to physical stimuli.

- **History of tattoos**
- **Diet and lifestyle diary**: date and time foods are eaten, major activities, bowel and urine habits, and stress to characterize temporal relations of urticaria with foods and activities.
- **Comprehensive physical examination**: to uncover clues and comorbidities.

## Laboratory Testing

- No relation exists between numbers of identified diagnoses and numbers of performed tests.
- Systemic diseases (excluding physical urticaria, allergens, infections, and psychologic causes) were identified and believed to be related causally to urticaria in only 1.6% of patients. These diseases included vasculitis, thyroid disease, lupus, other rheumatic disease, hereditary angioedema, and hematologic or oncologic conditions.
- Screening skin testing for food allergies is controversial. Skin testing for foods in patient with chronic urticaria is fraught with false-positive and false-negative results. Without a specific history suggesting a particular food allergen (exposure and time course of subsequent symptoms consistent with food allergy), skin testing can be counterproductive, particularly in patients with dermatographism and "twitchy mast cells."
- If symptoms do not remit after proper history, physical examination, and the following therapies, run complete blood count with differential, urinalysis, erythrocyte sedimentation rate, liver function tests, antinuclear antibody titers, and thyroid panel with antithyroid autoantibodies to ferret out uncommon cases with detectable but unsuspected underlying cause (e.g., infectious and parasitic conditions, rheumatic conditions, thyroid conditions, hematologic conditions).
- Skin biopsy can rule out urticarial vasculitis when suspected. Research labs can focus on autoimmune urticaria and detect anti-FcεRIα autoantibodies, but these tests are not standardized or routinely or widely available.
- Some specialists use autologous serum skin testing; patient's serum is centrifuged and used for skin prick testing in this form of a semiquantitative functional assay for auto-immunity to IgE or IgE receptors bound to cutaneous mast cells. This test is 75% sensitive and 74% specific for presence autoantibodies.

## Supplements

- **Vitamin $B_{12}$**: anecdotal reports indicate value in acute and chronic urticaria. Although serum $B_{12}$ is normal in most patients, additional $B_{12}$ is helpful. When injectable $B_{12}$ is used, placebo effect cannot be ruled out (*Textbook,* "Placebo and the Power to Heal").
- **Quercetin**: in vitro, it is a mast cell stabilizer and inhibitor of many pathways of inflammation (*Textbook,* "Flavonoids—Quercetin, Citrus Flavonoids, and Hydroxyethylrutosides"). Sodium cromoglycate (200-400 mg q.d.) is a compound similar to quercetin, which confers excellent protection against urticaria and angioedema in response to ingested food allergens.

## THERAPEUTIC APPROACH

**Conventional management of chronic urticaria**: patients often respond incompletely to antihistamines and often are uncomfortable and frustrated by chronic pruritus. Some patients respond to systemic steroids, but serious side effects preclude safe long-term use. A wide variety of drugs used singly or in combination testifies to the inability of pharmaceuticals to address and treat symptoms and underlying causes of urticaria fully.

Identify and control all factors that promote a patient's urticarial response. Thorough history is paramount. Acute urticaria are usually self-limiting, especially after eliciting agent is removed or reduced. Chronic urticaria respond to removal of eliciting agent(s). In severe anaphylaxis, emergency measures are imperative.

- **Diet**: elimination or oligoantigenic diet is paramount in chronic urticaria (*Textbook,* "Food Allergy Testing" and "Food Reactions"). Eliminate suspected allergens and all food additives.
  —Strictest elimination diets allow only water, lamb, rice, pears, and vegetables. Avoid foods most commonly linked to urticaria (milk, eggs, chicken, fruits, nuts, additives). Avoid foods containing vasoactive amines, even if no direct allergy to them is noted. Primary foods to eliminate are cured meat, alcohol, cheese, chocolate, citrus fruits, and shellfish.
  —Control arachidonic acid–dependent prostaglandins with a diet low in animal fat.
- **Supplements**
  —Vitamin C: 1 g t.i.d.
  —Vitamin $B_{12}$: 1000 mg IM per week
  —Quercetin: 250 mg 20 minutes before meals

- **Psychological**: relaxation techniques daily, including audiotaped relaxation programs.

## Physical Medicine

- Daily sunbathing for 15-20 minutes or ultraviolet A solarium, especially in chronic physical urticaria.
- Tepid oatmeal baths.
- CAUTION: with physical modalities when symptoms have physical triggers such as heat, cold, or water.

# Uterine Fibroids

## DIAGNOSTIC SUMMARY

- Majority are asymptomatic.
- When symptomatic: vague feeling of discomfort, pressure, congestion, bloating, heaviness; pain with vaginal sexual activity, urinary frequency, backache, abdominal enlargement, and abnormal bleeding.
- Abnormal bleeding occurs in 30% of women with fibroids.
- Fibroids can degenerate with necrosis, resulting in cystic degeneration.
- Calcification can occur.
- Examination by pelvic palpation and/or pelvic ultrasound.
- Main diagnostic consideration: differentiating fibroid from ovarian malignant tumor, abscess in fallopian tube/ovarian region, diverticulum of colon, pelvic kidney, endometriosis, adenomyosis, congenital anomalies, or uterine sarcoma.

## GENERAL CONSIDERATIONS

- Uterine fibroids consist of smooth muscle cells and connective tissue. Growth is stimulated by estrogen. They arise during reproductive years, grow during pregnancy, and regress after menopause. Growth spurt can happen in perimenopausal years—anovulatory cycles with irregular relative estrogen excess.
- Incidence is 20%-25% of women by age 40 years; >50% of women overall; African-American women have higher incidence. Fibroids are the most common indication for major surgery in women and the most common solid tumor in women.
- Cause is poorly understood. Factors include increased local estradiol concentration within fibroid itself, higher estrogen receptor density in fibroid tissue than in surrounding myometrium but lower than endometrium.
- From 50%-80% of fibroids are asymptomatic. Abnormal bleeding occurs in 30% of women with fibroids (menorrhagia and

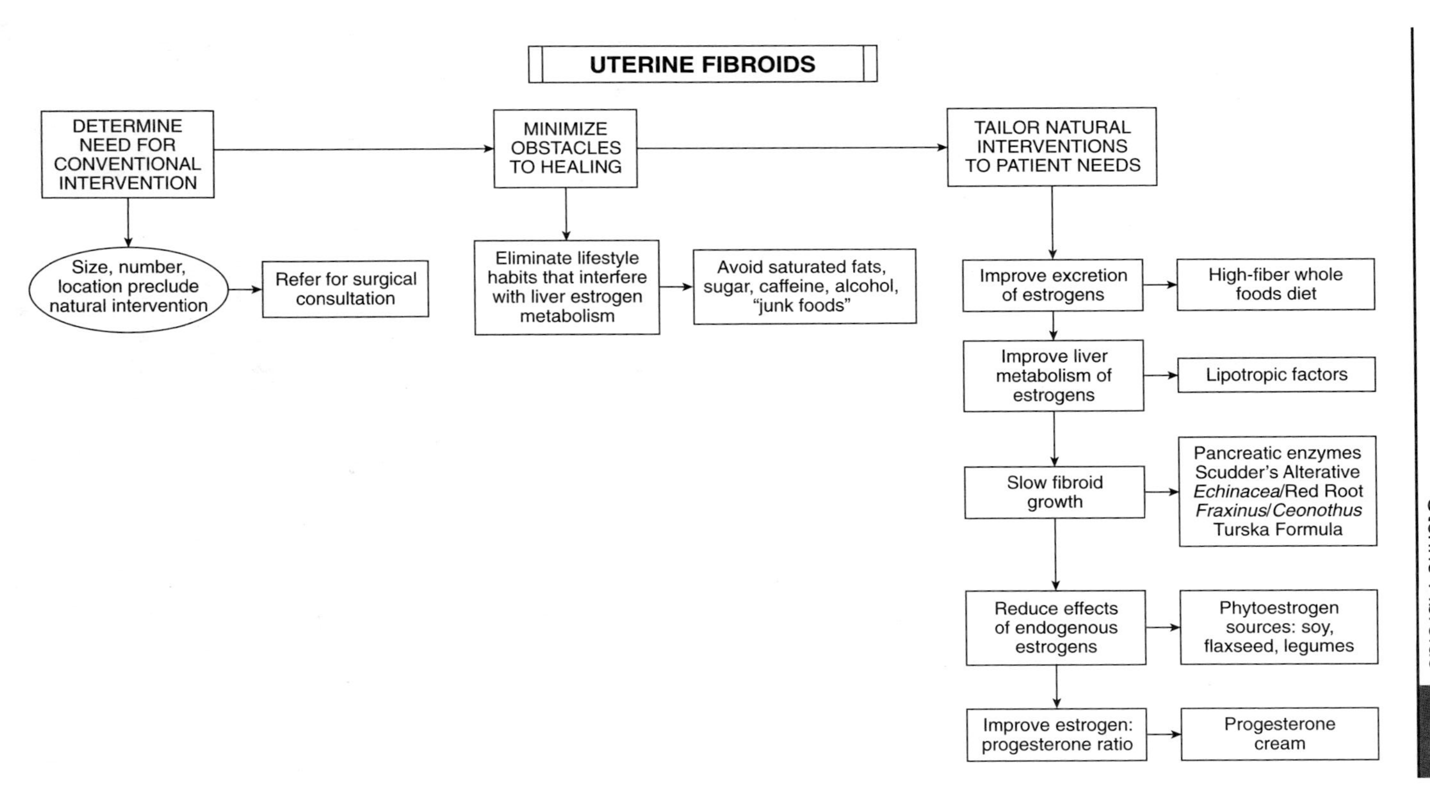
UTERINE FIBROIDS
DETERMINE NEED FOR CONVENTIONAL INTERVENTION
Size, number, location preclude natural intervention
Refer for surgical consultation
MINIMIZE OBSTACLES TO HEALING
Eliminate lifestyle habits that interfere with liver estrogen metabolism
Avoid saturated fats, sugar, caffeine, alcohol, "junk foods"
TAILOR NATURAL INTERVENTIONS TO PATIENT NEEDS
Improve excretion of estrogens
High-fiber whole foods diet
Improve liver metabolism of estrogens
Lipotropic factors
Slow fibroid growth
Pancreatic enzymes
Scudder's Alterative
Echinacea/Red Root
Fraxinus/Ceonothus
Turska Formula
Reduce effects of endogenous estrogens
Phytoestrogen sources: soy, flaxseed, legumes
Improve estrogen: progesterone ratio
Progesterone cream

metrorrhagia). Hydronephrosis can occur from compression of ureter. Fibroids cause of 2%-10% of infertility cases. Large fibroids can interfere with pregnancy by interfering with fetal growth and being associated with premature rupture of membranes, retained placenta, postpartum hemorrhage, abnormal labor, or abnormal lie of fetus. Incidence of miscarriage from fibroids is two to three times greater than normal.
- Degenerative changes: fibroid outgrows blood supply; cellular detail is lost from decreased vascularity of tumor. Necrosis results in cystic degeneration. Calcification can occur over time, especially in postmenopausal women.

## DIAGNOSIS

- Based on mitotic count, nuclear atypia, and other morphologic features, uterine smooth muscle tumors can be classified as leiomyomas, smooth muscle tumors of uncertain malignant potential, and leiomyosarcomas.
- Presumptive diagnosis of fibroids: thorough history and pelvic exam. Palpation findings: enlarged, firm uterus or uterus with irregular edges.
- Differentiate possible fibroid from ovarian malignant tumor, fallopian tube or ovarian region abscess, diverticulum, pelvic kidney, endometriosis, congenital anomaly, pelvic adhesions, or rare retroperitoneal tumors. Not all of these can be distinguished by medical history, physical examination, and pelvic ultrasound. Submucosal pedunculated fibroids can be visualized with laparoscopy. Laparoscopy can visualize intramural and subserous fibroids.
- Uterine fibroids are classified by location: submucosal (just under endometrium), intramural (within uterine muscle wall), subserosal (from outer wall of uterus), interligamentous (in cervix between the two layers of broad ligament), and pedunculated (on stalk either submucous or subserous).

## THERAPEUTIC CONSIDERATIONS

Natural therapies manage troublesome symptoms. No reliable alternative to surgery shrinks fibroids. Natural therapies help keep fibroid from growing larger and usually resolve or improve most symptoms. Do not expect size reduction despite individual case reports. Fibroids shrink as a result of the drop in estrogen after menopause.

## Diet

- Natural therapies work best in context of healthy lifestyle and diet. These changes can decrease heavy bleeding or pain and discomfort.
- Liver metabolizes estradiol for elimination by converting it to estrone, then to estriol, a weaker estrogen with little influence on the uterus.
- Saturated fats, sugar, caffeine, alcohol and junk foods are problematic because they interfere with metabolism of estradiol to estrone to estriol and are deficient in B vitamins or interfere with B-vitamin metabolism. B vitamins facilitate metabolic processes and help regulate estrogen levels.
- Whole grains are excellent sources of B vitamins and help excrete estrogens through the bowel. Vegetarian women who eat a high-fiber, low-fat diet have lower blood estrogen than omnivores with low-fiber diets. Fiber may prevent and perhaps reduce fibroids by reducing estrogen influence on uterine tissue.
- High-fiber diet may relieve bloating and congestion. Bulking stool and regulating bowel movements may improve bloating.
- Uterine fibroids are linked to a fourfold increased risk of endometrial cancer. Three dietary imperatives are to increase fiber, lower dietary fat, and increase soy products and other legumes. Higher fat intake is linked to increased risk for endometrial cancer, higher fiber intake reduces risk for endometrial cancer, and higher soy and legume intake decreases risk of endometrial cancer.
- Increase intake of other sources of phytoestrogens (whole grains, vegetables, fruits, seaweeds).
- Soy phytoestrogens do not have estrogenic effect on uterus. They are selective of tissues estrogenically affected. In the uterus, soy isoflavones have antiestrogen effect.

## Nutritional Supplements

Supplement recommendations are based on tradition, theory, logic, and clinical experiences rather than scientific evidence of clinical trials.

- **Lipotropic factors**: inositol and choline exert lipotropic effect, promoting removal of fat from the liver. Lipotropics combine vitamins, herbals, and animal liver extract to support liver function in metabolizing and excreting estrogens.

- **Pancreatic enzymes**: treat pancreatic insufficiency with symptoms of abdominal bloating, gas, indigestion, undigested food in stool, and malabsorption. Pancreatic enzymes help digest fibrous and smooth muscle tissue and dissolve fibroids. Supplement must be taken between meals rather than with meals when used for this purpose.

## Botanical Medicines

### Traditional Herbs

Attempt to reduce uterine fibroids or slow their growth as prescribed based on anecdotal reports of modest success reducing size and number of fibroids.

- **Scudder's alterative**
  —*Dicentra canadensis* (corydalis tubers)
  —*Alnus serrulate* (black alder bark)
  —*Podophyllum peltatum* (mayapple root)
  —*Scrophularia nodosa* (figwort flowering herb)
  —*Rumex crispus* (Yellow dock root)
  —30-40 drops to a small amount of warm water t.i.d.
- **Compounded *Echinacea*/red root**
  —*Echinacea* spp.
  —*Ceanothus americanus* (red root)
  —*Baptisia tinctoria* (Baptisia root)
  —*Thuja occidentalis* (thuja leaf)
  —*Stillingia sylvatica* (stillingia root)
  —*Iris versicolor* (blue flag root)
  —*Zanthoxylum clava-herculis* (prickly ash bark)
- **Compounded *Fraxinus*/*Ceanothus***
  —*Fraxinus americanus* (mountain ash bark)
  —*Ceanothus americanus* (red root)
  —*Senecio aureus* (life root)
  —*Podophyllum peltatum* (mayapple root)
  —*Chamaelirium luteum* (helonias root)
  —*Hydrastis canadensis* (goldenseal root)
  —*Lobelia inflate* (lobelia)
  —*Zingiber officinalis* (ginger root)
- **Compounded *Gelsemium*/*Phytolacca* (Turska's formula)**
  —*Gelsemium sempervirens* (*Gelsemium* root)
  —*Phytolacca americana* (poke root)
  —*Aconitum napellus* (aconite)
  —*Bryonia dioica* (bryonia root)

- Other herbal extracts to consider:
  —*Vitex agnus-castus* (chaste tree)
  —*Urtica dioica* (nettles)
  —*Arctium lappa* (burdock root)
  —*Taraxacum officinalis* (dandelion root)
  —*Berberis aquifolium* (Oregon grape)

### Topical Applications

- **Poke root oil**: rub on belly over uterus nightly before bed
- **Castor oil packs**: apply over pelvis three to five times per week

### Herbal Phytoestrogens

- Three types of phytoestrogens are found in medicinal plants: resorcylic acid lactones, steroids and sterols, and phenolics.
  —**Resorcylic acid lactones**: not true phytoestrogens because they are from plant mold contamination.
  —**Steroids**: classic steroidal estrogens estradiol and estrone are found in very minute amounts in apple seed, date palm and pomegranate—1 to 10 parts per billion. Diosgenin is a steroid derivative found in 20 plants (e.g., wild yam species). Beta-sitosterol is the most common phytosterol; found in plant oils such as wheat germ oil, cottonseed oil, and soybean oil. Beta-sitosterol is the dominant phytosterol in garlic and onions. Herbal sources include licorice root, saw palmetto, and red clover. Stigmasterol is related to beta-sitosterol. Soybean oil is a source of stigmasterol and a better source for lab synthesis of progesterone than is beta-sitosterol. Herbal sources include burdock, fennel, licorice, alfalfa, anise, and sage.
  —**Phenolic phytoestrogens**: are flavonoids. Phenolics include isoflavones, which are highest in legumes, especially soybeans. Coumestans have one estrogenic member, coumestrol, which is six times more estrogenic than isoflavones. Lignans are high in grains and highest in flaxseed.
- Phytoestrogens reduce incidence of uterine cancer.
- Red clover contains the highest concentrations of phytoestrogens. Both coumestans and isoflavones change typical stimulation with steroidal hormones (e.g., estradiol) in all target organs. Coumestrol temporarily enhances uptake of estradiol by the

uterus and vagina but inhibits uptake of estradiol by the uterus long term by competing with estradiol for receptor sites.
- Estrogenic effect of phytoestrogens is dose dependent. Given in high enough doses, they have estrogenic effects on all the same target tissues of estradiol.
- Soy phytoestrogens are not estrogen stimuli for endometrium; they are estrogen antagonists associated with low rates of endometrial cancer in countries where soy phytoestrogen intake is high.
- *Tripterygium wilfordii* Hook f.: traditional Chinese herbal therapy for uterine fibroids. A clinical study showed that treatment was effective and time dependent; 28% responded in 3-4 months and 52% in 5-6 months. Therapy induced an increase in luteinizing hormone and follicle-stimulating hormone and a decrease in estradiol and progesterone. Treatment effect may be caused by a reversible inhibitory effect on the ovary.

## Natural Progesterone

- Progesterone may inhibit growth of uterine fibroids. Progesterone administered to guinea pigs prevents formation of tumors induced by estrogen. Clinically diagnosed uterine fibroids have regressed after progesterone therapy.
- Dr. John Lee: Many women in their mid-30s have nonovulating cycles, producing less progesterone but normal (or more) estrogen. Indications of estrogen dominance and progesterone deficiency: retention of water and salt, fibrocystic swollen breast tissue, weight gain (hips and torso), depression, decreased libido, bone mineral loss, and fibroids. Natural progesterone replacement causes fibroid growth to cease (generally decrease in size) until menopause, after which they atrophy.
- Preferred form of natural progesterone for treating fibroids (unless heavy bleeding is present): topical cream with 400 mg progesterone per ounce. Apply ¼ tsp q.d. or b.i.d. for 1 week after menses, and ¼ to ½ tsp b.i.d. for next 2 weeks (second half of cycle). Progesterone cream is not used for 1 week during menstrual flow. Apply cream to inner arms, chest, inner thighs, and/or palms.
- Dr. Mitchell Rein: no evidence shows that estrogen directly stimulates myoma growth, but progesterone and progestins promote fibroids. Development and growth of myomas involves multistep chain of events.

## THERAPEUTIC APPROACH

Diet: High fiber, low fat, whole grains, high flaxseeds and soy foods; avoid saturated fats, sugar, caffeine, alcohol.

### Nutritional Supplements

- **Lipotropic factors**: 1-4 tablets q.d. with meals
- **Pancreatic enzymes**: 2-4 capsules t.i.d. between meals
- **Scudder's alterative**: 30-40 drops in small amount of warm water t.i.d.

### Herbal Medicines

- ***Echinacea*/red root compound**: 30 drops in small amount of warm water t.i.d.
- ***Fraxinus/Ceanothus* compound**: 30 drops in small amount of warm water t.i.d.
- **Turska's formula**: 5 drops in small amount of warm water t.i.d.

### Topical

- Natural progesterone cream: ¼ tsp b.i.d. from day 15 to day 26

Consider surgical options based on size, number, and location of fibroids.

- Myomectomy
- Laparoscopic surgery for subserous and subserous pedunculated fibroids
- Uterine embolization
- Hysteroscopic resection
- Supracervical hysterectomy
- Laparoscopic assisted vaginal hysterectomy

# Vaginitis and Vulvovaginitis

## DIAGNOSTIC SUMMARY

- Increased volume of vaginal secretions.
- Abnormal color, consistency, or odor of vaginal secretions.
- Vulvovaginal itching, burning, or irritation.
- Introitus may show patchy erythema, and vaginal mucosa may exhibit congestion or petechiae.
- Dysuria or dyspareunia may be present.

## GENERAL CONSIDERATIONS

Vaginitis is a common female complaint, accounting for 7% of all visits to gynecologists and being the most common gynecologic problem encountered by primary care providers for women. Seventy-two percent of young, sexually active women have one or more forms of vulvovaginitis. Vaginal infections are six times more common than urinary tract infections (UTI); dysuria is more likely caused by vaginitis than a UTI. Most women can distinguish "internal" dysuria of UTI from "external" dysuria felt when urine passes over inflamed labial tissues; question patients with dysuria more specifically about symptoms of vaginal discharge or irritation. Medical importance of vaginitis is as follows:

- Symptoms could overlie serious problem (e.g., chronic cervicitis or sexually transmitted disease). If infectious, agent may ascend the genital tract, leading to endometritis, salpingitis, and pelvic inflammatory disease (PID), leading to tubal scarring, infertility, or ectopic pregnancies.
- Implicated in recurrent UTIs by acting as reservoir of infectious agents.
- Some vaginal infections during pregnancy increase the risk of miscarriage and, if present at delivery, cause neonatal infections.
- Some forms of vaginitis are linked to cervical cellular abnormalities and increased risk of cervical dysplasia.

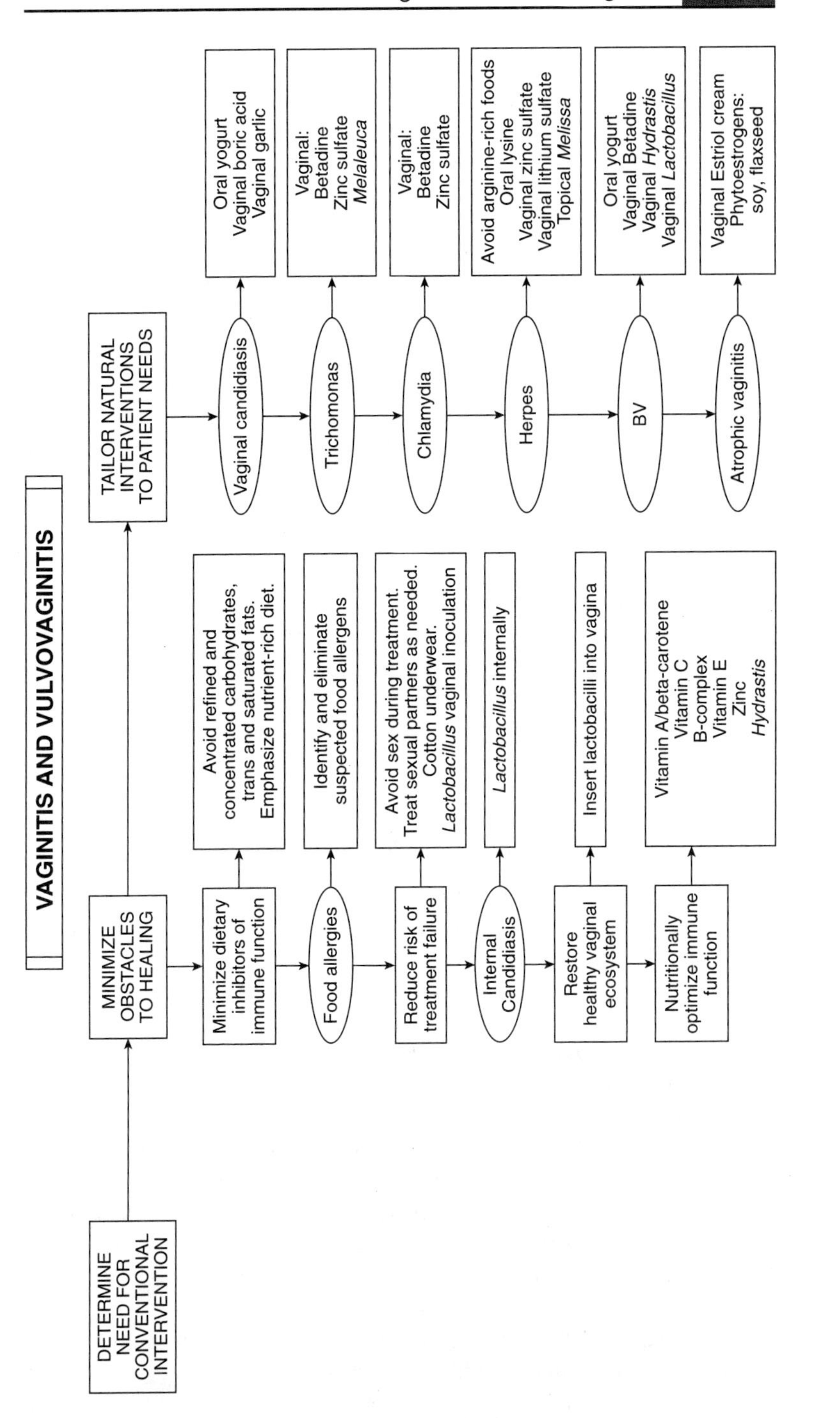
VAGINITIS AND VULVOVAGINITIS
DETERMINE NEED FOR CONVENTIONAL INTERVENTION
MINIMIZE OBSTACLES TO HEALING
TAILOR NATURAL INTERVENTIONS TO PATIENT NEEDS
Minimize dietary inhibitors of immune function
Avoid refined and concentrated carbohydrates, trans and saturated fats. Emphasize nutrient-rich diet.
Food allergies
Identify and eliminate suspected food allergens
Reduce risk of treatment failure
Avoid sex during treatment. Treat sexual partners as needed. Cotton underwear. *Lactobacillus* vaginal inoculation
Internal Candidiasis
*Lactobacillus* internally
Restore healthy vaginal ecosystem
Insert lactobacilli into vagina
Nutritionally optimize immune function
Vitamin A/beta-carotene
Vitamin C
B-complex
Vitamin E
Zinc
*Hydrastis*
Vaginal candidiasis
Oral yogurt
Vaginal boric acid
Vaginal garlic
Trichomonas
Vaginal:
Betadine
Zinc sulfate
*Melaleuca*
Chlamydia
Vaginal:
Betadine
Zinc sulfate
Herpes
Avoid arginine-rich foods
Oral lysine
Vaginal zinc sulfate
Vaginal lithium sulfate
Topical *Melissa*
BV
Oral yogurt
Vaginal Betadine
Vaginal *Hydrastis*
Vaginal *Lactobacillus*
Atrophic vaginitis
Vaginal Estriol cream
Phytoestrogens:
soy, flaxseed

Vaginal ecosystem is governed by the relations of normal endogenous microflora, metabolic products of microflora and host, estrogen, and pH. Normal microflora include *Candida, Lactobacillus* spp., gram-negative aerobic bacteria, facultative bacteria (*Mycoplasma* spp. and *Gardnerella vaginalis*), and obligate anaerobic bacteria (*Prevotella, Peptostreptococcus* spp., *Eubacterium* spp., *Mobiluncus*). *Lactobacillus* dominate a healthy vagina: *Lactobacillus plantarum, Lactobacillus fermentum, Lactobacillus acidophilus*. Other species of *Lactobacillus* may be more significant because of the production of $H_2O_2$: *Lactobacillus rhamnosus, Lactobacillus casei, Lactobacillus bulgaricus*. $H_2O_2$ and lactic acid from *Lactobacillus* maintain acidic environment of vagina.

## TYPES OF VAGINITIS

Hormonal, irritant, and infectious; each is divided into subgroups based on etiology.

- **Hormonal vaginitis**
  - —**Atrophic vaginitis**: affects perimenopausal and postmenopausal women. The structure and function of vaginal tissues undergo change with declining estrogenic stimulation, including estrogen loss after oophorectomy. Vaginal epithelium atrophies from a lack of estrogenic stimulation; this may cause a decrease in *Lactobacillus* in the vagina, more alkaline pH, vaginal thinning, less lubrication, more easily irritated and inflamed tissue, adhesions, dyspareunia, and increased susceptibility to infection. Most common symptoms are itching or burning and thin, watery discharge, occasionally blood tinged (any vaginal bleeding in postmenopausal women requires complete workup to rule out endometrial hyperplasia and endometrial carcinoma; see baseline evaluation in the chapter on menopause).
  - —**Increased vaginal discharge**: increased normal secretions in the absence of other symptoms. Diagnosis of physiologic vaginitis often is applied but is inappropriate because no inflammation exists. Increased discharge often reflects increased hormonal stimulation (pregnancy or some stages of menstrual cycle). This is primarily a diagnosis of exclusion after ruling out other causes. Usually no further treatment is required other than reassurance. Overly zealous douching or washing briefly alleviates symptoms but may aggravate the condition by causing irritant vaginitis.

- **Irritant vaginitis**
  - —Caused by physical or chemical agents damaging delicate vaginal membranes. Identified by careful history and examination.
  - —**Chemical vaginitis**: medications or hygiene products can irritate vaginal mucosa. Allergic vaginitis is damage elicited by immunologic reaction to a product rather than direct toxic reaction. Perfumed toilet paper, douches, spermicides, condoms, and lubricants can be irritating agents.
  - —**Traumatic vaginitis**: injury caused by physical agents or sexual activity.
  - —**Foreign body vaginitis**: foul discharge may indicate foreign body in vagina. Most common are forgotten tampons, contraceptive devices, and pessaries. Very young girls and adolescents may leave foreign bodies in their vaginas from exploring their bodies; they either forget or are too embarrassed to tell someone that they cannot retrieve the item. Also, semen may be an irritant in some women.
- **Infectious vaginitis**
  - —Ninety percent of vaginitis in reproductive-aged women is caused by bacterial vaginosis (BV), candidiasis, or trichomoniasis. BV is most common. Less-common causes include herpes simplex virus, gonorrhea (GC), and chlamydia. Infections of the vulva can cause local itching and/or discharge: folliculitis, hydradenitis, scabies, condyloma, herpes, syphilis, candida. Rare conditions of vulva causing itching and/or discharge include chancroid, lymphogranuloma venereum inguinale, and molluscum contagiosum.
  - —May be sexually transmitted or a result of a disturbance of the delicate ecosystem of the healthy vagina. It often involves common organisms found in the cervix and vagina of healthy, asymptomatic women.
  - —Unifying factor in pathogenesis of pelvic infections is not which microbes are present, but rather the cause of patient susceptibility.
  - —Factors influencing vaginal environment are pH, glycogen content, glucose level, presence of other microbes (lactobacilli), natural flushing action of vaginal secretions, presence of blood, and presence of antibodies and other compounds in vaginal secretions; all are affected by a woman's internal milieu and general health.

—Immune dysfunction predisposes increased vaginal infections: nutritional deficiencies, medicines (e.g., steroids), pregnancy, or serious illness.
—Other predisposing factors are diabetes mellitus, hypothyroidism, leukemia, Addison's disease, Cushing's syndrome, pregnancy, and *Candida* infections.
—Predisposing factors for sexually transmitted disease: increased number of sexual partners, unusual sexual practices, type of birth control (barriers reduce risk), unsafe sex, birth control pills, steroids, antibiotics, tight-fitting garments, occlusive materials, douches, chlorinated pools, perfumed toilet paper, and decrease in *Lactobacillus* in vagina.

- ***Trichomonas vaginalis***: flagellated protozoan found in the lower genitourinary tract of men and women. Human beings are the only host. Sexual intercourse is the primary mode of dissemination. *Trichomonas* do not invade tissues and rarely cause serious complications.
  —Most frequent symptoms are leukorrhea, itching, and burning. Discharge is malodorous, greenish yellow, and frothy.
  —"Strawberry cervix" with punctate hemorrhages is found only in a small percentage of *Trichomonas* cases.
  —Grows optimally at pH = of 5.5-5.8. Conditions elevating pH (e.g., increased progesterone) favor *Trichomonas* growth. Vaginal pH of 4.5 in women with vaginitis suggests agent other than *Trichomonas*.
  —Saline wet mount of fresh vaginal fluid shows small motile organisms, confirming diagnosis in 80%-90% of symptomatic carriers.
- ***Candida albicans***: 2.5-fold increase in candidal vaginitis has occurred in the past 20 years, paralleling the declining incidence of GC and *Trichomonas*. Contributing factors are increased use of antibiotics, which changes the vaginal ecosystem to favor *Candida*.
  —One hundred percent correlation between genital and gastrointestinal *Candida* cultures: significant intestinal colonization with *Candida* may be the single most significant predisposing factor in vulvovaginal candidiasis. However, this has not been confirmed by adequate research. Steroids, oral contraceptives, and diabetes mellitus contribute. Candidiasis is 10-20 times more frequent during pregnancy

because of elevated vaginal pH, increased vaginal epithelial glycogen, elevated blood glucose, and intermittent glycosuria.

—Candidiasis is three times more prevalent in women wearing pantyhose than in those wearing cotton underwear; pantyhose prevents drying of area.

—Four or more episodes of vulvovaginal candidiasis in 1 year classify the patient as having recurrent disease. Cause may be non-*albicans* strains of *Candida*—resistant strains generated by antifungals. Three main theories of why women get recurring yeast vaginitis: (1) intestinal reservoir migrating into vagina, (2) sexual partner is source of recurrence, and (3) vaginal relapse forms small residual numbers of yeast after treatment. Research supports this last theory. Women with recurrent infections have an abnormal immune response, increasing susceptibility.

—Allergies can cause recurrent candidiasis, which resolves after allergies treated.

—Primary symptom of candidiasis is vulvar itching (sometimes severe). Burning of vulva, exacerbated by urination or vaginal sexual activity, also occurs. Thick, curdy or "cottage cheese" discharge that adheres to vaginal walls may be present. Such discharge is strong evidence of yeast infection, but its absence does not rule out *Candida*. Less than 20% of symptomatic candidiasis displays classic thrush patches. In addition, an increase or change in the consistency of the vaginal discharge is common.

—Other clues include erythema of vulva and excoriations from scratching. Vaginal pH is not usually altered.

—Neither the character of discharge nor the symptoms are sufficient alone for diagnosis of *Candida*. Wet mount in saline or 10% KOH; mycelia are confirmatory. Budding forms of yeast are found in normal and symptomatic vaginas, but mycelial stage is only found in symptomatic women.

- **Nonspecific vaginitis (NSV)**: vaginitis not caused by *Trichomonas*, GC, or *Candida*.
- **Bacterial vaginosis (BV)**: shift in flora predominance from lactobacilli to anaerobes and facultative bacteria that degrade mucins of natural gel barrier on vaginal epithelium, causing characteristic vaginal discharge. Destruction of mucins exposes cervical epithelium and allows other organisms to affect cervix, resulting in appearance of clue cells. Epithelial surface disruption causes

immunologic shifts: upregulation of interleukin-1-beta and decrease in protectant molecules (e.g., secretory leukocyte protease inhibitor).

—Three factors shift dominance from lactobacilli to anaerobes and facultative bacteria: sexual activity, douching, and absence of peroxide-producing lactobacilli. A new sexual partner or frequent sexual activity increases incidence of BV. Routine douching is linked to loss of vaginal lactobacilli and occurrence of BV. Women who regularly douche for hygiene purposes have BV twice as often as women who do not routinely douche. Women lacking vaginal peroxide–producing lactobacilli may not have had normal lactobacilli at menarche, or lactobacilli were eliminated by broad-spectrum antibiotics.

—Other factors increasing risk for BV: cigarette smoking suppresses immune response. Racial background: Hispanic women have a 50% greater risk and African-American women have twice the risk. African-American women practice douching twice as often as white women; African-American women also are less likely to have vaginal lactobacilli.

—Examination for BV: medical history; observe discharge to determine vaginal pH. Symptomatic BV releases fishy odor. Discharge is thin, dark, or dull grey. Itching is uncommon in BV unless discharge is profuse. Perform whiff test and wet mount to detect clue cells and observe vaginal flora. Abundance of various bacteria and absence or decrease of lactobacilli suggests BV. Numbers of bacteria increase from 100-fold to 1000-fold. Diagnosis of BV requires three of four criteria:
  1. Thin, dark, or dull grey, homogeneous, malodorous discharge that adheres to vaginal walls
  2. pH >4.5
  3. Positive KOH (whiff/amine test)
  4. Clue cells on wet mount microscopic exam.

  pH is elevated to 5.0-5.5; correlation exists between elevated pH and presence of odor.

—Patient having four or more BV episodes per year (recurrent BV) has an underlying problem—the inability to reestablish normal lactobacilli vaginal ecosystem. Thirty percent of women have recurrence of symptomatic BV within 1 to 3 months; 70% have recurrence within 9 months. Whether this is a relapse or reinfection is unclear. One possibility includes chronic underlying abnormal vaginal ecosystem, sometimes asymptomatic, sometimes symptomatic. Asymptomatic women lacking lactobacilli have a four times greater risk for BV. No proven treatment benefit exists for asymptomatic women.

- Other potential consequences of altered vaginal flora:
  —Increased susceptibility to HIV and GC. PID is linked to BV. Organisms in pregnant women with BV can ascend the genital tract, causing preterm delivery and postpartum endometritis. BV increases risk for infection after gynecologic surgery.
  —*Neisseria gonorrhea*: an uncommon cause of vaginitis, responsible for <4% of cases. GC vaginitis is more common in young girls because the vaginal epithelium is thinner prepubertally.
  —Mucopurulent cervicitis is a primary symptom. Spread of infection causes urethritis, bartholinitis, or salpingitis.
  —GC, alone or with other microbes, is cultured in 40%-60% of PID cases, a major cause of infertility.
  —Eighty percent of GC infections in women are asymptomatic; therefore GC cultures are imperative. Culture and microscopically examine any purulent discharge from the cervical os. Three or more polymorphonuclear leukocytes with gram-negative intracellular diplococci per high-power field are highly suggestive of GC, with a less than 2% false-positive rate.
- **Herpes simplex**: most common cause of genital ulcers in the United States. Other causes to be ruled out are syphilis, chancroid, lymphogranuloma venereum, and granuloma inguinale (see the chapter on herpes simplex).
- ***Chlamydia trachomatis***: an obligate intracellular parasite rarely causing vaginitis but frequently found with other common etiologic agents. It infects 5%-10% of women.
  —Usually asymptomatic until complications appear: cervicitis, salpingitis, or urethritis.
  —Organism is most frequently recovered from patients with PID. Tubal scarring is more frequent after *Chlamydia* infection than after GC; *Chlamydia* is a more important cause of infertility and ectopic pregnancy.
  —Infection during pregnancy increases risk of prematurity and neonatal death. There is a 50% chance that a healthy, term

infant will have chlamydial conjunctivitis and a 10% chance of pneumonia.

—Test for this agent in all vaginitis patients, particularly if pregnant.

## THERAPEUTIC CONSIDERATIONS

### Dietary Considerations

Vaginal secretions are continuously released and contain water, nutrients, electrolytes, and proteins (secretory immunoglobulin A) and are altered by hormonal and dietary factors. Prescribe a well-balanced diet low in fats, sugars, and refined foods. Nutrients for proper immune function are zinc, vitamin A, vitamin C, vitamin E, manganese, and vitamin B complex. Diet high in lysine and low in arginine reduces number and severity of herpetic outbreaks, but many foods high in lysine are animal products high in fats. A low-arginine diet plus lysine supplements is a viable alternative.

- ***Lactobacillus* yogurt**: the most specific medicinal food for BV. Daily ingestion of 8 oz *Lactobacillus acidophilus* yogurt by women with recurrent candidal vaginitis induced a threefold decrease in infections and candidal colonization compared with women who do not eat yogurt.

### Nutritional Supplements

A high-quality multivitamin/mineral supplement is a low-cost compensation for dietary inadequacies.

- **Vitamin A and beta-carotene**: are necessary for epithelial tissues of the vaginal mucosa. Vitamin A is needed for adequate immune response and resistance to infection. Secretory immunoglobulin A is a major factor in resistance to infection. Beta-carotene is a nontoxic vitamin A precursor that enhances T-cell number and ratio. Excessive vitamin A is toxic and teratogenic; use caution in women of reproductive age. Limit total vitamin A intake to 5000 IU q.d. Use mixed carotenoids rather than synthetic beta-carotene.
- **B vitamins**: needed for carbohydrate metabolism, protein catabolism and synthesis, cell replication, and immune function. $B_2$ and $B_6$ have estrogenlike effects and act synergistically with estradiol. $B_1$ and pantothenic acid enhance estradiol activity without estrogenic activity themselves. B vitamins are useful in estrogen deficiency (atrophic vaginiti), especially if combined with phytoestrogens.

- **Vitamin C and bioflavonoids**: vitamin C deficiency reduces phagocytic activity of leukocytes. Vitamin C and bioflavonoids improve connective tissue integrity, reducing spread of infection and frequency and severity of herpetic outbreaks.
- **Vitamin E**: supplemental vitamin E increases resistance to *Chlamydia*. It regulates retinol in human beings; an inadequacy of vitamin E hinders utilization of vitamin A. It is used to treat atrophic vaginitis. Excess vitamin E intake may be immunosuppressive (>1200 IU q.d.) and transiently elevate blood pressure. It improves glycogen storage and tone of heart muscle. Use extra caution in patients with diabetes, hypoglycemia, hypertension, or heart disease. In high-risk patients, begin with a daily dose of 100 IU. Monitor blood sugar and/or blood pressure while increasing dosage slowly over time (e.g., 50 IU q.d.).
- **Zinc (Zn)**: all DNA and RNA polymerases and repair and replication enzymes require Zn. It enhances prostaglandin $E_1$ synthesis, normalizes lymphocyte activity, and enhances epithelial growth. Zn deficiency is linked to depressed immunity and thymic atrophy, which are corrected when Zn is replenished. Zn is essential for utilization of vitamin A. Topical and oral Zn reduces duration and severity of herpes outbreaks because of its antiviral activity. High levels are toxic to *Chlamydia* and *Trichomonas* and are effective in some cases unresponsive to antibiotics.
- **Lysine**: decreases frequency and severity of herpes outbreaks but may not shorten healing time. It becomes incorporated into the virus capsule in place of arginine, generating an inactive virus. It is taken at low doses prophylactically and higher doses at first sign of prodrome, the time of greatest viral replication. Efficacy is dose related. It works best when combined with a low-arginine diet.
- **Lithium**: lithium ointment interferes with replication of DNA viruses without affecting host cells. Lithium succinate (8% solution) may be combined with Zn in topical ointment or used alone.

## Botanical Medicines

- ***Glycyrrhiza glabra***: licorice is antiviral against RNA and DNA viruses. It is effective in treating herpes. The number and severity of recurrences are reduced by the repeated application of gel to active lesions. Isoflavonoids in licorice are effective against *Candida* (*Textbook, "Glycyrrhiza glabra* [Licorice]").

- **Chlorophyll**: has a bacteriostatic and soothing action. Water-soluble chlorophyll added to douching solutions offers symptomatic relief.
- ***Allium sativum***: garlic is antibacterial, antiviral, and antifungal and is effective against some antibiotic-resistant organisms. Major growth inhibitory component is allicin; therefore garlic products with the highest amount of allicin are preferred. A garlic clove may be carefully peeled, so as not to knick the clove, pierced with thread, and inserted into the vagina. Garlic capsules may also be inserted into the vagina.
- ***Hydrastis canadensis* (goldenseal) and *Berberis vulgaris* (barberry)**: contain berberine, a broad-range antibacterial. Berberine enhances immune function when taken internally and offers symptomatic relief when used in douching solutions; it soothes inflamed mucous membranes (*Textbook, "Hydrastis canadensis* [Goldenseal] and Other Berberine-Containing Botanicals").
- **Estrogenic plants:** atrophic vaginitis is best treated by vaginal estrogen: cream, suppository, tablet, or vaginal ring as used in conventional medicine. A few plants taken orally have very modest effects on vaginal epithelium, although not studied as true treatments for atrophic vaginitis. These include soy, ginseng, black cohosh, and flaxseed (see the chapter on menopause).
- ***Melaleuca alternifolia***: alcoholic extract of tea tree oil diluted to 1% in water is a strong antibacterial and antifungal. It is effective in treating trichomoniasis, candidiasis, and cervicitis. Use daily as a douche and weekly as saturated tampons. No adverse reactions have been reported. It has soothing effect. Tea tree oil preparations have antimicrobial activity against *Staphylococcus aureus* and *Candida albicans* (*Textbook, "Melaleuca alternifolia* [Tea Tree]").
- ***Melissa officinalis***: member of the mint family. It is effective in controlling herpetic symptoms and reducing frequency and severity of oral and genital herpes. It is taken orally as a water extract or applied topically as a cream.
- **Botanical mixture**: cream containing *Azadirachta indica* (neem) seed oil, *Sapindus mukerossi* (reetha) saponin extract, and quinine—effective and proven better than placebo. It is applied intravaginally at bedtime for 14 days for *Chlamydia trachomatis* vaginitis and BV. It offers no benefit for candidal or trichomonal infections.

## Other Agents

- ***Lactobacillus acidophilus***: helps maintain healthy vaginal ecosystem by preventing overgrowth of undesirable species. Produce lactic acid, acidic pH, natural antibiotic substances, and peroxides. They compete with other bacteria by consuming glucose and interfering with adherence and colonization of pathogenic bacteria on vaginal cells. Insert live *Lactobacillus* culture unflavored yogurt (read labels carefully). A more efficient and less messy method is to insert 1 capsule *Lactobacillus* into vagina b.i.d. for 1-2 weeks. *Lactobacillus* orally and intravaginally may be one of the most important aspects of effectively treating yeast and bacterial vaginitis. Use whenever antibiotics are used to reduce risk of complications (*Candida*) (see the chapter on candidiasis).

- **Iodine**: used as douche, it is effective against many organisms (*Trichomonas, Candida, Chlamydia*), and nonspecific vaginitis. Povidone-iodine (Betadine) does not sting or stain. It is effective in treating 100% of cases of candidal vaginitis, 80% of *Trichomonas*, and 93% of combination infections. Although douching in recent years is not as recommended, one study used a douching solution diluted to 1 part iodine to 100 parts water (1.5-3 tsp Betadine to 1 quart water) used b.i.d. for 14 days.
- **Boric acid**: capsules of boric acid treat candidiasis almost as well as nystatin. Women with chronic resistant yeast vaginitis who did not respond to extensive, prolonged conventional therapy were treated with 600 mg boric acid vaginal suppositories b.i.d. for 2 or 4 weeks. This regimen cured 98% of these women. Boric acid is inexpensive and accessible.
- **Gentian violet**: swabbing vagina with gentian violet is "as close to a specific treatment for *Candida* as exists."

## DIAGNOSTIC APPROACH

Question women directly regarding pruritus, vaginal discharge, dysuria, etc.

- Complete gynecological and sexual history: sexual activity and practices of patient and partner(s), method of contraception, personal hygiene, self-medication. Rule out associated symptoms suggesting PID or systemic infection. Ascertain previous occurrences: diagnosis, treatment, and resolution.
- Identify causative agent; avoid douching, intercourse, and vaginal medications for 1-2 days before office visit.
- Determine by speculum examination whether discharge emanates from vagina or cervix, condition of vaginal mucosa, and character of discharge. Collect specimens and place on slides for saline and KOH examination.

- Culture if diagnosis remains in question or if screening for GC or *Chlamydia*.
- Best time to test for low-level persistent infection (*Candida*) is just before menstrual period.

## THERAPEUTIC APPROACH

Focus of this protocol is on *Candida, Trichomonas,* and BV. (For atrophic vaginitis, see the chapter on menopause; for herpes simplex, see the chapter on herpes simplex.)

- **Diet**: nutrient-dense diet; avoid refined foods and simple carbohydrates. Minimize trans and saturated fats. Determine and eliminate suspected food allergens.
- **Supplements**:
  —Vitamin A: 5000 IU q.d. or beta-carotene 50,000 IU q.d.
  —Vitamin C: 500-1000 mg q4h
  —Vitamin B complex: balanced B complex averaging 20-50 mg of each major component
  —Zn: 10-15 mg q.d. (picolinate is best; 30-50 mg if using other forms)
  —Vitamin E (mixed tocopherols): 200 IU q.d. of D-alpha-tocopherol
  —*Lactobacillus* spp.: 0.5 tsp b.i.d.
- **Botanical medicines**
  —Hydrastis + *Echinacea* + *Phytolacca* (2:2:1): tincture, 20-60 drops q2-4 h; tea, 1 tsp/cup q2-4h
- **Topical treatment**: douches and saturated tampons; choose one or more of agents below; do not try to include all at once; variety provides alternatives for resistant cases.
  —Betadine: 1:100 dilution in retention douche kills most organisms within 30 seconds.
  —Boric acid: acute, 600 mg in capsules b.i.d. for 3-7 days; chronic, 600 mg vaginal suppositories b.i.d. for 2 weeks (4 weeks if not symptom free and wet mount free at 2 weeks); prevention, 600 mg vaginal suppository q.d., 4 days per month during menses for 4 consecutive months. To prevent vulvar irritation from boric acid dispensed from dissolved capsule, apply vitamin E oil or petroleum jelly to external genitalia.
  —Allium sativum: peel clove and pierce with thread as a tampon, wrapped in gauze, insert as suppository; if irritation occurs, remove immediately.

—Gentian violet swab: sensitivity reactions are common; stains clothes if sanitary pad is not used.
—*Hydrastis canadensis*: insert capsule or make into a suppository in cocoa butter.
—*Glycyrrhiza glabra*: insert capsule or apply gel locally to vulva.
—Lithium sulfate: 8% solution.
—*Melaleuca alternifolia*: 1% dilution as douche, plus insertion of saturated tampon for 24 hours once a week (repeated use may result in sensitivity in some women). Douching is no longer a recommended method of delivering medication.
—Zinc sulfate: 1 tbsp of 2% solution in 1 pint water douche or combined with galvanic therapy.

### Other Botanicals

Traditional texts and modern practitioners find efficacy in treating vaginitis with the following herbs, used alone or with other agents as capsules or suppositories placed into vagina: *Hydrastis canadensis* (goldenseal); *Eucalyptus; Calendula officinalis* (marigold; use succus); and chlorophyll.

### General Recommendations

- *Lactobacillus* capsules or yogurt with active cultures: use daily, at least orally, if not vaginally, to reinoculate vagina.
- Treatment failures: incorrect diagnosis, reinfection, untreated predisposing factors, resistance to treatment.
- Sexual activity: avoid during treatment to avoid reinfection and reduce trauma. At least use condoms, because semen is alkaline and acidic pH is optimal for vagina.
- *Trichomonas* infections in women also require concurrent treatment of male partner.
- Wear cotton underwear, especially with candidal vaginitis.
- Early symptomatic relief of pruritus and burning: warm sitz baths, plain or with herbs or Epsom salts.
- Severe cases: cleanse vagina of microbe-infested discharge with calendula succus–soaked cotton swabs.
- In recurrent or chronic BV or yeast vaginitis, consider treating male or female partners as vectors for recurrent disease.

### Specific Recommendations

- ***Candida***: treat internal candidiasis simultaneously to prevent recurrences

**Diagnostic Differentiation of Common Causes of Infectious Vaginitis**

| | *Candida* | NSV | *Trichomonas* | GC | Herpes | *Chlamydia* |
|---|---|---|---|---|---|---|
| Keynote symptoms | Itching | Odor | Odor and itching | Asymptomatic or cervicitis | Vesicles or ulcers | Asymptomatic |
| Discharge | | | | | | |
| pH | <4.5 | >4.5 | >5.0 | <4.5 | <4.5 | <4.5 |
| Odor | None | Fishy/amines | May be fishy | None | None | None |
| Appearance | Curdy, adherent, scant to thick | Gray, homogeneous | Greenish-yellow, frothy | Mucopurulent cervicitis | None | None |
| Pelvic examination | Adherent white patches with an erythematous border | Unremarkable | May show petechial lesion on cervix or vagina mucosa, a "strawberry cervix" | Cervical discharge, may have adnexal tenderness | Small, multiple vesicles or ulcers on cervix or vulva | Unremarkable or may show signs of PID |
| Microscopic | Mycelia (10% KOH) examination | "Clue cells," few white blood cells | Motile, flagellated organisms, few white blood cells | Many white blood cells with gram-negative intracellular diplococci | Unremarkable | Unremarkable |
| Culture media | Sauerbaud's | CNAF | Diamond's | Thayer-Martin | Live cell | Live cell or antibody test |

—Boric acid capsules inserted daily into vagina for 3-7 days
—Daily ingestion of 8 oz. of acidophilus yogurt
—One garlic capsule or raw clove daily

- ***Trichomonas***
  —Betadine: b.i.d.
  —Zn sulfate: daily
  —*Melaleuca alternifolia*: oil daily
- ***Chlamydia***
  —Betadine: daily
  —Zn sulfate: daily
- **Herpes**
  —Avoid arginine-rich foods
  —Lysine: 1000-2000 mg/day maintenance dose, double during outbreak
  —Zn sulfate: daily
  —Lithium sulfate: add to the Zn sulfate douching solution
  —*Melissa officinalis*: ointment or cream t.i.d.
- **BV**
  —Betadine: daily
  —*Hyrastis canadensis*: daily
  —*Lactobacillus* yogurt: 8 oz q.d. and/or *Lactobacillus* spp. capsules 1 to 2 q.d.
- **Atrophic vaginitis**
  —Intravaginal estriol cream: 1 mg/g. Insert 1 g q.d. for 2 weeks, then 1 g twice weekly as maintenance
  —Increase soy foods and flax meal in diet

# Varicose Veins

## DIAGNOSTIC SUMMARY

- Dilated, tortuous, superficial veins in the lower extremities.
- May be asymptomatic or associated with fatigue, aching discomfort, feeling of heaviness, or pain.
- Edema, pigmentation, and ulceration of the skin of the distal leg may develop.
- Women are affected four times as often as men.

## GENERAL DISCUSSION

Veins are frail structures. Defects in the venous wall allow dilation of vein and damage to valves. Valve damage increases static pressure, causing bulging known as varicose veins.

- Fifty percent of middle-aged adults are affected.
- Subcutaneous veins of legs are most commonly affected because of gravitational pressure that standing exerts on veins. Sanding for long periods increases pressure up to 10 times. Occupations requiring long periods of standing are greatest risk for varicose veins.
- Women are affected four times as often as men. Obesity greatly increases risk. Risk increases with age because of the loss of tissue tone and muscle mass, weakening vein walls. Pregnancy increases risk by increasing venous pressure in legs.
- Pose little harm if involved vein is near surface, but they are cosmetically unappealing. Significant symptoms are uncommon, but legs may feel heavy, tight, and tired.
- If varicose veins are associated with chronic venous insufficiency, leg ulcers may form that are often difficult to resolve.
- Serious varicosities involve obstruction and valve defects of deeper veins of the leg. This can lead to thrombophlebitis, pulmonary embolism, myocardial infarction, and stroke. Phlebography and Doppler ultrasonography are the most accurate methods of diagnosing deep vein involvement.

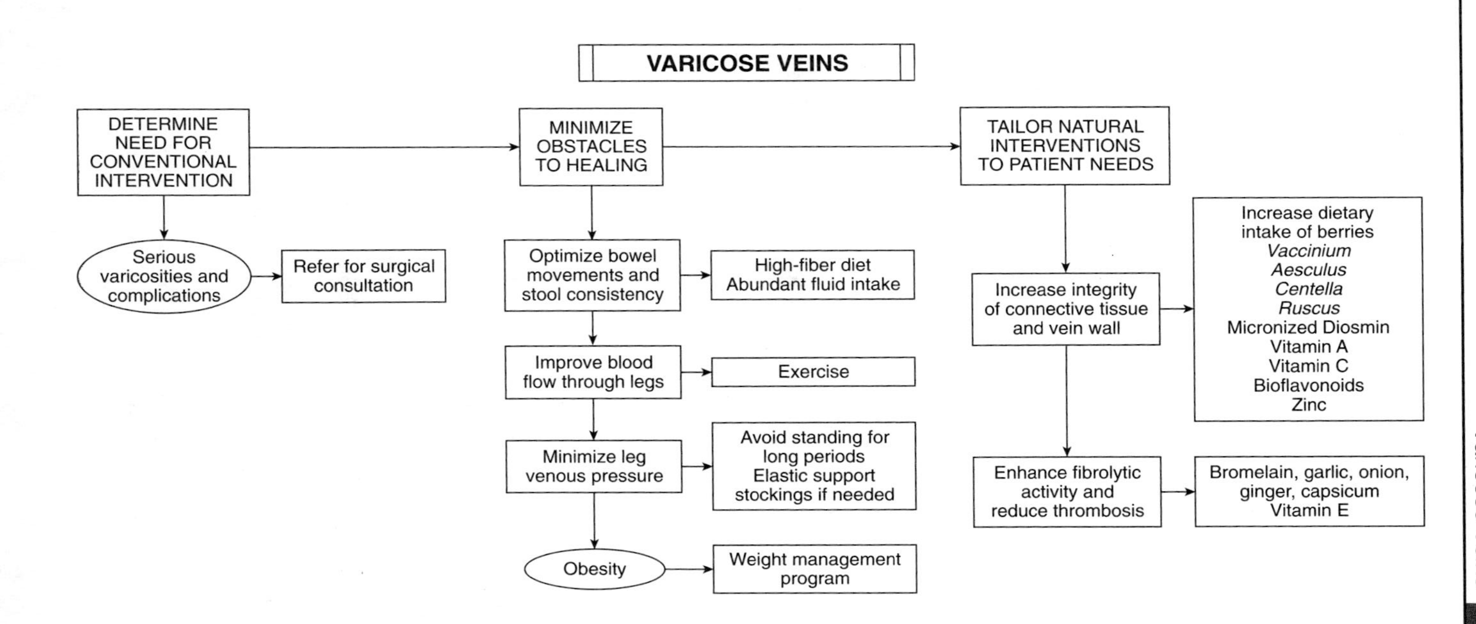
VARICOSE VEINS
DETERMINE NEED FOR CONVENTIONAL INTERVENTION
Serious varicosities and complications
Refer for surgical consultation
MINIMIZE OBSTACLES TO HEALING
Optimize bowel movements and stool consistency
High-fiber diet Abundant fluid intake
Improve blood flow through legs
Exercise
Minimize leg venous pressure
Avoid standing for long periods Elastic support stockings if needed
Obesity
Weight management program
TAILOR NATURAL INTERVENTIONS TO PATIENT NEEDS
Increase integrity of connective tissue and vein wall
Increase dietary intake of berries Vaccinium Aesculus Centella Ruscus Micronized Diosmin Vitamin A Vitamin C Bioflavonoids Zinc
Enhance fibrolytic activity and reduce thrombosis
Bromelain, garlic, onion, ginger, capsicum Vitamin E

### Etiology

- Genetic weakness of veins or venous valves.
- Excess venous pressure from increase in straining during defecation because of a low-fiber diet.
- Long periods of standing and/or heavy lifting.
- Damage to veins or venous valves as a result of thrombophlebitis.
- Weakness of vascular walls from abnormalities in proteoglycans of interendothelial cement substance or excessive release of lysosomal enzymes, which break down ground substance, increasing capillary permeability and loss of integrity of the venous structure.

## THERAPEUTIC CONSIDERATIONS

### Dietary Factors

- **Fiber**: varicose veins are rarely seen in parts of world with high-fiber, unrefined diets. A low-fiber diet contributes to the development of varicose veins because of the need to strain more during bowel movements (smaller, harder stools are more difficult to pass). Straining increases abdominal pressure, obstructing return of blood through the legs. Long-term increased pressure may weaken the vein wall, causing varicosities or hemorrhoids, or may weaken wall of large intestine, producing diverticuli. A high-fiber diet is the most important treatment and preventive measure for varicose veins (and hemorrhoids).
- **Bulking agents**: psyllium seed, pectin, and guar gum have a mild laxative action. They attract water and form a gelatinous mass, keeping feces soft, promoting peristalsis, and reducing straining during defecation.

### Physical Measures

Exercise and the avoidance of standing for long periods reduce risk. Walking, riding a bike, and jogging are particularly beneficial. Contraction of leg muscles pushes pooled blood back into circulation. Elastic compression stockings occasionally are beneficial. Surgical stripping of veins is performed in severe cases.

### Botanical Medicines

*Centella asiatica*: extract containing 70% triterpenic acids (asiatic acid, madecassic acid, asiatoside) is impressive in treating cellulite, venous insufficiency of lower limbs, and varicose veins. It exerts normalizing action on metabolism of connective tissue. It enhances tissue integrity by stimulating glycosaminoglycan (GAG) synthesis without promoting excessive collagen synthesis or cell growth. GAGs are major components of amorphous intercellular matrix (ground substance) in which collagen fibers are embedded. Net effect is normal tissue. Effect in venous insufficiency and varicose veins is to enhance connective tissue structure, reducing sclerosis and improving blood flow through affected limbs.

***Aesculus hippocastanum* (Horse chestnut)**: seeds of the horse chestnut tree were traditionally used to improve hemorrhoids and varicose veins. Horse chestnut seed extract (HCSE) contains escin (a triterpenic saponin), proanthocyanidin A2, and esculin. All three active components are vasoprotective and venotonic—provide antioxidant effects combined with the ability to inhibit enzymes that destroy venous structures (collagenase, hyaluronidase, beta-glucoranidase, elastase), thus shifting equilibrium between degradation and synthesis of proteoglycans and other venous structures toward net synthesis. HCSE prevents accumulation of leucocytes in varicose vein–affected limbs and their subsequent activation. Ultimate effect of HCSE-treatment is prevention of vascular leakage and increasing venous tone.

- **Venotonic**: substance improving venous tone by increasing contractile potential of elastic fibers in the vein wall. HCSE's venotonic activity is confirmed in the treatment of varicose veins and thrombophlebitis.
- HCSEs standardized for escin are as effective as compression stockings without the nuisance.
- Can be given orally, or escin/cholesterol complex can be applied topically. Topical formula is beneficial in treatment of bruises by decreasing capillary fragility and swelling.

***Ruscus aculeatus* (butcher's broom)**: a subshrub of the lily family native to the Mediterranean region. Active ingredients are ruscogenins, with antiinflammatory and vasoconstrictive effects. Extracts are used internally and externally in Europe for treating varicose veins and hemorrhoids. Clinical trials have confirmed benefits in both symptomatic relief and improved venous blood flow.

Flavonoid-rich extracts:

- Berries (hawthorn berries, cherries, blueberries, blackberries) are beneficial in preventing and treating varicose veins. Berries are rich sources of proanthocyanidins and anthocyanidins.

Bioflavonoids give berries their blue-red color. Proanthocyanidins and anthocyanidins improve integrity of ground substance and vascular system.

- **Buckwheat (*Fagopyrum esculentum*)** is high in rutin. Tea standardized to 5% total flavonoids, yielding a daily dosage of 270 mg of rutin, decreased total leg volume from edema of chronic venous insufficiency.
- Efficacy of these extracts is related to their ability to:
  —Reduce capillary fragility
  —Increase the integrity of the venous wall
  —Inhibit the breakdown of the compounds composing ground substance
  —Increase the muscular tone of the vein
- **Micronized diosmin**: the most useful single flavonoid for varicose veins. Micronization reduces size of particles for superior absorption, increased bioavailability, and greater clinical efficacy. Micronized diosmin improves signs and symptoms of chronic venous insufficiency. It decreases levels of some plasma markers of endothelial activation—soluble endothelial adhesion molecules. It promotes healing of venous ulcers and hemorrhoids.

**Bromelain and other fibrinolytic compounds**: persons with varicose veins have a decreased ability to break down fibrin. Fibrin is deposited in tissue near the varicosity. Skin then becomes hard and "lumpy" from fibrin and fat. Decreased fibrinolysis increases risk of thrombi and thrombophlebitis, myocardial infarction, pulmonary embolism, or stroke. Herbs increasing fibrinolytic activity of blood are capsicum (cayenne), garlic, onion, ginger; all increase fibrin breakdown. Use them liberally in food. Bromelain (proteolytic enzyme from pineapple) is also indicated. Vein walls are an important source of plasminogen activator, which promotes breakdown of fibrin. Varicose veins have decreased plasminogen activator. Bromelain acts in a similar manner to plasminogen activator, causing fibrin breakdown. It may help prevent hard and lumpy skin (lipodermatosclerosis) found around varicose veins.

## THERAPEUTIC APPROACH

Consume a diet high in fiber. Exercise regularly. Avoid standing in one place for long periods (use elastic support stocking if standing is necessary). Avoid obesity. Use measures that increase the integrity of the connective tissue and vein wall. Enhance fibrinolytic activity.

- **Diet**: rich in dietary fiber; liberal amounts of proanthocyanidin- and anthocyanidin-rich berries; garlic, onions, ginger, and cayenne liberally
- **Supplements**:
  —Vitamin A: 10,000 IU q.d.
  —Vitamin B complex: 10-100 mg q.d.
  —Vitamin C: 500-3000 mg q.d.
  —Vitamin E (mixed tocopherols): 200-600 IU q.d.
  —Bioflavonoids: 100-1000 mg q.d.
  —Zinc: 15-30 mg q.d.
- **Botanical medicines**:
  —*Aesculus hippocastanum*: bark of root, 500 mg t.i.d.
  —Escin: 50 mg t.i.d.; an escin/cholesterol complex may be applied topically in a 1% concentration
  —*Centella asiatica* extract (70% triterpenic acid content): 30 mg t.i.d.
  —*Ruscus aculeatus* extract (9%-11% ruscogenin content): 100 mg t.i.d.
  —*Vaccinium myrtillus*: fresh berries, 55-110 g t.i.d., extract containing 25% anthocyanoside, 80-160 mg t.i.d.
- **Micronized diosmin**: 500-1000 mg q.d.
  —Bromelain (minimum 1500 MCU): 500-750 mg t.i.d. between meals

## Additional Recommendations

For severely affected veins, sclerotherapy with segmental phlebectomy (stripping of vein) or surgical phlebectomy may be necessary. Sclerotherapy with segmental phlebectomy: sclerosing agent is injected at the highest portion of vein that is causing clot to form and pinch off vein. Only the most badly diseased segments of vein are stripped away with segmental phlebectomy.

# Index


**A**

AAs. *See* Amino acids.
Abraham, Guy, 654
Abscess, anal, 666f, 671-672
Acarbose, 376
ACE inhibitors. *See* Angiotensin-converting enzyme inhibitors.
Acetyl-L-carnitine. *See* L-carnitine.
*Achillea millefolium*, 683
Acne conglobata, 3-7
Acne vulgaris, 3-7
Acupressure
  asthma and, 71, 72
  nausea and vomiting of pregnancy and, 536
Acupuncture
  angina pectoris and, 54
  asthma and, 71, 72
  diabetes mellitus and, 221
  HIV/AIDS and, 333
  hyperthyroidism and, 359
  migraine headaches and, 512-13
  nausea and vomiting of pregnancy and, 536
Acute glaucoma, 275
Acyclovir, 327
AD. *See* Alzheimer's disease.
ADHD. *See* Attention deficit hyperactivity disorder in children.
Adiponectin, 543-544
Adrenal gland
  asthma and, 63
  chronic fatigue syndrome and, 172-73
  stress and, 13-14
Adrenocortical hypofunction and fibromyalgia syndrome, 263-264
Adriamycin, 131
*Aesculus hippocastanum*, 151, 683, 775, 777
Affective disorders
  bipolar (manic) depression and hypomania, 22-24
  conventional versus natural interventions, 9-10f
  depression, 8, 11-22
  diagnosis, 8-11
  seasonal affective disorder, 24-25
Age
  diabetes mellitus and, 203
  gallstones and, 270
  hair cycle and, 289


Page numbers followed by f indicate figures; t, tables.


Age *(Continued)*
  macular degeneration and, 459
  peptic ulcers and, 618
  senile cataracts and, 717
*AIDS and Complementary & Alternative Medicine, Current Science and Practice*, 316
AIDSInfo Web site, 315
Alanine
  benign prostatic hyperplasia and, 118
  gout and, 286
Al-Anon, 33
Ala-Teen, 33
Alcohol and alcoholism
  angina pectoris and, 55
  benign prostatic hyperplasia and, 115, 117
  botanical medicines, 34
  consequences, 26, 28
  conventional versus natural interventions, 27f
  depression and, 15, 22, 33-34
  diagnosis, 26
  effect on fetus, 28
  etiology, 28-29
  gout and, 285
  HIV/AIDS and, 331
  hypoglycemia and, 373
  intoxication and withdrawal symptoms, 29
  macular degeneration and, 462
  metabolic effects, 29-30
  nutrition and, 30-33
  osteoporosis and, 567
  porphyrias and, 646
  psychosocial aspects, 33-34
  senile dementia and, 40t
  therapeutic approach, 34-35
  therapeutic considerations, 30-33
  uterine fibroids and, 751
  *See also* Red wine.
Alcoholics Anonymous, 33
Alkylating chemotherapy agents, 128
Alkylglycerols, 134
Allergic rhinitis, 107
Allergies
  bacterial sinusitis and, 107, 109
  food
    aphthous stomatitis and, 56, 58
    asthma and, 64, 65-66, 71
    atopic dermatitis and, 92-93
    attention deficit hyperactivity disorder and, 101-102
    celiac disease and, 142, 144-146

Allergies (*Continued*)
chronic candidiasis and, 163
chronic fatigue syndrome and, 172
depression and, 18, 22
dermatitis herpetiformis and, 193
epilepsy and, 239
gallstones and, 271
infectious diarrhea and, 404
inflammatory bowel disease and, 409
irritable bowel syndrome and, 439
migraine headaches and, 508-509, 515, 518-519t
multiple sclerosis and, 530
otitis media and, 584-585
peptic ulcers and, 621
rheumatoid arthritis and, 699
rosacea and, 711, 712
seborrheic dermatitis and, 713
urticaria and, 741
glaucoma and, 278
HIV/AIDS and, 321
Allium family
asthma and, 69-70
atherosclerosis and, 81, 85, 89
chronic candidiasis and, 165
cystitis and, 189
diabetes mellitus and, 218, 224, 225
HIV/AIDS and, 320, 325, 333
hypertension and, 344, 349, 350
intestinal protozoan infestation and, 435
pneumonia and, 638, 639
vaginitis and, 766, 768
Allopathic treatment
hyperthyroidism, 360
multiple sclerosis, 525-526
Aloe vera, 70, 225
kidney stones and, 447, 449
psoriasis and, 691
seborrheic dermatitis and, 715-716, 716
Alpha-lipoic acid, 220, 221, 224
hepatitis and, 298
HIV/AIDS and, 324, 329
multiple sclerosis and, 529
*Althea officinalis*, 418, 683
Aluminum and Alzheimer's disease, 38, 42-43, 46
Alzheimer's disease
botanical medicines, 45-46, 47
conventional versus natural interventions, 37f
diagnosis, 36, 39-42
etiology, 36, 38, 39t
fingerprint patterns in, 42
hormone replacement therapy and, 481
imaging tests, 41-42
lab tests in, 41
neuropathology, 36
therapeutic approach, 46-47
therapeutic considerations, 42-46
*See also* Senile dementia.
Amalgam restorations and periodontal disease, 628
Amantadine, 604
American Heart Association, 87
Amines, dietary, 509-510
Amino acids
alcoholism and, 31-32
benign prostatic hyperplasia and, 115
HIV/AIDS and, 330
senile cataracts and, 721-722
*Ammi visnaga*, 53-54, 55, 447, 449
Anabolic steroids, 332
Anal abscess, 666f, 671-672
Anal cryptitis, 666f, 672
Anal fissure, 665f, 672-674
Anal fistula, 666f, 671-672
Analgesic rebound headache, 507-508
Androgenic female pattern hair loss, 291
Androgens
acne vulgaris/conglobata and, 3-5
dependent disorder of metabolism, 112
*Andrographis paniculata*, 332
Anemia
gout and, 287
inflammatory bowel disease and, 413
macrocytic, 329
rheumatoid arthritis and, 698
*Angelica sinensis*, 660, 662
trichomoniasis and, 735
Angina pectoris
acupuncture for, 54
angiograms, 50-51
antioxidant supplements, 52-53
botanical methods, 53-54, 55
causes of, 48
conventional versus natural interventions, 49f
coronary artery surgery study, 51
diagnosis, 48, 50
EDTA chelation therapy for, 54
hypoglycemia and, 371
relaxation and breathing exercises for, 54, 55
therapeutic approach, 55
therapeutic considerations, 50-54
Angiograms, coronary, 50-51, 88
Angioplasty, 50, 88
Angiotensin-converting enzyme inhibitors, 341, 342-343
Animal fat and macular degeneration, 462
Animal proteins
atherosclerosis and, 79
benign prostatic hyperplasia and, 115
osteoporosis and, 567, 569, 573
premenstrual syndrome and, 654
Anorectal anatomy, 663, 671
Anterior cortical cataracts, 719
Anterior subcapsular cataracts, 717
Anthraquinones, 447
Anti-ACE peptides, 348
Antiangiogenic agents, 128
Antibiotics
bacterial sinusitis and, 107, 109
hair loss in women and, 292t
infectious diarrhea and, 399, 400, 403

Antibiotics *(Continued)*
inflammatory bowel disease and, 409
otitis media and, 581, 583
pelvic inflammatory disease, 612-613
pneumonia and, 639
rosacea, 710
streptococcal pharyngitis and, 725, 727
trichomoniasis, 731, 732-733
urticaria and, 740
Anticholinergic drugs, 604
Antidepressants
bipolar depression and, 23
depression and, 12, 19
fibromyalgia syndrome and, 264
Antifungal griseofulvin therapy, 457
Antigliadin antibodies, 293
Antimetabolites, 128
Antinuclear antibodies, 698
Antioxidants
alcoholism and, 31
Alzheimer's disease and, 42, 43
angina pectoris and, 52-53
asthma and, 65, 67
cancer and, 134
chemotherapy and, 134-135
chronic candidiasis and, 164
diabetes mellitus and, 204, 220
epilepsy and, 242
hepatitis and, 300-301
hyperthyroidism and, 356-357
hypothyroidism and, 383
inflammatory bowel disease and, 416-417
leukoplakia and, 453
macular degeneration and, 462
male infertility and, 471-472
multiple sclerosis and, 529
osteoarthritis and, 558
Parkinson's disease and, 595, 596-597
porphyrias and, 648
rheumatoid arthritis and, 702
senile cataracts and, 719-21
Antisperm antibodies, 469
Antitumor antibiotics, 128
Anxiety
irritable bowel syndrome and, 440-441
trichomoniasis and, 733
Aphthous stomatitis
causes of, 56
conventional versus natural interventions, 57f
diagnosis, 56
therapeutic approach, 59
therapeutic considerations, 56, 58-59
Apnea, sleep, 426-27
Apoptosis and Parkinson's disease, 590-591
Appetite regulating hormones, 544-545
Arachidonic acid, 510-511, 689
*Arctium lappa,* 96, 753
*Arctostaphylos uva ursi,* 188, 190
Arnica, 126
*Artemisia*
*annua,* 435
*douglasiana,* 623-624
Artery bypass surgery, 50, 88
Arthritis, inflammatory bowel disease and, 412
Ascorbic acid. *See* Vitamin C.
Ashwaganda. *See Withania somnifera.*
Aspartic acid, 286
Aspirin
cancer and, 132
inflammatory bowel disease and, 411
myocardial infarction and, 87
osteoarthritis and, 556
peptic ulcers and, 620
urticaria and, 740-741
Asthma
botanical medicines, 69-71, 72
breastfeeding and, 63, 66
causes of, 62-64
conventional versus natural interventions, 61f
diagnosis, 60
food allergies and, 64, 65-66, 71-72
genetic factors, 60
hormones and, 64-65
inflammation and, 62-64
influenza vaccine and, 64
mild episodic versus moderate to severe sustained, 63
pertussis vaccine and, 63-64
supplements for, 66-69, 71-72
therapeutic approach, 71-72
therapeutic considerations, 64-71
*Astragalus,* 391-392, 393
Astringent herbs, 498-499
Atherosclerosis
angina pectoris and, 48
antioxidant status and, 83
botanical medicines, 81-83
conventional versus natural interventions, 74f
diabetes mellitus and, 75, 77, 89, 211
diagnosis, 73
diet and, 77-80, 83-85
fibrinogen and, 85
genetic factors, 76
HIV/AIDS and, 325
hypoglycemia and, 371
hypothyroidism and, 380
macular degeneration and, 459, 461
natural cholesterol-lowering agents and, 82-83
periodontal disease and, 625
phytochemicals and, 83
preventing recurrent heart attack and, 87-88
process of, 73, 75
risk factors, 75-77, 85-86
supplements for, 80-81, 83-86, 86, 89
therapeutic approach, 88-89
therapeutic considerations, 77-88

Atkins diet, 547-548
Atopic dermatitis
botanical medicines, 95-96, 96
conventional versus natural interventions, 91f
diagnosis, 90
diet and, 92-94, 95
environmental considerations, 95
signs and symptoms, 90, 92
supplements for, 95
therapeutic approach, 95-96
*See also* Dermatitis herpetiformis.
*Atractylis gummifera,* 301
Atrophic "dry" ARMD, 459, 461
Atrophic vaginitis, 486, 758, 771
Attention deficit hyperactivity disorder in children
botanical medicines, 106
challenges of, 97
cognitive behavior therapies, 104
conventional versus natural interventions, 98f, 104
diagnosis, 97
diet and, 100-103
drug therapy, 104
environmental toxins and, 99-100
executive control in, 97, 99
food allergies and, 101-102
gastrointestinal function and, 102-103
genetic factors, 99
immune system function and, 103
neurofeedback, 104
reward deficiency syndrome and, 99
supplements for, 105
therapeutic approach, 104-106
therapeutic considerations, 99-104
Autism, 100
Autoimmunity
diabetes mellitus and, 200-201
Hashimoto's disease, 354, 379, 380, 384-385
hyperthyroidism and, 351
urticaria, 739-740
Autonomic nervous system, 63
Azelaic acid, 6-7
*A-Z Guide to Drug-Herb-Vitamin Interactions,* 127
Azidothymidine/Zidovudine/Retrovir, 318
Azoospermia, 465, 469
AZT, 318

## B

*Bacopa monniera,* 46
Bacteria
acne, 3
atopic dermatitis and, 92
bacterial sinusitis and, 109-110
cystitis and, 189-190
glaucoma and, 280
infectious diarrhea and, 396-398
intestinal, 695
migraine headaches and, 510, 515
Bacteria *(Continued)*
pelvic inflammatory disease and, 605
periodontal disease and, 627
rosacea and, 711, 712
urticaria and, 743
Bacterial sinusitis
antibiotics for, 109
botanical medicines, 110
conventional versus natural interventions, 108f
diagnosis, 107
local treatments, 111
mucolytics for, 109
predisposing factors, 107
supplements for, 110
therapeutic approach, 110-111
therapeutic considerations, 107, 109-110
Bacterial vaginosis, 155, 761-763, 771
Bacteriotherapy and streptococcal pharyngitis, 727
Balneotherapy, 705-706
Balsam pear. *See Momordica charantia.*
*Baptista tinctoria,* 418
Barbiturates and senile dementia, 40t
Bartlett, John G., 315
Bartter's syndrome, 288
Bastyr's formula, 418, 420
B cells, 122
Bearberry. *See Arctostaphylos uva ursi.*
Behavioral therapy
attention deficit hyperactivity disorder, 104
obesity, 547
Benign prostatic hyperplasia
botanical medicines, 116-117, 118
conventional versus natural interventions, 113f
diagnosis, 112, 114
dietary and nutritional factors, 115-116
genetic factors, 112
prevalence, 112
supplements for, 118
surgery, 114
therapeutic approach, 117-118
therapeutic considerations, 114-117
Benzoates, 742
Berberine-containing plants
chronic candidiasis and, 165
infectious diarrhea and, 403, 405
trichomoniasis and, 734
uterine fibroids and, 753
vaginitis and, 766
Berkson program, 300, 302
Beta-blockers, 342
Beta carotenes. *See* Carotenes.
Betadine
trichomoniasis and, 734, 735
vaginitis and, 768
Betaine
epilepsy and, 241
rheumatoid arthritis and, 707
Bilberry extract, 724

Bile
  gallstones and, 267, 269, 272, 273
  psoriasis and, 687-688
Biochemistry of porphyrias, 643
Bioelectrical impedance, 541-542
Biofeedback
  attention deficit hyperactivity disorder and, 104
  migraine headaches and, 513, 516
Bioflavonoids. *See* Flavonoids.
Biogenic amine model of depression, 11
Biological response modifiers, 128-129
Biotin
  depression and, 16
  diabetes mellitus and, 216, 223
  seborrheic dermatitis and, 713, 715, 716
Bipolar (manic) depression
  antidepressants, 23
  botanical medicines, 23-24
  conventional versus natural interventions, 10f
  diagnosis, 8, 10f, 22-23
  therapeutic approach, 24
  therapeutic considerations, 23-24
Bismuth salts, 399, 622, 624
Bitter melon. *See Momordica charantia.*
Black cohosh. *See Cimicifuga racemosa.*
Bladder infections. *See* Cystitis.
Bladderwrack. *See Fucus vesiculosus.*
Bleeding
  dysfunctional uterine, 494
  uterine fibroids and, 748
Blindness and diabetes mellitus, 211
Blood
  heme formation, 643
  loss
    inflammatory bowel disease and, 413
    menorrhagia and, 492-501
  pressure, high. *See* Hypertension.
  tests
    Alzheimer's disease and, 41
    benign prostatic hyperplasia and, 114
Blue-green algae, 333
BM. *See Bacopa monniera.*
BMI. *See* Body mass index.
Body fat composition, 550-551
Body mass index, 538, 540
Bone
  cancer, 122
  mineral density tests, 570-571
Boric acid and vaginitis, 767, 768
Boron
  osteoarthritis and, 560-561, 563
  osteoporosis and, 574-575, 580
*Boswellia,* 70, 139, 562, 564
Botanical medicines
  *Achillea millefolium,* 683
  *Aesculus hippocastanum,* 151, 683, 775, 777
  alcoholism, 34
  *Aloe vera,* 70, 225, 447, 449, 691, 715-716, 716
  *Althea officinalis,* 418, 683

Botanical medicines *(Continued)*
  Alzheimer's disease, 45-46, 47
  *Ammi visnaga,* 53-54, 55, 447, 449
  *Andrographis paniculata,* 332
  *Angelica sinensis,* 660, 662, 735
  angina pectoris, 53-54, 55
  anorectal diseases, 683
  anthraquinone, 447
  antiyeast, 164-165
  *Arctium lappa,* 96, 753
  *Arctostaphylos uva ursi,* 188, 190
  *Artemisia,* 435, 623-624
  asthma, 69-71, 72
  *Astragalus,* 391-392, 393
  atherosclerosis, 81-83
  atopic dermatitis, 94, 96
  attention deficit hyperactivity disorder, 106
  *Bacopa monniera,* 46
  bacterial sinusitis, 110
  benign prostatic hyperplasia, 116-117, 118
  berberine-containing plants, 165, 403, 405, 734, 753, 766
  bipolar (manic) depression, 23-24
  *Boswellia,* 70, 139, 562, 564
  *Bupleuri,* 243, 705, 707
  *Buxus sempervirens,* 332, 334, 336
  *Camellia sinensis,* 72, 202, 600
  cancer, 131, 134
  *Capsicum frutescens,* 69, 691
  carpal tunnel syndrome, 139
  cellulite, 150-151, 151
  *Centella asiatica,* 126, 150, 151, 632, 774-775, 777
  cernilton flower pollen extract, 117, 118
  chamomile preparations, 96, 537, 690-691
  Chinese herbal, 94, 242-243, 301, 440, 536
  chronic candidiasis, 164-165
  chronic fatigue syndrome, 174-175
  *Cimicifuga racemosa,* 489-90, 491, 660-661, 662
  *Coleus forskohlii,* 70, 72, 93, 96, 243
  *Collinsonia canadensis,* 683
  congestive heart failure, 182
  *Crataegus* spp., 53, 55, 182, 349, 350
  *Curcuma longa,* 274, 332, 334, 385, 704, 707, 723
  *Cynara scolymus,* 274
  cystitis, 188-189, 190
  depression, 21, 22
  diabetes mellitus, 202, 217-218
  *Echinacea,* 391, 392, 586, 637, 728, 735, 752, 755, 768
  *Eleutherococcus senticosus,* 174, 175, 475
  *Emblica officinalis,* 359
  endometriosis, 230-232
  *Ephedra sinica,* 69, 72
  epilepsy, 242-243
  escin, 151, 777
  fenugreek seeds, 218

Botanical medicines *(Continued)*
- flavonoid, 68, 93-94
- *Fraxinus/Ceanothus,* 752, 755
- *Fucus vesiculosus,* 150, 151
- furanocoumarin-containing, 447
- *Galanthus nivalis,* 46
- gallstones, 274
- *Gelsemium/Phytolacca,* 752
- ginger, 243, 498, 513, 516, 535, 562-563, 623, 704-705
- ginseng, 106, 174, 175, 218, 318, 391, 392-393, 474, 475, 490, 707
- *Glycyrrhiza glabra,* 69, 72, 93, 96, 175, 299-300, 301, 332, 623, 639, 660, 662, 690, 707, 765, 769
- gout, 286, 287
- gugulipid, 81-82, 82
- *Gymnema sylvestre,* 217, 223
- *Hamamelis virginiana,* 683
- *Harpagophytum procumbens,* 286, 287, 562, 564
- hepatitis, 299-301
- herpes simplex, 306
- HIV/AIDS, 332-333, 336
- huperzine A, 46, 47
- *Hydrangea,* 447
- *Hydrastis,* 111, 189, 190, 403, 614, 616, 638, 683, 692, 727, 728, 735, 766, 768, 769
- hypertension, 349
- hyperthyroidism, 358-359, 360
- *Hyssopus officinalis,* 332
- immune system function, 391-392, 392-393
- infectious diarrhea, 403-404, 405
- inflammatory bowel disease, 417-419, 420
- insomnia, 431, 432
- intestinal protozoan infestation, 435
- irritable bowel syndrome, 440, 441
- *Juglans nigra,* 435
- kava kava, 21, 22, 301, 601
- kempo, 46
- kidney stones and, 447
- *Lentinus edodes,* 332, 334
- *Leonurus,* 230, 231
- *Leptotania,* 447
- lichen planus, 457-458
- *Lobelia inflata,* 69, 636
- *Lycopus,* 358-359
- macular degeneration, 464
- male infertility, 474, 475
- *Medicago sativa,* 564
- *Melissa officinalis,* 306, 327, 766
- menopause, 489-490
- menorrhagia and, 498-499, 501
- *Mentha piperita,* 535
- migraine headaches, 513-414, 516
- milk thistle, 34, 126, 131, 164, 229, 300, 301, 324, 332, 336
- *Mitchella repens,* 447
- *Momordica charantia,* 217-218, 332
- *Mucuna pruriens,* 601, 604
- multiple sclerosis, 530

Botanical medicines *(Continued)*
- nausea and vomiting of pregnancy, 535-536, 537
- obesity, 550
- olive leaf extract, 327, 332, 334, 349, 350
- osteoarthritis, 562-563, 564
- otitis media and, 586-587
- Parkinson's disease, 600-601, 604
- *Passiflora incarnata,* 431, 432
- pelvic inflammatory disease, 614
- pelvic inflammatory disease and, 616
- peptic ulcers, 623-624, 624
- periodontal disease, 631-632
- *Peucedanum,* 447
- *Peumus boldo,* 274
- *Phyllanthus amarus,* 300, 332, 334
- *Phytolacca americana,* 418, 753, 768
- pneumonia, 636-637, 639
- policosanol, 81, 82
- *Polygonum aviculare,* 447
- *Potentilla tormentilla,* 403-404, 405
- premenstrual syndrome, 659-661, 662-663
- proctologic conditions, 676
- *Prunella vulgaris,* 332
- psoriasis, 690-691, 692
- *Pterocarpus marsupium,* 202
- *Pygeum africanum,* 117, 118, 474
- *Rheum,* 447, 623
- rheumatoid arthritis, 704-705, 707
- *Rosmarinus officinalis,* 332
- *Rubia,* 447, 449
- *Rubus idaeus,* 535
- *Rumex,* 447, 449
- *Ruscus aculeatus,* 683, 775-776, 777
- *Sanguinaria canadensis,* 631-632
- Scudder's alterative, 752
- *Scutellaria,* 243, 333
- seasonal affective disorder, 25
- seborrheic dermatitis, 715-716
- senile cataracts, 722-723, 724
- senna, 447
- *Serenoa repens,* 116, 118
- *Silybum marianum,* 692
- *Smilax sarsaparilla,* 692
- *Spirulina platensis,* 333
- St. John's wort, 21, 22, 23, 25, 333, 661, 663
- streptococcal pharyngitis, 728
- stroke, 88
- *Symphytum officinale,* 301, 614, 616
- *Tanacetum parthenium,* 513, 516
- *Taraxacum officinale,* 96, 230, 231, 274, 753
- *Terminalia arjuna,* 182
- trichomoniasis, 733-34, 735
- *Trifolium pretense,* 489, 491
- Turska's formula, 230, 232, 755
- *Tylophora asthmatica,* 70
- *Urtica dioica,* 117, 118, 753
- uterine fibroids, 752-753, 755
- *Vaccinium myrtillus,* 93, 280, 287, 463, 464
- vaginitis and vulvovaginitis, 765-767

Botanical medicines *(Continued)*
*Valeriana officinalis*, 431, 432
varicose veins, 774-776, 777
*Viscum album*, 349
*Vitex agnus-castus*, 230, 498, 501, 661, 662, 753
*Xanthoxylum americanum*, 230, 231
yucca, 562, 564
*Zizyphi fructus*, 69
*See also* Allium family; Drugs; *Ginkgo biloba;* Grape seed extract; Green tea; *Lactobacillus acidophilus; Melaleuca; Silybum marianum.*
Bottle blowing, 636
Bovine cartilage, 559
Bovine spleen extracts, 638
Bowel permeability, 695
Bowel toxemia, 687
BPH. *See* Benign prostatic hyperplasia.
Brachytherapy, 132
Brain
attention deficit hyperactivity disorder and, 99
hypoglycemia and, 370
senile dementia and, 40-41
Branched-chain amino acids, 31
BRAT diet, 400
Breast cancer and hormone replacement therapy, 481
Breastfeeding
asthma and, 63, 66
atopic dermatitis and, 92
HIV/AIDS and, 329-30
otitis media and, 584
Breathing
exercises, 54, 174, 366, 536
patterns, normal, 363, 365
Bromelain
bacterial sinusitis and, 110
cancer and, 127
gout and, 285-286, 287
pelvic inflammatory disease and, 614, 616
pneumonia and, 635, 636
rheumatoid arthritis and, 701, 704
varicose veins and, 776
Brown fat cells, 545-546
Buckwheat, 271, 776
*Bupleuri*
*falcatum*, 705, 707
*radix*, 243
Bushite stones, 450
Butterbur, 513-614
Butylated hydroxyanisole, 742
Butylated hydroxytoluene, 742
Butyrate enemas, 418-419
*Buxus sempervirens*, 332, 334, 336

**C**

Cabbage and peptic ulcers, 621-622
Cadmium
benign prostatic hyperplasia and, 116
hyperthyroidism and, 353
senile cataracts and, 722
Caffeine
angina pectoris and, 55
atherosclerosis and, 79
benign prostatic hyperplasia and, 118
cellulite and, 150
depression and, 15, 21
glaucoma and, 278
hypertension and, 348-349
osteoporosis and, 569
premenstrual syndrome and, 655
uterine fibroids and, 751
Calabrese, C., 316
Calcium
attention deficit hyperactivity disorder and, 105
channel blockers, 341, 342-343
fibromyalgia syndrome and, 266
hypertension and, 347
hyperthyroidism and, 357
inflammatory bowel disease and, 415
kidney stones and, 447, 449
nausea and vomiting of pregnancy and, 537
osteoporosis and, 567, 568, 569, 573, 575-576, 580
premenstrual syndrome and, 658
stones, 449
trichomoniasis and, 733
*Callilepis laureola*, 301
*Camellia sinensis*, 72
diabetes mellitus and, 202
Parkinson's disease and, 600
CAMP. *See* Cyclic adenosine monophosphate.
*Campylobacter jejuni*, 397, 399
Cancer
antioxidants and, 134-135
botanical medicines and, 131, 134
breast, 481
cell cycle, 121
cervical, 155
chemotherapy, 121, 127-132
clinical care, 125
clinical trials, 135
colorectal, 479
conventional versus natural interventions, 120f
development stages, 121
diagnosis, 119
diet for patients, 135
endometrial, 479
hyperuricemia and, 287
natural therapy goals, 126, 130-132, 133
oral, 451
ovarian, 481-482
performance indexes and, 123-124
prevention, 119
radiation therapy, 132-133
radiopotentiation, 133-134
roles of naturopathy in, 119, 121, 125
staging, 122-123
surgery, 126-27
therapeutic considerations, 125-35
tumor markers, 123

Cancer *(Continued)*
tumor response criteria and terminology, 124-125
types, 122
*Candida albicans*
asthma and, 64
atopic dermatitis and, 93
chronic fatigue syndrome and, 171-172
HIV/AIDS and, 325
irritable bowel syndrome and, 440
urticaria and, 743
vaginitis, 760-761
*See also* Chronic candidiasis.
Canker sores. *See* Aphthous stomatitis.
Canola oil, 79
Capecitabine, 132
Caprylic acid, 165
Capsaicin, 221, 556
*Capsicum frutescens*, 69, 691
Carbohydrates
alcoholism and, 34
angina pectoris and, 55
atherosclerosis and, 78
benign prostatic hyperplasia and, 117
gallstones and, 270-271, 271
hypoglycemia and, 371-372
inflammatory bowel disease and, 409
kidney stones and, 446
nausea and vomiting of pregnancy and, 536-537
obesity and, 548
Carbon dioxide intoxication, 40t
Carbon monoxide intoxication, 40t
Carboplatin, 131
Cardiac catheterization. *See* Coronary angiograms.
Cardiac output, 179
Cardiovascular disease. *See* Atherosclerosis.
Carotenes
asthma and, 72
atherosclerosis and, 83
cancer and, 130
celiac disease and, 145
cervical dysplasia and, 156, 159-160
cystitis and, 190
endometriosis and, 229, 231
fibrocystic breast disease and, 254
fibromyalgia syndrome and, 266
HIV/AIDS and, 322, 336
immune system function and, 389
leukoplakia and, 451, 453
lichen planus and, 458
macular degeneration and, 464
male infertility and, 475
otitis media and, 586
pelvic inflammatory disease and, 614, 616
periodontal disease and, 632
porphyrias and, 648, 649
senile cataracts and, 722
Carpal tunnel syndrome
botanical medicine, 139
Carpal tunnel syndrome *(Continued)*
conventional versus natural interventions, 137f
diagnosis, 136, 138-139
etiology, 136
nutrition and, 139
physical medicine, 140
prevention, 141
risk factors and frequency of occurrence, 138
surgery, 140-141
therapeutic approach, 141
therapeutic considerations, 139-141
Carrageenans, 411
CASS. *See* Coronary artery surgery study.
Castor oil, 753
Catalase and senile cataracts, 721
Cataracts, 211, 220
Catecholamines, 342
Cayenne. *See Capsicum frutescens.*
CCK hormone, 544
CD4+ cells, 310-312
Celiac disease
aphthous stomatitis and, 58
causes of, 142
conventional versus natural interventions, 143f
diabetes mellitus and, 201
diagnosis, 142, 145
etiology, 144
hair loss in women and, 293
therapeutic approach, 146
therapeutic considerations, 145-146
Cell cycle and cancer, 121
prevention, 149
Cell-mediated immunity defects and atopic dermatitis, 92
Cellulite
botanical medicines, 150-51, 151
clinical features, 149
conventional versus natural interventions, 148f
diagnosis, 147
histologic features, 147, 149
stages, 149
therapeutic approach, 151
therapeutic considerations, 149-151
*Centella asiatica*, 126, 150, 151, 632, 774-775, 777
Cerebrovascular disease and senile dementia, 39t
Cernilton flower pollen extract, 117, 118
Cervical cancer, 155
Cervical dysplasia
conventional versus natural interventions, 153f
diagnosis, 152
epidemiology, 154
etiology, 152, 154
histology, 154
risk factors, 155
therapeutic approach, 158-160
therapeutic considerations, 155-158

Cervical manipulation and migraine headaches, 512
Chamomile preparations, 96, 537, 690-691
Chaste tree. *See Vitex agnus-castus.*
Chelation therapy, EDTA, 54, 88
Chemical sensitivities
  chronic fatigue syndrome and, 169
  porphyrias and, 644
  vaginitis, 759
Chemotherapy
  action of drugs used in, 121, 128
  antioxidants and, 134-135
  clinical uses of, 127-128
  drug families, 128-129
  effectiveness improvement, 130
  Kaposi's sarcoma and, 328
  recommendations for specific agents used in, 131-132
  resistance testing, 129
  side effects, 129, 130-131
Cherries, 286
Children
  headaches in, 517
  inflammatory bowel disease in, 419-420, 422-423
Chinese herbal medicine
  atopic dermatitis and, 94
  epilepsy and, 242-43
  hepatitis and, 301
  irritable bowel syndrome and, 440
  nausea and vomiting of pregnancy and, 536
Chlamydia, 155, 470
  pelvic inflammatory disease and, 605, 608
  vaginitis, 763-764, 771
Chlorophyll
  menorrhagia and, 497, 500
  pelvic inflammatory disease and, 613, 616
  vaginitis and, 766
Chlorpropamide, 376
Cholesterol
  benign prostatic hyperplasia and, 115-116
  diabetes mellitus and, 220, 224-225
  gallstones and, 267, 269
  hypothyroidism and, 380
  -lowering agents, natural, 82-83
Choline
  cystitis and, 190
  epilepsy and, 241
  fibrocystic breast disease and, 254
  gallstones and, 274
Cholinergic urticaria, 739
Chondroitin sulfate and osteoarthritis, 559
Chromium
  depression and, 17-18, 22
  diabetes mellitus and, 213
  glaucoma and, 278, 280
  hypoglycemia and, 373
  obesity, 550
  obesity and, 549
  psoriasis and, 689, 691
Chronic candidiasis
  botanical medicines, 164-165
  causes of, 161
  chronic fatigue syndrome and, 171
  conventional versus natural interventions, 162f
  diagnosis, 161, 163
  related syndromes, 161
  therapeutic approach, 165-166
  therapeutic considerations, 163-165
Chronic daily headaches, 504
Chronic fatigue syndrome
  botanical medicines, 174-175
  chronic candidiasis and, 171-172
  conventional versus natural interventions, 168f
  depression and, 170
  diagnosis, 167, 170
  diet and nutrition and, 173-174, 175
  environmental illness and, 170-171
  etiology, 167, 169-170
  fibromyalgia syndrome and, 169
  food allergies and, 172
  gastrointestinal function and, 171
  hypoadrenalism and, 172-173
  hypoglycemia and, 172
  hypothyroidism and, 172
  immune system function and, 169, 171
  lab tests, 170, 171
  liver function and, 170-171
  stress and, 170
  therapeutic approach, 175-176
  therapeutic considerations, 170-175
Chronic glaucoma, 275
Chronic meningitis and senile dementia, 39t
Chronic sinusitis, 109
Chu, Edward, 131
Chvostek's sign, 364
*Cimicifuga racemosa,* 489-490, 491
  premenstrual syndrome and, 660-661, 662
Cinnamomum, 683
Cinnamon oil, 501
Circadian rhythms, 24
Cisplatin, 131, 133
Citrate and kidney stones, 447
Clinical Global Impressions Scale, 46
Clinical trials, cancer, 135
*Clostridium difficile,* 397, 400
Clozapine, 604
Cluster headaches, 504
Coffee and gallstones, 271-272
Cognitive function
  behavior therapies and attention deficit hyperactivity disorder, 104
  hormone replacement therapy and, 481
  menopause and, 486
*Cola vera,* 151
Colchicine and gout, 284
Cold urticaria, 739

*Coleus forskohlii*
  asthma and, 72
  atopic dermatitis and, 93, 96
  epilepsy and, 243
Collagen
  glaucoma and, 275, 277
  periodontal disease and, 628-629
*Collinsonia canadensis*, 683
Colon function
  fibrocystic breast disease and, 253
  porphyrias and, 649
  rheumatoid arthritis and, 699-700
Colorants, food, 741-742
Colorectal cancer, 479
Colposcopy, 152, 158
Comedones, 3-7
Comfrey. *See Symphytum offinale.*
Complement system in periodontal disease, 627-628
Comprehensive stool and digestive analysis, 163
Computed tomography. *See* CT (computed tomography).
Condoms, 615
Condyloma lata, 679
Condylomata acuminata, 678-679
Congestive heart failure
  botanical medicines, 182
  causes of, 177, 179
  conventional versus natural interventions, 178f
  diagnosis, 177, 179
  nutritional supplements for, 180-181
  signs and symptoms, 179
  stages, 177
  therapeutic approach, 182
  therapeutic considerations, 179-182
Conjunctivitis, acute, 279t
Copper
  HIV/AIDS and, 323
  hypothyroidism and, 383
  osteoarthritis and, 560-561, 563
  periodontal disease and, 630
  rheumatoid arthritis and, 703, 707
  /zinc ratio, 157-158
CoQ10
  angina pectoris and, 51-52, 53, 55
  atherosclerosis and, 79
  cancer and, 131
  congestive heart failure and, 181
  epilepsy and, 242
  HIV/AIDS and, 324, 325, 329
  hypertension and, 348, 350
  hyperthyroidism and, 358, 360
  Parkinson's disease and, 597-598, 604
  periodontal disease and, 630-631
Corneal trauma, 279t
Coronary angiograms, 50-51
Coronary artery surgery study (CASS), 51
Coronary heart disease and hormone replacement therapy, 479-481
Corticosteroids, 95
  glaucoma and, 277
  inflammatory bowel disease and, 410, 413
  multiple sclerosis and, 526
Cortisol
  depression and, 13, 15
  seasonal affective disorder and, 25
  smoking and, 15
Counseling
  alcoholism, 35
  asthma, 72
  chronic fatigue syndrome and, 175-176
  depression, 12-13
  diabetes mellitus and, 212
  HIV/AIDS and, 321
  hyperventilation syndrome/breathing pattern disorders, 366
  irritable bowel syndrome and, 441
C-peptide determination, 207
Cranberry juice, 187, 450
Cranioelectrical stimulation, 333
*Crataegus*, 53, 55
  hypertension and, 349, 350
  *oxyacantha*, 182
  *pentagyna*, 93
C-reactive protein and pelvic inflammatory disease, 611-612
Creatine and Parkinson's disease, 599-600
Crohn's disease, 269, 406, 408, 410-412, 419, 421t
  proctologic conditions and, 673, 674
  *See also* Inflammatory bowel disease.
Cryosurgery, 676
Cryptitis, anal, 666f, 672
*Cryptosporidium parvum*, 398
CSDA. *See* Comprehensive stool and digestive analysis.
CT (computed tomography), and Alzheimer's disease, 42
CTS. *See* Carpal tunnel syndrome.
*Curcuma longa*, 274, 332, 334, 385, 704, 707, 723
Cyclic adenosine monophosphate, 92
Cyclooxygenase inhibitors, 556, 688-689
Cyclophosphamide, 131
*Cynara scolymus*, 274
Cystic fibrosis, 269
Cystine stones, 450
Cystitis
  botanical medicines, 188-189, 190
  causes of, 183, 185
  conventional versus natural interventions, 184f
  diagnosis, 183, 185-186
  menopause and, 486
  nutritional supplements for, 188, 190
  risk factors, 185
  therapeutic approach, 189-190
  therapeutic considerations, 186-189
Cysts, acne, 3-7
Cytokine abnormalities, 331
Cytomegalovirus, 294, 303, 396

Cytostatic chemotherapy drugs, 128
Cytotoxic chemotherapy drugs, 128, 288
Cytoxan, 131

## D

Dairy products
celiac disease and, 146
chronic candidiasis and, 163
senile cataracts and, 722
Dandelion root. *See Taraxacum officinale.*
DASH diet, 344-349
Dead Sea spa therapy, 705-706
Deep brain stimulation, 594
Deglycyrrhizinated licorice, 59
Dehydroepiandrosterone. *See* DHEA.
Dementia. *See* Alzheimer's disease; Senile dementia.
*Demodex folliculorum,* 711
Dennie's sign, 90
Dental amalgams and lichen planus, 457
Depression
alcoholism and, 15, 22, 33-34
botanical medicines, 21, 22
chronic fatigue syndrome and, 170
conventional versus natural interventions, 9f
diabetes mellitus and, 212
diagnosis, 8, 9f
environmental toxins and, 14
epilepsy and, 244
fibromyalgia syndrome and, 263
hormonal factors in, 13-14
hypothyroidism and, 380
irritable bowel syndrome and, 440
lifestyle factors in, 14-15, 22
models, 11-12
monoamine metabolism and precursor therapy for, 18-21
nutrition and, 16-18, 21-22
premenstrual syndrome and, 657
supplements for, 16-18, 22
therapeutic approach, 21-22
therapeutic considerations, 12-13
trichomoniasis and, 733
Dermatitis herpetiformis
causes of, 191
conventional versus natural interventions, 192f
diagnosis, 191
hypothyroidism and, 381
therapeutic approach, 193
therapeutic considerations, 191, 193
*See also* Atopic dermatitis.
Dermographism, 738-39
Dessiccated thyroid, 383-384
Detoxification
dysfunction, 592
porphyrias and, 649
Devil's claw. *See Harpagophytum procumbens.*
DeVita, Vincent, Jr., 131
DGL. *See* Deglycyrrhizinated licorice.
DHA, attention deficit hyperactivity disorder and, 100-101
DHEA
Alzheimer's disease and, 45
asthma and, 65
depression and, 13
Hashimoto's disease, 385
HIV/AIDS and, 323, 331
rheumatoid arthritis and, 696, 700
DHT. *See* Dihydrotestosterone.
Diabetes insipidus, 288
Diabetes mellitus
atherosclerosis and, 75, 77, 89, 211
causes of and risk factors, 200-205, 203-205
celiac disease and, 144
classification, 194, 195f, 197f, 198-99
complications of, 194, 196f, 198, 209-212, 220-221
conventional versus natural interventions, 195f, 197f
diagnosis, 194, 199-200
diet therapy and, 212
early treatment and possible reversal of, 202
flavonoids and, 219-220
gestational, 199
hypoglycemia and, 367
insulin function and sensitivity improvement, 217-218
nutritional and herbal supplements, 213-217
obesity and, 542-543
patient monitoring, 205-207, 208t
pre-, 199
preventing nutritional and oxidative stress in, 218-220
secondary, 199
senile dementia and, 40t
supplements for, 222-225
therapeutic approach, 222-225
therapeutic considerations, 212-221
Diabetic nephropathy, 211, 221, 225
Diabetic neuropathy, 211, 221
Diabetic retinopathy, 211, 220, 225
Diagnosis
acne vulgaris/conglobata, 3
affective disorders, 8-11, 22-23
alcoholism, 26
Alzheimer's disease, 36, 39-42
angina pectoris, 48, 50
aphthous stomatitis, 56
asthma, 60
atopic dermatitis, 90
attention deficit hyperactivity disorder in children, 97
bacterial sinusitis, 107
benign prostatic hyperplasia, 112, 114
cancer, 119
carpal tunnel syndrome, 136, 138-139
celiac disease, 142, 145
cellulite, 147
cervical dysplasia, 152

Diagnosis *(Continued)*
chronic candidiasis, 161, 163
chronic fatigue syndrome, 167, 170
congestive heart failure, 177, 179
cystitis, 183, 185-186
dermatitis herpetiformis, 191
diabetes mellitus, 194, 199-200
endometriosis, 226, 228
epilepsy, 233, 236-237
erythema multiforme, 246
fibrocystic breast disease, 249, 251
fibromyalgia syndrome, 255
gallstones, 267
glaucoma, 275, 277
gout, 281
hair loss in women, 289
hepatitis, 294, 296
herpes simplex, 303, 305
HIV/AIDS, 308, 312-315
hypertension, 337
hyperthyroidism, 351, 353-355
hyperventilation syndrome/breathing pattern disorders, 361, 363-364
hypoglycemia, 367, 369-370
hypothyroidism, 377, 380-381
infectious diarrhea, 394, 398-399
inflamed eye, 279t
inflammatory bowel disease, 406
insomnia, 424
intestinal protozoan infestation, 433
irritable bowel syndrome, 436
kidney stones, 442, 444-45
leukoplakia, 451
macular degeneration, 459
menopause, 476
menorrhagia, 492
migraine headaches, 502, 504
multiple sclerosis, 521, 525
obesity, 538
osteoarthritis, 552, 554-55
osteoporosis, 565, 570-572
otitis media, 581
Parkinson's disease, 588, 592-594
pelvic inflammatory disease, 605, 609-612
peptic ulcers, 618
periodontal disease, 625
pneumonia, 633, 637-638, 639
porphyrias, 640
premenstrual syndrome, 650, 652
psoriasis, 684
rheumatoid arthritis, 693, 696-699
rosacea, 708
seborrheic dermatitis, 713
senile cataracts, 717
streptococcal pharyngitis, 725
trichomoniasis, 729, 731-732
urticaria, 744-46
uterine fibroids, 748, 750
vaginitis and vulvovaginitis, 756, 767-768, 770f
varicose veins, 772
*See also* Laboratory tests.
Diamine oxidase and migraine headaches, 509
Diarrhea. *See* Infectious diarrhea.
Diathermy
bacterial sinusitis and, 111
pelvic inflammatory disease and, 613, 616
*Dictamnus dasycarpus*, 301
Diet and nutrition
acne vulgaris/conglobata and, 5-6, 7
alcoholism and, 30-33, 34
Alzheimer's disease and, 42, 46-47
angina pectoris and, 51, 52-53, 55
aphthous stomatitis and, 58, 59
asthma and, 65-66, 71
atherosclerosis and, 77-80
atopic dermatitis and, 95
attention deficit hyperactivity disorder and, 100-101
benign prostatic hyperplasia and, 115-116, 117-118
bipolar (manic) depression and, 24
cancer and, 126-27, 135
carpal tunnel syndrome and, 139, 141
celiac disease and, 145
cellulite and, 151
cervical dysplasia and, 155-158, 159
chronic candidiasis and, 163
chronic fatigue syndrome and, 173-174, 175
congestive heart failure and, 180-181, 182
cystitis and, 189
depression and, 16, 21-22
dermatitis herpetiformis and, 193
diabetes mellitus and, 203, 212
endometriosis and, 228-29, 231
epilepsy and, 237-38, 237-239, 244
fibrocystic breast disease and, 254
fibromyalgia syndrome and, 263
gallstones and, 270-272, 273-274
glaucoma and, 277-278
gout and, 281, 284, 287
hair loss in women and, 292-293
hepatitis and, 298-299, 301
herpes simplex and, 307
HIV/AIDS and, 322-324, 336
hypertension and, 343-344, 349-350
hyperthyroidism and, 355-359
hyperventilation syndrome/breathing pattern disorders and, 365
hypoglycemia and, 371-373, 374
hypothyroidism and, 382-383
immune system function, 389-390
infectious diarrhea and, 400-402
inflammatory bowel disease and, 409, 412-417, 420
irritable bowel syndrome and, 438-439, 441
kidney stones and, 445-447, 449
macular degeneration and, 461-463, 463-464
male infertility and, 471-473, 475
Mediterranean, 77-78, 85, 88
menopause and, 487-488, 491
menorrhagia and, 500

Diet and nutrition *(Continued)*
migraine headaches and, 508-512, 515-516
multiple sclerosis and, 526-527, 530-531
nausea and vomiting of pregnancy and, 535, 536-537
obesity and, 545-551
osteoarthritis and, 557-558
osteoporosis and, 573-575, 579-580
otitis media and, 586
Parkinson's disease and, 595-596, 596-597, 603-604
pelvic inflammatory disease and, 616
peptic ulcers and, 621-623, 624
periodontal disease and, 632
porphyrias and, 648-49, 649
premenstrual syndrome and, 654-655, 661-662
psoriasis and, 688-89, 691-692
rheumatoid arthritis and, 699-700, 701-703, 706
seborrheic dermatitis and, 716
senile cataracts and, 719-722, 723
senile dementia and, 40t
trichomoniasis and, 733, 735
urticaria and, 745, 746-747
uterine fibroids and, 751-752
vaginitis and, 764-765, 768
varicose veins and, 774, 776-77
*See also* Supplements.
Dietary Approaches to Stop Hypertension, 344-349
Dietary fats
saturated
Alzheimer's disease and, 38
diabetes mellitus and, 204
male infertility and, 472-473
obesity and, 549-550
premenstrual syndrome and, 654, 655
rheumatoid arthritis and, 700
uterine fibroids and, 751
trans fatty acids
Alzheimer's disease and, 38
atherosclerosis and, 79
diabetes mellitus and, 204
male infertility and, 472-473
rheumatoid arthritis and, 700
Diethylstilbestrol, 116
Dihydrotestosterone, 112
Dimethyl sulfoxide, 328
Dioxin and endometriosis, 231
Disturbances of electrolyte metabolism and senile dementia, 40t
Diuretics, 342, 343
D-Mannose, 188, 190
Docetaxel, 132
Docosahexanoic acid. *See* DHA.
Dopamine activity in attention deficit hyperactivity disorder, 97, 99
Douching, 615
Down's syndrome, 36, 42
Doxorubicin, 131
*Drosera rotundifolia*, 69
Drugs
acne vulgaris/conglobata, 7
antibiotic, 107, 109, 399, 400, 403, 581, 583, 612-613, 639, 710, 725, 727, 731, 732-733, 740
antidepressant, 12, 264
antihypertensive, 342-343
antiviral, 327
atherosclerosis, 78-79
attention deficit hyperactivity disorder, 104
bacterial sinusitis, 107, 109
bipolar (manic) depression, 23
chemotherapy, 121
hair loss in women and, 291, 292t
hyperthyroidism and, 353
induced headaches, 507-508
-induced parkinsonism, 594
infectious diarrhea, 399, 403
mucolytic, 109
multiple sclerosis, 525-526
oral hypoglycemic, 376
osteoarthritis, 556
osteoporosis, 572-573
osteoporosis and, 569
otitis media, 581
Parkinson's disease, 604
pelvic inflammatory disease, 612-613
pneumonia, 639
porphyrias and, 647
rosacea, 710
streptococcal pharyngitis, 725, 727
tamoxifen, 132, 269
thyroid, 383-384
trichomoniasis, 731
urticaria and, 740-741
*See also* Botanical medicines.
Duodenal ulcers, 618
Dust mites, 95
Dysbiosis, 695
Dysfunctional uterine bleeding, 494
Dyspareunia, 608


## E


*E. coli*, 396-397, 399, 400, 605
Ear drops, herbal, 583, 585, 587
Eastern Cooperative Oncology Group (ECOG) score, 123-124
*Echinacea*, 391, 392, 418
otitis media and, 586
pneumonia and, 637
streptococcal pharyngitis and, 728
trichomoniasis and, 735
uterine fibroids and, 752, 755
vaginitis and, 768
Ectomorph body type, 540
Eczema. *See* Atopic dermatitis.
Edetate calcium disodium. *See* EDTA (edetate calcium disodium).
EDTA (edetate calcium disodium)
bipolar (manic) depression and, 24
chelation therapy, 54, 88
depression and, 14

EEG (electroencephalogram), senile dementia and, 41-42
EFAs. *See* Essential fatty acids.
Egger theory, 509
Ehlers-Danlos syndrome, 275, 277
Eicosanoid metabolism, 410
Eicosapentaenoic acid, 285
Electroencephalogram. *See* EEG (electroencephalogram).
Electrolyte replacement
  alcoholism and, 35
  infectious diarrhea and, 400
Elemental diet, 414
*Eleutherococcus senticosus,* 174, 175, 475
Elimination diet, 414
EM. *See* Erythema multiforme.
*Emblica officinalis,* 359
EMS. *See* Eosinophiliamyalgia syndrome.
Emulsifiers, food, 743
Encephalomyelitis and senile dementia, 39t
Endocrine disorders
  acne and, 3-5
  affective disorders and, 13-14
  atherosclerosis and, 83
  atopic dermatitis and, 94
  depression and, 13-14
  HIV/AIDS and, 331
  senile dementia and, 40t
Endometrial cancer, 479
Endometriosis
  botanical medicines, 230-232
  conventional versus natural interventions, 227f
  diagnosis, 226, 228
  risk factors, 226
  supplements for, 229-231, 231
  therapeutic approach, 231-232
  therapeutic considerations, 228-229
Endomorph body type, 540
Endorphins, 15, 656
Endothelial cells, 73
Endotoxemia and inflammatory bowel disease, 411-412
Enemas, butyrate, 418-419
Entacapone, 604
*Entamoeba histolytica,* 398
  intestinal protozoan infestation and, 433
Enteric-coated volatile oils, 440
Enteroviruses, 201
Environmental toxins
  asthma and, 71
  atopic dermatitis and, 96
  attention deficit hyperactivity disorder and, 99-100
  chronic fatigue syndrome and, 170-171
  depression and, 14
  epilepsy and, 237
  multiple sclerosis and, 525
  osteoporosis and, 569
  Parkinson's disease and, 591-592
  porphyrias and, 646-647
Enzymes
  cancer and, 131
  celiac disease and, 145-146
  HIV/AIDS and, 321
  hyperuricemia and, 287
  migraine headaches and, 509-510
  porphyrias and, 645
  uterine fibroids and, 752, 755
Eosinophiliamyalgia syndrome, 18-19
EPA
  gout and, 287
  rheumatoid arthritis and, 700
*Ephedra sinica,* 69, 72, 301
Epicatechin and diabetes mellitus, 202
Epidemiology
  cervical dysplasia, 154
  epilepsy, 233
  lichen planus, 456
  multiple sclerosis, 523
  periodontal disease, 625, 627
Epididymitis, 729
Epilepsy
  botanical medicines, 242-243
  causes of, 235
  classification, 235-236
  conventional versus natural interventions, 234f
  diagnosis, 233, 236-37
  dietary considerations, 237-239, 244
  environmental toxins and, 237
  epidemiology, 233
  etiology, 235
  genetic factors, 233
  nutritional considerations, 239-242, 244-245
  pathophysiology, 237
  spiritual healing and, 243-244
  therapeutic approach, 244-45
  therapeutic considerations, 237-44
Epileptic dementia, 39t
Epinephrine and asthma, 63
Epstein-Barr virus, 167, 169, 294, 303, 396
  rheumatoid arthritis and, 698
Ergotamine rebound headache, 507-508
Erythema multiforme
  conventional versus natural interventions, 247f
  diagnosis, 246
  manifestations, 246
  therapeutic approach, 248
  therapeutic considerations, 248
Erythropoietic porphyrias, 642
*Escherichia coli,* 396-397, 399, 400, 605
Escin, 151, 777
Essential fatty acids
  alcoholism and, 32-33
  Alzheimer's disease and, 44
  atherosclerosis and, 85
  atopic dermatitis and, 93
  attention deficit hyperactivity disorder and, 100-101
  benign prostatic hyperplasia and, 115
  chronic fatigue syndrome and, 174

Essential fatty acids *(Continued)*
endometriosis and, 229
epilepsy and, 242
hair loss in women and, 292
HIV/AIDS, 321
HIV/AIDS and, 324, 325, 329, 330, 336
menorrhagia and, 497
migraine headaches and, 510-511
nausea and vomiting of pregnancy and, 537
premenstrual syndrome and, 659
Essential hypertension, 339
Essential oils
atopic dermatitis and, 95
chronic candidiasis and, 165
trichomoniasis and, 734
Estradiol, 482, 501
Estrogen
Alzheimer's disease and, 42
asthma and, 64-65
environmental, 654
forms of, 485
male infertility and, 470-471
menopause and, 476
metabolism, 652-53, 654-655
migraine headaches and, 514-515
natural, 482-83
osteoarthritis and, 556-557
osteoporosis and, 569
Parkinson's disease and, 602
porphyrias and, 644
premenstrual syndrome and, 663
replacement therapy, 478-486
uterine fibroids and, 748
vitamin B and, 653
Ethanol metabolism, 29-30
Etiology
alcoholism, 28-29
Alzheimer's disease, 36, 38, 39t
carpal tunnel syndrome, 136
celiac disease, 144
cervical dysplasia, 152, 154
chronic fatigue syndrome, 167, 169-170
epilepsy, 235
hypertension, 341
inflammatory bowel disease, 408-409
lichen planus, 456
menorrhagia, 494
multiple sclerosis, 524-525
nausea and vomiting of pregnancy, 533
Parkinson's disease, 590
pelvic inflammatory disease, 607-608
porphyrias, 644-645
premenstrual syndrome, 650
rosacea, 710
senile cataracts, 719
senile dementia, 39-40t
varicose veins, 774
ETOH. *See* Alcohol and alcoholism.
Eucalyptus packs, 111
*Euphorbia hirta,* 69
European boxwood. *See Buxus sempervirens.*
Evening primrose oil
atopic dermatitis and, 95
fibrocystic breast disease and, 252
multiple sclerosis and, 528
rheumatoid arthritis and, 701
Excessive platelet aggregation and atherosclerosis, 85
Executive control in attention deficit hyperactivity disorder, 97, 99
Exercise
alcoholism and, 34, 35
angina pectoris and, 55
atherosclerosis and, 75, 77, 79
benign prostatic hyperplasia and, 114-115, 117
breathing, 54, 174, 366, 536
cellulite and, 150, 151
chronic fatigue syndrome and, 174
depression and, 15
diabetes mellitus and, 212-213
fibromyalgia syndrome and, 259, 263, 266
glaucoma and, 279
HIV/AIDS and, 333-334, 336
hypertension and, 344
hypoglycemia and, 373, 374
hypothyroidism and, 383, 386
insomnia and, 428
irritable bowel syndrome and, 441
isometric, 561
macular degeneration and, 463, 464
multiple sclerosis and, 530, 532
nausea and vomiting of pregnancy and, 536
osteoarthritis and, 557-58, 564
osteoporosis and, 569, 579
premenstrual syndrome and, 656
rheumatoid arthritis and, 705
varicose veins and, 774
wrist, 141
Expectorants, 635
External hemorrhoids, 677-678
Eye
differential diagnosis of inflamed, 279t
*See also* Macular degeneration.

## F

Fasting blood glucose, 199-200
Fasting hypoglycemia, 367
Fat cells
brown, 545-546
engorgement, 543-544
number and size, 542
Fatty liver, 30
FBD. *See* Fibrocystic breast disease.
Fecal calprotectin, 419
Fenugreek seeds, 218
Ferulic acid, 488
Fetal alcohol syndrome, 28
Feverfew. *See Tanacetum parthenium.*

Fiber intake
alcoholism and, 34
angina pectoris and, 55
atherosclerosis and, 79
chronic candidiasis and, 164
depression and, 21
diabetes mellitus and, 204, 216, 222
endometriosis and, 228-229
fibrocystic breast disease and, 252, 253, 254
gallstones and, 270-271, 274
hypoglycemia, 372-373
hypothyroidism and, 384
irritable bowel syndrome and, 438-439, 441
male infertility and, 471
peptic ulcers and, 621
premenstrual syndrome and, 655
proctologic conditions and, 672, 674, 675
psoriasis and, 687, 692
supplements for obesity, 548-549, 550
uterine fibroids and, 751
varicose veins and, 774, 776-777
Fibrinogen and atherosclerosis, 85
Fibrocystic breast disease
conventional versus natural interventions, 250f
diagnosis, 249, 251
diet and, 254
methylxanthines and, 251-252
signs and symptoms, 249, 251
supplements for, 252-253, 254
therapeutic approach, 254
therapeutic considerations, 251-253
Fibromyalgia Impact Questionnaire, 263
Fibromyalgia syndrome
chronic fatigue syndrome and, 169
conventional versus natural interventions, 256f
depression and, 263
diagnosis, 255
integrated metabolic therapies, 263
mechanisms, 257
metabolism-regulating therapies for, 258-259
patient status assessment, 262-263, 264-265
rehabilitation, 262-264
signs and symptoms, 257-258
supplements for, 265-266
therapeutic approach, 264-266
therapeutic considerations, 259-264
thyroid function and, 259-261, 263, 265
FibroQuest Symptoms Survey, 262-263
Fingerprint patterns and Alzheimer's disease, 42
Fish oil. *See* Omega-3 fatty acids.
Fissure, anal, 665f, 672-674
Fistula, anal, 666f, 671-672
Fitz-Hugh-Curtis syndrome, 608, 611
Flavonoids
asthma and, 68
atopic dermatitis and, 93
bacterial sinusitis and, 110
cancer and, 134
cystitis and, 190
diabetes mellitus and, 219-220
glaucoma and, 278, 280
herpes simplex and, 307
immune system function and, 392
inflammatory bowel disease and, 417
macular degeneration and, 463
menorrhagia and, 497, 501
osteoporosis and, 578-579
otitis media and, 586
peptic ulcers and, 622, 624
periodontal disease and, 631, 632
pneumonia and, 636
proctologic conditions and, 675
senile cataracts and, 722-723
streptococcal pharyngitis and, 728
uterine fibroids and, 753
vaginitis and, 765
varicose veins and, 777
Flavorings, food, 742
Flaxseed oil
Alzheimer's disease and, 47
atopic dermatitis, 93
atopic dermatitis and, 95
benign prostatic hyperplasia and, 118
depression and, 22
endometriosis and, 229
fibrocystic breast disease and, 254
hypertension and, 350
menopause and, 488
menorrhagia and, 497
psoriasis and, 691
seborrheic dermatitis and, 716
Floxuridine, 132
Fluconazole and HIV/AIDS, 325
Fluids. *See* Water intake.
Fluoride and osteoporosis, 578
Fluorouracil (5-Fu), 132, 133
Folate
Alzheimer's disease and, 38
atherosclerosis and, 86
cancer and, 130, 131, 132
cervical dysplasia and, 157, 159-160
depression and, 16-17, 22
epilepsy and, 240, 244
gout and, 285, 287
HIV/AIDS and, 318, 322
hypertension and, 347
infectious diarrhea and, 401, 404
inflammatory bowel disease and, 416
kidney stones and, 449
macrocytic anemia and, 329
male infertility and, 475
Parkinson's disease and, 597
periodontal disease and, 631, 632
seborrheic dermatitis and, 715

Folic acid. *See* Folate.
Folliculitis, 672
Food
  additives
    asthma and, 64
    urticaria and, 741-742
  allergies
    aphthous stomatitis and, 56, 58
    asthma and, 64, 65-66, 71
    atopic dermatitis and, 92-93
    attention deficit hyperactivity disorder and, 101-102
    celiac disease and, 142, 144-146
    chronic candidiasis and, 163
    chronic fatigue syndrome and, 172
    depression and, 18, 22
    dermatitis herpetiformis and, 193
    epilepsy and, 239
    gallstones and, 271
    infectious diarrhea and, 404
    inflammatory bowel disease and, 409
    irritable bowel syndrome and, 439
    migraine headaches and, 508-509, 515, 518-519t
    multiple sclerosis and, 530
    otitis media and, 584-585
    peptic ulcers and, 621
    rheumatoid arthritis and, 699
    rosacea and, 711, 712
    seborrheic dermatitis and, 713
    urticaria and, 741
  colorants, 741-742
  emulsifiers, 743
  flavorings, 742
  hypothyroidism and, 386
  preservatives, 742-743
  stabilizers, 743
  yeast-containing, 163, 164-165
Foot ulcers and diabetes mellitus, 211, 221, 225
Fractionated citrus pectin, 126
*Fraxinus/Ceanothus,* 752, 755
Free radicals
  Alzheimer's disease and, 38
  angina pectoris and, 54
  atherosclerosis and, 78
  diabetes mellitus and, 204, 210
  diet and, 77
  macular degeneration and, 459, 463
  male infertility and, 471, 474
  multiple sclerosis and, 524
  senile cataracts and, 723
  sleep and, 428
Fruits and vegetables
  Alzheimer's disease and, 42-43
  atherosclerosis and, 78, 88
  endometriosis and, 228-229
  fibromyalgia syndrome and, 265
  gallstones and, 270-271
  HIV/AIDS and, 318, 321
  hypertension and, 344
Fruits and vegetables *(Continued)*
  macular degeneration and, 461-462
  osteoporosis and, 567, 574
  Parkinson's disease and, 595
*Fucus vesiculosus,* 150, 151, 229
Fumaric acid and psoriasis, 689
Functional hypothyroidism, 379
Fusion inhibitors, 317, 320


## G


GAGs, 87-88
*Galanthus nivalis,* 46
Galantino, M. L., 316
Gallant, Joel E., 315
Gallbladder disease, 569
Gallstones
  botanical medicines, 274
  categories, 267
  chemical dissolution of, 272-273
  conventional versus natural interventions, 268f
  diagnosis, 267
  diet and, 270-72, 273-274
  hormone replacement therapy and, 481
  pathogenesis, 267, 269-270
  pigmented, 270
  risk factors, 269-270
  supplements for, 274
  therapeutic approach, 273-274
  therapeutic considerations, 270-273
Gamma linolenic acid, 701
Gamma-oryzanol, 488
Gargles, 728
Garlic. *See* Allium family.
Gastric acid
  osteoporosis and, 574
  peptic ulcers and, 618, 620
Gastric ulcers, 618, 620
Gastrointestinal function
  attention deficit hyperactivity disorder and, 102-103, 105
  chronic fatigue syndrome and, 171
  gallstones and, 269
  psoriasis and, 686-687
  *See also* Inflammatory bowel disease; Intestinal protozoan infestation.
*Gelsemium/Phytolacca,* 752
Gender
  gallstones and, 269
  hyperthyroidism and, 351
  hyperventilation syndrome/breathing pattern disorders and, 361
  kidney stones and, 442
Genetic factors
  Alzheimer's disease, 36, 38, 39t
  asthma, 60
  atherosclerosis, 76
  attention deficit hyperactivity disorder in children, 99
  benign prostatic hyperplasia, 112
  epilepsy, 233

Genetic factors *(Continued)*
- gallstones, 269
- hyperthyroidism, 353
- inflammatory bowel disease, 408
- multiple sclerosis, 524
- obesity, 542
- osteoporosis, 567, 568-569
- Parkinson's disease, 590
- porphyrias, 643
- rheumatoid arthritis, 695

Gentian violet, 767, 769
*Geranium maculatum,* 418
Gestational diabetes, 199
Ghrelin, 545
*Giardia intestinalis,* 398
- intestinal protozoan infestation and, 433

*Giardia lamblia,* 398
Ginger. *See Zingiber.*
Gingival sulcus, 627
*Ginkgo biloba*
- Alzheimer's disease and, 45-46, 47
- asthma and, 70
- atopic dermatitis and, 94
- attention deficit hyperactivity disorder and, 106
- depression and, 21, 22
- diabetes mellitus and, 225
- epilepsy and, 243
- macular degeneration and, 463, 464
- menopause and, 490, 491
- multiple sclerosis and, 530, 531
- Parkinson's disease and, 600-601, 604
- premenstrual syndrome and, 661, 663
- stroke and, 88

Ginseng
- attention deficit hyperactivity disorder and, 106
- chronic fatigue syndrome and, 174, 175
- diabetes mellitus and, 218
- epilepsy and, 243
- HIV/AIDS and, 318
- immune system function and, 391, 392-393
- male infertility and, 474, 475
- menopause and, 490
- rheumatoid arthritis and, 707

Glatiramer acetate, 525
Glaucoma
- collagen and, 275, 277
- conventional versus natural interventions, 276f
- diagnosis, 275
- nutrition and, 277-278
- therapeutic approach, 280
- therapeutic considerations, 277-280
- types of, 275

Gliadins, 142, 144, 146
- hair loss in women and, 293

Glibenclamide, 376
Gliclazide, 376
Glimepiride, 376
Glipizide, 376
GLP-1 hormone, 544
Glucocorticoids, 13, 556
Glucomannan, 224, 225
Glucosamine sulfate and osteoarthritis, 558, 563
Glucose
- hair loss in women and, 291
- hypoglycemia and, 367
- -insulin tolerance test, 369
- levels, nocturnal, 428-429
- monitoring, 205-207, 224
- tolerance test, 199-200, 203, 369

Glucosidase inhibitors and diabetes mellitus, 216-217, 223, 224
Glutamic acid, 286
- kidney stones and, 446

Glutathione
- HIV/AIDS and, 323
- Parkinson's disease and, 592, 597, 604
- psoriasis and, 689
- senile cataracts and, 720

Gluten sensitivity, 58, 142, 145
- dermatitis herpetiformis and, 191, 193
- diabetes mellitus and, 201
- hair loss in women and, 293

Glycemic index and glycemic load, 203-204, 212, 372
Glycine
- benign prostatic hyperplasia and, 118
- gout and, 286
- senile cataracts and, 724

Glycosylated hemoglobin, 200
Glycosylation of proteins, 210
*Glycyrrhiza glabra*
- asthma and, 69, 72
- atopic dermatitis and, 93, 94, 96
- chronic fatigue syndrome and, 175
- epilepsy and, 243
- hepatitis and, 299-300, 301
- HIV/AIDS and, 332
- peptic ulcers and, 623
- pneumonia and, 639
- premenstrual syndrome and, 660, 662
- psoriasis and, 690
- rheumatoid arthritis and, 707
- vaginitis and, 765, 769

Glycyrrhizin and lichen planus, 458
Goiters, 354, 379
Goitrogens, 382, 386
Goldenseal. *See Hydrastis.*
Gonorrhea. *See Neisseria gonorrhea.*
Gotu kola, 126, 150
Gout
- botanical medicines, 286, 287
- causes of, 281, 283
- conventional versus natural interventions, 282f
- diagnosis, 281
- diet and, 281, 284-285, 287
- signs and symptoms, 283
- supplements for, 285-286
- therapeutic approach, 286-288
- therapeutic considerations, 284-286

Granule matrix-derived mediators, 738

Grape seed extract
asthma and, 72
atherosclerosis and, 84-85
attention deficit hyperactivity disorder and, 105
diabetes mellitus and, 224
macular degeneration and, 463
Graves' disease, 351, 353, 354, 356, 359
Green tea, 69, 106
cancer and, 130
diabetes mellitus and, 222
Parkinson's disease and, 600, 604
*Grindelia camporum,* 69
Growth hormone, 428
Guar gum, 548-549
Gugulipid, 81-82
Guided imagery, 516
Gut
-derived appetite regulators, 544-545
-derived hormone applications, 544
microecology and premenstrual syndrome, 653
permeability and attention deficit hyperactivity disorder, 102
*Gymnema sylvestre,* 217, 223

## H

Hachimijiogan, 723, 724
*Haemophilus influenzae*
bacterial sinusitis and, 107
pelvic inflammatory disease and, 605
Hair
loss in women
causes of, 289
conventional versus natural interventions, 290f
diagnosis, 289
hypothyroidism and, 380
nutritional deficiency and, 292-293
physiology of hair cycle and, 289
as a side effect of drugs, 291, 292t
therapeutic considerations, 289, 291-293
mineral analysis, 448
Hair mineral analysis, 14
*Hamamelis virginiana,* 683
Hamster egg penetration test, 468
*Harpagophytum procumbens,* 286, 287, 562, 564
Hashimoto's thyroiditis, 354, 379, 380, 384-385
Hawthorn. *See Crataegus.*
Headache. *See* Migraine headache.
*Headache Alternative, The,* 517
*Headache and Diet,* 517
*Headache Free,* 517
*Headache Help,* 516
*Headache Relief for Women,* 516
Headaches, migraine, 371
*Headaches in Children,* 517
Head injury and Alzheimer's disease, 38, 39t
Heart attack. *See* Myocardial infarction.
Heavy metals
depression and, 14
male infertility and, 471
Parkinson's disease and, 591-592, 595, 596
porphyrias and, 647
senile cataracts and, 722
*Helicobacter pylori,* 109-110, 280, 510, 515, 620
rosacea and, 711, 712
Heme formation, 643
Hemorrhoids, 674-678
Hepatic porphyrias, 642
Hepatitis
antioxidants and, 300-301
botanical medicines, 299-301
causes of, 294
conventional versus natural interventions, 295f
diagnosis, 294, 296
nutritional considerations, 298-299, 301
prevention, 297-298
symptoms, 296
therapeutic approach, 301-302
therapeutic considerations, 297-301
types, 294
Herbal ear drops, 583, 585, 587
Herbal tincture, 327
Herpes simplex
botanical medicines, 306
conventional versus natural interventions, 304f
diagnosis, 303, 305
hepatitis and, 294
HIV/AIDS and, 326-327
immunologic aspects, 303, 305
proctologic conditions and, 679-680
recurrence rate, 303
supplements for, 305-6, 307
therapeutic approach, 306-307
therapeutic considerations, 305-306
topical preparations, 306, 307
vaginitis and, 763, 771
viruses included in, 303
Herxheimer reaction, 164-165
Hesperidin, 488, 491
High-complex carbohydrate, high-fiber diet, 414
Histamine, 93-94
migraine headaches and, 509, 520
HIV/AIDS
alternative treatments, 334-336
botanical medicines, 332-333, 336
*Candida albicans* and, 325
cardiovascular disease and, 325
CDC 1993 surveillance case definition of, 310-312
clinical history of patient with, 313-314
conventional versus natural interventions, 309f
diagnosis, 308, 312-315
diarrhea and, 325-326, 331
diet and, 336
fusion inhibitors and, 317, 320

HIV/AIDS *(Continued)*
herpes simplex and, 326-327
Kaposi's sarcoma and, 327-328
lipodystrophy and, 328
macrocytic anemia and, 329
medical management of, 315-316
movement therapies, 333-334
naturopathic medical management of, 316-317
neuropathy, 329
NNRTIs and, 317, 319
NRTIs and, 317-318
nutrient deficiencies and, 322-324
pathogenesis, 310
physical medicine and acupuncture for, 333
pregnancy and, 329-330
protease inhibitors and, 317, 319-320
psychological conditions and, 330
side effects and complications associated with, 324-332
structured treatment interruptions, 334-336
wasting syndrome, 330-332
Hodgkin's disease, 122
Homeopathy, 646
Homocysteine
Alzheimer's disease and, 38, 44
atherosclerosis and, 86
diabetes mellitus and, 210
Parkinson's disease and, 597
Hormonal vaginitis, 486, 758
*Hormone Headache, The,* 516-17
Hormones
Alzheimer's disease and, 42
appetite regulating, 544-545
asthma and, 64-65
depression and, 13-14, 19
inhibitors, 129
migraine headaches and, 514-515
natural, 231, 232, 482-483, 499-500
osteoarthritis and, 556-557
osteoporosis and, 568
premenstrual syndrome and, 656
replacement therapy
advantages of combined continuous, 485
benefits and risks of, 478-484
migraine headaches and, 514-515
osteoporosis and, 572-573
types of, 484-485
thyroid, 13-14, 260-261, 263, 265, 383-384, 384-386
Hot packs and bacterial sinusitis, 111
*How to Prevent and Treat Cancer with Natural Medicine,* 135
HPV. *See* Human papilloma virus.
5-HTP
depression and, 19, 22
insomnia and, 429
migraine headaches and, 506-507, 510, 516
obesity and, 548
5-HTP *(Continued)*
Parkinson's disease and, 596, 603
seasonal affective disorder, 25
Human papilloma virus, 154-155
Human recombinant interferon-beta, 525
Humidifiers, 586
Huntington's chorea, 39t
HupA. *See* Huperzine A.
Huperzine A, 46, 47
Hyaluronic acids, 556
*Hydrangea,* 447
*Hydrastis*
cystitis and, 189, 190
infectious diarrhea and, 403
inflammatory bowel disease and, 418
pelvic inflammatory disease and, 614, 616
pneumonia and, 638, 639
proctologic conditions and, 683
psoriasis and, 692
streptococcal pharyngitis and, 727, 728
tea, 111
trichomoniasis and, 735
vaginitis and, 766, 768, 769
Hydronephrosis, 750
Hydrotherapy, 140, 141, 359, 360, 676
Hydroxycitrate, 550
5-Hydroxy-L-tryptophan. *See* 5-HTP.
Hygiene and periodontal disease, 632
Hyperbaric oxygen and multiple sclerosis, 530
Hypercalciuria, 445
Hypercholesterolemia and atherosclerosis, 75-76
Hyperemesis gravidarum, 533
Hyperhomocysteinemia, 86
*Hypericum perforatum. See* St. John's Wort.
Hyperinsulinemia, 199
Hyperkeratinization, 3
Hyperketoacidemia, 288
Hyperlacticemia, 288
Hyperlipidemia, 76
Hyperplastic-hypertrophic obesity, 542
Hyperplastic obesity, 542
Hypertension
angina pectoris and, 48
atherosclerosis and, 75, 76, 77
botanical medicines, 349
classification, 337, 339-341
conventional versus natural interventions, 338f
DASH diet for, 344-349
diabetes mellitus and, 203, 210-211
diagnosis, 337
diet and, 349-350
drugs, 342-343
essential, 339
etiology, 341
lifestyle and dietary factors, 343-344
macular degeneration and, 459
stroke and, 76
therapeutic approach, 349-350
therapeutic considerations, 341-349
white coat, 340-41

Hyperthyroidism
botanical medicines, 358-359, 360
conventional versus natural interventions, 352f
diagnosis, 351, 353-355
diet and, 355-356, 360
disease risk, 351, 353
exercise and, 383
menorrhagia and, 494
supplements for, 356-359
therapeutic approach, 359-360
therapeutic considerations, 355-359
Hypertriglyceridemia, 76
Hypertrophic obesity, 542
Hyperuricemia, 287-288, 445
Hyperventilation syndrome/breathing pattern disorders
conventional versus natural interventions, 362f
diagnosis, 361, 363-364
diet and, 365
gender and, 361
organic causes of, 364
prevalence, 361
symptoms, 363-364
therapeutic approach, 365-366
therapeutic considerations, 365
Hypnosis and Parkinson's disease, 602-603
Hypoadrenalism and chronic fatigue syndrome, 172-173
Hypochlorhydria
asthma and, 64
chronic candidiasis and, 163
rosacea and, 710-711
Hypoglycemia
alcoholism and, 30
angina pectoris and, 55
categories, 367
chronic fatigue syndrome and, 172
conventional versus natural interventions, 368f
depression and, 16
diabetes mellitus and, 209
diagnosis, 367, 369-370
dietary factors, 371-373, 374
drugs, 376
epilepsy and, 237-238
health impact of, 370-371
lifestyle factors, 373, 374
migraine headaches and, 510
questionnaire, 369-370, 375f
senile dementia and, 40t
symptoms, 367, 369
therapeutic approach, 373-376
Hypoglycemic index, 369
Hypomania. *See* Bipolar (manic) depression.
Hypometabolism and fibromyalgia syndrome, 257
Hyponatremia and senile dementia, 40t
Hypothalamic-pituitary functions and depression, 14
Hypothyroidism
affective disorders and, 13-14
atherosclerosis and, 83
atopic dermatitis and, 94
causes of, 379
chronic fatigue syndrome and, 172
conventional versus natural interventions, 378f
diagnosis, 377, 380-381
diet and nutrition and, 382-383, 386
fibromyalgia syndrome and, 255, 258, 259-261
functional assessment, 381
hair loss in women and, 293
laboratory tests, 381
menorrhagia and, 494
osteoarthritis and, 557
premenstrual syndrome and, 656
prevalence, 377
senile dementia and, 40t
therapeutic approach, 384-386
therapeutic considerations, 382-384
thyroid hormone replacement for, 383-384
*Hyssopus officinalis,* 332

**I**

Imagery, guided, 516
Imaging tests and Alzheimer's disease, 41-42
Immobilization for carpal tunnel syndrome, 140
Immune modulators, 128-129
Immune system function
attention deficit hyperactivity disorder and, 103
botanical medicines, 391-392, 392-393
chronic candidiasis and, 164
chronic fatigue syndrome and, 169, 171
conventional versus natural interventions, 388f
diabetes mellitus and, 211
diagnosis of poor, 387
diet and, 389-390
herpes simplex and, 303, 305
HIV/AIDS and, 324
lifestyle and, 389
psoriasis and, 684, 686
psychoneuroimmunology and, 387
rheumatoid arthritis and, 695-696
streptococcal pharyngitis and, 727-728
therapeutic approach, 392-393
therapeutic considerations, 389-392
vaginitis and, 762
Immunoglobulin, 399, 457, 628
pneumonia and, 633, 635
urticaria and, 741
Impaired glucose tolerance, 199
Impedance, bioelectrical, 541-542
Indian tobacco. *See Lobelia inflata.*

Infection
  chronic fatigue syndrome and, 167, 169
  corneal, 279t
  diabetes mellitus and, 201
  genitourinary, 155, 470
  herpes simplex, 303, 305
  inflammatory bowel disease and, 408-409
  intestinal protozoan infestation, 433-435
  proctologic conditions and, 681
  urticaria and, 743
  vaginitis and, 759-764, 769-771
Infectious diarrhea
  bacterial agents, 396-398
  botanical medicines, 403-404, 405
  conventional medicines, 399
  conventional versus natural interventions, 395f
  diagnosis, 394, 398-399
  diet and, 400
  HIV/AIDS and, 325-326, 331
  hydration/electrolyte balance in, 400
  infectious agents and symptoms, 394, 396-398
  lab tests, 398-99
  parasitic agents, 398, 404
  probiotics and, 402-403
  supplements for, 400-402, 404-405
  therapeutic approach, 404-405
  therapeutic considerations, 399-404
  underlying and predisposing factors, 399-400
  viral agents in, 394, 396
Infertility
  endometriosis and, 226, 228
  trichomoniasis and, 729
  *See also* Male infertility.
Inflammation
  asthma and, 62-64
  atherosclerosis and, 77
  rheumatoid arthritis and, 695-696
Inflammatory bowel disease
  antibiotic exposure and, 409
  botanical medicines, 417-419, 420
  butyrate enemas and, 418-419
  in children, 419-20, 422-23
  clinical manifestations, 406, 408
  conventional versus natural interventions, 407f
  definition, 406
  diagnosis, 406
  dietary factors, 409, 420
  etiology, 408-409
  extra-gastrointestinal manifestations, 412
  genetic factors, 408
  infection and, 408-409
  malnutrition and, 412-414
  nutritional deficiencies, 412-417
  supplements for, 420
  therapeutic approach, 420-423
  therapeutic considerations, 410-419
  therapeutic monitoring and evaluation, 419-420
Influenza vaccine and asthma, 64
Infrared coagulation, 677
Inositol hexaniacinate
  atherosclerosis and, 89
  diabetes mellitus and, 215
  kidney stones and, 448
Insomnia
  botanical medicines, 431, 432
  causes of, 424, 426, 430-431
  conventional versus natural interventions, 425f
  diagnosis, 424
  nocturnal myoclonus and, 430-431
  normal sleep patterns and, 427-428
  restless leg syndrome and, 430-431
  sleep apnea and, 426-427
  therapeutic approach, 432
  therapeutic considerations, 428-431
  *See also* Sleep.
Insulin
  acne vulgaris/conglobata and, 5
  atherosclerosis and, 77
  celiac disease and, 144
  -dependent diabetes mellitus, 194, 195f, 198
  function and sensitivity improvement, 217-218
  glycemic index and glycemic load and, 203-204
  hypoglycemia and, 367
Intercourse during menses, 615
Intermittent claudication, 371
Internal hemorrhoids, 674-677
Intestinal flora
  alcoholism and, 34
  inflammatory bowel disease and, 411
  kidney stones and, 446
  rheumatoid arthritis and, 699-700
Intestinal hyperpermeability and attention deficit hyperactivity disorder, 102
Intestinal protozoan infestation
  botanical medicines, 435
  conventional versus natural interventions, 434f
  diagnosis, 433
  protozoans involved in, 433
  therapeutic approach, 435
  therapeutic considerations, 435
Intoxication and withdrawal symptoms, 29, 35
Intrauterine devices, 608-609, 615
Iodine
  deficiency
    fibrocystic breast disease and, 252-253, 254
    goiters and, 379
  hyperthyroidism and, 353, 355, 357
  hypothyroidism and, 382
  vaginitis and, 767
Iontophoresis, 673-674
Ipriflavone and osteoporosis, 578-579
Iritis, acute, 279t

Iron
attention deficit hyperactivity disorder and, 101, 105
hair loss in women and, 292-293
immune system function and, 390
inflammatory bowel disease and, 415
menorrhagia and, 496, 500
Parkinson's disease and, 592
porphyrias and, 649
rheumatoid arthritis and, 698
trichomoniasis and, 733
Irritable bowel syndrome
botanical medicines, 440, 441
conventional versus natural interventions, 437f
counseling for, 441
diagnosis, 436
dietary fiber and, 438-439, 441
supplements for, 439, 441
therapeutic approach, 441
therapeutic considerations, 438-441
Irritant vaginitis, 759
Isometric exercise, 561
*Isospora belli*, 398
Itching. *See* Pruritus.

**J**

Jin Bu Huan, 301
Johns Hopkins AIDS Service and AIDS Guide, 315
*Juglans nigra*, 435
Jujube plum. *See Zizyphi fructus.*

**K**

Kaposi's sarcoma, 327-328
Karnofsky score, 123-124
Kava kava, 21, 22, 301, 601
Kempo, 46
Ketoacidosis, diabetic, 205, 209
Ketogenic diet, 238, 595
Khella. *See Ammi visnaga.*
Kidney(s)
disease and osteoporosis, 569
gout and, 283, 288
stones
botanical medicines, 447
calcium, 449
causes of, 442
conventional versus natural interventions, 443f
diagnosis, 442, 444-445
dietary factors, 445-446, 449
lifestyle factors, 448
supplements for, 449
surgery, 449
therapeutic approach, 448-450
therapeutic considerations, 445-448
uric acid, 449-450
Korsakoff syndrome, 40t
Kynurenine, 19

**L**

Laboratory tests
Alzheimer's disease, 41

Laboratory tests *(Continued)*
benign prostatic hyperplasia, 114
chronic candidiasis, 163
chronic fatigue syndrome, 170, 171
cystitis, 185-86
diabetes mellitus, 199-200
epilepsy, 236-237
HIV/AIDS, 312-315
hyperthyroidism, 355
hypoglycemia, 369-370
hypothyroidism, 381
infectious diarrhea, 398-399
osteoporosis, 571-572
pelvic inflammatory disease, 611-612
porphyrias, 645-646
rheumatoid arthritis, 698-699
thyroid function, 259-260
urticaria, 745
*See also* Diagnosis.
LAC. *See* L-Acetylcarnitine and Alzheimer's disease.
L-Acetylcarnitine and Alzheimer's disease, 45, 47
*Lactobacillus acidophilus*
alcoholism and, 35
atopic dermatitis and, 93, 95
fibrocystic breast disease and, 254
infectious diarrhea and, 402-403, 405
intestinal protozoan infestation and, 435
irritable bowel syndrome and, 439, 441
trichomoniasis and, 735
vaginitis and, 764, 766-767, 769
Lactoferrin and streptococcal pharyngitis, 728
Lactose intolerance and migraine headaches, 510
L-Arginine
cancer and, 126
congestive heart failure and, 181
herpes simplex and, 305-306
HIV/AIDS and, 324, 325
hypertension and, 348, 350
male infertility and, 473
*Laribacter hongkongensis*, 398
*Larrea tridentata*, 301
L-Carnitine
alcoholism and, 31, 35
angina pectoris and, 52, 55
chronic fatigue syndrome and, 174, 175
congestive heart failure and, 181
HIV/AIDS and, 318, 323, 325, 328, 329, 331, 336
hyperthyroidism and, 357-358, 360
male infertility and, 473
L-Cysteine and senile cataracts, 724
Lead
attention deficit hyperactivity disorder and, 100
gout and, 284, 288
mobilization test, 14
Leaky gut
asthma and, 64
atopic dermatitis and, 92
diabetes mellitus and, 201

Learned helplessness model of depression, 12
Lecithin. *See* Phosphatidylcholine.
Lee, John, 754
Left-handedness, 353
Lemon balm. *See Melissa officinalis.*
*Lentinus edodes,* 332, 334
*Leonurus,* 230, 231
*Leptotania,* 447
Leukemia, 122
Leukocytes, 92
Leukoplakia
  conventional versus natural interventions, 452f
  diagnosis, 451
  oral cancer and, 451
  therapeutic approach, 453
  therapeutic considerations, 451, 453
Levodopa, 594, 595
Levothyroid, 384
Lewy bodies, 593
L-Glutamine
  alcoholism and, 33, 35
  benign prostatic hyperplasia and, 118
  cancer and, 126, 132, 134
  HIV/AIDS and, 326, 328, 331
  infectious diarrhea and, 401-402, 405
  peptic ulcers and, 624
  senile cataracts and, 724
Lichen planus
  botanical medicines, 457-458
  conventional versus natural interventions, 455f
  course of oral, 456
  diagnosis, 454
  epidemiology, 456
  etiology, 456
  incidence, 456
  onset, 456
  signs and symptoms, 454
  supplements, 457-458
  therapeutic considerations, 457-458
  variants, 456
Licorice root. *See Glycyrrhiza glabra.*
Lifestyle factors
  Alzheimer's disease and, 38, 46
  angina pectoris and, 51, 55
  atherosclerosis and, 79, 88
  benign prostatic hyperplasia and, 114-115, 117
  cellulite and, 150
  chronic fatigue syndrome and, 175
  depression and, 14-15, 22
  diabetes mellitus and, 203
  epilepsy and, 244
  gallstones and, 273
  HIV/AIDS and, 336
  hypertension and, 343-344
  hypoglycemia and, 373, 374
  hypothyroidism and, 384
  immune system function, 389
  insomnia and, 432
  kidney stones and, 448
Lifestyle factors *(Continued)*
  macular degeneration and, 463, 464
  menopause and, 490-491, 491
  osteoporosis, 567
  osteoporosis and, 569, 573
  Parkinson's disease and, 603
  peptic ulcers, 621
  trichomoniasis and, 733
  urticaria and, 745
Light therapy
  Alzheimer's disease and, 47
  bipolar (manic) depression and, 24
  psoriasis and, 690, 692
  seasonal affective disorder and, 25
  urticaria and, 744, 747
Liotrix, 384
Lipodystrophy, 328
Lipotropics
  endometriosis and, 230, 231
  fibrocystic breast disease and, 254
  gallstones and, 272
  uterine fibroids and, 751-752, 755
Lithium, 23
  vaginitis and, 765, 769
Lithotripsy, 449
Liver
  alcohol dehydrogenase, 29-30
  atherosclerosis and, 76, 80, 82
  attention deficit hyperactivity disorder and, 100
  chronic candidiasis and, 164
  chronic fatigue syndrome and, 170-171
  damage and alcoholism, 31-32
  detoxification, 653-654
  endometriosis and, 230
  extracts, 298, 301
  fibrocystic breast disease and, 253
  hepatitis and, 296, 298, 301
  hypothyroidism and, 382
  inflammatory bowel disease and, 412
  nausea and vomiting of pregnancy and, 535
  porphyrias and, 649
  premenstrual syndrome and, 653-654
  psoriasis and, 687-88
  uterine fibroids and, 751
*Lobelia inflata,* 69, 636
Loss of neuronal redundancy, 39t
Low-level laser therapy for carpal tunnel syndrome, 140
Low-protein diet, 595-596
LP. *See* Lichen planus.
L-Tryptophan
  alcoholism and, 33-34
  asthma and, 67
  bipolar (manic) depression and, 23
  depression and, 13-14, 15
  eosinophiliamyalgia syndrome and, 18-19
  insomnia and, 429, 432
  irritable bowel syndrome and, 439
Lutein, 462, 464, 719-720, 723
Lycopene and male infertility, 472

*Lycopus,* 358-59
Lymphocytes, 627
Lymphogranuloma venereum, 679
Lymphoma, 122
Lysine
  herpes simplex and, 305-306, 307
  HIV/AIDS and, 327
  vaginitis and vulvovaginitis and, 765

**M**

Macrocytic anemia, 329
Macrophages and monocytes, 627
Macular degeneration
  atherosclerosis and, 459, 461
  botanical medicines, 463, 464
  conventional versus natural interventions, 460f
  diagnosis, 459
  dietary fruits and vegetables and, 461-462
  lifestyle factors, 463, 464
  risk factors, 459
  therapeutic approach, 463-464
  therapeutic considerations, 461-463
  types of, 459, 461
Magnesium
  alcoholism and, 32, 35
  Alzheimer's disease and, 42-43
  ammonium phosphate stones, 450
  angina pectoris and, 53, 55
  asthma and, 68-69, 72
  atherosclerosis and, 86
  attention deficit hyperactivity disorder and, 101, 105
  chronic fatigue syndrome and, 173-174, 175
  congestive heart failure and, 180
  diabetes mellitus and, 215, 221, 225
  epilepsy and, 241, 244
  fibromyalgia syndrome and, 266
  glaucoma and, 278, 280
  HIV/AIDS and, 323
  hypertension and, 346-347, 350
  inflammatory bowel disease and, 415
  insomnia and, 432
  insufficiency and angina pectoris, 48
  kidney stones and, 446, 449
  migraine headaches and, 511-512, 516
  osteoporosis and, 577, 580
  premenstrual syndrome and, 658, 662
  trichomoniasis and, 733
Magnetic resonance imaging. *See* MRI (magnetic resonance imaging).
Magnetic therapies, 561
Ma huang, 69, 301
Malabsorption
  HIV/AIDS and, 326, 331
  multiple sclerosis and, 530
Male infertility
  avoiding estrogens and, 470-471
  botanical medicines, 474, 475
  causes of, 467-69
Male infertility *(Continued)*
  conventional versus natural interventions, 466f
  diagnosis, 465
  genitourinary infections and, 470
  incidence, 465
  nutritional considerations, 471-473, 475
  scrotal temperature and, 469, 474
  therapeutic approach, 474-475
  therapeutic considerations, 469-474
Malnutrition and inflammatory bowel disease, 412-414
*Managing Your Migraine,* 516
Manganese
  diabetes mellitus and, 215
  epilepsy and, 241, 244
  rheumatoid arthritis and, 702, 707
Manual manipulation for carpal tunnel syndrome, 140, 141
Marfan's syndrome, 277
Marshmallow root. *See Althea officinalis.*
Massage
  cellulite and, 150, 151
  HIV/AIDS and, 333
  rheumatoid arthritis and, 707
Mastalgia, 249
Mast cells
  aphthous stomatitis and, 58
  asthma and, 62
  periodontal disease and, 628
  urticaria and, 738
Maternal drug use and attention deficit hyperactivity disorder, 99-100
Meal replacement formulas, 548
*Medicago sativa,* 564
*Medical Management of HIV Infection,* 315
Medications. *See* Botanical medicines; Drugs.
Mediterranean diet, 77-78, 85, 88
Medium-chain triglycerides, 549-550
Melaleuca
  alternifolia
    acne vulgaris/conglobata and, 6
    chronic candidiasis and, 165
    trichomoniasis and, 734, 735
    vaginitis and, 766, 769
  leucadendron and HIV/AIDS, 333
Melatonin
  Alzheimer's disease and, 45
  asthma and, 65
  cancer and, 130, 134
  depression and, 19
  epilepsy and, 242, 245
  HIV/AIDS and, 331
  insomnia and, 430, 432
  migraine headaches and, 514, 516
  Parkinson's disease and, 598
  peptic ulcers and, 622-623
  seasonal affective disorder and, 25
  senile cataracts and, 722
*Melissa officinalis,* 306, 327, 766

Menopause
 benefits and risks of conventional and natural HRT, 478-484
 botanical medicines, 489-490, 491
 causes of, 476
 conventional versus natural interventions, 477f
 coronary heart disease and, 479-481
 diagnosis, 476
 diet and nutrition and, 487-488
 estrogen replacement therapy and, 478
 gallstones and, 481
 lifestyle factors, 490-491, 491
 natural hormones and, 482-483
 osteoporosis and, 478, 479
 as social construct, 478
 stroke and, 480-481
 symptoms of, 485-486
 task force recommendations for treating, 483
 therapeutic approach, 491
 therapeutic considerations, 486-491
 topical preparations, 490
 types of hormone replacement therapy for, 484-485
Menorrhagia
 botanical medicines, 498-499, 501
 conventional versus natural interventions, 493f
 diagnosis, 492
 diet and, 500
 estimating menstrual blood loss and, 495
 etiology, 494
 natural hormones and, 499-500
 patterns, 492
 supplements for, 496-498, 500
 therapeutic approach, 500-501
 therapeutic considerations, 496-500
Mental attitude and chronic fatigue syndrome, 173
*Mentha piperita,* 535
Menthol, 111
Mercury exposure and hyperthyroidism, 353
Mesomorph body type, 540
Metabolism
 androgen-dependent disorder of, 112
 effects of alcohol, 29-30
 eicosanoid, 410
 estrogen, 652-653, 654-655
 HIV/AIDS and, 331
 hypothyroidism and, 380
 -impairing medicines, 264, 266
 obesity and, 547
 uric acid, 447
Metformin, 376
Methionine
 fibrocystic breast disease and, 254
 gallstones and, 274
 kidney stones and, 450
Methotrexate, 132
3-methoxy-4-hydroxyphenethylene glycol (MHPG), 20
Methylcobalamin, 47
Methylxanthines and fibrocystic breast disease, 251-252
Metronidazole, 731, 732-33
MHPG. *See* 3-methoxy-4-hydroxyphenethylene glycol.
MI. *See* Myocardial infarction
Michigan alcoholism screening test, 28
Microcurrent therapy for carpal tunnel syndrome, 141
Micronized diosmin, 776, 777
*Microsporidia,* 398
Microtubule and chromatin inhibitors, 128
Microwaves, 95
*Migraine: Everything You Need to Know...,* 517
Migraine headaches
 botanical medicines, 513-514
 causes of, 502, 518f
 classification, 504, 517f
 conventional versus natural interventions, 503f
 diagnosis, 502, 504
 diet and, 508-510, 515-516, 518-519t
 histamine-induced, 509, 520
 hormones and, 514-515
 hypoglycemia and, 371
 neuronal disorder theory, 506
 pain, 502
 pathophysiology, 505-507
 patient resources, 516-517
 physical medicine, 512-513, 516
 platelet disorder theory, 505-506
 as a serotonin deficiency syndrome, 506-507
 stages, 507
 supplements for, 510-512, 516
 symptoms, 502, 504
 therapeutic approach, 515-520
 therapeutic considerations, 507-515
 vasomotor instability theory, 505
Milk. *See* Dairy products.
Milk thistle, 34, 126
 cancer and, 131
 chronic candidiasis and, 164
 endometriosis and, 229
 hepatitis and, 300, 301
 HIV/AIDS and, 320, 324, 332, 336
Mint, 537
Mistletoe. *See Viscum album.*
*Mitchella repens,* 447
Mold, 163
*Momordica charantia,* 217-218, 332
Monoamine metabolism and precursor therapy for depression, 18-21
Monoclonal antibodies, 128-129
Monolaurin, 327
Monopolar direct current technique, 676-677
Morning sickness. *See* Nausea and vomiting of pregnancy.
*Morus indica,* 217
Mother wort. *See Leonurus.*

Mouth. *See* Aphthous stomatitis; Lichen planus.
Movement therapies and HIV/AIDS, 333-334
MRI (magnetic resonance imaging), Alzheimer's disease and, 42
MS. *See* Multiple sclerosis.
Mucin defects, 410-411
Mucolytics and bacterial sinusitis, 109
*Mucuna pruriens,* 601, 604
Mulberry plant, 217
Multiple sclerosis
  botanical medicine, 530
  conventional versus natural interventions, 522f
  diagnosis, 521, 525
  diet therapy, 526-527, 530-531
  epidemiology, 523
  etiology, 524-525
  pathogenesis, 523-524
  relapsing/remitting, 521, 523
  supplements for, 527-29, 531
  therapeutic approach, 530-532
  therapeutic considerations, 525-529
Murray, Michael, 135
Muscle weakness and hypothyroidism, 380
Mushroom extracts and cancer, 131
*Mycoplasma hominis,* 605
Mycoplasmal pneumonia, 637
Mycotoxins, 40t
Myocardial infarction
  excessive platelet aggregation and, 85
  fibrinogen and, 85
  hyperhomocysteinemia and, 86
  preventing recurring, 87-88
  "type A" personality and, 86
Myoclonus, nocturnal, 430-431
Myxedema, 377

## N

*N*-acetyl-cysteine
  bacterial sinusitis and, 110
  HIV/AIDS and, 324
Nateglinide, 376
Naturopathic medicine
  chemotherapy support, 130-132
  gout and, 284
  HIV/AIDS and, 316-317
  radiation therapy support, 133
  roles in cancer, 119, 121, 125
  therapeutic order in, 1-2f
Nausea and vomiting of pregnancy
  botanical medicines, 535-536, 537
  conventional versus natural interventions, 534f
  diagnosis, 533
  etiology, 533
  nutrition and, 535, 536-537
  psychological, emotional, and lifestyle aspects, 533, 536
  supplements for, 537
  therapeutic approach, 536-537
  therapeutic considerations, 533, 535-536
*Neisseria gonorrhea,* 605, 607-608, 729
Neovascular "wet" ARMD, 461
Nephropathy, diabetic, 211, 221, 225
Neurofeedback and attention deficit hyperactivity disorder, 104
Neuromusculoskeletal lesion and fibromyalgia syndrome, 264
Neuronal disorder theory, 506
Neuropathology, Alzheimer's disease, 36
Neuropathy
  diabetic, 211, 221
  HIV/AIDS and, 329
Neurotransmitters
  depression and, 17, 20
  premenstrual syndrome and, 650
New-breed chemotherapy agents, 129
Niacin
  atherosclerosis and, 80, 82
  depression and, 16
  diabetes mellitus and, 214-215, 225
  gout and, 286
  insomnia and, 432
Niacinamide
  diabetes mellitus and, 202, 214-215, 222
  osteoarthritis and, 559, 563
  rheumatoid arthritis and, 700, 703
Nicotinamide deficiency
  chronic fatigue syndrome and, 174, 175
  diabetes mellitus and, 214-215
  Parkinson's disease and, 599
  senile dementia and, 40t
Nicotine. *See* Smoking.
Nitrates and diabetes mellitus, 202
NNRTIs, 317, 319
Nocturnal glucose levels, 428-429
Nocturnal myoclonus, 430-431
Nodules, acne, 3-7
Non-Hodgkin's lymphoma, 122, 144
Non-insulin-dependent diabetes mellitus, 197f, 198
Nonketogenic hyperosmolar hyperglycemia, 209
Non-nucleoside reverse transcriptase inhibitors, 317, 319
Non-REM sleep, 427-428
Nonspecific vaginitis, 761
Nonsteroidal antiinflammatory drugs, 292t
  osteoarthritis and, 556
  peptic ulcers and, 620
  rheumatoid arthritis and, 695
  urticaria and, 740-741
Norepinephrine and attention deficit hyperactivity disorder, 104
North American Menopause Society, 483
Norwalk virus, 396
NRTIs and HIV/AIDS, 317-318
Nuclear cataracts, 719
Nucleoside and nucleotide reverse transcriptase inhibitors, 317-318
Nutraceuticals, 106
Nutrition. *See* Diet and nutrition.
Nuts and seeds, 78
Nystatin and HIV/AIDS, 325

## O


OA. *See* Osteoarthritis.
Obesity
  atherosclerosis and, 77, 88
  body fat composition and, 550-551
  body mass index and, 538, 540
  botanical medicines, 550
  causes of, 542-546
  cellulite and, 149, 150, 151
  conventional versus natural interventions, 539f
  diabetes mellitus and, 203
  diagnosis, 538
  dietary strategies, 547-550
  diet-induced thermogenesis, 545-546
  gallstones and, 269
  gout and, 285
  hypertension and, 343, 344
  kidney stones and, 446
  natural weight loss aids for, 548-550
  physiologic features, 543-545
  prevalence, 540-542
  therapeutic approach, 550-551
  therapeutic considerations, 546-550
  types, 542
  varicose veins and, 772
Oil of bitter orange, 111
Olea. *See* Olive leaf extract.
Olive leaf extract, 327, 332, 334
  hypertension and, 349, 350
Olive oil, 77, 78, 79
  gallstones and, 272
  multiple sclerosis and, 527-528
OM. *See* Otitis media.
Omega-3 fatty acids
  Alzheimer's disease and, 42, 46
  angina pectoris and, 55
  asthma and, 66-67
  atherosclerosis and, 77, 78, 79, 88, 89
  atopic dermatitis and, 93
  attention deficit hyperactivity disorder and, 105
  bipolar (manic) depression and, 23
  cancer and, 131
  chronic fatigue syndrome and, 175
  depression and, 18, 22
  diabetes mellitus and, 201-202, 204, 222-225
  endometriosis and, 231
  gallstones and, 272
  glaucoma and, 278
  hypertension and, 347-348
  inflammatory bowel disease and, 409, 410
  multiple sclerosis and, 527, 531
  myocardial infarction and, 87
  osteoarthritis and, 563
  psoriasis and, 688
  rheumatoid arthritis and, 702, 707
Omega-6 fatty acids
  multiple sclerosis and, 527-528
  rheumatoid arthritis and, 701
Onions and garlic. *See* Allium family.
OP. *See* Osteoporosis.
Opioid activity and celiac disease, 144
Oral cancer, 451
Oral contraceptives
  cervical dysplasia and, 155
  migraine headaches and, 514-515
  pelvic inflammatory disease and, 609, 614-615
Oral erythema multiforme, 246
Oral lichen planus. *See* Lichen planus.
Oregano oil and HIV/AIDS, 325
Orexin A, 545
Ornish, Dean, 87
Osteoarthritis
  botanical medicines, 562-563, 564
  categories, 554
  conventional pharmacologic treatment, 556
  conventional versus natural interventions, 553f
  diagnosis, 552, 554-555
  dietary and exercise considerations, 557-558, 563, 564
  exercise considerations, 557-558
  hormonal considerations, 556-557
  hypothyroidism and, 557
  magnetic therapies, 561
  nutritional supplements, 558-561
  physical medicine, 561, 564
  risk factors, 567-569
  signs and symptoms, 552
  supplements for, 563
  therapeutic approach, 563-564
  therapeutic considerations, 555-563
Osteogenesis imperfecta, 275
Osteoporosis
  conventional versus natural interventions, 566f
  diagnosis, 565, 570-572
  dietary factors, 573-575, 579-580
  drug therapy, 572-573
  hormonal factors, 568
  hormone replacement therapy and, 479
  lab tests, 571-572
  menopause and, 478
  pathophysiology, 565
  risk factors, 567-568
  supplements for, 575-579, 580
  therapeutic approach, 579-580
  therapeutic considerations, 572-579
Otitis media
  acute, 581
  botanical medicines, 586-587
  causes of, 583-584
  chronic, 581, 585
  conventional versus natural interventions, 582f
  diagnosis, 581
  physical medicine, 587
  standard medical treatment, 581, 583
  supplements for, 586
  therapeutic approach, 586-587
  therapeutic considerations, 584-586
  types of, 581

Ovarian cancer, 481-482
*Oxalobacter formigenes,* 446
Oxidative stress and Parkinson's disease, 592
Ozone, 333, 334, 649

## P

Paclitaxel, 132, 133
*Paeoniae radix,* 243
Pain
  angina pectoris and, 48
  proctologic conditions, 673, 674
*Panax ginseng. See* Ginseng.
*Panax quinquefolium,* 218
Pancreatic enzymes
  celiac disease and, 145-146
  uterine fibroids and, 752, 755
Pancreatin and rheumatoid arthritis, 707
Pantethine. *See* Pantothenic acid.
Pantothenic acid
  acne vulgaris/conglobata and, 6
  angina pectoris and, 52-53, 55
  atherosclerosis and, 81, 83, 89
  chronic fatigue syndrome and, 175
  depression and, 16
  osteoarthritis and, 560, 563
  rheumatoid arthritis and, 700, 703
Pap smears, 152, 154, 158
Para-aminobenzoic acid, 193
Parasitic agents in infectious diarrhea, 398, 404
Parathyroid hormone, 568
Parkinson's disease, 39t, 43
  apoptosis, 590-591
  botanical medicines, 600-601, 604
  characteristics of, 588
  conventional drugs, 604
  conventional versus natural interventions, 589f
  detoxification dysfunction in, 592
  diagnosis, 588, 592-594
  dietary recommendations, 603
  etiology, 590
  genetic factors, 590
  lifestyle recommendations, 603
  nutritional considerations, 596-600
  oxidative stress and glutathione deficiency in, 592
  prevalence, 588
  smoking and, 601-602
  supplements for, 603-604
  therapeutic approach, 603-604
  therapeutic considerations, 594-596, 601-603
  toxic exposure and, 591-592
Paromomycin, 732
Particle radiation, 132
Parvovirus, 396
*Passiflora incarnata,* 431, 432
Pathophysiology and pathogenesis
  epilepsy, 237
  gallstones, 267, 269-270
  HIV/AIDS, 310
  migraine headaches, 505-507
Pathophysiology and pathogenesis *(Continued)*
  multiple sclerosis, 523-524
  osteoporosis, 565
  periodontal disease, 627-629
  rheumatoid arthritis, 693, 695-696
  urticaria, 736, 738
PEA. *See* Phenylethylamine.
Pediatric patients with inflammatory bowel disease, 419-420, 422-423
Pelvic inflammatory disease
  botanical medicines, 614, 616
  complications, 608
  conventional versus natural interventions, 606f
  diagnosis, 605
  drugs for, 612-613
  etiology, 607-608
  intercourse during menses and, 615
  lab tests, 611-612
  pathogen access to upper female tract in, 609
  physical medicine, 613, 616-617
  prevention of, 614-615
  risk factors, 608-609
  supplements for, 613-614, 616
  therapeutic approach, 616-617
  therapeutic considerations, 612-615
Penicillin, 740
Peptic ulcers
  botanical medicines, 623-624, 624
  complications, 624
  conventional versus natural interventions, 619f
  diagnosis, 618
  incidence, 618
  lifestyle factors, 621
  nutritional factors, 621-623
  symptoms, 618
  therapeutic approach, 624
  therapeutic considerations, 620-624
*Peptococcus,* 605
*Peptostreptococcus,* 605
Percutaneous transluminal coronary angioplasty, 50
Performance indexes and cancer, 123-124
Perianal dermatological disorders, 667f, 678-683
Pericardium 6, 536
Periodontal disease
  atherosclerosis and, 625
  botanical medicines, 631-632
  conventional versus natural interventions, 626f
  diagnosis, 625
  pathophysiology, 627-629
  prevalence and epidemiology, 625, 627
  supplements for, 629-631, 632
  therapeutic approach, 632
  therapeutic considerations, 629-632
Personality, type A, 86
Pertussis vaccine and asthma, 63-64

Pesticides
benign prostatic hyperplasia and, 115, 116, 118
Parkinson's disease and, 591
*Petasites hybridus. See* Butterbur.
*Peucedanum,* 447
*Peumus boldo,* 274
Phenylalanine and tyrosine, 19-20
Phenylethylamine, 19-20
Phosphatidylcholine
Alzheimer's disease and, 44
bipolar (manic) depression and, 23, 24
gallstones and, 269, 272, 274
Phosphatidylserine
Alzheimer's disease and, 44, 47
Parkinson's disease and, 599, 604
Phospholipids and depression, 18
Phosphorus and osteoporosis, 573, 574
Photocoagulation, 461
Photodynamic therapy and lichen planus, 457
Photon radiation, 132
*Phyllanthus amarus,* 300, 332, 334
Physical inactivity. *See* Exercise.
Physical medicine
acne vulgaris/conglobata, 7
fibromyalgia syndrome, 259, 266
HIV/AIDS, 333
irritable bowel syndrome, 441
migraine headaches, 512-513, 516
osteoarthritis, 561, 564
otitis media, 587
pelvic inflammatory disease, 613, 616-617
pneumonia and, 637
psoriasis, 690, 692
rheumatoid arthritis, 705-706, 707
urticaria, 747
*Physicians' Cancer Chemotherapy Drug Manual,* 131
Phytochemicals, 83
Phytoestrogens
endometriosis and, 229
herbal, 753-754
male infertility and, 471
menopause and, 487-488, 489-490
osteoarthritis and, 557
uterine fibroids and, 751, 753-754
*Phytolacca americana,* 418, 753, 768
Phytosterols and phytostanols, 80-81
Pick's disease, 39t
PID. *See* Pelvic inflammatory disease.
Pilonidal sinus, 668f, 680
Pine bark extracts and atherosclerosis, 84-85
*Pinelliae tuber,* 243
Pinworms, 682, 683
*Piper methysticum,* 21, 301, 601
Plantain banana, 623
Plant terpenes, 272-273
Platelet disorder theory, 505-506
Platinum compounds, 128
PMS. *See* Premenstrual syndrome.
Pneumococci
bacterial sinusitis and, 107
pneumonia, 637-638
Pneumonia
conventional versus natural interventions, 634f
diagnosis, 633, 637-638, 639
immunoglobulin respiratory system defenses and, 633, 635
mycoplasmal, 637
physical therapy, 637
pneumococcal, 637-638
supplements for, 639
therapeutic approach, 636-639
therapeutic considerations, 635-636, 638-639, 639
viral, 639
Podophyllum resin, 333
Poke root. *See Phytolacca americana.*
Policosanol, 81, 82
Polycystic ovary syndrome, 203
*Polygala senega,* 69
*Polygonum aviculare,* 447
Polylactic acid, 328
Polymorphonuclear leukocytes, 627
Porphyrias
biochemistry of, 643
causes of, 646-647
classifications of, 640, 642
conventional versus natural interventions, 641f
diagnosis, 640
etiology, 644-645
heme formation and, 643
hepatic, 642
lab tests, 645-646
manifestation of, 643-644
nutritional therapies, 648-649
signs and symptoms, 642
supplements for, 649
therapeutic approach, 649
therapeutic considerations, 646-649
Postcoital test, 468
Posterior cortical cataracts, 719
Posterior subcapsular cataracts, 719
Potassium. *See* Vitamin K.
*Potentilla tormentilla,* 403-404, 405
Prediabetes, 199
Prednisone, 556
Preformed mediators, 738
Pregnancy
HIV/AIDS and, 329-330
nausea and vomiting of, 533-537
Premenstrual dysphoric disorder, 650, 652
Premenstrual syndrome, 370-371
botanical medicines, 659-661, 662-663
causes of, 663
classifications, 652
conventional versus natural interventions, 651f
diagnosis, 650, 652
diet and, 654-655, 661-662
environmental estrogens and, 654

Premenstrual syndrome *(Continued)*
estrogen and, 652-653
etiology, 650
exercise and, 656
gut microecology and, 653
hormone therapy, 656
liver detoxification and, 653-654
prevalence, 650
supplements for, 657-659, 662
symptoms, 650, 663
therapeutic approach, 661-663
therapeutic considerations, 652-661
Preservatives, food, 742-743
Prickly ash. *See Xanthoxylum americanum.*
Prinzmetal's variant angina, 48
Proanthocyanidins and male infertility, 472
Probiotics
atopic dermatitis and, 95
chronic candidiasis and, 164-165
HIV/AIDS and, 325, 326, 336
infectious diarrhea and, 402-403
inflammatory bowel disease and, 419
Proctalgia fugax, 668f, 680-681
Proctitis, 669f, 681-682
Proctologic conditions
Abscess, anal, 666f
anal abscess, 666f, 671-672
anal cryptitis, 666f, 672
anal fissure, 665f, 672-674
anal fistula, 666f, 671-672
anorectal anatomy and, 663, 671
botanical medicines, 683
conventional versus natural interventions, 665-670f
cryptitis, anal, 666f
fissure, anal, 665f
fistula, anal, 666f
hemorrhoids, 674-678
perianal dermatological disorders, 667-669f, 678-683
pilonidal sinus, 668f
proctalgia fugax, 668f
proctitis, 669f
pruritis ani, 670f
Procyanidolic oligomers, 84-85
Progesterone
asthma and, 64-65
cream, 490, 501, 755
endometriosis and, 231, 232
HIV/AIDS and, 331
menorrhagia and, 501
natural, 231, 232, 482-483, 754, 755
oral micronized, 501
premenstrual syndrome and, 656, 663
uterine fibroids and, 754, 755
Propolis, 165, 734
Prostaglandin metabolism
atopic dermatitis and, 93, 95
inflammatory bowel disease and, 410
menorrhagia and, 495
Prostatitis, 729
Protease inhibitors, 317, 319-320
Protein
digestion, incomplete, 686-687
drinks and smoothies, 127
Prothrombotic state, 77
Proton pump inhibitors, 400, 404
*Prunella vulgaris,* 332
*Prunus spinosa,* 93
Pruritus
ani, 670f, 682-683
atopic dermatitis, 94
lichen planus and, 454
Psoriasis, 288
botanical medicines, 690-691, 692
conventional versus natural interventions, 685f
diagnosis, 684
gastrointestinal function and, 686-687
immune system and, 684, 686
liver function and, 687-688
nutrition and, 688-689, 691-692
physical therapeutics, 690
psychological aspects of, 689-690
therapeutic approach, 691-692
therapeutic considerations, 686-691
topical treatments, 690-691
Psychiatry, 12
Psychological factors. *See* Stress and psychological factors.
Psychoneuroimmunology, 387
Psychopharmacology, 12
Psychosocial aspects of alcoholism, 33-34
Psychotherapy and premenstrual syndrome, 657
Psychotropic drugs and senile dementia, 40t
*Pterocarpus marsupium,* 202
Pustules, acne, 3-7
*Pygeum africanum,* 117, 118
male infertility and, 474
Pyridoxine
acne vulgaris/conglobata and, 6
asthma and, 67
bipolar (manic) depression and, 24
carpal tunnel syndrome and, 141
cervical dysplasia and, 157, 159
epilepsy and, 239-240, 244
hypothyroidism and, 383
kidney stones and, 446
nausea and vomiting of pregnancy and, 535
osteoarthritis and, 560-561
Parkinson's disease and, 597
rheumatoid arthritis and, 703
seborrheic dermatitis and, 716
*See also* Vitamin B complex.

**Q**

Quercetin
aphthous stomatitis and, 58-59
asthma and, 72
atopic dermatitis and, 95
gout and, 286, 287
inflammatory bowel disease and, 417, 420

Quercetin *(Continued)*
periodontal disease and, 632
rheumatoid arthritis and, 700
urticaria and, 746
*See also* Flavonoids.

**R**

RA. *See* Rheumatoid arthritis.
Race/ethnicity
diabetes mellitus and, 203
uterine fibroids and, 748
vaginitis and, 762
Radiation therapy, 132-133
antioxidants and, 134-135
Radiography
osteoarthritis, 554, 555
osteoporosis, 570-571
rheumatoid arthritis, 698-699
Radioimmunotherapy, 133
Radiopotentiation, 133-134
Radioprotection, 134
Raspberry leaf, 537
Reactive hypoglycemia, 367
Recurrent aphthous stomatitis. *See* Aphthous stomatitis.
Red clover. *See Trifolium pretense.*
Red wine
atherosclerosis and, 78, 84
migraine headaches and, 509
Rein, Mitchell, 754
Relaxation
angina pectoris and, 54, 55
insomnia and, 428
migraine headaches and, 513
osteoarthritis and, 562
urticaria and, 747
REM sleep, 427-428
Renal/hepatic encephalopathy and senile dementia, 40t
Repaglinide, 376
Resistance testing, chemotherapy, 129
Restless leg syndrome, 430-431
Resveratrol, 306
Retinoic acid, 457-458
Retinol, 150
Retinopathy, diabetic, 211, 220, 225
Reward deficiency syndrome, 99
*Rhamnus alnus,* 447
*Rheum,* 447, 623
Rheumatoid arthritis
botanical medicines, 704-705, 707
conventional versus natural interventions, 694f
diagnosis, 693, 696-699
diet and, 699-700, 706
lab tests, 698-99
nutrition and, 701-703
pathogenesis, 693, 695-696
physical medicine, 705-706, 707
radiography, 698-699
supplements for, 700
therapeutic approach, 706
therapeutic considerations, 699-706
Riboflavin
alcoholism and, 35
carpal tunnel syndrome and, 141
depression and, 16
hypothyroidism and, 383
migraine headaches and, 511, 516
senile cataracts and, 721
*See also* Vitamin B complex.
Robert's formula, 440
Rosacea
conventional versus natural interventions, 709f
diagnosis, 708
etiology, 710
ocular, 710
stages, 708
supplements for, 712
therapeutic approach, 711-712
therapeutic considerations, 710-711
*Rosa damascena,* 93
*Rosmarinus officinalis,* 332
Rotavirus, 201, 396, 400
*Rubia tinctura,* 447, 449
*Rubus idaeus,* 535
*Rumex crispus,* 449
Ruscogenin, 150
*Ruscus aculeatus,* 683, 775-776, 777
*Ruta graveolens,* 93, 447

**S**

*Saccharomyces* and infectious diarrhea, 402-403, 405
SAD. *See* Seasonal affective disorder.
S-adenosyl-methionine
depression and, 17, 20-21
HIV/AIDS and, 330
osteoarthritis and, 559-560, 563
Saiko-Keishi-To, 242-243, 245
Salicylates, 742
*Salmonella,* 397, 399
Salt
asthma and, 64
hypertension and, 344, 346
kidney stones and, 448
migraine headaches and, 510
osteoporosis and, 569, 573
premenstrual syndrome and, 655
SAM. *See* S-adenosyl-methionine.
Sandalwood oil, 190
*Sanguinaria canadensis,* 631-632
Sarcomas, 122
Sarcosine and epilepsy, 241
Saw palmetto. *See Serenoa repens.*
Scarring, acne, 3-7
Schizophrenia
celiac disease and, 144
phenylethylamine and, 20
Scratching. *See* Pruritus.
Scrotal temperature, 469, 474
Scudder's alterative, 752, 755
*Scutellaria*
*baicalensis,* 333
*radix,* 243

Sea cucumber, 559
Seasonal affective disorder, 11, 24-25
Seborrheic dermatitis
  botanical medicines, 715-716
  clinical manifestations, 713
  conventional versus natural
    interventions, 714f
  diagnosis, 713
  diet and, 716
  supplements for, 716
  therapeutic approach, 716
  therapeutic considerations, 713, 715-716
  topical treatments, 716
Secondarily formed mediators, 738
Secondary diabetes, 199
Seizures. *See* Epilepsy.
Selenium
  alcoholism and, 32, 35
  asthma and, 68, 72
  atherosclerosis and, 84
  cervical dysplasia and, 157, 159-160
  depression and, 17, 22
  endometriosis and, 230, 231
  epilepsy and, 244
  hepatitis and, 298
  HIV/AIDS and, 323
  hyperthyroidism and, 357, 360
  hypothyroidism and, 383, 385
  immune system function and, 390
  macular degeneration and, 464
  multiple sclerosis and, 529, 531
  periodontal disease and, 630, 632
  psoriasis and, 692
  rheumatoid arthritis and, 702, 707
  senile cataracts and, 720-721, 724
Seligman, Martin, 11, 12
Senile cataracts
  botanical medicines, 722-723, 724
  causes of, 717
  classification of, 717, 719
  conventional versus natural
    interventions, 718f
  diagnosis, 717
  etiology, 719
  supplements for, 719, 723-724
  therapeutic approach, 723-724
  therapeutic considerations, 719-723
Senile dementia
  causes of and mechanisms of, 36, 39-40t
  hormone replacement therapy and, 481
  lab tests in, 41
  reversible causes of, 41
  signs of, 40-41
  *See also* Alzheimer's disease.
*Senna*, 447
*Serenoa repens*, 116, 118
  hair loss in women and, 291
Serotonin
  Alzheimer's disease and, 45
  deficiency and migraine, 506-507
  depression and, 15, 19, 33
  fibromyalgia syndrome and, 255, 257
  migraine headaches and, 510
Serotonin *(Continued)*
  obesity and, 546
  precursor and cofactor therapy, 429-430
  premenstrual syndrome and, 657
*Serratia* peptidase and bacterial sinusitis,
  110
Sertoli cells, 470-471
Serum bactericidal activity, 92
Sex steroid hormones and migraine
    headaches, 514-515
Sexual dysfunction and HIV/AIDS, 330
Shark cartilage, 559
*Shigella*, 397, 399
Shiitake mushrooms, 332
Shingles and HIV/AIDS, 326-327
Short-wave diathermy, 561
Sho-saiko-to, 301
Shy-Drager syndrome, 594
Sick building syndrome, 109
Side effects
  chemotherapy, 129
  HIV/AIDS, 324-332
  radiation therapy, 133
Silicon and osteoporosis, 578
*Silybum marianum*, 34, 274
  hepatitis and, 300, 301
  HIV/AIDS and, 324, 332, 336
  psoriasis and, 692
Silymarin, 164
Sinemet, 604
Sinusitis. *See* Bacterial sinusitis.
Sitz baths, 613, 616-617, 672, 674, 678
Skin
  acne conglobata, 3-7
  acne vulgaris, 3-7
  biopsy, 745
  fold thickness, 540, 541t
  hypothyroidism and, 380
  inflammatory bowel disease and, 412
  lichen planus and, 454-458
  porphyrias and, 644
Sleep
  Alzheimer's disease and, 38
  apnea, 426-427
  HIV/AIDS and, 321
  hyperventilation syndrome/breathing
    pattern disorders and, 366
  importance of adequate, 428
  irritable bowel syndrome and, 440
  kidney stones and, 448
  patterns, normal, 427-428
  *See also* Insomnia.
Slippery elm. *See Ulmus fulva.*
*Smilax sarsaparilla*, 692
Smoking, 76t
  angina pectoris and, 55
  atherosclerosis and, 75, 76t, 79
  attention deficit hyperactivity disorder
    and, 100
  cervical dysplasia and, 155
  depression and, 15, 21
  hyperthyroidism and, 353
  macular degeneration and, 459

Smoking *(Continued)*
male infertility and, 472
menopause and, 491
osteoporosis and, 567, 569
Parkinson's disease and, 601-602
peptic ulcers and, 621
periodontal disease and, 628
vaginitis and, 762
Snowdrop. *See Galanthus nivalis.*
Sodium. *See* Salt.
Soft drinks and osteoporosis, 574
Soft tissue cancer, 122
Solvents and Parkinson's disease, 591
Sorbitol accumulation, 210
Soy
benign prostatic hyperplasia and, 116, 118
diabetes mellitus and, 217
endometriosis and, 229
fibrocystic breast disease and, 252
male infertility and, 471
menopause and, 488
osteoporosis and, 575
uterine fibroids and, 751
Spermatogenesis, 467-468
Spirituality
epilepsy and, 243-44
rheumatoid arthritis and, 701
*Spirulina platensis*, 333
Splenic flexure syndrome, 436
Splint, wrist, 141
Squalene, 134
St. John's Wort
bipolar (manic) depression and, 23
depression and, 21, 22
HIV/AIDS and, 320, 330, 333
premenstrual syndrome and, 661, 663
seasonal affective disorder, 25
Stabilizers, food, 743
Staging, cancer, 122-123
Standish, L. J., 316
Staphylococcus aureus
atopic dermatitis and, 92
bacterial sinusitis and, 107
Statins, 78-79
Stimulant drugs and attention deficit hyperactivity disorder, 104
Streptococcal pharyngitis
botanical medicines, 728
conventional versus natural interventions, 726f
diagnosis, 725
immune system function and, 727-728
supplements for, 728
therapeutic approach, 728
therapeutic considerations, 727-728
Streptococcus
bacterial sinusitis and, 107
pelvic inflammatory disease and, 605
*See also* Streptococcal pharyngitis.
Stress and psychological factors
adrenal function, 13-14
angina pectoris, 55
Stress and psychological factors *(Continued)*
aphthous stomatitis, 58
chronic fatigue syndrome, 170
diabetes mellitus, 212
gallstones, 273
HIV/AIDS, 321-322, 330
hypertension, 343-344
hyperthyroidism, 351
infectious diarrhea, 404
inflammatory bowel disease, 409
irritable bowel syndrome, 440-441
kidney stones, 448
male infertility, 474
menorrhagia, 496
multiple sclerosis, 530-531, 532
nausea and vomiting of pregnancy, 536
oxidative, 592
peptic ulcers, 621, 624
premenstrual syndrome, 656
psoriasis, 689-690, 692
urticaria and, 744
Stretching for carpal tunnel syndrome, 140
Stroke
aspirin and, 87
botanical medicines, 88
excessive platelet aggregation and, 85
hormone replacement therapy and, 480-481
hypertension and, 76
preventing subsequent, 88
*Strongyloides*, 398
Struvite stones, 450
Subclinical hypothyroidism, 379
Substance abuse
attention deficit hyperactivity disorder and, 99-100
HIV/AIDS and, 330
Sugar intake
acne vulgaris/conglobata and, 5
alcoholism and, 34
attention deficit hyperactivity disorder and, 105
chronic candidiasis and, 163
depression and, 16
gallstones and, 271
hypoglycemia and, 371-372
immune system function and, 392
infectious diarrhea and, 404
irritable bowel syndrome and, 439
obesity and, 548
osteoporosis and, 574
premenstrual syndrome and, 655
uterine fibroids and, 751
Sulfasalazine, 410
Sulfites, 742-743
Sulfur and rheumatoid arthritis, 703
Sunbathing, 273
Superoxide dismutase, 560, 721

Supplements
acne vulgaris/conglobata, 7
alcoholism, 35
Alzheimer's disease, 47
aphthous stomatitis, 59
asthma, 66-69, 71-72
atherosclerosis, 80-81, 83-86, 86, 89
atopic dermatitis, 95
attention deficit hyperactivity disorder, 105
bacterial sinusitis, 110
benign prostatic hyperplasia, 118
bipolar (manic) depression, 24
cancer, 130-131
carpal tunnel syndrome, 139, 141
celiac disease, 145
cervical dysplasia, 159
chronic fatigue syndrome, 173-174, 175
congestive heart failure, 180-181, 182
cystitis, 188, 190
depression, 16-18, 22
dermatitis herpetiformis, 193
diabetes mellitus, 213-217, 222-225
endometriosis, 229-231, 231
epilepsy, 239-242, 244-245
fibrocystic breast disease, 252-253, 254
fibromyalgia syndrome, 259, 263, 265-266
gallstones, 274
glaucoma, 280
gout, 285-286
herpes simplex, 305-306, 307
hypertension, 350
hyperthyroidism, 356-359, 360
hypoglycemia, 374
hypothyroidism, 386
infectious diarrhea, 400-402
infectious diarrhea and, 404-405
inflammatory bowel disease, 420
insomnia and, 432
irritable bowel syndrome and, 441
kidney stones, 449
lichen planus, 457-458
macular degeneration, 464
male infertility, 475
menopause, 488, 491
menorrhagia and, 496-498, 500
migraine headaches, 510-512, 516
multiple sclerosis, 527-529, 531
nausea and vomiting of pregnancy and, 537
obesity, 550
osteoarthritis, 558-561, 563-564
osteoporosis, 575-579, 580
otitis media, 586
Parkinson's disease, 603-604
pelvic inflammatory disease, 613-614
pelvic inflammatory disease and, 616
peptic ulcers, 624
periodontal disease, 629-631, 632
pneumonia, 639
pneumonia and, 636
porphyrias and, 649

Supplements *(Continued)*
premenstrual syndrome, 657-659
premenstrual syndrome and, 662
rheumatoid arthritis, 700
rosacea, 712
seborrheic dermatitis, 716
senile cataracts, 719, 723-724
streptococcal pharyngitis, 728
trichomoniasis, 733, 735
urticaria, 746
uterine fibroids, 751-752, 755
vaginitis and, 764-765
varicose veins, 777
*See also* Diet and nutrition.
Surgery
anal fissure, 673
artery bypass, 50
benign prostatic hyperplasia, 114
cancer, 126-127
carpal tunnel syndrome, 140-141
hemorrhoid, 676
kidney stone, 449
osteoporosis and, 569
otitis media, 581, 583
pelvic inflammatory disease, 612
renal abscess, 672
Swank Diet, 526-527, 530-531
Swimming, 561
*Symphytum offinale,* 301, 418, 614, 616
Syndrome X, 199, 371
Synovial fluid and rheumatoid arthritis, 698-699
Synthroid, 384

## T

Tai chi, 333
*Taking Control of Your Headaches,* 517
Tamoxifen, 132, 269
*Tanacetum parthenium,* 513, 516
*Taraxacum officinale,* 96, 230, 231
gallstones and, 274
uterine fibroids and, 753
Tartrazine, 742
Tattoos, 745
Taurine and epilepsy, 240-241, 244
Taxotere, 132
T cells, 122, 144, 229
*astragalus* and, 391-392
HIV/AIDS and, 314
immune system function and, 390
Tea tree oil, 6
Temporomandibular joint dysfunction syndrome and migraine headaches, 512
*Terminalia arjuna,* 182
Terpenes, plant, 272-73
Testosterone and HIV/AIDS, 323, 332
Tetrahydrobiopterin and senile cataracts, 721
Tetrahydrobiopterin and depression, 17
*Teucrium chamaedrys,* 301
Thalidomide, 332
*Thea sinensis. See* Green tea.

T-helper cells, 56, 693
Therapeutic touch, 333
Thermogenesis, diet-induced, 545-546
Thiamin
  Alzheimer's disease and, 43, 47
  aphthous stomatitis and, 58
  congestive heart failure and, 180-181
  depression and, 16
  epilepsy and, 240
Thiazolidinediones, 376
Thromboembolism, venous, 479
Thrombophlebitis, 774
Th1/Th2 balances, 62-64
Thymus
  extract
    bacterial sinusitis and, 110
    chronic fatigue syndrome and, 175
    hepatitis and, 298-299, 301
    herpes simplex and, 307
    otitis media and, 585, 586
    pneumonia and, 636
  function and chronic candidiasis, 164
Thyroid
  antibodies, 260-261
  cancer, 354
  celiac disease and, 144
  fibrocystic breast disease and, 252-253
  fibromyalgia syndrome and, 255, 257, 260-261, 263, 265
  function tests, 259-260
  hormones and depression, 13-14
  hormone therapy, 260-261, 263, 265, 383-384, 384-386
  menorrhagia and, 494
  premenstrual syndrome and, 656
  storm, 359
  surgery, 569
  urticaria and, 744
Thyrolar, 384
Tibetan herbal formula Padma Lax, 440
Tinidazole, 732-733
TNM score, 122-23
Tobacco. *See* Smoking.
Tolazamide, 376
Tolbutamide, 376
Tolcapone, 604
Topical treatments
  acne vulgaris/conglobata, 6-7, 7
  herpes simplex, 306, 307
  lichen planus, 457-458
  menopause and, 490
  proctologic conditions, 673, 675
  psoriasis, 690-691, 692
  seborrheic dermatitis, 716
  trichomoniasis, 734, 735
  uterine fibroids, 753, 755
  vaginitis, 768-769
Tormentil root. *See Potentilla tormentilla.*
Touchi, 217
Transcutaneous electrical stimulation and migraine headaches, 512, 516
Transient ischemic attack, migraine headaches and, 505
Transurethral resection of the prostate, 114
Trauma
  corneal, 279t
  vaginitis, 759
Traumeel, 126
Trichomoniasis
  botanical medicines, 733-734, 735
  complications of, 729
  conventional therapy, 732-733
  conventional versus natural interventions, 730f
  diagnosis, 729, 731-732
  in men, 732
  supplements for, 733, 735
  therapeutic approach, 734-735
  therapeutic considerations, 732-734
  topical treatments, 734, 735
  vaginitis, 760, 771
  in women, 731-732
*Trifolium pretense*, 489, 491, 753
Trigeminovascular neurons, 506
Triglycerides and hypothyroidism, 380
*Trigonella foenum-graecum*, 218
*Tripterygium wilfordii*, 754
Trousseau's sign, 364
Tuberculosis and senile dementia, 39t
Tumor markers, 123
Turmeric, 229, 332, 385, 704
Turska's formula, 230, 232, 755
*Tylophora asthmatica*, 70
Type 1 diabetes, 194, 195f, 198, 222-223
  causes of and risk factors, 200-202
  early treatment and possible reversal of, 202
  risk factors, 203-205
Type 2 diabetes, 197f, 198, 222
Tyrosine
  hypothyroidism and, 382
  phenylalanine and, 19-20

## U

Ubiquinone. *See* CoQ10.
Ulcerative colitis, 406, 408, 410-411, 410-412, 418-419
  *See also* Inflammatory bowel disease.
Ulcerative stomatitis. *See* Aphthous stomatitis.
*Ulmus fulva*, 418
Ultrasound
  endometriosis and, 228
  psoriasis and, 692
  therapy for carpal tunnel syndrome, 140
*Ureaplasma urealyticum*, 605
Uric acid
  metabolism, 287-288, 447
  stones, 449-50
  *See also* Gout.
Urinary tract infection, 183

Urine
  tests
    benign prostatic hyperplasia, 114
    cystitis, 185-186
  *See also* Kidney(s), stones.
*Urtica dioica,* 117, 118, 753
Urticaria
  autoimmune, 739-740
  causes of, 738-743
  celiac disease and, 144
  conventional versus natural
      interventions, 737f
  dermographism and, 738-39
  diagnosis, 736, 744-746
  drugs and, 740-741
  infections and, 743
  lab tests, 745
  pathophysiology, 736, 738
  physical medicine, 747
  supplements for, 746-747
  therapeutic approach, 746-747
  therapeutic considerations, 744
Uterine fibroids
  botanical medicines, 752-753
  causes of, 748
  conventional versus natural
      interventions, 749f
  diagnosis, 748, 750
  diet and, 751
  incidence, 748
  natural progesterone and, 754, 755
  phytoestrogens and, 753-754
  supplements for, 751-752, 755
  therapeutic considerations, 750-754
  topical treatments, 753, 755

**V**

VA. *See* Vanadium.
Vaccines, 128-129
*Vaccinium myrtillus,* 93, 280, 287, 463, 464
Vaginal depletion pack, 158, 614, 616
Vaginitis and vulvovaginitis
  atrophic, 486, 758, 771
  bacterial, 155, 761-763, 771
  botanical medicines, 765-767
  *Candida albicans,* 760-61
  *Chlamydia* and, 763-764, 771
  conventional versus natural
      interventions, 757f
  diagnosis, 756, 767-768, 770f
  herpes simplex and, 763, 771
  hormonal, 486, 758
  irritant, 759
  nonspecific, 761
  prevalence, 756
  supplements for, 764-765
  therapeutic approach, 768-771
  therapeutic considerations, 764-767
  topical treatments, 768-769
  *Trichomonas,* 760, 771
  types of, 758-764
Valcyclovir, 327
*Valeriana officinalis,* 431, 432
Valproate, 23
Vanadium, 24
Varicella zoster, 303
Varicose veins
  botanical medicines, 774-776, 777
  conventional versus natural
      interventions, 773f
  diagnosis, 772
  dietary factors, 774, 776-777
  etiology, 774
  physical measures and, 774
  supplements for, 777
  therapeutic approach, 776-777
  therapeutic considerations, 774-776
Vasomotor instability theory, 505
Vegetarian diets, 66, 271
  kidney stones and, 445
  osteoporosis and, 573-574
  premenstrual syndrome and, 654-655
Venous thromboembolism, 479
Vincristine intoxication, 40t
Viral agents
  infectious diarrhea, 394, 396
  rheumatoid arthritis, 696
  urticaria, 743
Viral encephalopathy and senile
    dementia, 39t
Viral hepatitis, acute, 296
Viral pneumonia, 639
*Viscum album,* 349
Vitamin A
  acne vulgaris/conglobata and, 5
  alcoholism and, 31, 35
  atopic dermatitis and, 95
  bacterial sinusitis and, 110
  cancer and, 126, 130, 131
  celiac disease and, 145
  cervical dysplasia and, 156
  cystitis and, 190
  fibrocystic breast disease and, 252
  hair loss in women and, 292
  HIV/AIDS and, 322
  hyperthyroidism and, 356, 360
  hypothyroidism and, 382
  immune system function and, 389, 392
  infectious diarrhea and, 400-401, 404
  inflammatory bowel disease and,
    415-416
  leukoplakia and, 451, 453
  lichen planus and, 457-458
  menorrhagia and, 496-497, 500
  osteoarthritis and, 560-561, 563
  otitis media and, 586
  peptic ulcers and, 622, 624
  periodontal disease and, 629-630
  pneumonia and, 635, 636
  proctologic conditions and, 673
  psoriasis and, 689, 691
  rheumatoid arthritis and, 700
  senile cataracts and, 722
  trichomoniasis and, 735
  vaginitis and, 764
  varicose veins and, 777

Vitamin B complex
alcoholism and, 32, 35
Alzheimer's disease and, 38, 43-44
aphthous stomatitis and, 58
asthma and, 67, 68, 71
atherosclerosis and, 85
attention deficit hyperactivity disorder and, 101
cancer and, 126, 130, 132
carpal tunnel syndrome and, 139
cervical dysplasia and, 157, 159
depression and, 16-17, 22
diabetes mellitus and, 215
endometriosis and, 229, 231
epilepsy and, 244
fibrocystic breast disease and, 254
fibromyalgia syndrome and, 265
HIV/AIDS and, 322-323
infectious diarrhea and, 405
insomnia and, 432
kidney stones and, 449
macrocytic anemia and, 329
male infertility and, 473, 475
menorrhagia and, 498
migraine headaches and, 510, 516
multiple sclerosis and, 529-530
nausea and vomiting of pregnancy and, 535, 537
osteoarthritis and, 563
osteoporosis and, 577-578
Parkinson's disease and, 597, 604
porphyrias and, 648
premenstrual syndrome and, 653, 657, 662
rheumatoid arthritis and, 703
rosacea and, 711
seborrheic dermatitis and, 715, 716
senile dementia and, 40t
trichomoniasis and, 735
uterine fibroids and, 751
vaginitis and, 764-765
varicose veins and, 777
Vitamin C
alcoholism and, 32, 35
Alzheimer's disease and, 43, 47
angina pectoris and, 51, 55
aphthous stomatitis and, 59
asthma and, 66, 67-68, 72
atherosclerosis and, 81, 84, 89
bacterial sinusitis and, 110
bipolar (manic) depression and, 24
cancer and, 126, 130, 131, 134
cervical dysplasia and, 156-157, 159-160
chronic fatigue syndrome and, 173, 175
cystitis and, 190
depression and, 15, 16, 22
diabetes mellitus and, 213-214, 222-225
endometriosis and, 229, 231
fibrocystic breast disease and, 254
fibromyalgia syndrome and, 265
gallstones and, 274
glaucoma and, 277-278, 280
gout and, 286
Vitamin C *(Continued)*
hair loss in women and, 291
hepatitis and, 298, 301
herpes simplex and, 305, 307
HIV/AIDS and, 324
hypertension and, 347, 350
hyperthyroidism and, 356, 360
hypothyroidism and, 383
immune system function and, 389-390, 392
inflammatory bowel disease and, 416, 417
kidney stones and, 448
leukoplakia and, 453
macular degeneration and, 464
male infertility and, 475
menopause and, 488, 491
menorrhagia and, 497, 500, 501
multiple sclerosis and, 529
nausea and vomiting of pregnancy and, 535, 537
osteoarthritis and, 560, 563
otitis media and, 586
Parkinson's disease and, 596-597, 604
pelvic inflammatory disease and, 613-614, 616
peptic ulcers and, 624
periodontal disease and, 629, 632
pneumonia and, 635, 636
rheumatoid arthritis and, 700, 703
senile cataracts and, 720, 723
streptococcal pharyngitis and, 727, 728
trichomoniasis and, 735
vaginitis and, 765
varicose veins and, 777
Vitamin D
cancer and, 130
diabetes mellitus and, 201
epilepsy and, 241-242
inflammatory bowel disease and, 416
multiple sclerosis and, 530, 531
osteoarthritis and, 560
osteoporosis and, 567, 569, 576, 577, 580
psoriasis and, 689, 691
Vitamin E
acne vulgaris/conglobata and, 6
alcoholism and, 35
Alzheimer's disease and, 43, 47
angina pectoris and, 51, 55
asthma and, 67, 72
atherosclerosis and, 83-84, 89
atopic dermatitis and, 94, 95
bipolar (manic) depression and, 24
cancer and, 127, 130, 131, 132
cervical dysplasia and, 159-160
chronic fatigue syndrome and, 175
depression and, 22
diabetes mellitus and, 214, 221, 222-225
endometriosis and, 229, 231
epilepsy and, 242, 244
fibrocystic breast disease and, 252, 254
fibromyalgia syndrome and, 265
gallstones and, 274

Vitamin E *(Continued)*
gout and, 285, 287
hair loss in women and, 291
HIV/AIDS and, 318, 323
hypertension and, 350
hyperthyroidism and, 356, 360
hypothyroidism and, 382
immune system function and, 390
inflammatory bowel disease and, 416, 417
leukoplakia and, 453
macular degeneration and, 464
male infertility and, 472, 475
menopause and, 488
menorrhagia and, 497, 500
multiple sclerosis and, 529, 531
osteoarthritis and, 560, 563
Parkinson's disease and, 604
pelvic inflammatory disease and, 616
peptic ulcers and, 622, 624
periodontal disease and, 630, 632
pneumonia and, 636
porphyrias and, 649
premenstrual syndrome and, 659, 662
proctologic conditions and, 673
psoriasis and, 691
rheumatoid arthritis and, 700
senile cataracts and, 723
trichomoniasis and, 733, 735
vaginitis and, 765
Vitamin K
atherosclerosis and, 86
cancer and, 134
hypertension and, 344, 346
inflammatory bowel disease and, 415, 416
iodide and erythema multiforme, 248
kidney stones and, 447, 449
menorrhagia and, 497
nausea and vomiting of pregnancy and, 535, 537
osteoporosis and, 574
*Vitex agnus-castus*
endometriosis and, 230, 231
menorrhagia and, 498, 501
premenstrual syndrome and, 661, 662
uterine fibroids and, 753
*Vitis vinifera. See* Grape seed extract.
Vulvovaginitis. *See* Vaginitis and vulvovaginitis.

**W**

Wasting and HIV/AIDS, 330-332
Waterborne infections, 398
Water intake
gallstones and, 274
gout and, 285
HIV/AIDS and, 320, 326
immune system function and, 392
infectious diarrhea and, 400
nausea and vomiting of pregnancy and, 535
Weak electromagnetic fields and Parkinson's disease, 602
Weight reduction
cellulite, 150, 151
dietary strategies, 547-550
gout and, 285
HIV/AIDS and, 330-332
hypertension and, 349
inflammatory bowel disease and, 412
natural aids, 548-550
Wernicke-Korsakoff syndrome, 32
Whey protein shakes, 131
White coat hypertension, 340-341
Whole foods
Alzheimer's disease and, 42, 43, 46
angina pectoris and, 55
asthma and, 66
fibromyalgia syndrome and, 258-259, 265
HIV/AIDS and, 318, 336
hyperthyroidism and, 355, 360
hypoglycemia and, 371-372
nausea and vomiting of pregnancy and, 535
uterine fibroids and, 751
Whooping cough, 64
Wickham's striae, 454
Wild indigo. *See Baptista tinctoria.*
Wilson's syndrome, 385
*Withania somnifera,* 134
World Health Organization, 26
Wound healing and diabetes mellitus, 211, 213-214, 221, 225
Wrist splinting and exercise, 141

**X**

*Xanthoxylum americanum,* 230, 231
Xeloda, 132
Xenobiotics, 100
Xenoestrogens, 654
Xylitol, 585, 587

**Y**

Yeast-containing foods, 163, 164-165
*Yersinia enterocolitica,* 397-398
Yoga and HIV/AIDS, 334
Yucca, 562, 564

**Z**

Zinc
acne vulgaris/conglobata and, 5-6
alcoholism and, 30, 35
Alzheimer's disease and, 44
aphthous stomatitis, 58
atopic dermatitis and, 94, 95
attention deficit hyperactivity disorder and, 101, 105
bacterial sinusitis and, 110
benign prostatic hyperplasia and, 118
cancer and, 126
cervical dysplasia and, 157-158, 159
copper ratio, 157-158
cystitis and, 190

Zinc *(Continued)*
depression and, 17, 22
diabetes mellitus and, 215, 221
epilepsy and, 241, 244
erythema multiforme and, 248
fibrocystic breast disease and, 254
hair loss in women and, 292
herpes simplex and, 305, 307
HIV/AIDS and, 318, 323, 330
hyperthyroidism and, 357
hypothyroidism and, 382, 383
immune system function and, 390, 392
infectious diarrhea and, 401, 405
inflammatory bowel disease and, 414-415
macular degeneration and, 462, 464
male infertility and, 473, 475
osteoarthritis and, 560-561, 563
otitis media and, 586
peptic ulcers and, 622, 624
periodontal disease and, 630, 632
pneumonia and, 636
premenstrual syndrome and, 658-659
psoriasis and, 689, 692
rheumatoid arthritis and, 702, 707
seborrheic dermatitis and, 716
senile cataracts and, 722
streptococcal pharyngitis and, 728
trichomoniasis and, 733, 735
vaginitis and, 765, 769
varicose veins and, 777
*Zingiber officinale*
menorrhagia and, 498
migraine headaches and, 513, 516
nausea and vomiting of pregnancy and, 535, 537
osteoarthritis and, 562-63
peptic ulcers and, 623
rheumatoid arthritis, 704-705
*rhizoma*, 243
Zing's Self-Rating Depression Scale, 263
*Zizyphi fructus*, 69, 243